CLINICAL DERMATOLOGY TEXTBOOK 2026

AF872748

Evidence-Based Approaches to Cutaneous Diagnosis, Therapeutics, and Procedural Management for Board Review Candidates

Ramon C. Henson, MD

Trademark Disclaimer

All brand names, product names, drug names, certification names, and registered trademarks mentioned in this textbook are the property of their respective owners. Their use in this publication does not imply endorsement, affiliation, or sponsorship by the trademark owner, nor does it imply that the trademark owner has reviewed, approved, or is in any way associated with this work. All trademarked names and registered marks appearing in this textbook are used solely for purposes of identification and educational reference, without any intent of trademark infringement.

Medical Disclaimer

This textbook is intended solely for educational and informational purposes and is designed to support the continuing professional development of licensed healthcare providers. The clinical content presented herein reflects information believed to be accurate and current at the time of publication; however, medicine evolves rapidly, and readers are advised that new research findings, updated clinical practice guidelines, and revised regulatory approvals may alter or supersede information contained in this work after its publication date.

Nothing in this publication constitutes medical advice, clinical guidance specific to any individual patient, or a substitute for the independent professional judgment of a licensed and qualified healthcare provider. No clinician-patient relationship is established, implied, or intended by the use of this textbook or any portion thereof. All clinical decisions, including but not limited to diagnosis, therapeutic selection, drug dosing, and patient monitoring, must be individualized based on thorough and direct assessment of the patient, the totality of current published evidence, applicable clinical practice guidelines, institutional protocols, and the informed professional judgment of the responsible clinician.

Drug information, dosages, treatment protocols, and therapeutic recommendations presented in this publication are offered for educational reference only and must be independently verified against current prescribing information, pharmacopeial references, and applicable regulatory approvals prior to clinical application. The author and publisher have made every reasonable effort to ensure the accuracy and completeness of the information presented; nevertheless, they expressly disclaim all liability for any adverse outcomes, clinical errors, patient harm, loss, or injury alleged to arise, directly or indirectly, from the use, misuse, or application of any information, recommendation, protocol, or clinical guidance contained in this publication.

TABLE OF CONTENT

Contents

PREFACE

Dermatology is, at its core, a discipline of visual pattern recognition. The clinician's eye moves across the skin surface, registers morphology, maps distribution, assesses configuration, and within seconds generates a differential diagnosis that determines whether a lesion is biopsied, treated, or observed. That visual reflex is what makes dermatology one of the most intellectually satisfying specialties in medicine, and it is also what makes it one of the most treacherous. When the pattern is right, the diagnosis is instantaneous. When the pattern deceives, the consequences range from unnecessary treatment to missed malignancy.

This textbook was written to serve that clinical moment, the moment when the clinician looks at a lesion and asks: what is this, what does it look like, and what else could it be? Every chapter in this book delivers comprehensive, evidence-based clinical content organized by the standard architecture of a medical reference: pathophysiology, clinical presentation, diagnostic workup, and management. But woven into that architecture is something that most dermatology textbooks discuss in passing but rarely formalize: a systematic framework for recognizing the conditions that mimic one another and the cognitive traps that drive misdiagnosis.

The Cutaneous Mimicker Recognition Atlas

Every major condition in this textbook carries a branded Mimicker Recognition callout that names the clinical pattern, identifies the most dangerous or common look-alike, exposes the cognitive bias or morphologic shortcut that leads to the diagnostic error, and anchors the clinical decision on the single finding that separates the two. These are not afterthoughts appended to the end of a section. They are embedded inside the clinical narrative at the point where the differential matters most, because that is where misdiagnosis actually happens: not at the end of the chapter, but in the middle of the clinical encounter.

At the back of the book, The Cutaneous Mimicker Master Atlas consolidates every mimicker pair from every chapter into an indexed reference organized by morphologic category, body site, and skin-tone considerations. It is designed to be the scannable navigator that a resident reaches for on consult, in clinic, or before a rotation, the quick-lookup tool that answers the question: this looks like X, but what else could it be, and how do I tell them apart?

Scope and Approach

This book covers the full breadth of clinical dermatology across twenty-four chapters organized into eight parts: foundational skin science and the diagnostic approach, inflammatory and papulosquamous dermatoses, vesiculobullous and granulomatous disorders, infectious dermatology, cutaneous oncology, disorders of skin appendages, connective tissue diseases and vasculitis, and special topics including pediatric dermatology, cutaneous manifestations of systemic disease, pigmentary disorders, and dermatologic therapeutics and procedures.

The content is written for dermatology residents, medical students on dermatology rotations, primary care clinicians who manage skin conditions, and nurse practitioners and physician assistants in dermatology practice. It is grounded in current clinical guidelines from the American Academy of Dermatology, the British Association of Dermatologists, the European Academy of Dermatology and Venereology, the National Comprehensive Cancer Network, and major specialty societies, synthesized with evidence from peer-reviewed dermatology literature and landmark clinical trials.

The visual content reflects the Enhanced level: comprehensive algorithms rendered as structured decision-tree prose, annotated dermoscopic and histopathologic images, clinical photography across skin types, anatomical illustrations, and comparative tables for classification systems, drug dosing, and scoring instruments. Every image placeholder in this textbook specifies its visual type from a locked specialty inventory, its rendering style, and its labeling requirements, so that each figure belongs to the professional visual vocabulary of dermatology publishing rather than generic infographic conventions.

What This Book Does Not Contain

This textbook contains no practice questions, review questions, board-style items, multiple-choice drills, mock examinations, or any content in question-and-answer format. It is a clinical reference, not an exam-prep workbook. Clinical cases appear as narrative scenarios with guided diagnostic and management reasoning, teaching the thought process rather than testing recall. The Mimicker Recognition Atlas teaches pattern discrimination through clinical decision anchors, not through stems and answer choices. Readers seeking question-bank resources will find them in dedicated board-review products; this book's purpose is to build the clinical foundation that makes those questions answerable.

A Note on Skin of Color

Dermatologic disease does not present uniformly across skin phototypes. Inflammation that appears pink or red in lightly pigmented skin may present as violaceous, hyperpigmented, or subtle in darker skin tones, and reliance on color-dependent diagnostic cues is a well-documented source of diagnostic error. Throughout this textbook, clinical descriptions include presentation features across the Fitzpatrick phototype spectrum, and the Mimicker Recognition Atlas flags skin-tone-dependent discriminating features where they alter the differential. This is not a separate chapter or an addendum. It is integrated into the clinical content because it belongs there.

It is my hope that this textbook serves as both a comprehensive clinical reference and a practical diagnostic companion, one that respects the complexity of cutaneous medicine while making its patterns visible, its mimickers named, and its traps avoidable.

CHAPTER 1: STRUCTURE AND FUNCTION OF THE SKIN

Learning Objectives

1. Describe the embryologic origin of each major skin compartment and its clinical significance in genodermatoses and developmental anomalies.
2. Explain the layered architecture of the epidermis, including the role of each stratum in barrier function, keratinization, and immune surveillance.
3. Distinguish the structural and functional roles of collagen, elastin, and ground substance within the papillary and reticular dermis.
4. Identify the anatomy and secretory function of the major adnexal structures and their relevance to common dermatologic conditions.
5. Describe the cutaneous immune system, including innate and adaptive components, and explain how immune dysregulation underlies inflammatory, autoimmune, and neoplastic skin disease.

Embryology and Development of the Skin

Ectodermal and Mesodermal Origins

The skin is the largest organ of the human body, spanning approximately 1.5 to 2.0 square meters in the average adult and accounting for roughly 15 percent of total body weight. Its clinical significance extends far beyond its role as a physical barrier: the skin functions simultaneously as an immunologic organ, a sensory interface, a thermoregulatory system, and a metabolic site for vitamin D synthesis. Understanding the structure and function of each compartment is foundational to every diagnostic and therapeutic decision in dermatology.

The skin derives from two embryonic germ layers. The epidermis, including melanocytes and Merkel cells, originates from surface ectoderm, while the dermis and hypodermis arise from mesoderm (lateral plate mesoderm for the limb and body wall skin, and neural crest mesoderm for the head and neck). Melanocytes and peripheral nerve components migrate from the neural crest, which is why neural crest disorders such as neurofibromatosis and Waardenburg syndrome manifest with both pigmentary and neurologic abnormalities. The epidermis begins as a single layer of ectodermal cells during the third week of gestation, stratifies into the periderm and basal layer by the fourth week, and progressively differentiates into the full stratified squamous epithelium by the end of the second trimester.

Clinical Significance of Developmental Anomalies

Adnexal structures begin to form between weeks 9 and 15 as epithelial downgrowths from the basal layer into the underlying mesenchyme, guided by reciprocal epithelial-mesenchymal signaling through the Wnt, Hedgehog, and Notch pathways. Disruption of these signaling cascades during development produces the genodermatoses, including the ectodermal dysplasias (which affect hair, nails, teeth, and sweat glands simultaneously because all share an ectodermal origin) and Gorlin syndrome, in which constitutive activation of the Hedgehog pathway drives both developmental anomalies and basal cell carcinomas. Blaschko lines, the V-shaped and S-shaped patterns visible on the trunk and extremities in conditions such as linear epidermal nevi and incontinentia pigmenti, trace the migration pathways of epidermal progenitor cells during embryogenesis and do not follow dermatomes, vascular territories, or lymphatic drainage.

Mosaicism is the developmental principle that underlies the clinical appearance of Blaschko-linear dermatoses. When a somatic mutation occurs in a single epidermal progenitor cell during embryogenesis, the mutant clone expands along the migration pathway and produces a stripe of genetically distinct skin visible as a linear or whorled lesion that follows Blaschko lines. This mechanism explains why linear epidermal nevi, linear morphea, and linear lichen planus all share the same distribution pattern despite having entirely different pathologic processes: the pattern reflects the embryonic clone, not the disease mechanism. Recognition of this mosaic distribution is clinically actionable because it separates genetic mosaicism conditions (which carry a risk of systemic involvement if the same mutation is present in non-cutaneous tissues) from acquired inflammatory conditions that may incidentally follow a linear distribution.

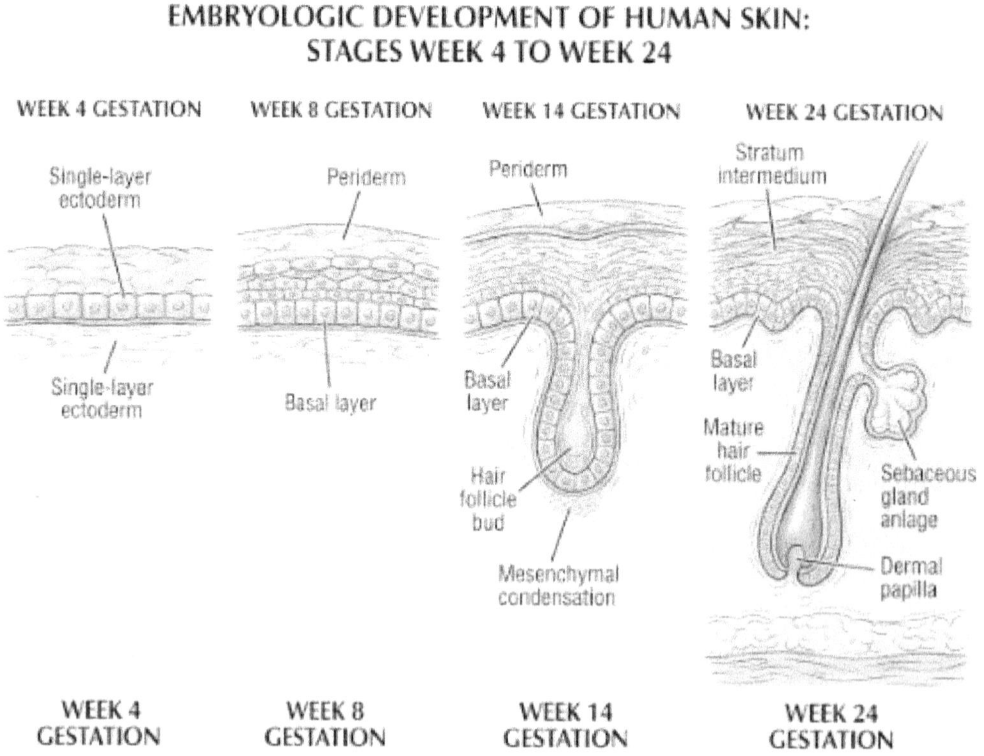

Epidermis: Layers, Keratinization, and Barrier Function

Stratified Architecture

The epidermis is a self-renewing stratified squamous epithelium approximately 0.05 to 1.5 millimeters thick, thinnest on the eyelids and thickest on the palms and soles. It consists of four layers in thin skin (stratum basale, stratum spinosum, stratum granulosum, and stratum corneum) and five layers in thick skin, where the stratum lucidum interposes between the granulosum and corneum. The entire epidermal transit time from basal cell division to corneocyte desquamation averages 40 to 56 days in normal skin but accelerates dramatically in hyperproliferative conditions such as psoriasis, where the transit time drops to as few as 4 to 7 days because of accelerated keratinocyte turnover driven by IL-17 and TNF-alpha signaling.

Keratinization and Terminal Differentiation

The stratum basale is a single layer of columnar to cuboidal keratinocytes anchored to the basement membrane zone by hemidesmosomes, which connect intracellular keratin filaments (keratins 5 and 14) to the extracellular matrix through integrin-laminin interactions. Mutations in keratins 5 or 14 cause epidermolysis bullosa simplex because the structural scaffold that resists mechanical shear is compromised at the basal layer, producing intraepidermal blistering with minimal trauma. The stratum spinosum consists of several layers of polyhedral keratinocytes connected by desmosomes, which are the intercellular junctions targeted by autoantibodies in pemphigus vulgaris and pemphigus foliaceus. Desmoglein 3 predominates in the lower epidermis and mucosae, while desmoglein 1 predominates in the upper epidermis and skin surface, which is why pemphigus vulgaris (anti-desmoglein 3) causes mucosal erosions and deeper blistering, while pemphigus foliaceus (anti-desmoglein 1) causes superficial cutaneous blistering without mucosal involvement. This desmoglein compensation theory directly determines clinical phenotype and biopsy level.

In the stratum granulosum, keratinocytes contain keratohyalin granules rich in profilaggrin, which is processed into filaggrin monomers that aggregate keratin filaments into dense macrofibrils. Loss-of-function mutations in the filaggrin gene (FLG) are the strongest known genetic risk factor for atopic dermatitis, because the resulting deficiency in filaggrin disrupts both the structural integrity of the cornified envelope and the composition of natural moisturizing factor, leading to transepidermal water loss and impaired barrier function. Lamellar bodies in the granulosum release their lipid contents (ceramides, cholesterol, and free fatty acids) into the intercellular space, forming the lipid lamellae of the stratum corneum, a hydrophobic barrier organized in a brick-and-mortar model where corneocytes are the bricks and the lipid lamellae are the mortar.

CLINICAL PEARL: The brick-and-mortar model explains why emollient therapy in atopic dermatitis targets lipid replacement (ceramide-containing moisturizers) rather than simply occluding the surface: the barrier deficit is in the mortar, not on top of the wall.

Resident Cell Populations

The epidermis contains four resident cell populations: keratinocytes (approximately 90 percent), melanocytes (approximately 5 to 10 percent), Langerhans cells (2 to 5 percent), and Merkel cells (less than 1 percent). Melanocytes reside in the basal layer and transfer melanin-containing melanosomes to surrounding keratinocytes via dendritic processes, forming the epidermal melanin unit. Differences in skin pigmentation across Fitzpatrick phototypes reflect differences in melanosome size, distribution, and degradation rate rather than melanocyte number, which is roughly constant across all skin types. Langerhans cells are bone-marrow-derived dendritic cells that function as antigen-presenting cells, capturing antigens in the epidermis and migrating to regional lymph nodes to activate T-cell responses; they are central to the pathogenesis of allergic contact dermatitis. Merkel cells, concentrated in the fingertips, lips, and hair follicle bulge, function as slowly adapting mechanoreceptors and are the cell of origin for Merkel cell carcinoma, a rare but aggressive cutaneous malignancy driven by Merkel cell polyomavirus integration in approximately 80 percent of cases.

The Basement Membrane Zone

The basement membrane zone is the specialized interface between the epidermis and dermis, and its structural integrity determines whether the skin resists mechanical separation. Ultrastructurally, the zone consists of four layers from superficial to deep: the hemidesmosomal plaque on the basal keratinocyte, the lamina lucida, the lamina densa, and the sub-lamina densa zone containing anchoring fibrils. Each layer contains distinct structural proteins, and autoimmune or genetic targeting of any one of them produces a specific blistering disease. Bullous pemphigoid autoantibodies target BP180 (type XVII collagen) and BP230 at the hemidesmosome, producing subepidermal blisters with eosinophilic infiltrates. Linear IgA bullous dermatosis targets the extracellular domain of BP180 after it is cleaved and shed into the lamina lucida. Anti-laminin-332 mucous membrane pemphigoid targets anchoring filaments in the lamina lucida and carries an association with occult malignancy. Epidermolysis bullosa acquisita autoantibodies target type VII collagen in the anchoring fibrils of the sub-lamina densa zone, producing a mechanobullous phenotype with skin fragility, scarring, and milia formation. The level of the split, identifiable on direct immunofluorescence with salt-split skin technique, is the diagnostic discriminator among subepidermal blistering diseases because the clinical morphology of a tense blister is often identical regardless of the target antigen.

KEY POINT: Salt-split skin direct immunofluorescence is the definitive technique for localizing autoantibodies within the basement membrane zone. Antibodies binding the epidermal side of the split (roof pattern) indicate bullous pemphigoid or linear IgA disease. Antibodies binding the dermal side (floor pattern) indicate epidermolysis bullosa acquisita or anti-laminin-332 pemphigoid. The technique separates conditions that are clinically and histologically indistinguishable.

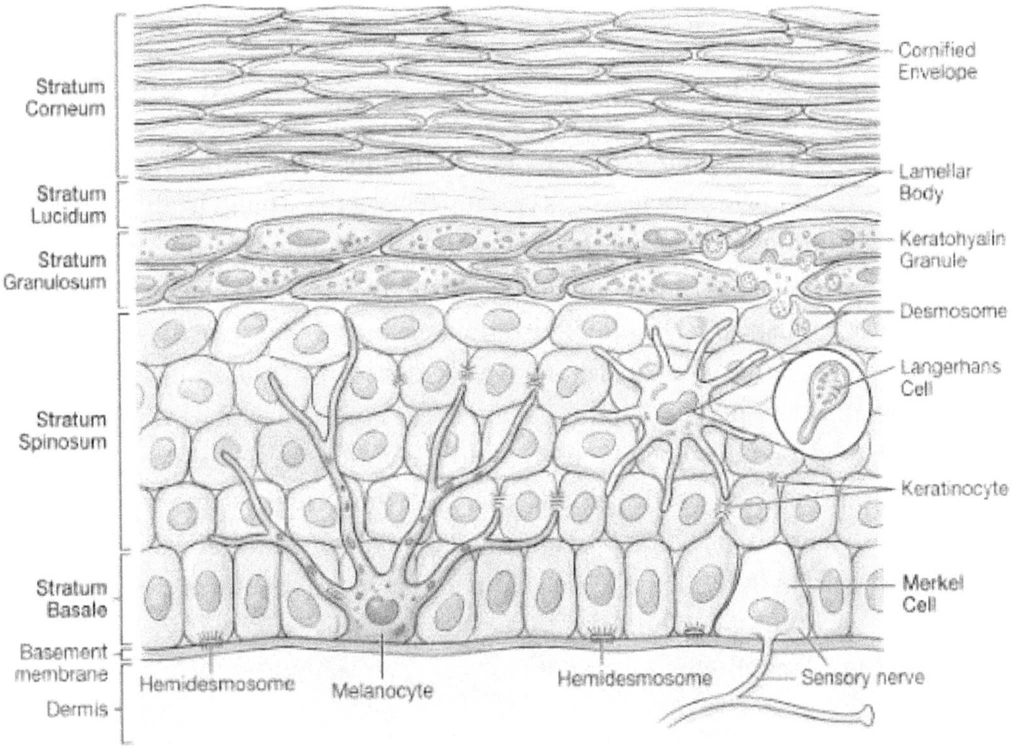

Dermis: Collagen, Elastin, and Ground Substance

Papillary and Reticular Dermis

The dermis is a connective tissue layer ranging from 0.3 millimeters on the eyelids to over 3 millimeters on the back, composed predominantly of type I and type III collagen (approximately 80 and 15 percent of total dermal collagen, respectively), elastic fibers, and ground substance. It is divided into the papillary dermis, a thin zone of loose connective tissue with fine collagen fibrils and capillary loops that interdigitates with the epidermis via dermal papillae, and the reticular dermis, a thicker zone of dense irregular connective tissue with coarse collagen bundles arranged in a basketweave pattern that provides tensile strength and mechanical resilience. The ratio of type III to type I collagen is higher in the papillary dermis and in fetal skin, which is why fetal wounds heal without scarring: the collagen architecture of the fetal dermis favors regenerative remodeling over fibrosis.

Extracellular Matrix Components

Elastic fibers in the dermis form a network of oxytalan fibers (in the papillary dermis, oriented perpendicular to the epidermis), elaunin fibers (at the papillary-reticular junction), and mature elastic fibers (in the reticular dermis). Ultraviolet radiation degrades elastic fibers through matrix metalloproteinase activation and reactive oxygen species generation, producing the disorganized elastotic material visible histologically as solar elastosis, the hallmark of photoaged skin. Ground substance fills the extracellular space and consists primarily of glycosaminoglycans (hyaluronic acid, dermatan sulfate, chondroitin sulfate) and proteoglycans (decorin, versican). Hyaluronic acid is the most abundant glycosaminoglycan in the dermis, capable of binding up to 1,000 times its weight in water, which is why dermal fillers based on cross-linked hyaluronic acid restore tissue volume and hydration.

Dermal Fibroblasts and Wound Healing

Dermal fibroblasts are the principal effector cells of the dermis, responsible for synthesizing collagen, elastin, and ground substance during homeostasis and for driving the wound healing response after injury. Wound healing proceeds through three overlapping phases: inflammation (neutrophil and macrophage infiltration, lasting 1 to 3 days), proliferation (fibroblast migration and collagen deposition, granulation tissue formation, angiogenesis, and re-epithelialization, lasting 3 days to 3 weeks), and remodeling (collagen cross-linking and scar maturation, lasting weeks to months). Abnormal wound healing produces either hypertrophic scars, which remain within the boundaries of the original wound and tend to regress, or keloids, which extend beyond the wound margins and recur after excision. The distinction is clinically important because keloids carry a strong genetic predisposition (highest prevalence in individuals of African, Asian, and Hispanic descent), require multimodal therapy (intralesional corticosteroids, silicone sheeting, pressure therapy, and in refractory cases radiation), and recur at rates exceeding 50 percent after excision alone, whereas hypertrophic scars often respond to simpler interventions and flatten spontaneously over 12 to 18 months.

KEY POINT: Solar elastosis on histopathology is the definitive marker of cumulative UV damage, not chronologic aging. Its presence in a skin biopsy specimen confirms that the site has sustained significant UV exposure regardless of the patient's reported sun history.

Collagen Type	Dermal Location	Clinical Significance
Type I	Reticular dermis (80% of dermal collagen)	Primary structural protein; deficient in Ehlers-Danlos syndrome (classic type)
Type III	Papillary dermis, perivascular (15%)	Predominates in fetal skin and early wound healing; excess in hypertrophic scars
Type IV	Basement membrane zone	Forms the scaffold of the lamina densa; targeted in Goodpasture syndrome (renal) and bullous pemphigoid (skin)
Type VII	Anchoring fibrils below lamina densa	Targeted by autoantibodies in epidermolysis bullosa acquisita; mutated in dystrophic EB

Hypodermis and Subcutaneous Tissue

Structure and Function

The hypodermis (subcutis) lies deep to the reticular dermis and consists of lobules of mature white adipocytes separated by fibrous septa containing blood vessels, lymphatics, and nerves. It functions as a thermal insulator, mechanical cushion, and metabolic reserve, and it is the site of pathology in the panniculitides, a group of inflammatory disorders classified histologically by whether inflammation is predominantly septal (as in erythema nodosum) or lobular (as in pancreatic panniculitis and lupus profundus). The subcutis also contains the deep portion of hair follicles and eccrine sweat glands, which is clinically relevant because deep shave biopsies and punch biopsies must reach the subcutis to capture pathology arising at the level of the hair bulb or deep glandular coil.

Panniculitis Classification

The septal-versus-lobular distinction is the first branch point in the histopathologic classification of panniculitis and directly determines the differential diagnosis. Septal panniculitis with lymphocytic inflammation points to erythema nodosum; septal panniculitis with granulomatous inflammation points to necrobiosis lipoidica. Lobular panniculitis with neutrophilic inflammation raises concern for pancreatic panniculitis, alpha-1-antitrypsin deficiency panniculitis, or infectious panniculitis; lobular panniculitis with lymphocytic inflammation suggests lupus profundus or subcutaneous panniculitis-like T-cell lymphoma. Vasculitis within the septa or lobules adds a further layer of diagnostic specificity.

Adipocyte Biology and Endocrine Function

Subcutaneous adipocytes are not simply passive energy storage depots. They function as endocrine cells that secrete adipokines, including leptin (which regulates appetite and energy expenditure), adiponectin (which modulates insulin sensitivity and has anti-inflammatory properties), and a range of pro-inflammatory cytokines (TNF-alpha, IL-6) that contribute to the systemic inflammatory state associated with obesity. This endocrine activity of subcutaneous fat is clinically relevant in dermatology because adipokine dysregulation has been linked to the increased prevalence and severity of psoriasis in obese patients: elevated TNF-alpha from visceral and subcutaneous fat amplifies the Th17-driven inflammatory cascade in psoriatic skin, which is one reason why weight loss has been shown to improve psoriasis severity scores and enhance the efficacy of biologic therapy. Lipodystrophy syndromes, in which subcutaneous fat is regionally or globally lost, produce both metabolic complications (insulin resistance, hypertriglyceridemia, hepatic steatosis) and distinctive cutaneous findings that may be the presenting feature, including localized lipoatrophy at insulin injection sites, HIV-associated lipodystrophy from antiretroviral therapy, and the rare inherited conditions such as Berardinelli-Seip congenital generalized lipodystrophy.

Adnexal Structures: Hair Follicles, Sebaceous Glands, and Sweat Glands

Hair Follicle Anatomy and the Hair Cycle

The hair follicle is a complex mini-organ extending from the epidermis into the dermis or subcutis, composed of the infundibulum (above the sebaceous gland duct insertion), the isthmus (between the sebaceous duct and the arrector pili muscle insertion), and the inferior segment (below the isthmus, including the bulb and dermal papilla). The follicular bulge, located at the isthmus level near the arrector pili insertion, contains the multipotent epithelial stem cells that regenerate the hair follicle and can repopulate the epidermis after wounding, which is why superficial wounds that spare the follicle re-epithelialize rapidly from the follicular reserve while full-thickness burns that destroy the follicle require grafting.

The hair cycle consists of three phases: anagen (active growth, lasting 2 to 7 years for scalp hair), catagen (involution, lasting 2 to 3 weeks), and telogen (resting, lasting 2 to 4 months before the hair is shed and replaced by a new anagen hair). Approximately 85 to 90 percent of scalp hairs are in anagen at any time. Telogen effluvium, the most common cause of diffuse hair shedding, occurs when a physiologic stressor (febrile illness, surgery, postpartum hormonal shift, nutritional deficiency) synchronizes a large proportion of anagen follicles into premature telogen, producing diffuse shedding 2 to 4 months after the inciting event. The temporal lag between the stressor and the onset of shedding is the diagnostic hallmark.

Sebaceous and Sweat Glands

Sebaceous glands are holocrine glands associated with hair follicles that produce sebum, a lipid-rich secretion composed of triglycerides, wax esters, squalene, and free fatty acids. Sebaceous gland activity is androgen-dependent, which is why acne vulgaris peaks during puberty and why anti-androgen therapy (spironolactone, combined oral contraceptives) is effective in adult female acne. Eccrine sweat glands are distributed across nearly the entire body surface and are the primary effectors of thermoregulation, producing a hypotonic sweat that cools the body through evaporation. Apocrine sweat glands are limited to the axillae, anogenital region, and periareolar area; their secretion is initially odorless but produces body odor when metabolized by resident bacteria. The apocrine glands are the target structures in hidradenitis suppurativa, a chronic inflammatory condition driven by follicular occlusion and secondary immune activation rather than primary infection.

Clinical Correlates of Adnexal Pathology

The clinical importance of the follicular bulge stem cell niche extends beyond wound healing. Destruction of the bulge in scarring alopecias (lichen planopilaris, frontal fibrosing alopecia, central centrifugal cicatricial alopecia) produces permanent hair loss because the stem cell reservoir that would otherwise regenerate the follicle in each new anagen cycle has been obliterated by inflammation. This is the biological basis for the clinical distinction between scarring and non-scarring alopecias: non-scarring alopecias (androgenetic alopecia, alopecia areata, telogen effluvium) preserve the bulge and therefore retain the potential for regrowth, while scarring alopecias destroy it and are irreversible. Dermoscopy of the scalp aids in this distinction by identifying the absence of follicular ostia in scarring alopecia (smooth, white, featureless scarred scalp) versus preserved ostia in non-scarring forms. Sebaceous gland hyperplasia, a common benign condition in middle-aged and older adults, presents as yellowish papules with a central dell on the face and must be distinguished from basal cell carcinoma, which can share a similar translucent, lobulated appearance; dermoscopy revealing crown vessels surrounding pale lobules is diagnostic for sebaceous hyperplasia.

THE CUTANEOUS MIMICKER RECOGNITION ATLAS — Hidradenitis Suppurativa versus Recurrent Furunculosis

The Clinical Pattern: Hidradenitis suppurativa presents with recurrent painful nodules, abscesses, and draining sinus tracts in the axillary, inguinal, and anogenital folds, often with double-ended comedones and rope-like scarring. The distribution is apocrine-gland-bearing skin, and the chronicity with sinus tract formation distinguishes the pattern from isolated infection.

The Mimicker: Recurrent furunculosis (staphylococcal abscesses) overlaps morphologically with early hidradenitis suppurativa: both present as painful, fluctuant nodules in intertriginous areas. The overlap is strongest in Hurley stage I hidradenitis, where sinus tracts and scarring have not yet developed, and a single abscess in the groin or axilla may be treated as a boil without further evaluation.

Trap Logic: Anchoring bias drives this misdiagnosis. The clinician anchors on the first presentation (a single abscess), incises and drains it, prescribes antibiotics, and closes the encounter. When the patient returns with a second abscess, the clinician anchors again on the prior diagnosis of furunculosis rather than reconsidering the pattern. Recurrence in apocrine-bearing sites is the signal that anchoring has overridden pattern recognition.

The Decision Anchor: The discriminating finding is **recurrence in apocrine-gland-bearing skin with architectural change**: double-ended comedones, sinus tracts connecting separate nodules, or rope-like bridging scars. Furunculosis produces discrete, independent abscesses without architectural interconnection. If the nodules recur in the same anatomical distribution and develop sinus tracts or scarring, the diagnosis is hidradenitis suppurativa regardless of culture results.

Cutaneous Vasculature and Lymphatics

Vascular Architecture

The cutaneous blood supply is organized into two horizontal plexuses: the superficial (subpapillary) plexus at the junction of the papillary and reticular dermis, and the deep plexus at the dermal-subcutaneous junction. Capillary loops arise from the superficial plexus and extend into each dermal papilla, forming the functional unit for thermoregulation through arteriolar shunting. Arteriovenous anastomoses, or glomus bodies, are concentrated in the digits, ears, nose, and lips, where they regulate blood flow for heat conservation. The glomus tumor, a benign but exquisitely painful neoplasm of the glomus body, characteristically presents as a small blue-red nodule beneath the nail with the classic triad of paroxysmal pain, point tenderness, and cold sensitivity.

Lymphatic Drainage and Dermal Edema

The cutaneous lymphatic network begins as blind-ended lymphatic capillaries in the papillary dermis that drain into collecting lymphatic vessels in the reticular dermis and subcutis, ultimately emptying into regional lymph nodes. Lymphatic drainage is critical in the pathogenesis of inflammatory edema (urticaria, angioedema), lymphedema (primary or secondary to lymph node dissection, radiation, or filariasis), and metastatic spread of cutaneous malignancies. Sentinel lymph node biopsy in melanoma staging relies on the principle that cutaneous lymphatic drainage from any given site follows a predictable pathway to the first echelon lymph node, which is the most likely site of initial metastatic deposition.

Vascular Pathology and Diagnostic Significance

The two-plexus vascular architecture is directly relevant to the histopathologic classification of cutaneous vasculitis. Small-vessel vasculitis (leukocytoclastic vasculitis, IgA vasculitis, urticarial vasculitis) affects the postcapillary venules of the superficial plexus, producing palpable purpura, urticarial lesions, or hemorrhagic vesicles in the skin. Medium-vessel vasculitis (polyarteritis nodosa) affects the muscular arterioles of the deep plexus and the arteries at the dermal-subcutaneous junction, producing livedo reticularis, subcutaneous nodules, and ulceration. This size-based classification predicts the clinical morphology, the depth of the biopsy required for diagnosis (a superficial shave will miss medium-vessel disease), and the systemic associations: small-vessel disease associates with ANCA, cryoglobulins, and drug reactions, while medium-vessel cutaneous polyarteritis nodosa is typically limited to the skin and follows a chronic relapsing course without the renal or gastrointestinal involvement seen in systemic polyarteritis.

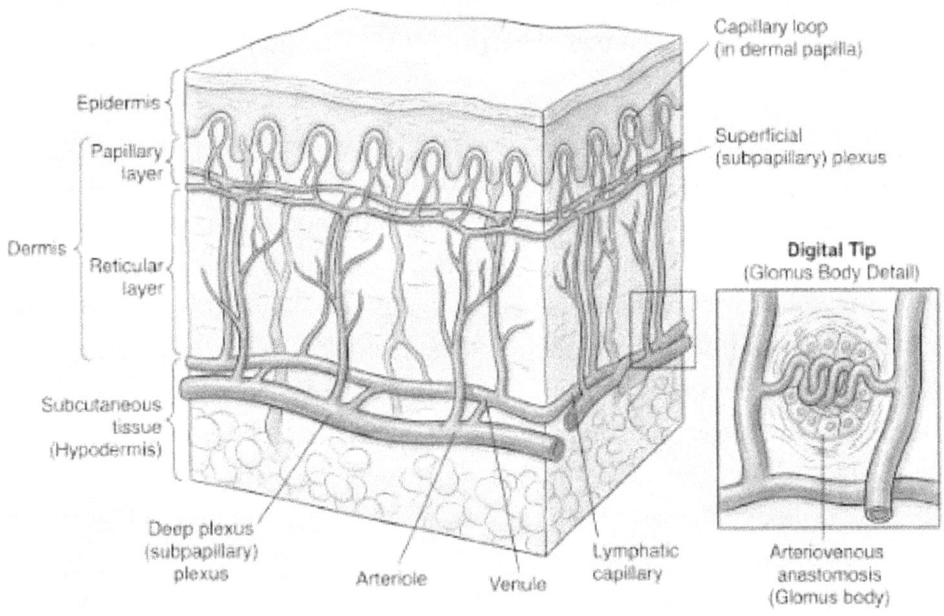

Cutaneous Innervation and Sensory Receptors

Sensory Nerve Supply

The skin is densely innervated by both somatic sensory and autonomic nerve fibers. Free nerve endings in the epidermis and papillary dermis mediate pain, temperature, and itch (pruritus) and are the most numerous cutaneous receptor type. Itch, the cardinal symptom of dermatologic disease, is transmitted by unmyelinated C fibers that are distinct from pain-transmitting fibers, which is why pain and itch can coexist but also antagonize each other (scratching relieves itch by activating pain pathways that suppress itch signaling). Histamine was long considered the primary pruritogen, but the discovery of non-histaminergic itch pathways mediated by IL-31, IL-4, IL-13, and thymic stromal lymphopoietin has explained why antihistamines fail to control pruritus in many inflammatory dermatoses, particularly atopic dermatitis, and why JAK inhibitors and anti-IL-31 antibodies (nemolizumab) are effective antipruritics in these conditions.

Encapsulated Receptors and Dermatome Mapping

Encapsulated mechanoreceptors include Meissner corpuscles (light touch, concentrated in the fingertips and lips), Pacinian corpuscles (deep pressure and vibration, located in the deep dermis and subcutis), Ruffini corpuscles (sustained pressure and skin stretch), and Merkel cell-neurite complexes (fine touch discrimination). The distribution and density of these receptors vary by body site, which is why two-point discrimination is finest on the fingertips and poorest on the back. Cutaneous sensory innervation follows a dermatomal pattern for the trunk and limbs, which is clinically exploited in the diagnosis of herpes zoster: the restriction of the vesicular eruption to a single dermatome is the pathognomonic distribution pattern that separates zoster from disseminated herpes simplex, varicella, and other vesicular eruptions.

Autonomic Innervation and Neuropeptide Signaling

Autonomic nerve fibers in the skin innervate blood vessels, arrector pili muscles, and eccrine sweat glands, and mediate the sympathetic vasomotor, pilomotor, and sudomotor responses that are clinically tested during the autonomic neuropathy workup. Sympathetic cholinergic fibers innervate eccrine glands (explaining why generalized hyperhidrosis is a sympathetically driven condition amenable to anticholinergic therapy or endoscopic thoracic sympathectomy), while sympathetic adrenergic fibers innervate blood vessels and arrector pili muscles (explaining the vasoconstriction and goosebumps of the fight-or-flight response). Cutaneous sensory nerves also release neuropeptides, including substance P and calcitonin gene-related peptide, which mediate neurogenic inflammation: vasodilation, plasma extravasation, and mast cell degranulation triggered by nerve fiber activation rather than by immunologic stimuli. Neurogenic inflammation explains the wheal-and-flare response to histamine skin testing, the pathogenesis of notalgia paresthetica (a localized pruritic patch on the upper back caused by dorsal rami neuropathy), and the contribution of stress and emotional triggers to inflammatory dermatoses such as rosacea and psoriasis, in which neuropeptide release amplifies the vascular and inflammatory components of the disease.

THE CUTANEOUS MIMICKER RECOGNITION ATLAS — Herpes Zoster versus Zosteriform Herpes Simplex

---

The Clinical Pattern: Herpes zoster presents as grouped vesicles on an erythematous base distributed along a single dermatome, preceded by a prodrome of dermatomal pain, burning, or tingling. The vesicles do not cross the midline, and new vesicle formation typically ceases within 5 to 7 days. The eruption follows VZV reactivation from a single dorsal root ganglion.

The Mimicker: Zosteriform herpes simplex virus (HSV) infection mimics herpes zoster both morphologically and distributionally: it produces grouped vesicles in a dermatomal or pseudodermatomal pattern, most commonly on the trunk, buttocks, or extremities. It is caused by HSV-1 or HSV-2 reactivation from ganglia, and can present with prodromal pain identical to zoster. The morphologic overlap is so close that clinical distinction is unreliable without laboratory confirmation.

Trap Logic: Premature closure is the cognitive trap. The clinician sees grouped vesicles in a dermatomal pattern, diagnoses herpes zoster, and stops the diagnostic workup. Zosteriform HSV is not considered because the distribution pattern has already satisfied the clinician's diagnostic script. The trap is reinforced by the fact that both conditions respond to valacyclovir, so even an incorrect diagnosis produces a clinical response, preventing the error from being corrected by treatment failure.

The Decision Anchor: The discriminating finding is **recurrence in the same distribution**. Herpes zoster virtually never recurs in the same dermatome in immunocompetent patients, while zosteriform HSV characteristically recurs repeatedly in the same area. A patient with a second episode of dermatomal vesicles in the same distribution almost certainly has zosteriform HSV, not recurrent zoster. Viral culture, direct fluorescent antibody testing, or PCR-based typing confirms the distinction on the first episode when recurrence has not yet been observed.

Skin Immunology: Innate and Adaptive Cutaneous Immunity

The Skin as an Immune Organ

The skin is one of the largest immunologic organs in the body, containing a resident population of immune cells that continuously surveys the cutaneous environment for pathogens, allergens, and neoplastic transformation. The concept of skin-associated lymphoid tissue encompasses the interacting network of keratinocytes (which function as non-professional antigen-presenting cells and secrete a broad array of cytokines, chemokines, and antimicrobial peptides), Langerhans cells (the sentinel dendritic cells of the epidermis), dermal dendritic cells, resident memory T cells, mast cells, macrophages, innate lymphoid cells, and the draining lymph nodes.

Innate Immunity and Antimicrobial Defense

Innate cutaneous immunity begins with the physical barrier of the stratum corneum and its acidic surface (pH 4.5 to 5.5, the acid mantle), which inhibits colonization by pathogenic bacteria while supporting the commensal microbiome. Keratinocytes produce antimicrobial peptides including human beta-defensins, cathelicidin (LL-37), and psoriasin (S100A7), which provide direct bactericidal, antiviral, and antifungal activity. Deficiency of cathelicidin is implicated in the increased susceptibility to eczema herpeticum in atopic dermatitis patients, because atopic skin produces less LL-37 in response to viral challenge, which is why widespread herpes simplex superinfection is a recognized complication of atopic dermatitis but not of psoriasis, despite both being chronic inflammatory dermatoses.

Mast Cells and Innate Lymphoid Cells

Mast cells are long-lived tissue-resident cells found predominantly in the perivascular dermis, where they function as sentinels of innate immunity and effectors of immediate hypersensitivity. Upon activation — by IgE cross-linking (type I hypersensitivity), complement fragments (C3a, C5a), neuropeptides (substance P), or direct physical stimuli — mast cells degranulate and release preformed mediators (histamine, tryptase, heparin), lipid mediators (prostaglandins, leukotrienes), and a broad panel of cytokines (TNF-alpha, IL-4, IL-13). This mediator release produces the clinical triad of urticaria: vasodilatation (erythema), increased vascular permeability (edema, the wheal), and pruritus. Mastocytosis, the clonal proliferation of mast cells carrying activating KIT mutations (most commonly D816V), produces urticaria pigmentosa (the cutaneous form characterized by red-brown macules and papules that urticate on stroking, the Darier sign) and systemic mastocytosis, in which mast cell infiltration of bone marrow, liver, and spleen causes constitutional symptoms, anaphylaxis risk, and cytopenias. Innate lymphoid cells (ILCs) are tissue-resident lymphocytes that mirror T-helper subsets without antigen-specific receptors: ILC1s produce IFN-gamma (parallel to Th1), ILC2s produce IL-5 and IL-13 (parallel to Th2), and ILC3s produce IL-17 and IL-22 (parallel to Th17). ILC2s are particularly abundant in the skin and are activated early in atopic dermatitis by epithelial alarmins (TSLP, IL-25, IL-33) released from damaged keratinocytes, providing a bridge between barrier disruption and the Th2-skewed adaptive immune response that sustains the disease.

Adaptive Immunity and T-Cell Polarization

Adaptive cutaneous immunity is orchestrated by T cells, which are recruited to the skin through addressin-mediated homing and retained as tissue-resident memory T cells in the dermis and epidermis. The T-helper cell polarization pattern determines the clinical phenotype of inflammatory skin disease: Th2-dominant inflammation (IL-4, IL-13, IL-31) drives atopic dermatitis, characterized by spongiotic dermatitis, eosinophilic infiltrates, and pruritus; Th1-dominant inflammation (IFN-gamma, TNF-alpha) drives allergic contact dermatitis and graft-versus-host disease; Th17-dominant inflammation (IL-17A, IL-17F, IL-22) drives psoriasis, characterized by epidermal hyperproliferation, neutrophilic microabscesses, and the classic silvery scale. This polarization framework directly explains why biologic therapies targeting specific cytokine axes are effective in one disease but not another: dupilumab (anti-IL-4R-alpha) treats atopic dermatitis but not psoriasis, while secukinumab (anti-IL-17A) treats psoriasis but not atopic dermatitis.

KEY POINT: The Th2/Th17 polarization dichotomy is not merely academic: it is the molecular basis for the entire modern biologic formulary in dermatology. Prescribing a Th17-targeted biologic for a Th2-driven disease, or vice versa, is not just ineffective but potentially harmful, as seen in the risk of paradoxical psoriasiform eruptions with TNF-alpha inhibitors and the risk of accelerating cutaneous T-cell lymphoma with Th2-targeted biologics.

Immune Privilege and Tolerance in the Skin

Certain anatomic sites within the skin maintain relative immune privilege, a state in which immune responses are actively suppressed to protect structures that cannot regenerate. The hair follicle bulge, which contains the epithelial stem cells necessary for follicular regeneration, is one such site. The bulge maintains immune privilege through downregulation of MHC class I expression and local production of immunosuppressive factors including alpha-melanocyte-stimulating hormone and TGF-beta. Collapse of follicular immune privilege, triggered by IFN-gamma-mediated upregulation of MHC class I on bulge cells, is the proposed mechanism for alopecia areata: autoreactive CD8+ T cells that were previously excluded from the bulge gain access and attack the follicular stem cells, producing the characteristic well-demarcated patches of non-scarring hair loss with exclamation-point hairs at the periphery. Regulatory T cells (Tregs) expressing the transcription factor FoxP3 reside in the dermis and hair follicle and actively maintain peripheral tolerance by suppressing autoreactive effector T cells. Loss of Treg function, as occurs in the IPEX syndrome (immune dysregulation, polyendocrinopathy, enteropathy, X-linked), produces severe multisystem autoimmunity with prominent cutaneous manifestations including eczematous dermatitis, psoriasiform eruptions, and alopecia.

SCHEMATIC DIAGRAM OF T-HELPER CELL POLARIZATION PATHWAYS IN CUTANEOUS INFLAMMATION

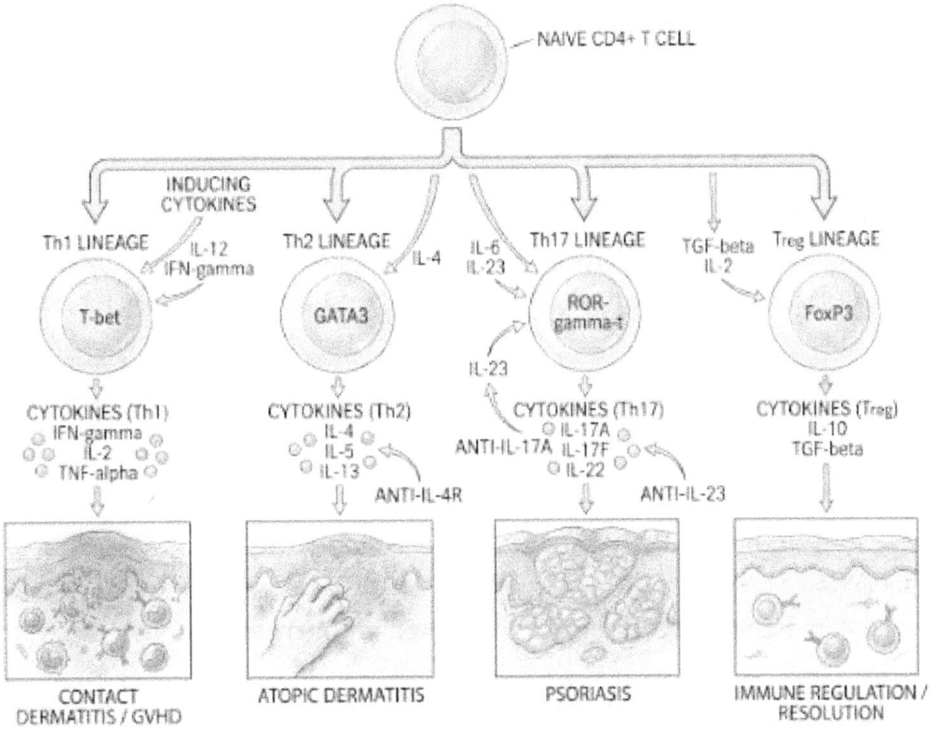

T-Helper Subset	Key Cytokines	Transcription Factor	Associated Dermatosis	Targeted Biologic
Th1	IFN-gamma, TNF-alpha	T-bet	Allergic contact dermatitis, GVHD	TNF-alpha inhibitors
Th2	IL-4, IL-13, IL-31	GATA3	Atopic dermatitis	Dupilumab (anti-IL-4R-alpha), tralokinumab (anti-IL-13)
Th17	IL-17A, IL-17F, IL-22	ROR-gamma-t	Psoriasis	Secukinumab, ixekizumab (anti-IL-17A); guselkumab, risankizumab (anti-IL-23)
Treg	IL-10, TGF-beta	FoxP3	Immune homeostasis (loss leads to autoimmunity)	Under investigation

Hidradenitis Suppurativa vs. Recurrent Furunculosis: The discriminating finding is recurrence in apocrine-gland-bearing skin with architectural change (double-ended comedones, sinus tracts, bridging scars). Furunculosis produces discrete, independent abscesses. Cognitive trap: anchoring bias on initial abscess diagnosis.

Herpes Zoster vs. Zosteriform Herpes Simplex: The discriminating finding is recurrence in the same dermatomal distribution. Zoster virtually never recurs in the same dermatome in immunocompetent patients; zosteriform HSV characteristically does. Cognitive trap: premature closure on the dermatomal vesicle pattern.

Summary and Key Concepts

The skin is a multilayered organ derived from ectoderm (epidermis, melanocytes, Merkel cells) and mesoderm (dermis, hypodermis), with neural crest contributions (melanocytes, peripheral nerves). Embryologic signaling through Wnt, Hedgehog, and Notch pathways governs adnexal development; disruption produces the genodermatoses. Mosaicism along Blaschko lines reflects clonal expansion of somatically mutated epidermal progenitor cells during embryogenesis.

The epidermis self-renews through basal keratinocyte division, terminal differentiation through the spinous and granular layers, and cornification into the stratum corneum barrier. Filaggrin mutations (FLG) disrupt barrier function and are the strongest genetic risk factor for atopic dermatitis. Desmoglein compensation theory explains the clinical phenotypes of pemphigus vulgaris versus foliaceus. The basement membrane zone, composed of hemidesmosomes, lamina lucida, lamina densa, and anchoring fibrils, is the target of autoimmune and genetic blistering diseases classifiable by salt-split skin immunofluorescence.

The dermis provides structural support through type I and III collagen, elastic fibers, and ground substance. Solar elastosis is the histopathologic hallmark of cumulative UV damage. Collagen type VII anchoring fibrils are targeted in epidermolysis bullosa acquisita. Abnormal wound healing produces hypertrophic scars (confined to wound boundaries, self-resolving) or keloids (extending beyond boundaries, recurrent after excision).

Adnexal structures include hair follicles (with the stem cell-rich bulge region whose destruction causes permanent scarring alopecia), sebaceous glands (androgen-dependent, central to acne pathogenesis), eccrine glands (thermoregulation), and apocrine glands (the target in hidradenitis suppurativa).

The cutaneous immune system integrates innate defense (barrier, antimicrobial peptides, mast cells, innate lymphoid cells) with adaptive immunity (Langerhans cell antigen presentation, T-cell polarization, tissue-resident memory T cells). The Th2/Th17 dichotomy is the molecular basis of the modern biologic formulary: Th2-targeted therapies treat atopic dermatitis, Th17-targeted therapies treat psoriasis, and mismatching the axis to the disease is clinically harmful. Immune privilege at the hair follicle bulge, maintained by MHC class I downregulation and Treg activity, is lost in alopecia areata.

CHAPTER 2: APPROACH TO THE DERMATOLOGIC PATIENT

Learning Objectives

1. Obtain a focused dermatologic history that identifies the key features of onset, evolution, distribution, symptoms, exacerbating and alleviating factors, and relevant medical and medication history.
2. Identify and accurately describe primary and secondary skin lesions using standardized morphologic terminology.
3. Recognize major distribution patterns and configurations and apply them to generate a morphology-based differential diagnosis.
4. Describe the principles and clinical applications of dermoscopy, including the two-step algorithm for pigmented lesion assessment.
5. Select the appropriate biopsy technique and special diagnostic procedure for a given clinical scenario and interpret the major histopathologic reaction patterns.

The Dermatologic History

Core Elements of the Cutaneous History

The dermatologic history follows the same systematic approach as the general medical history but focuses on the temporal and morphologic evolution of the skin complaint. The onset of the eruption, its rate of progression, whether it is stable or changing, and whether it is recurrent or a first episode are the first data points that stratify the differential. Acute onset (hours to days) suggests urticaria, drug eruption, acute contact dermatitis, or infection; subacute onset (days to weeks) raises concern for eczematous dermatitis, pityriasis rosea, or secondary syphilis; chronic duration (weeks to months) points to psoriasis, lichen planus, dermatophytosis, or cutaneous malignancy. The distribution of the eruption at onset versus its current extent reveals whether the process is localizing or generalizing, which further refines the differential.

Symptom Characterization

Symptom characterization is critical because the presence, character, and severity of pruritus, pain, or burning narrow the differential independently of morphology. Pruritus is the dominant symptom in eczematous dermatitis, urticaria, dermatitis herpetiformis, prurigo nodularis, and scabies; its absence in a condition that looks eczematous should prompt reconsideration (mycosis fungoides in the patch and plaque stage may mimic eczema but is often less pruritic, or conversely, intensely pruritic in later stages). Pain suggests herpes zoster, cellulitis, vasculitis, calciphylaxis, or pyoderma gangrenosum. Burning without visible skin change raises the possibility of neuropathic pruritus or small-fiber neuropathy.

Medication, Occupational, and Social History

The medication history is essential because drug eruptions are among the most common mimickers in dermatology. The temporal relationship between drug initiation and eruption onset is the diagnostic anchor: morbilliform drug eruptions typically appear 7 to 14 days after the first exposure to the offending agent or within 1 to 3 days on re-exposure, while drug reaction with eosinophilia and systemic symptoms (DRESS) characteristically presents 2 to 8 weeks after drug initiation, and Stevens-Johnson syndrome or toxic epidermal necrolysis may appear 1 to 3 weeks after exposure. The occupational history identifies exposures to contactants, irritants, and photoactive agents that cause occupational dermatitis. The social history addresses sun exposure habits, tanning bed use, sexual history (relevant to secondary syphilis, genital herpes, and anogenital condylomata), travel history (relevant to cutaneous leishmaniasis, larva migrans, and imported mycoses), and pet exposure (relevant to dermatophytosis and flea-borne diseases).

Review of Systems and Cutaneous Clues to Systemic Disease

The dermatologic review of systems extends beyond the skin itself because cutaneous findings frequently serve as the first visible manifestation of systemic disease. Joint symptoms in a patient with psoriatic plaques raise suspicion for psoriatic arthritis and alter the treatment algorithm toward systemic agents that address both domains. Photosensitivity, oral ulcers, arthritis, and malar erythema constitute the mucocutaneous and musculoskeletal criteria for systemic lupus erythematosus. Dysphagia, proximal muscle weakness, and a heliotrope rash or Gottron papules point toward dermatomyositis, which in adults mandates age-appropriate malignancy screening because of the well-established paraneoplastic association. Weight loss, night sweats, and progressive patches or plaques that fail to respond to topical corticosteroids raise concern for cutaneous T-cell lymphoma (mycosis fungoides), particularly when the patient is older and the lesions involve non-sun-exposed sites such as the buttocks and bathing-trunk distribution. A systematic review of systems that screens for these associations prevents the clinician from treating the skin in isolation when the eruption is the surface marker of an internal process that requires its own evaluation and management.

Morphologic Description of Skin Lesions: Primary and Secondary Lesions

Primary Lesions

Accurate morphologic description is the foundation of dermatologic diagnosis. Primary lesions are those that arise de novo from previously normal skin and represent the earliest manifestation of the disease process. The standard terminology distinguishes flat lesions from raised lesions and solid lesions from fluid-filled lesions. A macule is a flat, circumscribed area of color change less than 1 centimeter in diameter; a patch is the same lesion exceeding 1 centimeter. A papule is a solid, elevated lesion less than 1 centimeter; a plaque is a broad, elevated lesion greater than 1 centimeter, often formed by the coalescence of papules. A nodule is a solid lesion greater than 1 centimeter that extends into the dermis or subcutis and can be palpated as a three-dimensional mass. A vesicle is a fluid-filled blister less than 1 centimeter; a bulla is a fluid-filled blister greater than 1 centimeter. A pustule is a vesicle containing purulent exudate, which may be infectious (staphylococcal folliculitis) or sterile (pustular psoriasis). A wheal (hive) is a transient, edematous, pink papule or plaque caused by dermal edema, characteristic of urticaria; its hallmark is resolution within 24 hours without residual change.

Secondary Lesions and Surface Changes

Secondary lesions result from the evolution, manipulation, or regression of primary lesions and provide essential diagnostic information. Scale represents excess stratum corneum and is classified by its character: fine and powdery in pityriasis versicolor, silvery and micaceous in psoriasis, greasy and yellowish in seborrheic dermatitis, and collarette-shaped in pityriasis rosea. Crust is dried serum, blood, or purulent exudate on the surface; honey-colored crusts are the hallmark of impetigo. Erosion is a loss of the epidermis that heals without scarring; ulceration extends through the epidermis into the dermis or deeper and heals with a scar. Excoriation is a linear erosion produced by scratching and is the physical sign of pruritus. Lichenification is the thickening of skin with accentuation of skin markings produced by chronic rubbing or scratching, seen most characteristically in chronic atopic dermatitis and lichen simplex chronicus. Atrophy refers to thinning of the epidermis (seen as cigarette-paper wrinkling), dermis, or subcutis, and is an important sign of potent topical corticosteroid overuse, morphea, and lipodermatosclerosis.

Color as a Diagnostic Feature

The color of a skin lesion is an independent diagnostic variable that stratifies the differential beyond morphology alone. Violaceous (purple) coloration suggests lichen planus, dermatomyositis, lupus erythematosus, or vascular compromise. Yellow coloration raises consideration for xanthoma, xanthelasma, necrobiosis lipoidica (with a waxy, yellowish atrophic center), or sebaceous hyperplasia. Blue or blue-gray coloration indicates deep melanin (blue nevus, dermal melanocytosis), hemosiderin deposition (stasis dermatitis), or foreign body (tattoo pigment, amalgam tattoo). White lesions prompt a differential including vitiligo, morphea, lichen sclerosus, idiopathic guttate hypomelanosis, and post-inflammatory hypopigmentation. Color assessment must account for the patient's baseline skin phototype: erythema that is readily visible as pink or red in Fitzpatrick phototype I-II may present as violaceous, dusky, or hyperpigmented in phototype V-VI, and the clinician who uses redness as a diagnostic criterion without adjusting for skin tone will systematically underdiagnose inflammatory conditions in patients with darker skin. Palpation, warmth, and tenderness become critical substitute signs for inflammation when erythema is not visually apparent.

CLINICAL PEARL: The distinction between a vesicle and a bulla is not merely semantic: it determines the differential diagnosis. Vesicular eruptions point to herpes simplex, herpes zoster, dyshidrotic eczema, or dermatitis herpetiformis. Bullous eruptions point to bullous pemphigoid, pemphigus (when flaccid), bullous drug eruption, or bullous impetigo. The size of the blister is the first branch point.

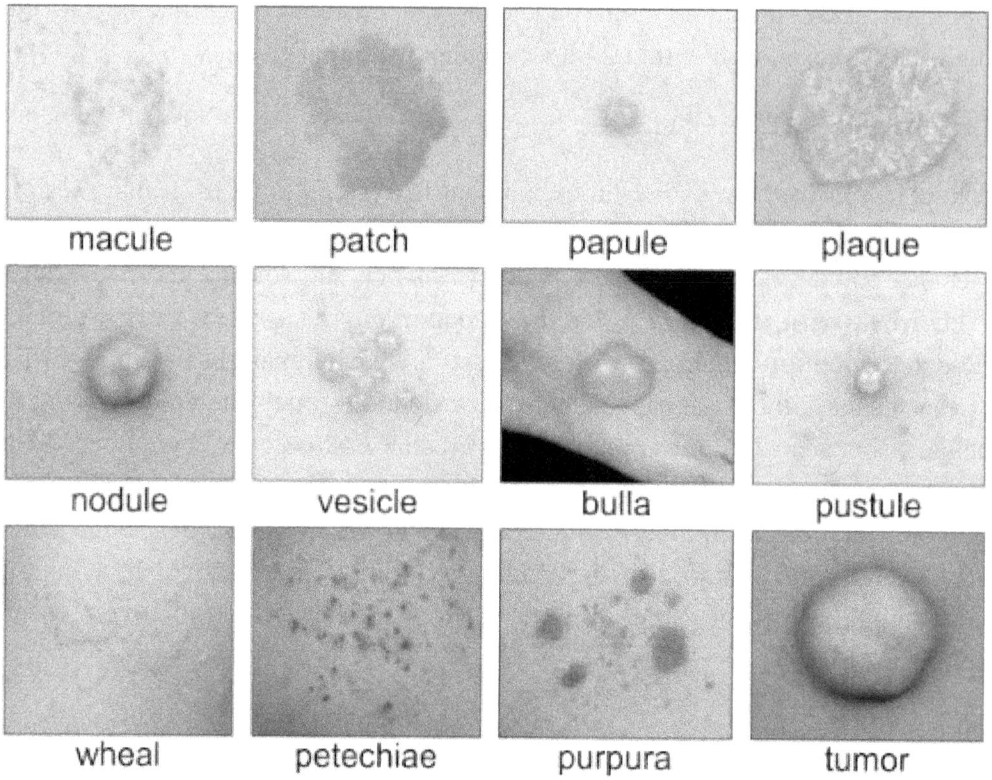

Distribution Patterns and Configuration

Anatomic Distribution as a Diagnostic Clue

The distribution of skin lesions across the body surface is often more diagnostically valuable than the morphology of the individual lesion, because many diseases produce similar-appearing papules, plaques, or patches but distribute them in characteristic patterns that are disease-specific. Extensor-surface involvement (elbows, knees, scalp, sacrum) is the hallmark of psoriasis. Flexural involvement (antecubital and popliteal fossae, neck, wrists) characterizes atopic dermatitis in older children and adults. Sun-exposed distribution (face, dorsal hands, V-neck, forearms) suggests photodermatosis, phototoxic drug eruption, lupus erythematosus, or actinic keratosis. Intertriginous distribution (axillae, groin, inframammary folds, interdigital spaces) points to intertrigo, inverse psoriasis, candidiasis, or erythrasma. Dermatomal distribution indicates herpes zoster. Blaschko-linear distribution suggests mosaicism or an inflammatory dermatosis following embryonic clones.

Configuration and Arrangement

Configuration refers to the arrangement of individual lesions relative to one another. Grouped (herpetiform) vesicles suggest herpes simplex or herpes zoster. Annular (ring-shaped) lesions have an extensive differential including granuloma annulare, tinea corporis, erythema annulare centrifugum, subacute cutaneous lupus erythematosus, and secondary syphilis. Linear lesions suggest an external cause (contact dermatitis along a streak of allergen, koebnerization in psoriasis or lichen planus along a line of trauma) or Blaschko-linear mosaicism. Targetoid (iris) lesions with three concentric zones of color change are the morphologic signature of erythema multiforme. Reticular (net-like) patterning is characteristic of livedo reticularis, which may be physiologic (cutis marmorata) or pathologic (associated with antiphospholipid syndrome, cholesterol embolization, polyarteritis nodosa, or calciphylaxis). Recognizing these configurations converts a list of individual findings into a diagnostic pattern that directs the workup.

Skin-Tone Considerations in Distribution Assessment

Distribution assessment requires particular attention to how skin color modifies the visual signal of disease. Post-inflammatory hyperpigmentation, which is more pronounced and persistent in Fitzpatrick phototype III-VI skin, may be the most prominent finding in a resolving eruption, causing the clinician to focus on pigmentary change rather than the underlying inflammatory process that produced it. Conversely, post-inflammatory hypopigmentation in darker skin tones may mimic vitiligo or pityriasis alba, leading to unnecessary workup when the pigmentary alteration is simply the aftermath of a treated or spontaneously resolving dermatitis. The Koebner phenomenon (isomorphic response), in which lesions arise at sites of trauma, is diagnostically useful in psoriasis, lichen planus, and vitiligo; in darker skin tones, the koebnerized lesion may present predominantly as hyperpigmented or hypopigmented rather than erythematous, altering its clinical appearance but preserving its diagnostic significance if the distribution pattern is recognized.

CAUTION: Annular morphology is one of the most overtreated patterns in dermatology. Not every ring-shaped lesion is tinea. Granuloma annulare, nummular dermatitis, erythema annulare centrifugum, and annular psoriasis all produce annular plaques that are routinely misdiagnosed as tinea and treated with topical antifungals without confirmatory KOH or culture. The result is either treatment failure (the lesion is not fungal) or diagnostic obscuration (application of topical antifungal-corticosteroid combination creams partially suppresses inflammation, creating tinea incognito that delays correct diagnosis).

Dermoscopy: Principles and Clinical Application

Optical Principles and Technique

Dermoscopy (dermatoscopy, epiluminescence microscopy) is a noninvasive, in-vivo technique that uses a handheld device with magnification (typically 10x) and a light source to visualize subsurface structures of the epidermis, dermoepidermal junction, and papillary dermis that are not visible to the naked eye. By eliminating surface reflection through either a liquid interface (contact dermoscopy) or cross-polarized light (polarized dermoscopy), the technique renders the pigment network, vascular patterns, and structural features that underlie clinical morphology. Polarized dermoscopy is now the dominant modality in clinical practice because it requires no contact fluid, permits faster examination, and enhances the visualization of vascular structures (which appear more prominently under polarization) while slightly reducing the visibility of superficial structures such as milia-like cysts.

The Two-Step Algorithm

Dermoscopic assessment of a pigmented lesion follows the two-step algorithm. Step 1 determines whether the lesion is melanocytic or non-melanocytic. Melanocytic structures include the pigment network (a grid-like pattern of brown lines corresponding to melanin in the rete ridges), globules (round or oval brown-black structures corresponding to nests of melanocytes), and homogeneous blue pigmentation (corresponding to deep dermal melanin or melanophages). Non-melanocytic structures include comedo-like openings and milia-like cysts (seborrheic keratosis), leaf-like areas and blue-gray ovoid nests (basal cell carcinoma), and red lacunae (hemangioma). If the lesion is melanocytic, Step 2 evaluates it for malignancy using one of several validated algorithms: pattern analysis, the ABCD rule of dermoscopy, the 7-point checklist, or the Menzies method. Dermoscopic features of melanoma include an atypical pigment network (irregular, thickened, interrupted lines), irregular streaks (pseudopods and radial streaming at the periphery), blue-white structures (regression or deep melanin), atypical vascular patterns (dotted, linear-irregular, or polymorphous vessels), and negative pigment network (serpiginous lighter lines surrounding darker clods, associated with Spitz and desmoplastic melanoma).

Dermoscopy of Non-Pigmented Lesions and Inflammatory Dermatoses

Although dermoscopy was originally developed for pigmented lesion assessment, its applications have expanded substantially to include non-pigmented tumors, inflammatory dermatoses, and scalp and hair disorders (trichoscopy). In non-pigmented basal cell carcinoma, dermoscopy reveals arborizing telangiectasia (branching, tree-like vessels), shiny white structures (chrysalis-like structures visible only under polarized light), and short fine telangiectasia, features that distinguish it from dermatofibroma (central white scar-like patch with peripheral delicate pigment network) and from squamous cell carcinoma (glomerular vessels, white structureless areas, and keratin). In inflammatory dermatoses, dermoscopy characterizes the vascular morphology that reflects the underlying histopathology: dotted vessels arranged in a regular pattern over a light-red background in psoriasis (correlating with dilated capillaries in elongated dermal papillae), glomerular vessels in Bowen disease, and linear-irregular or polymorphous vessels in amelanotic melanoma. In scalp dermoscopy, the presence or absence of follicular ostia, perifollicular scaling, yellow dots, black dots, and broken hairs differentiates scarring from non-scarring alopecias and distinguishes alopecia areata (exclamation-point hairs, black dots, yellow dots) from trichotillomania (broken hairs at different lengths, flame hairs, V-sign, absence of exclamation-point hairs).

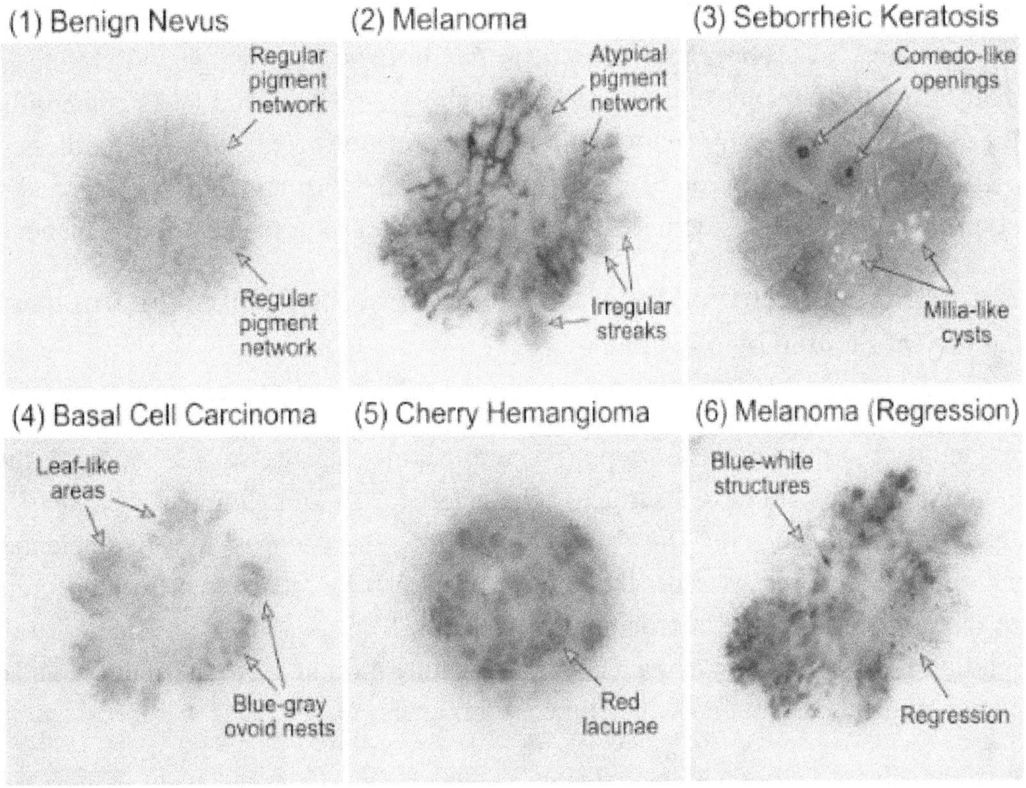

THE CUTANEOUS MIMICKER RECOGNITION ATLAS — Melanoma versus Seborrheic Keratosis

The Clinical Pattern: Seborrheic keratoses are the most common benign cutaneous neoplasms in adults, presenting as well-demarcated, stuck-on, waxy papules and plaques with a verrucous surface. They are typically symmetric with uniform pigmentation and a characteristic dull, matte surface. Dermoscopy reveals comedo-like openings (crypts), milia-like cysts, and a brain-like or cerebriform pattern. The clinical impression of a benign, sharply demarcated, warty lesion is usually correct.

The Mimicker: Melanoma, particularly nodular melanoma and melanoma arising within a seborrheic keratosis (collision tumor), can closely resemble a darkly pigmented seborrheic keratosis. Both may present as dark brown to black papules or plaques with irregular surface contour. The overlap is most treacherous when a melanoma develops a verrucous surface (verrucous melanoma) or when a rapidly growing seborrheic keratosis becomes irritated and partially denuded, producing an asymmetric, irregularly pigmented lesion.

Trap Logic: Satisfaction of search is the cognitive trap. The clinician identifies a pigmented lesion in a patient with multiple seborrheic keratoses and automatically categorizes the new lesion as another keratosis without performing dermoscopy or noting features that deviate from the rest of the patient's keratoses. The trap is reinforced by base rate reasoning: seborrheic keratoses outnumber melanomas by a ratio exceeding 1,000 to 1, so the prior probability favors benignity, and the clinician unconsciously adjusts the threshold for concern.

The Decision Anchor: The discriminating finding is the **ugly duckling sign combined with dermoscopic absence of seborrheic keratosis structures**. A pigmented lesion that differs morphologically from the patient's other keratoses (the ugly duckling) and lacks comedo-like openings and milia-like cysts on dermoscopy cannot be classified as a seborrheic keratosis regardless of its clinical appearance. The presence of any melanocytic dermoscopic feature (pigment network, streaks, blue-white structures, atypical vessels) in a lesion initially presumed to be a seborrheic keratosis mandates biopsy.

The Dermatologic Differential Diagnosis: A Morphology-Based Framework

Constructing the Differential by Morphology

The dermatologic differential diagnosis is constructed by working outward from the primary lesion morphology: identify the primary lesion type (macule, papule, plaque, vesicle, nodule), then refine by distribution, configuration, color, surface characteristics, and clinical context (age, sex, immunocompetence, medications). This morphology-first approach is the fundamental diagnostic algorithm of clinical dermatology because the same disease can present differently on different body sites, and different diseases can produce morphologically identical lesions. The clinician who diagnoses by pattern recognition alone, without systematically interrogating morphology, distribution, and context, will consistently miss atypical presentations and clinical mimickers.

Differential Diagnosis by Primary Lesion Type

Papulosquamous lesions (papules and plaques with scale) generate a differential anchored by psoriasis, lichen planus, pityriasis rosea, secondary syphilis, dermatophytosis, and mycosis fungoides. Each can be separated by the character and color of the scale, the distribution, and associated findings: silvery scale on extensor surfaces with Auspitz sign suggests psoriasis; violaceous, polygonal, flat-topped papules with Wickham striae suggest lichen planus; a herald patch followed by a Christmas-tree distribution of oval patches suggests pityriasis rosea; generalized symmetric papulosquamous eruption with mucous patches and lymphadenopathy in a sexually active patient demands serologic evaluation for syphilis. Vesiculobullous lesions generate a separate differential stratified by blister level: intraepidermal blistering (pemphigus), subepidermal blistering (bullous pemphigoid, linear IgA disease, epidermolysis bullosa acquisita, dermatitis herpetiformis), or subcorneal blistering (subcorneal pustular dermatosis, staphylococcal scalded skin syndrome). Nodular lesions prompt consideration of benign neoplasms (dermatofibroma, epidermoid cyst, lipoma), malignant neoplasms (basal cell carcinoma, squamous cell carcinoma, melanoma, cutaneous metastasis), and inflammatory processes (erythema nodosum, foreign body granuloma, sarcoidosis).

The Ugly Duckling Concept and Pattern Recognition Heuristics

Beyond the formal morphology-distribution-configuration algorithm, experienced clinicians employ pattern recognition heuristics that accelerate diagnosis. The ugly duckling sign is one of the most powerful: in a patient with multiple nevi, the lesion that does not look like the others is the one that warrants biopsy, even if it does not meet the individual criteria of the ABCDE rule when assessed in isolation. This comparative approach exploits the fact that a given patient's benign nevi tend to share a similar morphologic signature (size, color, border, symmetry), and a melanoma that deviates from that signature can be identified by its dissimilarity to the surrounding nevus population. The little red riding hood sign describes a lesion that looks benign clinically but has a dermoscopic pattern that raises concern, prompting biopsy of a lesion the clinician might otherwise have dismissed. Conversely, the wolf in sheep's clothing describes a melanoma that mimics a benign lesion so effectively that neither clinical nor dermoscopic assessment raises the appropriate alarm, which is most common in amelanotic and desmoplastic melanoma subtypes that lack the pigment-based features both algorithms rely on.

KEY POINT: Secondary syphilis is the great mimicker of dermatology. It produces papulosquamous, annular, nodular, macular, or pustular lesions that can simulate nearly any inflammatory dermatosis. Any generalized symmetric eruption in a sexually active patient that does not respond to initial treatment should prompt serologic testing for syphilis, regardless of the morphologic pattern.

Skin Biopsy: Indications, Techniques, and Specimen Handling

Indications for Biopsy

Skin biopsy is indicated when the clinical diagnosis is uncertain and histopathologic examination would change management, when malignancy is suspected and tissue confirmation is required before definitive treatment, or when an inflammatory dermatosis requires histopathologic classification to guide systemic therapy. The choice of biopsy technique depends on the clinical scenario, the depth of the pathology, and the cosmetic implications of the procedure. A biopsy should sample the most representative, fully developed lesion and should include the active border in annular or expanding lesions rather than the center, which may show only nonspecific changes.

Biopsy Techniques

The punch biopsy uses a circular blade (typically 3 to 6 millimeters in diameter) to obtain a cylindrical core of tissue extending from the epidermis through the dermis into the subcutis. It is the most versatile biopsy technique in dermatology, providing a full-thickness specimen suitable for routine histopathology, immunofluorescence, culture, and molecular studies. The shave biopsy (tangential excision) removes a disc of tissue at a depth chosen by the clinician, from superficial (saucerization) to deep (into the reticular dermis). Superficial shave biopsies are appropriate for epidermal and superficial dermal pathology (seborrheic keratosis, superficial basal cell carcinoma, actinic keratosis) but are inadequate for deep processes and should not be used for pigmented lesions suspicious for melanoma, because transection of the base prevents accurate measurement of Breslow thickness, which is the single most important prognostic factor in melanoma staging. The excisional biopsy removes the entire lesion with a margin of normal tissue and is the preferred technique for lesions suspicious for melanoma, providing the complete specimen needed for accurate Breslow depth, ulceration assessment, and mitotic rate.

Specimen Handling and Orientation

Proper specimen handling is essential for diagnostic accuracy. Routine biopsy specimens are placed in 10 percent neutral buffered formalin for fixation and standard hematoxylin and eosin processing. Specimens for direct immunofluorescence (required for autoimmune blistering diseases, lupus erythematosus, and vasculitis) must be placed in Michel transport medium or fresh-frozen in liquid nitrogen, because formalin fixation destroys the immunoglobulin and complement deposits that DIF detects. Specimens for culture (bacterial, fungal, mycobacterial, or viral) should be submitted fresh in sterile saline, not formalin. The clinician must anticipate the specimen's destination before the biopsy is performed: a punch biopsy for suspected bullous pemphigoid that is inadvertently placed entirely in formalin cannot be retroactively used for the DIF studies that are essential for diagnosis.

Orientation and site marking are critical when excisional biopsies are performed for malignancy. Marking the specimen with a suture at a defined anatomic landmark (typically 12 o'clock or the superior pole) allows the dermatopathologist to map positive margins precisely, so that Mohs micrographic surgery or re-excision can be directed to the involved margin rather than requiring circumferential re-excision. For melanoma excisions, the specimen should be submitted whole, intact, and without bisection, so that Breslow depth can be measured at the thickest point of the tumor rather than from a fragment that may not contain the deepest invasion. When multiple biopsies are taken from the same patient during a single visit, each specimen must be placed in a separately labeled container with the anatomic site recorded on both the container and the requisition form; mislabeled specimens have produced well-documented diagnostic errors including wrong-patient melanoma diagnoses and unnecessary surgeries.

Principles of Dermatopathology: Histologic Reaction Patterns

Pattern-Based Approach to Dermatopathology

Dermatopathology uses a pattern-based approach to histologic diagnosis, recognizing that hundreds of clinically distinct skin diseases produce a limited number of histologic reaction patterns. The major patterns include spongiotic (intercellular edema of the epidermis with lymphocytic infiltrate, seen in eczematous dermatitis, allergic contact dermatitis, and nummular dermatitis), psoriasiform (regular elongation of the rete ridges with parakeratosis and neutrophilic collections, seen in psoriasis), interface (vacuolar degeneration or apoptosis at the dermoepidermal junction, seen in lupus erythematosus, dermatomyositis, lichen planus, erythema multiforme, and graft-versus-host disease), and vasculitic (fibrinoid necrosis of vessel walls with perivascular inflammatory infiltrate, seen in leukocytoclastic vasculitis and polyarteritis nodosa).

Granulomatous, Vesiculobullous, and Neoplastic Patterns

Granulomatous dermatitis is characterized by collections of epithelioid histiocytes with or without multinucleated giant cells and encompasses sarcoidal granulomas (naked, non-necrotizing granulomas with a sparse lymphocytic rim, as in sarcoidosis), palisading granulomas (histiocytes arrayed radially around a central zone of altered collagen or mucin, as in granuloma annulare and necrobiosis lipoidica), and caseating granulomas (granulomas with central necrosis, as in cutaneous tuberculosis and deep fungal infections). The granuloma type directly influences the differential: a biopsy showing naked granulomas should prompt evaluation for sarcoidosis (chest radiography, serum ACE, calcium), while caseating granulomas mandate culture for mycobacteria and fungi, tissue stains (acid-fast, GMS, PAS), and clinical correlation for endemic exposure or immunosuppression.

The vesiculobullous pattern is subclassified by the level of the split: subcorneal (pemphigus foliaceus, staphylococcal scalded skin syndrome), intraepidermal suprabasal (pemphigus vulgaris), intraepidermal spinous (spongiotic dermatitis with vesicle formation), subepidermal (bullous pemphigoid, dermatitis herpetiformis, linear IgA disease, epidermolysis bullosa acquisita). The level of the split, combined with the composition of the inflammatory infiltrate (eosinophils in bullous pemphigoid, neutrophils at dermal papillae in dermatitis herpetiformis, sparse inflammation in epidermolysis bullosa acquisita) and the results of direct immunofluorescence, allows precise classification of blistering diseases. Neoplastic patterns in dermatopathology require assessment of cytologic atypia, architectural disorder, invasion of the basement membrane (separating in-situ from invasive malignancy), and immunohistochemical profiling for melanocytic (S100, SOX10, Melan-A, HMB-45), epithelial (cytokeratins, EMA, BerEP4 for BCC), or lymphoid markers (CD3, CD4, CD20, CD30). Immunohistochemistry transforms dermatopathology from pattern recognition to molecular classification, enabling the distinction of histologically ambiguous lesions such as spindle cell melanoma from spindle cell squamous cell carcinoma, atypical fibroxanthoma, and dermatofibrosarcoma protuberans.

Histologic Pattern	Key Features	Representative Conditions
Spongiotic	Intercellular edema, lymphocytic infiltrate	Eczematous dermatitis, allergic contact dermatitis, nummular dermatitis
Psoriasiform	Regular rete ridge elongation, parakeratosis, neutrophils	Psoriasis, pityriasis rubra pilaris, chronic eczema
Interface	Vacuolar degeneration of basal layer, apoptotic keratinocytes	Lupus erythematosus, lichen planus, erythema multiforme, GVHD
Granulomatous	Epithelioid histiocytes, giant cells	Sarcoidosis, granuloma annulare, tuberculosis, foreign body

Vasculitic	Fibrinoid necrosis, perivascular neutrophils, nuclear dust	Leukocytoclastic vasculitis, IgA vasculitis, polyarteritis nodosa

Special Diagnostic Procedures: KOH, Tzanck, Wood Lamp, Patch Testing, and Direct Immunofluorescence

KOH Preparation

The potassium hydroxide (KOH) preparation is a rapid, low-cost bedside test for diagnosing superficial fungal infections. A sample of scale, hair, or nail is placed on a glass slide, covered with 10 to 20 percent KOH solution to dissolve keratin, gently heated to accelerate keratin dissolution, and examined under light microscopy with the condenser lowered to enhance contrast. Dermatophyte hyphae appear as branching, septate filaments that cross cell boundaries; Candida appears as pseudohyphae and budding yeast cells; Malassezia (the causative organism of pityriasis versicolor) appears as clusters of round yeast cells with short hyphae in the classic spaghetti-and-meatballs pattern. The sensitivity of the KOH preparation depends on the adequacy of the sample (scrape from the active, scaling border rather than the cleared center), the concentration of KOH used, and the experience of the examiner. Adding chlorazol black E or Parker blue-black ink to the KOH solution stains the fungal elements, improving their visibility against the background keratinocytes. The KOH preparation is the first-line test that should be performed before initiating antifungal therapy for any suspected fungal infection, because a negative KOH in a clinically suspicious lesion raises the possibility of a non-fungal mimicker (nummular dermatitis, psoriasis, contact dermatitis), while a positive KOH confirms the diagnosis and directs targeted therapy. When the KOH is negative but clinical suspicion remains high, fungal culture on Sabouraud dextrose agar or dermatophyte test medium provides definitive identification of the organism and is the reference standard for tinea capitis diagnosis, where KOH sensitivity is lower than in glabrous skin infections.

Tzanck Smear and Wood Lamp Examination

The Tzanck smear is a rapid cytologic test for herpesvirus infection. The base of an unroofed vesicle is scraped, the material is smeared on a glass slide, stained with Giemsa or Wright stain, and examined for multinucleated giant cells and ballooning degeneration, which confirm herpesvirus cytopathic effect. The test does not distinguish between herpes simplex and varicella-zoster virus; viral culture, direct fluorescent antibody, or PCR is required for that distinction. The Wood lamp emits long-wave ultraviolet A light (365 nanometers) and produces characteristic fluorescence patterns that aid diagnosis. Coral-red fluorescence is produced by porphyrins of Corynebacterium minutissimum in erythrasma. Bright green or yellow-green fluorescence of affected hairs indicates Microsporum canis infection (ectothrix). Pale white fluorescence of depigmented patches confirms vitiligo (because amelanotic skin fluoresces brighter than surrounding pigmented skin under UV light). Blue-white fluorescence suggests Pseudomonas infection. The Wood lamp examination is performed in a darkened room, and its sensitivity depends on the operator's experience and the adequacy of the dark environment.

Patch Testing

Patch testing is the gold-standard diagnostic procedure for identifying the causative allergen in allergic contact dermatitis. Standardized allergen panels (the baseline series contains 35 to 80 allergens depending on the region and organization) are applied to the upper back in small aluminum chambers (Finn chambers) or polypropylene chambers (TRUE Test), secured with hypoallergenic tape, and read at 48 hours and 72 to 96 hours. A positive reaction produces an eczematous papulovesicular response at the site of the offending allergen, graded from 1+ (erythema and edema) to 3+ (vesiculation extending beyond the chamber). Irritant reactions, which produce a sharply demarcated erythema without vesiculation confined exactly to the chamber area, must be distinguished from true allergic responses, which tend to produce a less sharply marginated reaction with vesiculation. The clinical significance of a positive patch test depends on its relevance to the patient's clinical presentation: a positive reaction to nickel in a patient with earlobe and periumbilical dermatitis is clinically relevant, while a positive reaction to an allergen the patient has no current exposure to may represent a past sensitization without current clinical significance.

THE CUTANEOUS MIMICKER RECOGNITION ATLAS — Allergic Contact Dermatitis versus Irritant Contact Dermatitis

---

The Clinical Pattern: Allergic contact dermatitis presents as pruritic, eczematous plaques (erythema, vesiculation, weeping, crusting in acute phase; lichenification in chronic phase) in a distribution corresponding to the area of allergen contact. The distribution often has sharp geometric borders that reflect the shape of the contactant (watchband, shoe, glove). There is typically a 24- to 72-hour delay between exposure and onset, reflecting the type IV delayed hypersensitivity mechanism.

The Mimicker: Irritant contact dermatitis produces erythema, dryness, fissuring, and a burning sensation in the area of irritant exposure and accounts for approximately 80 percent of all contact dermatitis. The morphology overlaps with allergic contact dermatitis, particularly in chronic cases where both produce lichenified, scaly plaques on the hands. The overlap is strongest in occupational hand dermatitis, where distinguishing the two is critical for workplace management and prognosis.

Trap Logic: Diagnostic momentum is the cognitive trap. The clinician sees hand dermatitis in an occupation with known irritant exposures (healthcare worker, hairdresser, food handler) and attributes the eruption to irritant contact dermatitis without performing patch testing. The diagnosis becomes self-reinforcing: the patient is counseled on irritant avoidance, the dermatitis partially improves (because any eczema improves with emollients and reduced exposure), and the underlying allergic sensitization is never identified. The patient presents repeatedly with recurrent hand dermatitis attributed to irritant exposure, and years may pass before patch testing reveals an allergic contact allergen that could have been eliminated.

The Decision Anchor: The discriminating finding is **patch testing**. There is no clinical feature, distribution, or morphologic detail that reliably separates allergic from irritant contact dermatitis in every case. In chronic hand dermatitis that is recurrent or refractory to irritant avoidance and topical corticosteroids, patch testing is the definitive diagnostic tool. A positive patch test to a relevant allergen changes management from generic irritant avoidance to specific allergen avoidance, which is curative when the allergen can be eliminated.

Direct Immunofluorescence

Direct immunofluorescence (DIF) detects in-vivo deposits of immunoglobulins (IgG, IgA, IgM), complement (C3), and fibrinogen in skin biopsy specimens using fluorescein-conjugated antibodies. The specimen must be taken from perilesional clinically uninvolved skin (not from the blister itself, which may show nonspecific findings due to tissue destruction) and submitted in Michel transport medium or snap-frozen. The pattern and composition of immune deposits are diagnostic: linear IgG and C3 at the basement membrane zone in bullous pemphigoid; intercellular (chicken-wire) IgG between keratinocytes in pemphigus vulgaris and pemphigus foliaceus; granular IgA at the dermal papillae in dermatitis herpetiformis; linear IgA at the basement membrane zone in linear IgA bullous dermatosis; granular IgG, IgM, IgA, and C3 at the basement membrane zone (full-house pattern) in lupus erythematosus. Indirect immunofluorescence, which detects circulating autoantibodies in the patient's serum, complements DIF and is used for monitoring disease activity and antibody titers in pemphigus and bullous pemphigoid.

CAUTION: A biopsy for direct immunofluorescence that is inadvertently placed in formalin rather than Michel medium is irretrievably lost for DIF purposes. Formalin fixation destroys the immunoglobulin and complement deposits that the test detects. When an autoimmune blistering disease is in the differential, the clinician must prepare the appropriate transport medium before the procedure and clearly label the specimen containers to prevent this error.

THE CUTANEOUS MIMICKER RECOGNITION ATLAS — Diagnostic Approach Arcs

Melanoma vs. Seborrheic Keratosis: The discriminating finding is the ugly duckling sign combined with dermoscopic absence of seborrheic keratosis structures (comedo-like openings, milia-like cysts). Any melanocytic dermoscopic feature in a lesion presumed to be a seborrheic keratosis mandates biopsy. Cognitive trap: satisfaction of search in patients with multiple keratoses.

Allergic Contact Dermatitis vs. Irritant Contact Dermatitis: The discriminating finding is patch testing. No clinical feature reliably separates the two in every case. Chronic, recurrent, or refractory hand dermatitis requires patch testing to identify an eliminable allergic sensitization. Cognitive trap: diagnostic momentum attributing all hand dermatitis to irritant exposure without testing.

Summary and Key Concepts

The dermatologic history focuses on onset, temporal evolution, distribution, symptoms (pruritus, pain, burning), medication history (with specific attention to drug eruption timelines), occupational and social exposures, and prior treatments. Acute, subacute, and chronic timelines each generate distinct differential diagnoses.

Accurate morphologic description using standardized terminology (macule, papule, plaque, vesicle, bulla, nodule, pustule, wheal) and recognition of secondary changes (scale character, crust, erosion, ulceration, lichenification, atrophy) is the foundation of dermatologic diagnosis. The primary lesion type is the first branch point in differential construction.

Distribution patterns (extensor, flexural, sun-exposed, intertriginous, dermatomal, Blaschko-linear) and configurations (grouped, annular, linear, targetoid, reticular) provide diagnostic specificity that morphology alone cannot deliver.

Dermoscopy uses magnification and elimination of surface reflection to visualize subsurface structures. The two-step algorithm first classifies a pigmented lesion as melanocytic or non-melanocytic, then evaluates melanocytic lesions for malignancy using validated scoring systems.

Biopsy technique selection (punch, shave, excisional) must match the clinical scenario: punch for full-thickness specimens and inflammatory disease, excisional for suspected melanoma (to preserve Breslow depth), and shave only for superficial pathology. Specimen handling must anticipate the destination: formalin for H and E, Michel medium for DIF, sterile saline for culture. The five major histopathologic reaction patterns (spongiotic, psoriasiform, interface, granulomatous, vasculitic) organize hundreds of diseases into a manageable diagnostic framework.

CHAPTER 3: ECZEMATOUS DERMATITIS AND ATOPIC DERMATITIS

Learning Objectives

1. Classify eczematous dermatoses by etiology and distinguish the major subtypes based on morphology, distribution, and clinical context.
2. Explain the pathophysiology of atopic dermatitis, including the roles of barrier dysfunction, immune dysregulation, and the atopic march.
3. Describe the age-specific clinical presentation of atopic dermatitis across Fitzpatrick phototypes and apply standardized diagnostic criteria.
4. Differentiate allergic contact dermatitis from irritant contact dermatitis and describe the role of patch testing in clinical management.
5. Select evidence-based topical, systemic, and biologic therapies for eczematous dermatitis based on disease severity, patient age, and comorbidity profile.

Classification of Eczematous Dermatoses

Definition and Unifying Features

Eczema, or eczematous dermatitis, is a clinical reaction pattern rather than a single disease. The term encompasses a group of inflammatory skin conditions that share a common histopathologic signature — spongiosis (intercellular edema of the epidermis) with a lymphocytic infiltrate — and a common clinical morphology that evolves through three phases. Acute eczema presents with erythema, vesiculation, weeping, and crusting. Subacute eczema presents with erythema, scale, and mild edema without active vesiculation. Chronic eczema presents with lichenification (thickened skin with accentuated skin markings), fissuring, and post-inflammatory pigmentary change. The recognition that all eczematous conditions share this spongiotic substrate allows the clinician to categorize a dermatitis as eczematous on the basis of morphology and histopathology, and then to determine the specific subtype by integrating distribution, clinical context, and exposure history.

Epidemiology and Global Variation

The collective burden of eczematous dermatoses is substantial. Atopic dermatitis alone affects an estimated 230 million people worldwide, with a striking geographic gradient: prevalence in industrialized and urban populations exceeds that in rural and low-income settings by a factor of two to three, supporting the hygiene hypothesis and its modern refinement, the biodiversity hypothesis. In the United States, the prevalence among children of African descent is approximately 20 percent, compared with 16 percent among white children, a disparity that persists after adjustment for socioeconomic factors and underscores the contribution of genetic and environmental modifiers beyond FLG mutations (which are less common in African and Asian populations). Contact dermatitis accounts for approximately 90 percent of occupational skin disease, with an estimated annual cost to the US economy exceeding several billion dollars in lost productivity, medical visits, and disability claims. Eczematous dermatoses collectively represent one of the most common reasons for dermatology referral, and the clinician who can systematically classify an eczematous eruption by subtype will provide more precise, cost-effective care than one who treats all eczema identically.

Etiologic Classification

Eczematous dermatoses are classified by etiology into endogenous and exogenous forms. Endogenous forms arise from intrinsic predisposition: atopic dermatitis (the prototypical endogenous eczema, driven by genetic barrier defects and Th2 immune dysregulation), nummular dermatitis (discoid eczema of uncertain etiology), dyshidrotic eczema (pompholyx, a vesicular dermatitis of the palms and soles), asteatotic eczema (eczema craquelé, associated with dry skin and low humidity), seborrheic dermatitis (driven by Malassezia yeast colonization and lipid composition changes), and stasis dermatitis (secondary to chronic venous insufficiency). Exogenous forms arise from external triggers: allergic contact dermatitis (a type IV delayed hypersensitivity reaction to a specific allergen) and irritant contact dermatitis (a direct cytotoxic response to a chemical or physical irritant without immunologic sensitization). The clinical approach to an eczematous eruption begins with establishing the spongiotic pattern and then determining the etiologic subtype, because the treatment of contact dermatitis (allergen or irritant avoidance) is fundamentally different from the treatment of atopic dermatitis (barrier restoration, immune modulation).

Atopic Dermatitis: Pathophysiology, Genetics, and the Atopic March

Genetic Basis and Barrier Dysfunction

Atopic dermatitis is a chronic, relapsing inflammatory dermatosis with a lifetime prevalence of 15 to 20 percent in children and 7 to 10 percent in adults in industrialized countries. Its pathogenesis rests on two converging mechanisms: epidermal barrier dysfunction and immune dysregulation. The strongest identified genetic risk factor is loss-of-function mutation in the filaggrin gene (FLG), present in approximately 20 to 30 percent of patients with atopic dermatitis in European populations. Filaggrin deficiency compromises the stratum corneum barrier through multiple mechanisms: loss of keratin filament aggregation weakens the structural integrity of the cornified envelope, deficiency of filaggrin breakdown products (urocanic acid, pyrrolidone carboxylic acid) reduces natural moisturizing factor and raises the stratum corneum pH, and increased transepidermal water loss allows penetration of allergens, irritants, and microbial products through the disrupted barrier, initiating the immune cascade. Beyond filaggrin, genome-wide association studies have identified susceptibility loci in genes governing ceramide synthesis (ELOVL1), tight junction integrity (claudin-1), and cornified envelope crosslinking (SPINK5, encoding the serine protease inhibitor LEKTI), underscoring that barrier dysfunction in atopic dermatitis is polygenic and extends beyond a single pathway.

Immune Dysregulation and the Th2 Axis

The immune component of atopic dermatitis is driven by Th2-polarized inflammation. Barrier disruption activates keratinocytes to release epithelial alarmins — thymic stromal lymphopoietin (TSLP), IL-25, and IL-33 — which activate dendritic cells and group 2 innate lymphoid cells (ILC2s), promoting Th2 differentiation and the production of IL-4, IL-13, and IL-31. IL-4 and IL-13 further impair barrier function by downregulating filaggrin and loricrin expression (creating a vicious cycle of barrier damage and inflammation), drive IgE class switching (explaining the elevated serum IgE seen in most atopic patients), and suppress antimicrobial peptide production (explaining the increased susceptibility to skin infections, including eczema herpeticum and staphylococcal superinfection). IL-31 is the primary pruritogenic cytokine in atopic dermatitis, acting directly on sensory neurons to induce itch through a non-histaminergic pathway, which is why antihistamines are largely ineffective for atopic itch and why anti-IL-31 therapy (nemolizumab) produces rapid itch reduction. In chronic lesions, the immune phenotype evolves toward a Th1/Th22 profile, with increased interferon-gamma and IL-22 driving epidermal hyperplasia and lichenification — a shift that explains why chronic atopic dermatitis appears clinically distinct from acute disease and why treatment strategies may need adjustment as lesions mature.

Microbiome Dysbiosis and Staphylococcal Colonization

The skin microbiome in atopic dermatitis is profoundly altered compared with healthy skin. Staphylococcus aureus colonizes the lesional skin of approximately 90 percent of patients with atopic dermatitis, compared with 5 percent of healthy individuals, and the density of colonization correlates directly with disease severity. The mechanistic basis for this selective colonization is multifactorial: the elevated stratum corneum pH (caused by filaggrin deficiency) favors S. aureus adhesion and growth over commensal species; Th2 cytokines (IL-4 and IL-13) suppress the expression of antimicrobial peptides (cathelicidin LL-37, beta-defensins) that normally limit pathogenic colonization; and the disrupted barrier exposes fibronectin and fibrinogen, which serve as ligands for S. aureus surface adhesins. S. aureus itself amplifies the inflammatory cycle through multiple virulence mechanisms: superantigens (staphylococcal enterotoxins A and B, toxic shock syndrome toxin-1) activate T cells polyclonally, delta-toxin degranulates mast cells directly, protein A induces Th2 polarization via TSLP, and biofilm formation creates a persistent reservoir resistant to topical antimicrobials. Disease flares are consistently preceded by a bloom of S. aureus and a concurrent decline in microbial diversity, particularly in Staphylococcus epidermidis and other protective commensals. This understanding has driven interest in microbiome-directed therapies, including topical application of commensal bacteria (S. hominis, Roseomonas mucosa) and targeted anti-staphylococcal strategies that spare the protective microbiome.

The Atopic March

The atopic march describes the natural history of atopic disease in which atopic dermatitis in infancy is followed sequentially by food allergy, allergic rhinitis, and asthma over the first decade of life. The epidemiologic data supporting this progression are robust: approximately 30 percent of children with moderate-to-severe atopic dermatitis develop asthma, and 60 to 70 percent develop allergic rhinitis. The mechanistic hypothesis holds that epicutaneous allergen sensitization through the disrupted skin barrier of atopic dermatitis initiates systemic Th2 priming, which subsequently manifests at mucosal sites (gut, nasal mucosa, bronchial epithelium) as the other atopic diseases. This hypothesis is supported by the observation that FLG mutations increase the risk not only of atopic dermatitis but also of allergic sensitization and asthma, even in individuals who never develop clinical eczema, suggesting that barrier-mediated sensitization is the upstream driver of the entire atopic cascade.

KEY POINT: The atopic march is not merely an epidemiologic observation — it identifies epidermal barrier disruption as the upstream event that initiates systemic atopic sensitization. Early aggressive barrier restoration and disease control in infantile atopic dermatitis may reduce the risk of subsequent allergic rhinitis and asthma, though prospective intervention trials are ongoing.

Clinical Presentation Across Age Groups and Skin Types

Infantile, Childhood, and Adult Patterns

Atopic dermatitis follows an age-dependent distribution pattern that reflects changes in skin physiology and environmental exposures across the lifespan. In infants (2 months to 2 years), the eruption typically involves the cheeks, forehead, scalp, and extensor surfaces of the extremities, with relative sparing of the diaper area (which is protected by the occlusive environment of the diaper). In children (2 to 12 years), the distribution shifts to the classic flexural pattern: antecubital fossae, popliteal fossae, neck, wrists, and ankles. In adolescents and adults, the eruption may persist in flexural sites or evolve to involve the face (particularly the periorbital area), neck, hands, and feet. Adult-onset atopic dermatitis, which is increasingly recognized as a distinct subset, may present with a more widespread eczematous pattern that overlaps with other dermatoses and poses diagnostic challenges.

Associated Clinical Stigmata

Beyond the primary eczematous eruption, atopic dermatitis is associated with a constellation of minor clinical features that aid diagnosis and reflect the underlying barrier and immune abnormalities. Dennie-Morgan infraorbital folds (an accentuated double or triple crease beneath the lower eyelid) and periorbital darkening (allergic shiners, resulting from venous congestion in the periorbital tissues) are among the most recognizable facial stigmata. Hertoghe sign (thinning or loss of the lateral third of the eyebrow from chronic rubbing) and anterior neck folds are additional facial clues. Keratosis pilaris — follicular keratotic papules on the lateral upper arms, anterior thighs, and cheeks — is present in a substantial proportion of atopic individuals and reflects the generalized keratinization defect. Ichthyosis vulgaris (fine, white, polygonal scales on the extensor extremities with palmar hyperlinearity) is present in up to 37 percent of patients with atopic dermatitis, reflecting the close genetic linkage between FLG mutations and both conditions. White dermographism (a paradoxical blanching response to stroking, rather than the red flare seen in non-atopic individuals) reflects altered vascular reactivity and heightened vasoconstrictor tone in atopic skin. These associated features, while individually non-specific, collectively contribute to the clinical diagnosis and are incorporated into the Hanifin and Rajka minor criteria.

Presentation in Skin of Color

In Fitzpatrick phototype IV-VI skin, the classic erythematous morphology of atopic dermatitis may be absent or difficult to detect because inflammation that presents as bright pink or red in lighter skin may appear as violaceous, hyperpigmented, or dusky brown in darker skin. Follicular accentuation (perifollicular papules and roughening) is more prominent in patients with darker skin tones and may be the dominant morphologic finding, sometimes described as a papular variant of atopic dermatitis. Post-inflammatory hyperpigmentation and hypopigmentation are more pronounced and persistent, and may be the primary concern for the patient, persisting for months after the active inflammation resolves. Lichenification develops readily and may be more pronounced. Clinicians trained predominantly on light-skin presentations may underdiagnose or underestimate the severity of atopic dermatitis in patients with darker skin because they rely on erythema-dependent assessment criteria. Scoring systems that weight erythema heavily (such as the original SCORAD) may systematically underestimate disease severity in these populations.

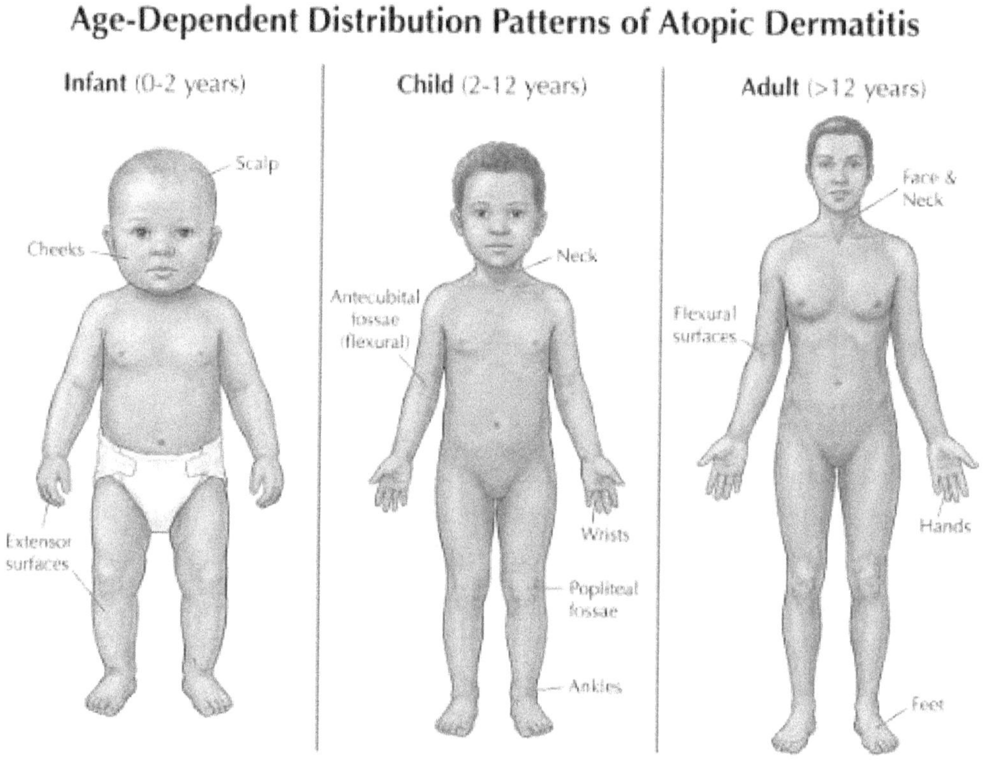

Diagnostic Criteria and Severity Assessment

Clinical Diagnostic Criteria

Atopic dermatitis is a clinical diagnosis. No single laboratory test confirms it, and biopsy shows nonspecific spongiotic dermatitis. The Hanifin and Rajka criteria (1980) remain the most widely cited diagnostic framework, requiring 3 of 4 major criteria (pruritus, typical morphology and distribution, chronic or relapsing course, personal or family history of atopy) plus 3 of 23 minor criteria (xerosis, ichthyosis, elevated serum IgE, early age of onset, Dennie-Morgan folds, facial pallor, keratosis pilaris, and others). The UK Working Party refinement simplified the criteria for epidemiologic use: an itchy skin condition in the last 12 months plus 3 of 5 features (onset before age 2, history of flexural involvement, history of dry skin, personal history of other atopic disease, or visible flexural dermatitis at the time of examination). In clinical practice, the diagnosis rests on the recognizable pattern of pruritic, eczematous dermatitis in a characteristic distribution with a chronic relapsing course.

Severity Scoring Instruments

Disease severity in atopic dermatitis is assessed using validated instruments that quantify the extent, intensity, and impact of the disease. The Eczema Area and Severity Index (EASI) scores four body regions (head/neck, upper limbs, trunk, lower limbs) for erythema, induration/papulation, excoriation, and lichenification on a 0-3 scale, multiplied by percentage body surface area involved, generating a composite score from 0 to 72. The Scoring Atopic Dermatitis (SCORAD) index incorporates extent (rule of nines), intensity (erythema, edema, oozing/crusting, excoriation, lichenification, dryness on a 0-3 scale), and subjective symptoms (pruritus and sleep loss on visual analog scales). The Investigator Global Assessment (IGA) is a single 0-to-4 ordinal scale used in clinical trials as the primary endpoint for regulatory approval of new therapies. Mild disease corresponds to EASI less than 7 or IGA 2; moderate disease to EASI 7 to 21 or IGA 3; severe disease to EASI greater than 21 or IGA 4.

Differential Diagnosis

The differential diagnosis of atopic dermatitis varies by age and presentation. In infants, seborrheic dermatitis (greasy, yellowish scale on the scalp and diaper area without prominent pruritus), scabies (papulovesicular eruption with burrows on the palms, soles, and genital area, with family members affected), and immunodeficiency-associated eczema (Wiskott-Aldrich syndrome, Hyper-IgE syndrome, IPEX syndrome — suggested by failure to thrive, recurrent infections, or unusual severity) must be considered. In adults, contact dermatitis (geometric or exposure-patterned distribution, resolving when the trigger is removed), nummular dermatitis (coin-shaped plaques without flexural predilection), dermatomyositis (heliotrope rash, Gottron papules, proximal muscle weakness), and cutaneous T-cell lymphoma (fixed patches with poikiloderma, poor treatment response, as discussed in the Mimicker Recognition block above) enter the differential. Drug eruptions, particularly from checkpoint inhibitors, can produce an eczematous pattern indistinguishable from atopic dermatitis and require a careful medication history. The systematic approach to an eczematous eruption integrates morphology (acute vs. chronic), distribution (flexural vs. exposed vs. acral), exposure history (occupational, recreational, cosmetic), family history (atopy), and response to therapy to narrow the differential and direct confirmatory testing.

Contact Dermatitis: Allergic and Irritant

Allergic Contact Dermatitis

Allergic contact dermatitis (ACD) is a type IV delayed hypersensitivity reaction that requires prior sensitization to a specific allergen. The sensitization phase occurs over 10 to 14 days during which Langerhans cells capture the hapten-protein complex, migrate to regional lymph nodes, and prime allergen-specific T cells. On subsequent re-exposure, the elicitation phase produces an eczematous reaction within 24 to 72 hours. The most common contact allergens include nickel sulfate (jewelry, belt buckles, mobile phone casings), fragrance mix (cosmetics, personal care products, household cleaners), methylisothiazolinone (preservative in water-based cosmetics and household products), p-phenylenediamine (hair dye), cobalt (jewelry, metal alloys), and potassium dichromate (leather tanning, cement). The distribution of the eruption provides the most important diagnostic clue: earlobe and periumbilical dermatitis suggests nickel, eyelid dermatitis suggests cosmetic or nail polish allergen (transferred by hand-to-face contact), and foot dermatitis in a shoe-shaped distribution suggests chromate or rubber accelerator allergy.

Irritant Contact Dermatitis and Occupational Considerations

Irritant contact dermatitis (ICD) accounts for approximately 80 percent of all contact dermatitis and results from direct cytotoxic injury to the epidermis without immunologic sensitization. The threshold for irritation depends on the concentration and duration of exposure, the integrity of the skin barrier, and individual susceptibility factors (atopic patients are more susceptible to irritants because their baseline barrier is compromised). Common irritants include water (wet work), soaps and detergents, solvents, acids and alkalis, and mechanical friction. Chronic ICD of the hands is the most common occupational dermatosis, with the highest incidence in healthcare workers, hairdressers, food handlers, cleaners, and construction workers. The clinical distinction between ACD and ICD on the hands is often impossible without patch testing, because both produce erythematous, scaly, fissured plaques with blurred borders. The economic and personal impact of occupational hand dermatitis is substantial: it causes more lost workdays than any other occupational skin disease, and chronic refractory cases may require job change.

Patch Testing: Technique and Interpretation

Patch testing is the gold standard for identifying the causative allergen in suspected allergic contact dermatitis, and its appropriate application distinguishes the dermatologist who manages contact dermatitis effectively from one who treats empirically and misses the diagnosis. The standard technique involves applying a series of allergens at standardized concentrations (the baseline series, such as the North American Contact Dermatitis Group or European standard series, typically containing 70 to 80 allergens) in individual Finn chambers or TRUE Test panels to the upper back. The patches are applied on day 0, removed on day 2 (48 hours), and readings are taken at day 2 and day 4 (96 hours) — the delayed second reading is critical because some reactions, particularly to neomycin, corticosteroids, and metals, may not peak until 72 to 96 hours. Reactions are graded using the International Contact Dermatitis Research Group scale: negative (no reaction), irritant (glazed erythema without infiltration), 1+ (erythema and edema), 2+

(erythema, edema, and papules), and 3+ (erythema, edema, and vesicles or bullae). The clinical relevance of a positive patch test must be established by correlating the identified allergen with the patient's clinical history, exposure pattern, and distribution of dermatitis — a positive reaction to an allergen the patient has never been exposed to represents past sensitization without current clinical relevance, and acting on it by imposing unnecessary avoidance measures reduces compliance with the avoidance regimen for the truly relevant allergen.

CLINICAL PEARL: Patch testing should be considered in any patient with hand eczema, facial eczema, or generalized eczema that fails to respond to standard topical therapy, even if the patient carries a longstanding diagnosis of atopic dermatitis. Up to 40 to 50 percent of patients with atopic dermatitis have at least one relevant positive patch test, and identifying and eliminating the contact allergen can convert treatment-refractory disease into manageable disease without escalation to systemic therapy.

THE CUTANEOUS MIMICKER RECOGNITION ATLAS — Atopic Dermatitis versus Cutaneous T-Cell Lymphoma (Mycosis Fungoides)

The Clinical Pattern: Atopic dermatitis presents with pruritic, eczematous patches and plaques in flexural distribution (antecubital and popliteal fossae, neck, wrists) with a chronic relapsing course, personal or family history of atopy, and onset typically before age 5. The morphology ranges from acute (vesiculation, weeping) to chronic (lichenification, excoriation) and responds, at least partially, to topical corticosteroids and moisturizers.

The Mimicker: Early-stage mycosis fungoides (patch and plaque stage) can closely mimic eczematous dermatitis: it presents as erythematous, scaly patches and thin plaques with pruritus, often in a bathing-trunk distribution (buttocks, lower trunk, proximal thighs) or in areas not typically affected by atopic dermatitis. The overlap is strongest in adults who present with a new-onset or recalcitrant eczematous eruption, particularly when lesions occur in non-classic atopic locations, vary in size and shape, and show a poor or inconsistent response to topical corticosteroids.

Trap Logic: Availability bias is the cognitive trap. Eczematous dermatitis is vastly more common than cutaneous T-cell lymphoma, so the clinician's diagnostic script defaults to eczema for any pruritic, scaly plaque, particularly in a patient who has ever carried an atopic dermatitis diagnosis. The bias is reinforced when topical corticosteroids produce partial improvement (which they can in early mycosis fungoides, because they suppress the T-cell infiltrate), confirming the clinician's initial impression without challenging it. The diagnostic delay for mycosis fungoides averages 3 to 6 years from the onset of skin findings.

The Decision Anchor: The discriminating findings are **persistent fixed patches in non-flexural distribution with poikiloderma (atrophy, telangiectasia, dyspigmentation) and biopsy showing epidermotropism of atypical lymphocytes**. Atopic dermatitis waxes and wanes with treatment and does not produce fixed, persistent patches that remain unchanged in the same location for months or years. Poikiloderma (the triad of atrophy, telangiectasia, and mottled hyper/hypopigmentation within the same patch) is a red flag for mycosis fungoides and is not a feature of eczematous dermatitis. Any eczematous eruption in an adult that is refractory to standard therapy, fixed in distribution, or shows poikilodermatous change requires biopsy with immunohistochemistry (CD3, CD4, CD8) and T-cell receptor gene rearrangement studies.

Nummular Dermatitis, Dyshidrotic Eczema, and Asteatotic Eczema

Nummular (Discoid) Dermatitis

Nummular dermatitis presents as coin-shaped (discoid), well-demarcated, erythematous plaques with overlying scale, crusting, and occasionally vesiculation, typically on the extremities and trunk. It is more common in men and tends to appear in middle age. The lesions are intensely pruritic and often become impetiginized with Staphylococcus aureus, which can obscure the underlying diagnosis. The differential includes tinea corporis (annular with central clearing and a raised border, KOH-positive), plaque-type psoriasis (silvery scale, extensor distribution, nail changes), and early mycosis fungoides (persistent, fixed patches that do not respond to topical therapy). KOH preparation is mandatory to exclude tinea before initiating corticosteroid treatment, because topical corticosteroids suppress the inflammatory response to dermatophytes, creating tinea incognito.

Dyshidrotic Eczema and Asteatotic Eczema

Dyshidrotic eczema (pompholyx) presents as recurrent crops of intensely pruritic, deep-seated vesicles on the lateral fingers, palms, and soles. The vesicles are firm, clear, and described as tapioca-like, and they resolve with desquamation over 2 to 3 weeks. Triggers include stress, heat, humidity, contact allergens (particularly nickel and cobalt), and dermatophyte infection at a distant site (an id reaction). Severe cases may present with large bullae and secondary infection. Asteatotic eczema (eczema craquelé) presents as a network of superficial fissures resembling cracked porcelain, typically on the anterior lower legs of elderly patients during winter months. The pathogenesis relates to reduced sebaceous gland activity, low ambient humidity, excessive bathing, and use of harsh soaps, all of which deplete the stratum corneum lipid barrier. Treatment is centered on barrier repair with emollients and reduction of bathing frequency and temperature, with low-potency topical corticosteroids for active inflammation.

Stasis Dermatitis and Seborrheic Dermatitis

Stasis dermatitis develops on the medial lower legs as a consequence of chronic venous insufficiency. The sustained venous hypertension drives erythrocyte extravasation, hemosiderin deposition (producing the characteristic orange-brown discoloration), perivascular inflammation, and progressive fibrosis. The clinical presentation evolves from erythematous, scaly, pruritic patches overlying the medial malleolus to confluent eczematous plaques, weeping, and crusting, and may eventually progress to lipodermatosclerosis (woody induration of the subcutaneous tissue that produces an inverted champagne bottle contour of the lower leg) and venous ulceration. The differential includes allergic contact dermatitis (patients with stasis dermatitis have a high rate of sensitization to topical medicaments, particularly neomycin, bacitracin, and fragrance mix, requiring patch testing in refractory cases), cellulitis (which is unilateral, rapidly progressive, and accompanied by systemic symptoms), and pretibial myxedema (bilateral, non-pitting, waxy plaques associated with Graves disease). Management addresses the underlying venous hypertension with compression therapy (graduated compression stockings, multilayer bandaging, or pneumatic compression) alongside emollients and topical corticosteroids for active dermatitis; patients who receive anti-inflammatory therapy without compression will invariably relapse. Seborrheic dermatitis, by contrast, is driven by the inflammatory response to Malassezia yeast colonization in sebum-rich areas. It presents as erythematous patches with greasy, yellowish scale on the scalp (dandruff), nasolabial folds, eyebrows, retroauricular area, and central chest. In infants, cradle cap is the prototypical presentation. The condition is chronic and relapsing, and management combines antifungal therapy (ketoconazole shampoo or cream, ciclopirox) with mild topical corticosteroids or calcineurin inhibitors for facial involvement.

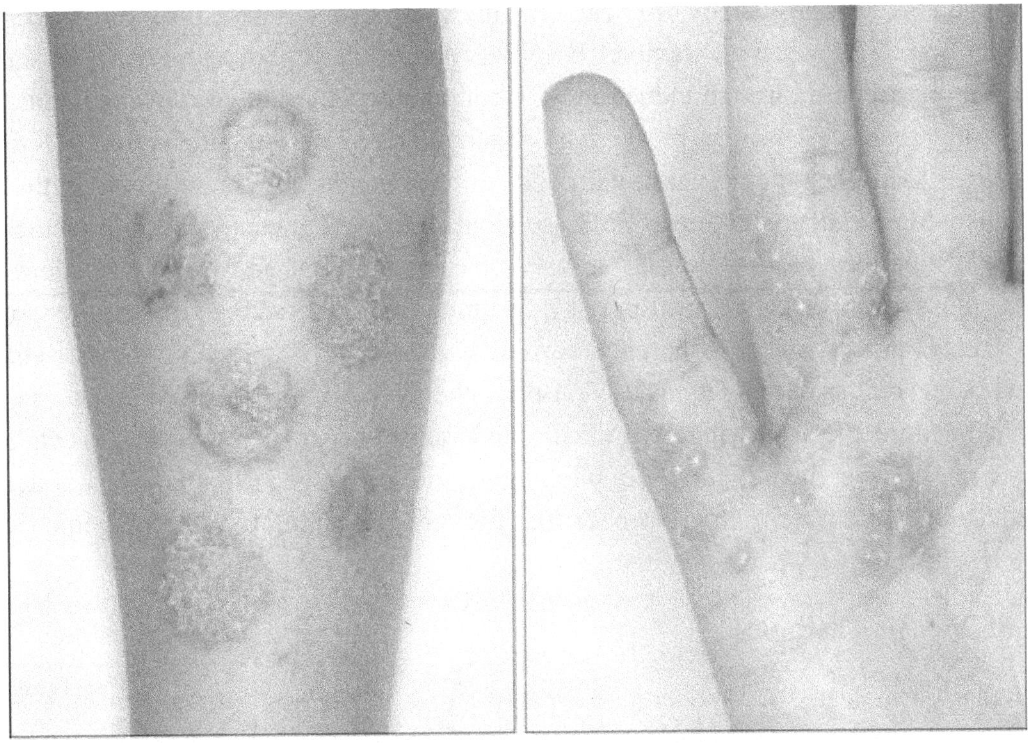

Nummular Dermatitis Dyshidrotic Eczema

Evidence-Based Management: Topical, Systemic, and Biologic Therapies

Topical Therapies

Topical corticosteroids remain the first-line anti-inflammatory therapy for eczematous dermatitis. They are classified by potency from class I (superpotent: clobetasol propionate) to class VII (least potent: hydrocortisone), and selection is guided by disease severity, body site, and patient age. Low-potency agents (class VI-VII) are appropriate for the face, eyelids, intertriginous areas, and infants. Mid-potency agents (class III-V) are appropriate for truncal and extremity involvement in adults and children. High-potency agents (class I-II) are reserved for thick, lichenified plaques on the trunk and extremities in adults and for short-duration rescue therapy. Proactive maintenance therapy with twice-weekly application of topical corticosteroids or calcineurin inhibitors to previously affected sites reduces flare frequency and is supported by randomized controlled trials as superior to reactive treatment only. Topical calcineurin inhibitors (tacrolimus ointment, pimecrolimus cream) are steroid-sparing alternatives that do not cause skin atrophy, making them particularly suitable for the face, eyelids, and intertriginous areas. Crisaborole, a topical phosphodiesterase-4 inhibitor, provides an additional non-steroidal option for mild-to-moderate atopic dermatitis in patients aged 3 months and older. Topical ruxolitinib, a JAK1/JAK2 inhibitor, was the first topical JAK inhibitor approved for atopic dermatitis and demonstrates rapid itch reduction within 12 hours of application.

Phototherapy

Phototherapy occupies an important position in the treatment algorithm for moderate atopic dermatitis that is inadequately controlled by topical therapy alone but does not yet warrant systemic immunosuppression. Narrowband ultraviolet B (NB-UVB) is the preferred modality: it suppresses the cutaneous immune response through induction of T-cell apoptosis, promotion of regulatory T cells, and reduction of Langerhans cell antigen-presenting capacity. Treatment is administered two to three times weekly in a supervised phototherapy unit, with dose titration guided by the minimal erythema dose and clinical response. Most patients require 20 to 30 sessions to achieve meaningful improvement. NB-UVB is effective, well-tolerated, steroid-sparing, and suitable for children and pregnant patients (for whom systemic immunosuppression carries greater risk). Its limitations are practical: the requirement for regular clinic visits creates an access and adherence barrier, particularly for patients in rural settings or with competing work and childcare obligations. UVA1 phototherapy (340 to 400 nm) is an alternative for acute flares and may be more effective than NB-UVB for moderate-to-severe disease, but it is available in fewer centers and carries a higher theoretical risk of photoaging with prolonged use. PUVA (psoralen plus UVA) is generally reserved for recalcitrant cases because of its greater cumulative carcinogenic risk compared with NB-UVB.

Systemic and Biologic Therapies

Systemic therapy is indicated for moderate-to-severe atopic dermatitis refractory to optimized topical management. Dupilumab, a monoclonal antibody targeting IL-4 receptor alpha (blocking both IL-4 and IL-13 signaling), was the first biologic approved for moderate-to-severe atopic dermatitis and has demonstrated sustained efficacy and safety in adults, adolescents, and children as young as 6 months. It produces clinically meaningful improvement in EASI scores, pruritus, and quality of life, with a favorable safety profile characterized primarily by conjunctivitis and injection-site reactions. Tralokinumab (anti-IL-13) provides an alternative biologic targeting the Th2 axis. Oral JAK inhibitors (abrocitinib and upadacitinib, targeting JAK1; baricitinib, targeting JAK1/JAK2) have emerged as rapid-acting oral options for moderate-to-severe disease, with onset of itch relief within days rather than the weeks required for biologics. Their safety profile requires monitoring for herpes zoster reactivation, laboratory abnormalities (lymphopenia, elevated creatine phosphokinase, lipid changes), and cardiovascular and thromboembolic risk, particularly in older patients and those with pre-existing cardiovascular risk factors. Conventional systemic immunosuppressives (cyclosporine, methotrexate, azathioprine, mycophenolate mofetil) remain options where biologics and JAK inhibitors are unavailable or contraindicated, though their evidence base is less robust and their toxicity profiles require closer monitoring.

Agent	Mechanism	Indication	Key Monitoring
Dupilumab	Anti-IL-4R-alpha (blocks IL-4 and IL-13)	Moderate-to-severe AD, age 6 months and older	Conjunctivitis, eosinophilia, injection-site reactions
Tralokinumab	Anti-IL-13	Moderate-to-severe AD, adults	Conjunctivitis, upper respiratory infections
Abrocitinib	JAK1 inhibitor (oral)	Moderate-to-severe AD, age 12 and older	CBC, lipids, CPK, herpes zoster risk, VTE risk
Upadacitinib	JAK1 inhibitor (oral)	Moderate-to-severe AD, age 12 and older	CBC, lipids, hepatic function, herpes zoster risk
Nemolizumab	Anti-IL-31R-alpha	Prurigo nodularis, atopic dermatitis (pruritus)	Musculoskeletal events, eczema worsening

Complications, Prognosis, and Long-Term Management

Infectious Complications

The disrupted epidermal barrier and impaired antimicrobial peptide production in atopic dermatitis predispose to bacterial, viral, and fungal superinfection. Staphylococcus aureus colonizes the skin of approximately 90 percent of patients with atopic dermatitis (compared with 5 percent of healthy controls), and clinical infection manifests as impetiginized eczema with honey-colored crusts, pustules, and rapid worsening despite anti-inflammatory therapy. Eczema herpeticum (Kaposi varicelliform eruption) is a disseminated herpes simplex infection that presents as a sudden eruption of monomorphic, punched-out erosions and vesicles, often with systemic symptoms (fever, malaise, lymphadenopathy). It is a dermatologic emergency requiring immediate systemic antiviral therapy because untreated cases can progress to viremia, keratoconjunctivitis, and multiorgan involvement. The risk of eczema herpeticum correlates with disease severity, early onset of atopic dermatitis, elevated IgE, and filaggrin mutation status.

Prognosis and Natural History

The natural history of atopic dermatitis is one of gradual improvement for the majority of affected children: approximately 60 to 70 percent of childhood-onset cases show significant improvement or complete resolution by adolescence, though a substantial minority persists into adulthood. Predictors of persistent disease include early onset before age 2, severe childhood disease (high SCORAD at baseline), filaggrin mutations, concomitant allergic rhinitis and asthma, and sensitization to multiple environmental allergens. Adult-onset atopic dermatitis, which accounts for approximately 25 percent of adult cases, follows a more chronic course with less spontaneous resolution and a higher rate of hand eczema. The concept of complete cure should be discussed carefully with patients: while many will achieve long periods of remission, the underlying atopic diathesis (barrier predisposition and immune tendency) persists, and flares can be triggered by environmental shifts, stress, hormonal changes, or new allergen exposures years after apparent resolution.

Psychosocial Impact and Quality of Life

The chronic, visible, and intensely pruritic nature of atopic dermatitis produces a disease burden that extends far beyond the skin surface. Sleep disruption from nocturnal pruritus is present in over 60 percent of affected children and results in daytime fatigue, impaired school performance, and behavioral disturbance. Adults with moderate-to-severe disease report quality-of-life impairment comparable to diabetes, chronic obstructive pulmonary disease, and heart disease when measured by generic instruments (EQ-5D, SF-36). Anxiety and depression are significantly more prevalent in patients with atopic dermatitis than in the general population, with a dose-response relationship between disease severity and psychiatric comorbidity. Addressing the psychosocial dimensions of atopic dermatitis — through validated instruments such as the Dermatology Life Quality Index (DLQI) and the Children's Dermatology Life Quality Index (CDLQI) — is an essential component of comprehensive management that influences treatment goals, systemic therapy decisions, and follow-up scheduling.

Prevention and Patient Education

Primary prevention of atopic dermatitis has been an area of intense investigation, driven by the recognition that barrier disruption is the upstream event in the atopic march. Prospective trials of early emollient application from birth to prevent the development of atopic dermatitis in high-risk infants have yielded mixed results: initial smaller trials (BEEP, Japanese cohort) suggested a protective effect, but the larger, adequately powered BEEP trial and subsequent meta-analyses did not confirm a statistically significant preventive benefit for emollients alone, tempering initial enthusiasm while emphasizing that emollient use remains the cornerstone of treatment once disease develops. Introduction of allergenic foods (particularly peanut) in the first year of life, guided by the LEAP trial findings, has been adopted into allergy prevention guidelines and is relevant to the dermatologist counseling families of infants with early atopic dermatitis and egg allergy. Patient education remains a therapeutic intervention in its own right: structured eczema education programs (eczema schools) that teach parents and patients about trigger avoidance, emollient application technique, topical corticosteroid use (including addressing corticosteroid phobia, which leads to undertreatment), and flare management have been shown to improve treatment adherence, reduce disease severity, and decrease healthcare utilization.

CAUTION: Eczema herpeticum is a dermatologic emergency. The presentation of monomorphic punched-out erosions and vesicles on a background of eczematous dermatitis, with or without fever, requires immediate systemic antiviral therapy (confirm against current formulary and guideline for dosing). Delay in treatment risks corneal involvement, viremia, and multiorgan dissemination. Do not mistake the vesicles for an eczema flare and intensify immunosuppressive therapy, which will worsen the viral infection.

THE CUTANEOUS MIMICKER RECOGNITION ATLAS — Nummular Dermatitis versus Tinea Corporis

---

The Clinical Pattern: Nummular dermatitis presents as well-demarcated, coin-shaped, erythematous plaques with overlying scale and crusting, typically on the extremities and trunk. The plaques are often intensely pruritic and may be multiple and bilateral. There is no central clearing, and the entire surface of the plaque is involved with inflammation and scale. Secondary impetiginization with Staphylococcus aureus is common and may produce honey-colored crusts overlying the eczematous base.

The Mimicker: Tinea corporis produces annular or arciform plaques with a raised, scaling, advancing border and relative central clearing. The morphologic overlap with nummular dermatitis occurs when tinea presents as a fully inflammatory, crusted plaque without obvious central clearing (particularly in immunosuppressed patients or when the lesion is secondarily infected) or when nummular dermatitis develops a slightly more active border, creating a pseudo-annular appearance. The overlap is further compounded when topical corticosteroids have been applied to a tinea lesion, suppressing the characteristic annular morphology and producing tinea incognito.

Trap Logic: Representativeness heuristic drives this error. The clinician sees a round, scaly plaque and automatically categorizes it as either eczema or tinea based on which prototype it most resembles, without performing the confirmatory test that distinguishes the two. The heuristic is especially dangerous when a clinician who sees primarily eczema defaults every round plaque to nummular dermatitis, or when a clinician in a high-tinea-prevalence practice defaults every round plaque to tinea. Both defaults produce diagnostic errors at a rate that reflects the prevalence mismatch.

The Decision Anchor: The discriminating test is the **KOH preparation**. Tinea corporis shows branching, septate hyphae on KOH; nummular dermatitis does not. No clinical or morphologic feature reliably distinguishes the two in every case, but KOH is a 5-minute bedside test that does. The KOH should be performed before initiating therapy for any round scaly plaque: if positive, antifungal therapy is indicated; if negative, topical corticosteroids are appropriate. Empiric use of combination antifungal-corticosteroid creams without a KOH delays diagnosis, creates tinea incognito, and is discouraged by all current guidelines.

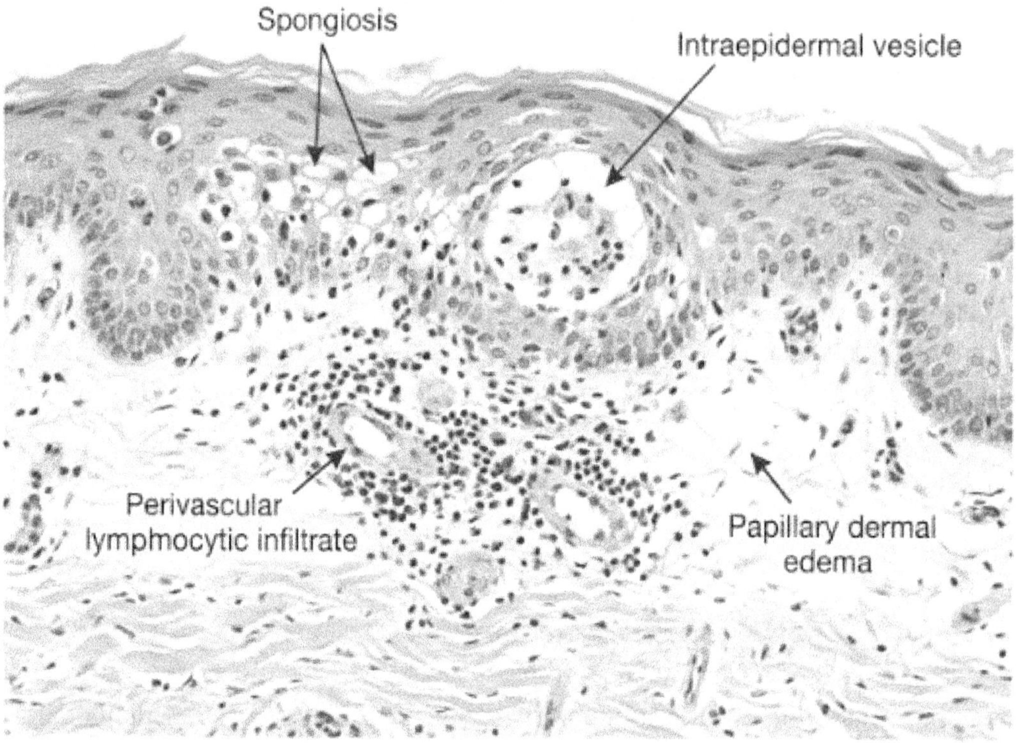

THE CUTANEOUS MIMICKER RECOGNITION ATLAS — Eczematous Diagnostic Arcs

Atopic Dermatitis vs. Cutaneous T-Cell Lymphoma: The discriminating findings are persistent fixed patches in non-flexural distribution with poikiloderma and biopsy showing epidermotropism of atypical lymphocytes with aberrant T-cell marker expression. Atopic dermatitis waxes and wanes; mycosis fungoides produces fixed patches that persist unchanged for months. Cognitive trap: availability bias defaulting every eczematous plaque to eczema.

Nummular Dermatitis vs. Tinea Corporis: The discriminating test is the KOH preparation showing branching, septate hyphae. No clinical feature reliably separates the two in every case. KOH before treatment is mandatory. Cognitive trap: representativeness heuristic categorizing every round plaque without confirmatory testing.

Summary and Key Concepts

Eczematous dermatitis is a spongiotic reaction pattern encompassing endogenous forms (atopic, nummular, dyshidrotic, asteatotic, seborrheic, stasis dermatitis) and exogenous forms (allergic and irritant contact dermatitis). The shared histopathologic substrate is spongiosis with lymphocytic infiltrate; the etiologic subtype determines management.

Atopic dermatitis is driven by the convergence of epidermal barrier dysfunction (FLG mutations, ceramide deficiency, transepidermal water loss) and Th2 immune dysregulation (IL-4, IL-13, IL-31, TSLP), compounded by microbiome dysbiosis with S. aureus dominance. The atopic march links infantile barrier disruption to subsequent food allergy, allergic rhinitis, and asthma through epicutaneous allergen sensitization.

Clinical presentation follows age-dependent distribution patterns (infantile facial/extensor, childhood flexural, adult face/hand/flexural). In skin of color (Fitzpatrick IV-VI), erythema may be absent, follicular accentuation is prominent, and post-inflammatory dyspigmentation is often the dominant finding. Severity scoring (EASI, SCORAD, IGA) quantifies disease for treatment decisions and clinical trial endpoints.

Treatment is stepwise: emollients and barrier restoration for all patients; topical corticosteroids and calcineurin inhibitors for mild-to-moderate disease; phototherapy for moderate disease inadequately controlled by topicals; systemic biologics (dupilumab, tralokinumab) and oral JAK inhibitors (abrocitinib, upadacitinib) for moderate-to-severe disease refractory to topical therapy. Proactive maintenance therapy reduces flare frequency.

Complications include staphylococcal superinfection (90% colonization rate), eczema herpeticum (a dermatologic emergency requiring immediate systemic antivirals), and significant psychosocial burden with sleep disruption, impaired quality of life, and increased prevalence of anxiety and depression. Patch testing should be considered in any refractory eczematous eruption to identify a treatable contact allergen component.

CHAPTER 4: PSORIASIS AND PSORIASIFORM DERMATOSES

Learning Objectives

1. Describe the immunopathogenesis of psoriasis, including the IL-23/Th17 axis, and explain the genetic basis of susceptibility.
2. Recognize the clinical variants of psoriasis and their distinguishing morphologic and distributional features across skin phototypes.
3. Screen for psoriatic arthritis and psoriasis-associated comorbidities using validated instruments and evidence-based criteria.
4. Differentiate psoriasis from its clinical mimickers, including pityriasis rosea, pityriasis rubra pilaris, and secondary syphilis.
5. Apply current treatment algorithms integrating topical therapy, phototherapy, conventional systemic agents, and biologic therapies based on disease severity, phenotype, and comorbidity profile.

Psoriasis: Immunopathogenesis and Genetic Susceptibility

Definition and Epidemiology

Psoriasis is a chronic, immune-mediated, systemic inflammatory disease that manifests primarily in the skin and joints. It affects approximately 2 to 3 percent of the global population, with prevalence highest in northern European and Scandinavian populations and lowest in East Asian and certain African populations. The age of onset follows a bimodal distribution: type I (early onset) peaks between 15 and 25 years and carries a stronger genetic component (HLA-Cw6 association), while type II (late onset) peaks between 50 and 60 years and is typically less familial. The disease has no sex predilection, but the impact on quality of life is substantial: patients with moderate-to-severe psoriasis report impairment in daily functioning comparable to that seen in diabetes, chronic heart failure, and depression, and the cumulative life course impairment from decades of visible skin disease, social stigma, and treatment burden produces measurable psychosocial harm that extends beyond any single severity score.

The IL-23/Th17 Immune Axis

The current understanding of psoriasis pathogenesis centers on the IL-23/Th17 axis. In genetically susceptible individuals, an initiating trigger (trauma, infection, stress, medication) activates dendritic cells and macrophages in the skin, which produce IL-12 and IL-23. IL-23 is the critical upstream cytokine: it drives the differentiation, expansion, and survival of Th17 and Th22 cells, which in turn produce effector cytokines — IL-17A, IL-17F, and IL-22 — that act on keratinocytes to induce the histopathologic hallmarks of psoriasis. IL-17A stimulates keratinocyte proliferation and accelerates the epidermal transit time from the normal 28 to 30 days to approximately 3 to 5 days, producing the characteristic acanthosis (epidermal thickening) and parakeratosis (retained nuclei in the stratum corneum). It also induces keratinocyte production of antimicrobial peptides (LL-37, beta-defensins, S100 proteins), chemokines (CXCL1, CXCL8) that recruit neutrophils to the epidermis (forming the Munro microabscesses that are the histopathologic signature of psoriasis), and additional pro-inflammatory mediators that sustain the inflammatory cycle. IL-22 synergizes with IL-17A to promote keratinocyte hyperproliferation and suppress terminal differentiation, further contributing to the disordered keratinization. TNF-alpha amplifies the entire cascade by promoting dendritic cell maturation, enhancing IL-23 production, and facilitating leukocyte trafficking through upregulation of endothelial adhesion molecules. This understanding of the IL-23/Th17/IL-17 axis has directly informed the development of biologic therapies that target each node in the cascade with remarkable clinical efficacy.

Genetic Susceptibility and HLA Associations

Psoriasis has a strong genetic component, with concordance rates of approximately 65 to 70 percent in monozygotic twins and 15 to 20 percent in dizygotic twins. The most strongly associated locus is PSORS1 on chromosome 6p21, which accounts for approximately 35 to 50 percent of the heritable risk and maps to HLA-Cw6 within the major histocompatibility complex. HLA-Cw6-positive patients are more likely to develop early-onset disease, guttate psoriasis triggered by streptococcal pharyngitis, and extensive plaque disease, while HLA-Cw6-negative patients are more likely to develop late-onset disease and nail involvement. Beyond PSORS1, genome-wide association studies have identified over 80 susceptibility loci in genes governing innate immunity (IL-23R, IL-12B, IL-23A, TRAF3IP2), adaptive immunity (TNFAIP3, TNIP1, NFKBIA), epidermal barrier function (LCE3B/3C deletions on the epidermal differentiation complex), and NF-kB signaling (CARD14, whose gain-of-function mutations cause familial pityriasis rubra pilaris-like psoriasis). The genetic overlap between psoriasis and other immune-mediated diseases — Crohn disease (IL-23R), ankylosing spondylitis (IL-23R, ERAP1), and type 1 diabetes (PTPN22) — reflects shared inflammatory pathways and partly explains the clustering of autoimmune comorbidities in psoriasis patients.

Clinical Variants: Plaque, Guttate, Inverse, Erythrodermic, and Pustular Psoriasis

Plaque Psoriasis

Chronic plaque psoriasis (psoriasis vulgaris) accounts for approximately 80 to 90 percent of all psoriasis cases. It presents as sharply demarcated, erythematous plaques covered with thick, silvery-white, micaceous scale, distributed symmetrically on the extensor surfaces of the elbows and knees, the scalp, the lumbosacral area, and the intergluteal cleft. The Auspitz sign (punctate bleeding upon removal of the scale, reflecting the thin suprapapillary plate overlying dilated capillaries in elongated dermal papillae) is characteristic but not pathognomonic. The Koebner phenomenon (isomorphic response) describes the development of new psoriatic lesions at sites of skin trauma and is seen in approximately 25 percent of patients. In Fitzpatrick phototype IV-VI skin, the classic silvery scale may be less prominent, and psoriatic plaques may appear violaceous, dark brown, or hyperpigmented rather than erythematous, making the diagnosis less immediately apparent to clinicians trained primarily on lighter skin presentations. Post-inflammatory hyperpigmentation or hypopigmentation persisting at resolved plaque sites may be more cosmetically distressing to the patient than the active disease itself and requires separate counseling about expected timelines for resolution.

Guttate, Inverse, and Erythrodermic Psoriasis

Guttate psoriasis presents as an acute eruption of numerous small (0.5 to 1.5 cm), drop-shaped, salmon-pink papules and plaques with fine scale, distributed predominantly on the trunk and proximal extremities. It is most common in children and young adults and is classically triggered by Group A streptococcal pharyngitis 2 to 3 weeks before onset — the mechanism involves molecular mimicry between streptococcal M protein and keratin, activating autoreactive T cells that traffic to the skin. Approximately one-third of guttate psoriasis cases progress to chronic plaque psoriasis; the remainder resolve spontaneously within 3 to 4 months. Inverse (flexural) psoriasis affects intertriginous sites — the axillae, inguinal folds, submammary folds, and intergluteal cleft — where the occlusive, moist environment modifies the morphology: plaques are erythematous and well-demarcated but smooth and shiny rather than scaly, because maceration prevents scale accumulation. The differential for inverse psoriasis includes candidal intertrigo (satellite pustules, KOH-positive), seborrheic dermatitis (greasy scale), and tinea cruris (annular advancing border, KOH-positive). Erythrodermic psoriasis is a severe, life-threatening variant in which erythema and scaling involve more than 90 percent of the body surface area, producing thermoregulatory failure (hypothermia from massive cutaneous heat loss), high-output cardiac failure (from cutaneous vasodilation and increased blood flow), hypoalbuminemia, and secondary infection. It may arise from unstable plaque psoriasis, abrupt withdrawal of systemic corticosteroids, or phototherapy burns, and requires inpatient management with hemodynamic monitoring and systemic therapy.

Pustular Psoriasis

Pustular psoriasis is characterized by sterile neutrophilic pustules and encompasses two major clinical forms. Generalized pustular psoriasis (von Zumbusch type) presents as an acute eruption of widespread, confluent sterile pustules on a background of fiery erythema, often accompanied by systemic toxicity (fever, malaise, leukocytosis, elevated inflammatory markers). It carries significant morbidity and mortality and may be triggered by withdrawal of systemic corticosteroids, infection, pregnancy, or hypocalcemia. Gain-of-function mutations in IL-36RN (encoding the IL-36 receptor antagonist) are identified in a proportion of cases, establishing generalized pustular psoriasis as an autoinflammatory disease distinct from classic plaque psoriasis in its genetic architecture and responsive to IL-36 blockade (spesolimab). Palmoplantar pustulosis presents as chronic, recurrent, sterile pustules on the palms and soles with erythema and scaling, is strongly associated with tobacco smoking, and is debated as either a variant of psoriasis or a distinct entity. Acrodermatitis continua of Hallopeau is a localized pustular variant affecting the distal digits, with pustules on the nail bed and surrounding skin, leading to nail destruction and onychodystrophy.

Nail Psoriasis and Scalp Psoriasis

Nail involvement occurs in approximately 50 percent of patients with plaque psoriasis and in up to 80 percent of patients with psoriatic arthritis, making psoriatic nail dystrophy both a clinical diagnostic feature and a risk marker for joint disease. The nail matrix and nail bed are affected by distinct pathologic processes that produce recognizable clinical signs. Matrix disease produces nail pitting (small, ice-pick-like depressions resulting from foci of parakeratosis in the proximal nail plate), leukonychia (white spots from incomplete keratinization), red spots in the lunula, and crumbling of the nail plate. Nail bed disease produces oil-drop (salmon patch) discoloration (translucent yellow-red patches visible through the nail plate, resulting from serum and glycoprotein accumulation), onycholysis (separation of the nail plate from the nail bed, often with an erythematous border), subungual hyperkeratosis (thickening of the hyponychium), and splinter hemorrhages (longitudinal red-brown lines from dilated, bleeding capillaries in the nail bed). The Nail Psoriasis Severity Index (NAPSI) scores each quadrant of each nail for matrix and bed features, providing a standardized severity measure for clinical trials. Nail psoriasis responds poorly to topical therapy alone and often requires systemic or biologic agents — IL-17 inhibitors (secukinumab, ixekizumab) and IL-23 inhibitors have demonstrated the most robust nail clearance rates. Scalp psoriasis, present in approximately 80 percent of psoriasis patients, produces erythematous, well-demarcated plaques with thick adherent scale that may extend beyond the hairline onto the forehead, retroauricular skin, and posterior neck. The differential includes seborrheic dermatitis (diffuse, greasy scale, typically less well-demarcated), tinea capitis (KOH and culture required to exclude, particularly in children), and discoid lupus (scarring alopecia with follicular plugging).

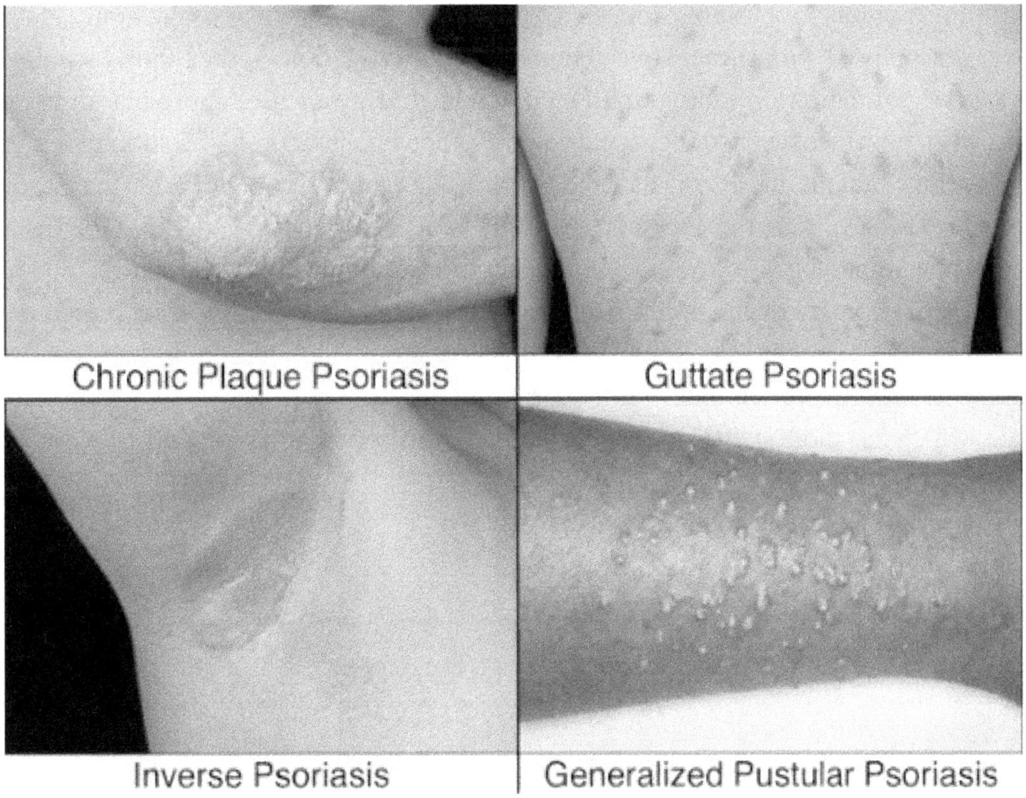

Psoriatic Arthritis: Screening, Classification, and Co-Management

Epidemiology and Clinical Patterns

Psoriatic arthritis (PsA) is a chronic inflammatory arthritis that occurs in approximately 30 percent of patients with psoriasis, though prevalence estimates range from 6 to 42 percent depending on the screening method and population studied. Skin disease precedes joint involvement in approximately 70 percent of cases, usually by 7 to 12 years, while concurrent onset (15 percent) and arthritis preceding skin disease (15 percent) are less common. PsA is classified into five clinical patterns: asymmetric oligoarthritis (the most common pattern, affecting fewer than 5 joints), symmetric polyarthritis (resembling rheumatoid arthritis but typically seronegative for rheumatoid factor), distal interphalangeal joint-predominant disease (strongly associated with psoriatic nail dystrophy), spondylitis and sacroiliitis (axial involvement resembling ankylosing spondylitis), and arthritis mutilans (a destructive, deforming pattern with telescoping digits, representing the most severe but least common variant). Dactylitis (sausage digit, resulting from tenosynovitis and synovitis of an entire digit) and enthesitis (inflammation at tendon and ligament insertion sites, particularly the Achilles tendon and plantar fascia) are hallmark extra-articular features of PsA that distinguish it from rheumatoid arthritis and aid classification.

Screening and Classification Criteria

Because early recognition and treatment of PsA prevents irreversible joint damage, systematic screening in the dermatology clinic is essential. The CASPAR criteria (Classification Criteria for Psoriatic Arthritis) are the accepted standard: a patient with inflammatory articular disease (joint, spine, or entheseal involvement) scores points for current psoriasis (2 points), history of psoriasis or family history (1 point), psoriatic nail dystrophy (1 point), negative rheumatoid factor (1 point), dactylitis (1 point), and juxta-articular new bone formation on radiograph (1 point) — a score of 3 or more classifies the patient as having PsA, with high sensitivity and specificity. Validated screening questionnaires applicable in dermatology settings include the Psoriasis Epidemiology Screening Tool (PEST), the Toronto Psoriatic Arthritis Screen (ToPAS), and the Psoriatic Arthritis Screening and Evaluation (PASE). Any patient presenting with new joint pain, stiffness, swelling, dactylitis, or enthesitis in the setting of psoriasis should be referred for rheumatologic evaluation. Co-management between dermatology and rheumatology is the standard of care, with treatment selection ideally addressing both skin and joint domains simultaneously — a consideration that favors biologics (anti-TNF, anti-IL-17, anti-IL-23) over conventional systemics (methotrexate, which has modest efficacy for peripheral arthritis and no proven efficacy for axial disease).

Psoriasis Comorbidities: Cardiovascular, Metabolic, and Psychiatric

Cardiovascular and Metabolic Risk

Psoriasis is now recognized as a systemic inflammatory disease whose impact extends far beyond the skin. The chronic systemic inflammation associated with moderate-to-severe psoriasis confers independent cardiovascular risk through multiple pathways: accelerated atherosclerosis (driven by the same Th1/Th17 cytokines that fuel the psoriatic plaque), insulin resistance (promoted by TNF-alpha and IL-6), dyslipidemia (with a characteristic pattern of elevated triglycerides, low HDL cholesterol, and small dense LDL particles), and endothelial dysfunction. Epidemiologic studies demonstrate that patients with severe psoriasis have a 50 percent increased relative risk of cardiovascular mortality and a mean reduction in life expectancy of approximately 5 years compared with the general population, independent of traditional cardiovascular risk factors. The concept of psoriasis as an independent cardiovascular risk factor has been incorporated into European cardiology guidelines and has led to recommendations for systematic cardiovascular risk assessment in all patients with moderate-to-severe disease. Metabolic syndrome (central obesity, hypertension, dyslipidemia, insulin resistance) is present in approximately 40 percent of psoriasis patients, compared with 25 percent of matched controls. Non-alcoholic fatty liver disease is increasingly recognized as a comorbidity, with prevalence estimates reaching 45 to 50 percent in psoriasis populations, and carries implications for systemic therapy selection (methotrexate hepatotoxicity risk, need for fibrosis assessment before initiating therapy).

Psychiatric Comorbidity and Quality of Life

The psychosocial burden of psoriasis is among the highest of any chronic medical condition. Depression affects 20 to 30 percent of patients with psoriasis (compared with approximately 7 percent of the general population), anxiety disorders affect 15 to 20 percent, and suicidal ideation is reported at rates significantly elevated above population baselines. The relationship between psoriasis and depression is bidirectional: inflammatory cytokines (TNF-alpha, IL-6, IL-17) cross the blood-brain barrier and modulate serotonergic and dopaminergic neurotransmission, contributing to neuroinflammation-driven depression, while psychological stress triggers the hypothalamic-pituitary-adrenal axis and sympathetic nervous system, releasing neuropeptides (substance P, nerve growth factor) that promote mast cell degranulation and neurogenic inflammation in the skin, potentially triggering flares. Alcohol use disorder is more prevalent among psoriasis patients and complicates disease management through multiple mechanisms: alcohol worsens psoriasis severity (through pro-inflammatory effects and impaired barrier function), reduces treatment adherence, and is a contraindication for methotrexate. Screening for depression (PHQ-2/PHQ-9), alcohol use (AUDIT-C), and psychosocial impact (DLQI) should be incorporated into routine psoriasis visits.

CLINICAL PEARL: A DLQI score of 10 or greater indicates that psoriasis is having a large or extremely large effect on the patient's quality of life and, in many treatment guidelines, independently qualifies the patient for systemic therapy even if the objective skin severity scores (BSA, PASI) fall below the traditional moderate-to-severe threshold. Treatment decisions should integrate both objective disease severity and patient-reported quality-of-life impact.

Pityriasis Rosea, Pityriasis Rubra Pilaris, and Other Papulosquamous Conditions

Pityriasis Rosea

Pityriasis rosea is an acute, self-limited papulosquamous eruption most common in adolescents and young adults. It begins with a single herald patch — an oval, salmon-colored plaque with a collarette of fine, inward-trailing scale — typically on the trunk, followed 1 to 2 weeks later by a generalized eruption of smaller, oval, salmon-pink papules and plaques oriented along the skin cleavage lines (Langer lines), producing the classic Christmas tree distribution on the posterior trunk. The peripheral collarette scale (the trailing edge of scale directed toward the center of the lesion) is the most reliable morphologic clue distinguishing pityriasis rosea from other papulosquamous conditions. The eruption is typically mildly pruritic and resolves spontaneously within 6 to 8 weeks. The etiology is presumed viral: human herpesvirus 6 (HHV-6) and HHV-7 reactivation have been implicated, though causation remains unproven. The critical differential is secondary syphilis, which can mimic pityriasis rosea closely (oval, coppery-red, scaly papules in a similar truncal distribution) and must be excluded with serologic testing (RPR or VDRL followed by confirmatory FTA-ABS) in any sexually active patient, because missing secondary syphilis has devastating consequences for the patient and public health.

Pityriasis Rubra Pilaris

Pityriasis rubra pilaris (PRP) is an uncommon papulosquamous disorder characterized by follicular keratotic papules, salmon-colored erythroderma with characteristic islands of sparing (areas of uninvolved, normal-appearing skin within the erythrodermic background), and waxy palmoplantar keratoderma. PRP is classified into six types: classic adult (type I, the most common, with cephalocaudal spread and a generally favorable prognosis over 1 to 3 years), atypical adult (type II, ichthyosiform with a more chronic course), classic juvenile (type III), circumscribed juvenile (type IV, well-defined plaques on the elbows and knees), atypical juvenile (type V, most common in HIV-associated PRP), and HIV-associated (type VI). The key clinical distinction from erythrodermic psoriasis is the presence of islands of sparing and the salmon-orange rather than red hue, though overlap exists and biopsy may be required. Histopathology shows alternating orthokeratosis and parakeratosis in both horizontal and vertical patterns (checkerboard pattern), which is distinct from the uniform parakeratosis of psoriasis. CARD14 gain-of-function mutations have been identified in familial PRP, linking it to the NF-kB signaling pathway that also underlies psoriasis and reinforcing the concept of a papulosquamous disease spectrum.

THE CUTANEOUS MIMICKER RECOGNITION ATLAS — Pityriasis Rosea versus Secondary Syphilis

---

The Clinical Pattern: Pityriasis rosea presents with a herald patch followed by an eruption of oval, salmon-pink papules and plaques with collarette scale, oriented along the skin cleavage lines (Christmas tree pattern on the posterior trunk), resolving spontaneously in 6 to 8 weeks. The patient is typically an otherwise healthy adolescent or young adult with mild pruritus and no systemic symptoms.

The Mimicker: Secondary syphilis produces a generalized eruption of oval, coppery-red, scaly papules and thin plaques in a similar truncal distribution that can closely resemble pityriasis rosea. Additional features of secondary syphilis include involvement of the palms and soles (which pityriasis rosea typically spares), mucous patches (painless, gray-white erosions on the oral or genital mucosa), condylomata lata (broad, flat, moist papules in intertriginous areas), diffuse lymphadenopathy, and constitutional symptoms (malaise, low-grade fever, weight loss, arthralgias).

Trap Logic: Premature closure is the cognitive trap. The clinician recognizes the Christmas tree pattern and collarette scale, diagnoses pityriasis rosea, and does not consider syphilis because the clinical pattern matched the expected prototype. The error is compounded by the assumption that sexually transmitted infections are unlikely in a patient who does not volunteer a sexual history, and by the fact that secondary syphilis may present without the mucocutaneous clues (palmar/plantar lesions, condylomata lata) that would trigger suspicion.

The Decision Anchor: The discriminating action is **serologic testing (RPR/VDRL with confirmatory FTA-ABS) in every sexually active patient presenting with a papulosquamous eruption that could be pityriasis rosea**. The clinical threshold for testing should be low: palm and sole involvement, mucous membrane lesions, lymphadenopathy, and constitutional symptoms increase suspicion, but their absence does not exclude secondary syphilis. Missing secondary syphilis allows progression to tertiary disease (cardiovascular, neurologic) and ongoing transmission. The cost of a screening RPR is negligible; the cost of a missed diagnosis is catastrophic.

Evidence-Based Therapeutics: Topical Agents, Phototherapy, Conventional Systemics, and Biologics

Topical Therapy

Topical therapy is the foundation of management for mild psoriasis (BSA less than 3 percent, or limited plaques) and remains an adjunct in moderate-to-severe disease. Topical corticosteroids are first-line, with potency selected by body site: mid-potency (triamcinolone acetonide, mometasone furoate) for truncal and extremity plaques, low-potency for the face and intertriginous areas, and superpotent (clobetasol propionate, halobetasol) for thick, lichenified plaques and the palms and soles, used for limited durations (2 to 4 weeks) to minimize the risk of skin atrophy, striae, and tachyphylaxis. Vitamin D3 analogs (calcipotriene, calcitriol) inhibit keratinocyte proliferation and promote differentiation, addressing the hyperproliferative component of psoriasis; they are most effective in combination with topical corticosteroids (fixed-combination calcipotriene/betamethasone dipropionate), which produces greater efficacy than either agent alone. Topical calcineurin inhibitors (tacrolimus, pimecrolimus) are used off-label for facial and inverse psoriasis where corticosteroid-induced atrophy is a concern. Tazarotene (a topical retinoid) normalizes keratinocyte differentiation and reduces scale but causes local irritation that limits tolerability; it is often combined with a topical corticosteroid to mitigate this. Topical roflumilast (a phosphodiesterase-4 inhibitor) represents a newer steroid-sparing option with demonstrated efficacy for plaque psoriasis including intertriginous areas.

Phototherapy

Phototherapy is appropriate for moderate psoriasis (BSA 3 to 10 percent, or widespread thin plaques) and for patients who prefer to avoid systemic immunosuppression. Narrowband UVB (311 to 313 nm) is the preferred modality: it induces T-cell apoptosis, suppresses the Th17 response, and promotes regulatory T-cell expansion in psoriatic skin. Treatment is administered 2 to 3 times weekly with dose titration based on the minimal erythema dose, and most patients achieve clearance or near-clearance within 20 to 30 sessions. Maintenance phototherapy (once to twice weekly after clearance) extends the remission period but must be weighed against cumulative UV exposure. Excimer laser (308 nm) delivers targeted high-dose UVB to individual plaques, allowing treatment of localized recalcitrant disease (particularly scalp, elbow, and knee plaques) while sparing uninvolved skin and reducing cumulative UV exposure; it achieves clearance in fewer sessions than whole-body NB-UVB for limited disease. Home NB-UVB units, prescribed and monitored by the dermatologist, provide a practical alternative for patients unable to attend clinic-based sessions three times weekly, and adherence data from registry studies suggest that home phototherapy achieves comparable outcomes when patients follow standardized dose-escalation protocols with regular teledermatology check-ins. PUVA (psoralen plus UVA) remains effective for thick plaque psoriasis and palmoplantar disease but is used less frequently due to the cumulative risk of squamous cell carcinoma and melanoma with prolonged use, and it is now generally reserved for cases refractory to NB-UVB.

Conventional Systemic Agents

Systemic therapy is indicated for moderate-to-severe psoriasis (BSA greater than 10 percent, or significant impact on quality of life, or involvement of difficult-to-treat sites including the scalp, nails, palms, soles, and genitalia). Methotrexate, the longest-established systemic agent, inhibits dihydrofolate reductase and suppresses lymphocyte proliferation, with efficacy demonstrated for both skin and peripheral joint disease. Hepatotoxicity is the primary concern with long-term use: current guidelines recommend assessment of liver fibrosis (by transient elastography or serum biomarkers such as the FIB-4 index and PIIINP procollagen peptide) rather than routine liver biopsy, with monitoring intervals guided by cumulative dose and risk factors (obesity, diabetes, alcohol use). Cyclosporine, a calcineurin inhibitor, provides rapid and reliable clearance of severe psoriasis but is limited to short-term use (generally 1 to 2 years) due to the risk of nephrotoxicity and hypertension. Acitretin, an oral retinoid, is most effective for pustular and erythrodermic psoriasis and is often combined with phototherapy (Re-PUVA or Re-UVB); its teratogenicity requires reliable contraception during and for 3 years after discontinuation in women of childbearing potential. Apremilast, an oral phosphodiesterase-4 inhibitor, has moderate efficacy for plaque psoriasis and psoriatic arthritis and does not require laboratory monitoring, making it a useful option for patients who cannot tolerate or who decline conventional immunosuppressives or biologics.

Biologic Therapies

Biologic therapies have transformed the management of moderate-to-severe psoriasis by targeting specific nodes of the IL-23/Th17/IL-17 axis with high efficacy and acceptable safety profiles. TNF-alpha inhibitors (etanercept, infliximab, adalimumab, certolizumab pegol) were the first biologic class approved for psoriasis and remain widely used; they are also effective for psoriatic arthritis, inflammatory bowel disease, and other TNF-driven conditions, making them first-line when these comorbidities coexist. IL-17A inhibitors (secukinumab, ixekizumab) and the IL-17A/F inhibitor bimekizumab achieve higher rates of skin clearance (PASI 90 and PASI 100 responses) than TNF inhibitors and are particularly effective for nail psoriasis and palmoplantar disease; the main safety consideration is an increased risk of candidal infections (oral and vulvovaginal), and IL-17 inhibition is relatively contraindicated in patients with inflammatory bowel disease due to the risk of exacerbation. IL-23 inhibitors (guselkumab, risankizumab, tildrakizumab) target the p19 subunit of IL-23, blocking the upstream driver of the Th17 response while preserving the IL-12/Th1 pathway and avoiding the immunosuppression associated with broader cytokine blockade. They offer high efficacy with infrequent dosing intervals (every 8 to 12 weeks after induction) and a favorable safety profile that makes them increasingly positioned as first-line biologics for moderate-to-severe plaque psoriasis. IL-12/23 inhibitors (ustekinumab, targeting the p40 subunit shared by IL-12 and IL-23) provided proof of concept for this pathway but are being superseded by the more selective p19 inhibitors that achieve higher clearance rates. Deucravacitinib, a selective TYK2 inhibitor, represents a novel oral option that targets the intracellular signaling downstream of IL-23 and IL-12 receptors while sparing JAK1/JAK2/JAK3, offering a potentially favorable cardiovascular and hematologic safety profile compared with non-selective JAK inhibitors.

Biologic Class	Key Agents	Target	PASI 90 Response (approx.)	Key Safety Considerations
TNF-alpha inhibitors	Adalimumab, infliximab, etanercept, certolizumab	TNF-alpha	40-55%	Infection risk, TB reactivation, demyelination (rare), heart failure exacerbation
IL-17 inhibitors	Secukinumab, ixekizumab, bimekizumab	IL-17A (and IL-17F for bimekizumab)	70-80%	Candidiasis, IBD exacerbation risk, neutropenia (uncommon)

IL-23 (p19) inhibitors	Guselkumab, risankizumab, tildrakizumab	IL-23 p19 subunit	70-85%	Favorable safety profile, upper respiratory infections
IL-12/23 (p40) inhibitor	Ustekinumab	IL-12 and IL-23 (p40 subunit)	45-60%	Infection, cardiovascular events (rare, debated)
TYK2 inhibitor (oral)	Deucravacitinib	TYK2	35-45%	Upper respiratory infections, CPK elevation, acne

Treatment Algorithms and Guideline-Directed Therapy

Severity-Based Treatment Selection

Current treatment guidelines from the American Academy of Dermatology, the European Academy of Dermatology and Venereology, and the British Association of Dermatologists all employ a stepwise, severity-based approach. Mild psoriasis (BSA less than 3 percent, DLQI less than 10) is managed with topical therapy alone. Moderate psoriasis (BSA 3 to 10 percent, or BSA less than 3 percent but involving high-impact sites such as the face, genitalia, palms, soles, or nails, or DLQI 10 or greater regardless of BSA) warrants consideration of phototherapy or systemic therapy. Severe psoriasis (BSA greater than 10 percent, or PASI greater than 10, or DLQI greater than 10) requires systemic therapy, with biologics generally preferred over conventional systemics based on superior efficacy and safety data from head-to-head trials and long-term registry data. The treat-to-target paradigm, borrowed from rheumatology, sets PASI 90 or IGA 0/1 (clear or almost clear) as the treatment goal, with escalation or switching if the target is not met within 16 weeks (for biologics with maintenance dosing) or 24 weeks (for biologics with longer time to maximal effect). This represents a shift from the historical acceptance of partial response (PASI 50 or PASI 75) as adequate.

Comorbidity-Driven Treatment Decisions

Treatment selection in psoriasis is increasingly guided not only by skin severity but by the patient's comorbidity profile. Patients with coexistent psoriatic arthritis are best served by agents with demonstrated joint efficacy (TNF inhibitors, IL-17 inhibitors, JAK inhibitors); IL-23 inhibitors have also shown efficacy for peripheral arthritis but less convincing data for axial disease. Patients with coexistent inflammatory bowel disease should avoid IL-17 inhibitors (which may worsen IBD) and are best served by TNF inhibitors (particularly infliximab and adalimumab, which are approved for both psoriasis and IBD) or IL-23 inhibitors (which have demonstrated efficacy in Crohn disease and ulcerative colitis). Patients with significant cardiovascular risk benefit from agents that reduce systemic inflammation broadly (TNF inhibitors and IL-23 inhibitors), and observational data suggest that sustained biologic therapy may reduce the incidence of major adverse cardiovascular events in severe psoriasis. Patients with chronic hepatitis B or latent tuberculosis require screening (HBsAg, anti-HBc, tuberculin skin test or interferon-gamma release assay) before initiating any biologic therapy, and latent TB must be treated before or concurrently with biologic initiation. The dermatologist managing moderate-to-severe psoriasis serves not only as the prescriber of skin-directed therapy but as the coordinator of a systemic disease that touches rheumatology, cardiology, hepatology, and psychiatry.

Special Populations and Drug-Triggered Psoriasis

Pregnancy requires special consideration: methotrexate and acitretin are absolutely contraindicated due to teratogenicity, cyclosporine may be continued under close monitoring as it has an established safety record in transplant recipients during pregnancy, and certolizumab pegol (a PEGylated anti-TNF with minimal placental transfer) is the biologic with the best pregnancy safety data. Pediatric psoriasis affects approximately 1 percent of children, and the therapeutic armamentarium has expanded with regulatory approvals of several biologics (etanercept, adalimumab, secukinumab, ixekizumab, ustekinumab) for children and adolescents with moderate-to-severe disease. Elderly patients with psoriasis require careful comorbidity screening (cardiovascular disease, renal impairment, hepatic dysfunction) and dose adjustments for conventional systemics; immunosenescence may alter both the risk-benefit ratio of biologic therapy and the response to phototherapy. Drug-triggered psoriasis is an important clinical entity in which certain medications provoke new-onset psoriasis or flare existing disease: beta-blockers, lithium, antimalarials (chloroquine, hydroxychloroquine), nonsteroidal anti-inflammatory agents (particularly indomethacin), interferons, and immune checkpoint inhibitors (anti-PD-1/PD-L1, anti-CTLA-4) are the most commonly implicated agents. The mechanism varies by drug class — lithium inhibits inositol monophosphatase and glycogen synthase kinase-3 beta, promoting neutrophil chemotaxis and keratinocyte proliferation, while checkpoint inhibitors remove the immune brakes that normally prevent autoreactive T-cell activation. Drug withdrawal resolves some cases, but checkpoint inhibitor-induced psoriasis may persist and require ongoing management.

KEY POINT: The treat-to-target paradigm in psoriasis sets PASI 90 or IGA 0/1 (clear or almost clear) as the treatment goal, replacing the older standard of PASI 75. Failure to achieve the target within the expected time frame should prompt treatment escalation or switching rather than acceptance of partial response, because the systemic inflammatory burden of under-treated psoriasis contributes to cardiovascular, metabolic, and psychiatric comorbidity.

THE CUTANEOUS MIMICKER RECOGNITION ATLAS — Plaque Psoriasis versus Nummular Dermatitis

The Clinical Pattern: Plaque psoriasis presents with sharply demarcated, erythematous plaques covered with thick, silvery-white, micaceous scale, symmetrically distributed on the extensor surfaces (elbows, knees), scalp, and lumbosacral area. The plaques are well-defined with a distinct border between involved and uninvolved skin. Removal of the scale may produce punctate bleeding (Auspitz sign). Nail changes (pitting, oil-drop discoloration, onycholysis, subungual hyperkeratosis) and scalp involvement support the diagnosis.

The Mimicker: Nummular dermatitis produces well-demarcated, coin-shaped plaques with scale and crusting on the extremities and trunk, overlapping morphologically with psoriasis — particularly when nummular lesions are on the extensor surfaces or when psoriatic plaques are exudative. The overlap is strongest in patients who present with a single or few well-demarcated scaly plaques without the classic psoriatic distribution or accessory findings. Secondary impetiginization of nummular dermatitis may mask the spongiotic morphology and produce a plaque that appears psoriasiform on initial examination.

Trap Logic: Pattern matching without integration is the cognitive trap. The clinician recognizes a round, scaly, well-demarcated plaque and assigns it to either psoriasis or nummular dermatitis based on which prototype the lesion most resembles in isolation, without synthesizing the full clinical picture: distribution pattern, bilateral symmetry, scalp and nail involvement, family history, and the character of the scale (silvery-white micaceous for psoriasis, crusted and often weeping for nummular dermatitis). Both conditions respond to topical corticosteroids, so an empiric trial without a definitive diagnosis delays recognition of the true underlying condition.

The Decision Anchor: The discriminating features are **the distribution pattern (extensor and symmetric for psoriasis, random or extremity-predominant for nummular), the scale character (thick silvery micaceous for psoriasis, crusted and occasionally weeping for nummular), and the presence of nail changes (psoriatic nail dystrophy has no equivalent in nummular dermatitis)**. When morphology alone is ambiguous, scalp examination (psoriasis involves the scalp in approximately 80 percent of cases; nummular dermatitis does not), nail examination (pitting, oil-drop spots, onycholysis), and biopsy (regular acanthosis with Munro microabscesses in psoriasis vs. spongiosis in nummular eczema) resolve the differential.

Dermoscopic Comparison: Plaque Psoriasis vs. Spongiotic Dermatitis

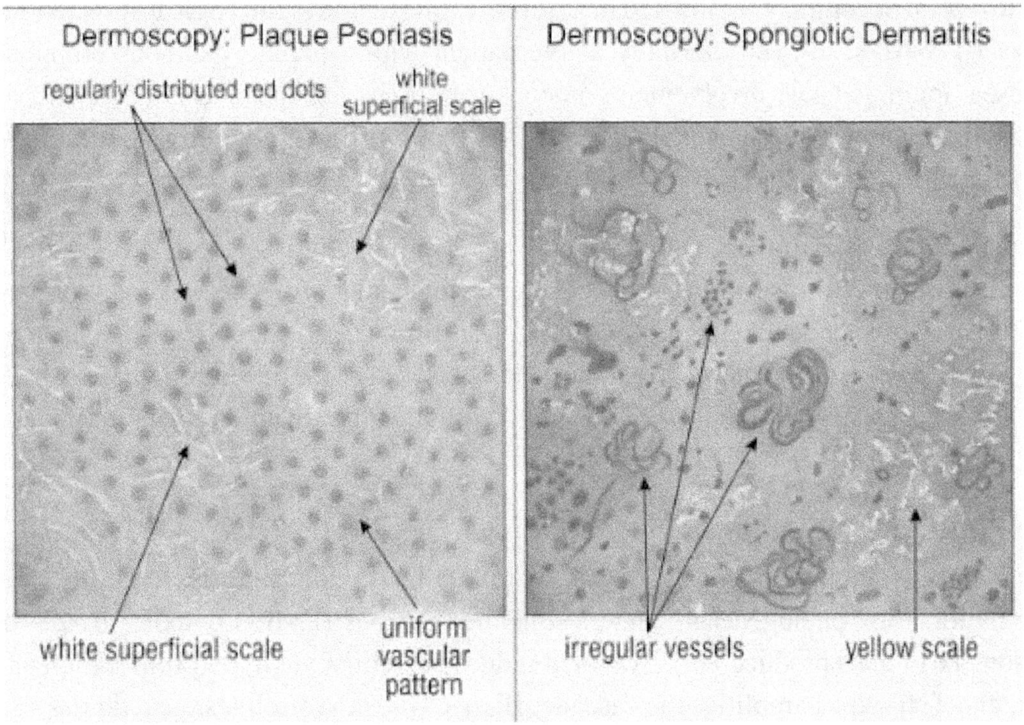

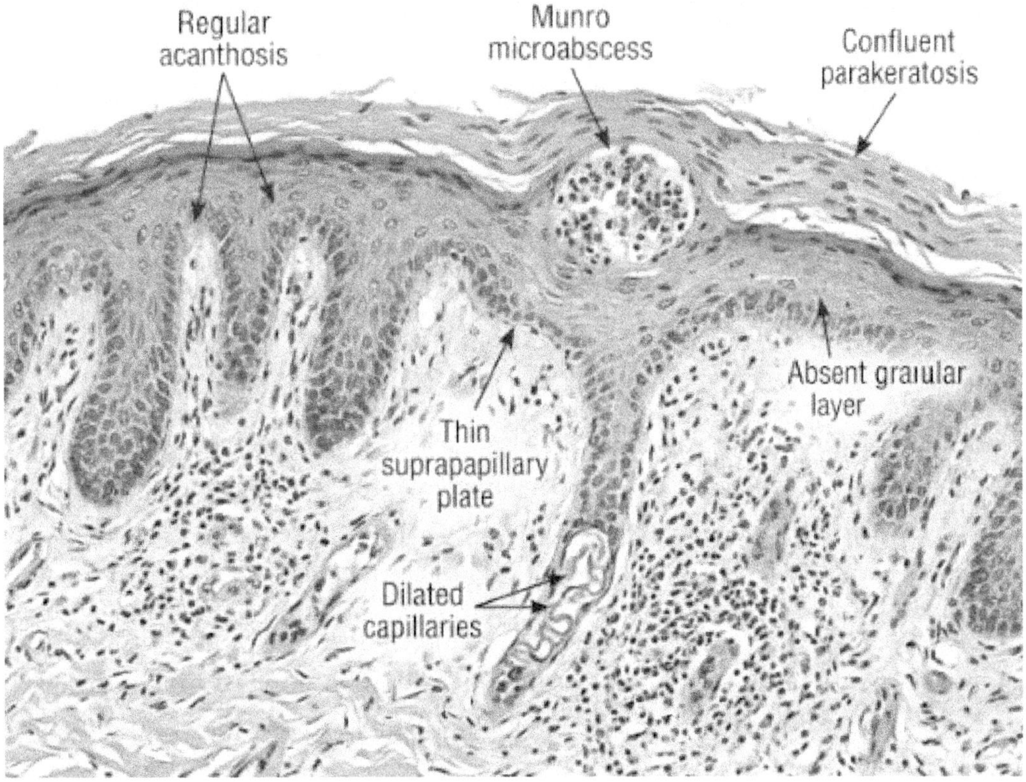

Pityriasis Rosea vs. Secondary Syphilis: The discriminating action is serologic testing (RPR/VDRL with confirmatory FTA-ABS) in every sexually active patient with a papulosquamous eruption resembling pityriasis rosea. Palm and sole involvement, mucous membrane lesions, and lymphadenopathy increase suspicion, but their absence does not exclude syphilis. Cognitive trap: premature closure after recognizing the Christmas tree pattern.

Plaque Psoriasis vs. Nummular Dermatitis: The discriminating features are distribution pattern (extensor and symmetric for psoriasis), scale character (thick silvery micaceous for psoriasis vs. crusted for nummular), and psoriatic nail changes (pitting, oil-drop spots, onycholysis) which have no nummular equivalent. Scalp involvement, biopsy (regular acanthosis with Munro microabscesses vs. spongiosis), and family history resolve ambiguous cases. Cognitive trap: pattern matching without integrating the full clinical picture.

Summary and Key Concepts

Psoriasis is a chronic, immune-mediated, systemic inflammatory disease affecting 2 to 3 percent of the global population. Its pathogenesis centers on the IL-23/Th17/IL-17 axis: IL-23 drives Th17 differentiation, Th17 cells produce IL-17A which induces keratinocyte hyperproliferation and neutrophil recruitment, and TNF-alpha amplifies the cascade. HLA-Cw6 is the strongest genetic risk factor.

Clinical variants include chronic plaque psoriasis (80 to 90 percent of cases: sharply demarcated, silvery-scaled plaques on extensors), guttate (streptococcal-triggered, drop-shaped, self-limited in two-thirds), inverse (flexural, smooth and shiny without scale), erythrodermic (life-threatening, thermoregulatory failure), and pustular psoriasis (generalized von Zumbusch or palmoplantar, with IL-36RN mutations identified in a subset).

Psoriatic arthritis affects approximately 30 percent of psoriasis patients and should be systematically screened for using validated instruments (PEST, ToPAS). Co-management with rheumatology and selection of agents with dual skin-joint efficacy (TNF inhibitors, IL-17 inhibitors, IL-23 inhibitors) is the standard of care.

Psoriasis-associated comorbidities include cardiovascular disease (50 percent increased relative risk of cardiovascular mortality in severe disease), metabolic syndrome (40 percent prevalence), NAFLD, depression (20 to 30 percent), and anxiety. Comorbidity screening and comorbidity-driven treatment selection are essential components of comprehensive psoriasis management.

Treatment follows a stepwise, severity-based algorithm: topical therapy for mild disease, phototherapy or systemic therapy for moderate disease, and biologics (IL-23 inhibitors, IL-17 inhibitors, TNF inhibitors) for severe disease. The treat-to-target paradigm sets PASI 90 or IGA 0/1 as the treatment goal, with treatment escalation if the target is not met within the expected time frame.

CHAPTER 5: URTICARIA AND ERYTHEMA

Learning Objectives

1. Describe the pathophysiology of urticaria, including the roles of mast cell degranulation, histamine, and non-histaminergic mediators.
2. Classify urticaria by duration, trigger, and mechanism and differentiate chronic spontaneous urticaria from inducible urticarias.
3. Recognize urticarial vasculitis as a distinct entity requiring biopsy and distinguish it from ordinary urticaria.
4. Differentiate erythema multiforme from Stevens-Johnson syndrome and identify the clinical and etiologic features of erythema nodosum and other reactive erythemas.
5. Apply current guidelines for the stepwise management of chronic urticaria, including second-generation antihistamines, omalizumab, and emerging biologic therapies.

Pathophysiology of Urticaria: Mast Cells, Histamine, and Beyond

Mast Cell Biology and Activation Pathways

Urticaria results from the degranulation of cutaneous mast cells, which release preformed and newly synthesized mediators into the surrounding dermis. Mast cells are tissue-resident immune cells derived from CD34+ hematopoietic progenitors that mature in peripheral tissues under the influence of stem cell factor (SCF) binding to the KIT receptor. In the skin, mast cells reside predominantly in the perivascular and perifollicular dermis and serve as sentinels of the innate immune system. Mast cell degranulation can be triggered through multiple pathways: IgE-mediated (the classic type I hypersensitivity mechanism, in which allergen cross-links IgE bound to the high-affinity IgE receptor FcepsilonRI), complement-mediated (C3a and C5a anaphylatoxins acting through complement receptors), neuropeptide-mediated (substance P acting through the MRGPRX2 receptor, a recently characterized pathway that explains non-allergic mast cell activation by drugs, neuropeptides, and physical stimuli), and autoimmune (autoantibodies against FcepsilonRI or against IgE itself, a mechanism central to the pathogenesis of chronic spontaneous urticaria). The distinction between IgE-dependent and IgE-independent activation pathways has direct therapeutic implications: IgE-dependent degranulation responds to allergen avoidance and anti-IgE therapy (omalizumab), while MRGPRX2-mediated degranulation explains the pseudoallergic reactions to opioids, fluoroquinolones, and radiocontrast media that occur without prior sensitization.

Histamine and Non-Histaminergic Mediators

Histamine is the dominant preformed mediator released during mast cell degranulation and is responsible for the hallmark clinical features of urticaria: vasodilation (producing erythema), increased vascular permeability (producing dermal edema, which manifests as the wheal), and sensory nerve stimulation (producing pruritus). Histamine acts through four receptor subtypes, of which H1 and H2 are most relevant to urticaria: H1 receptor activation drives vasodilation, vascular permeability, and pruritus, while H2 receptor activation contributes to vasodilation and gastric acid secretion. However, histamine alone does not account for the full spectrum of urticarial pathology. Mast cells also release lipid-derived mediators (prostaglandin D2, leukotriene C4, platelet-activating factor) that sustain vasodilation and edema, cytokines (TNF-alpha, IL-4, IL-5, IL-6, IL-13) that recruit eosinophils, basophils, and neutrophils to the site, and proteases (tryptase, chymase) that activate complement and coagulation cascades. The perivascular infiltrate in urticarial lesions contains eosinophils, basophils, and CD4+ T cells in addition to the degranulated mast cells, reflecting the broader immune activation that accompanies mast cell degranulation. Serum tryptase, released from mast cells during degranulation, is a clinically useful biomarker: a persistently elevated baseline tryptase (above the upper limit of normal) raises the possibility of mastocytosis or mast cell activation syndrome, while an acute elevation of tryptase (measured within 1 to 2 hours of symptom onset) confirms systemic mast cell degranulation in the evaluation of anaphylaxis.

KEY POINT: The discovery of the MRGPRX2 receptor on mast cells explains the mechanism of non-allergic (pseudoallergic) drug reactions — opioids, fluoroquinolones, vancomycin (red man syndrome), and neuromuscular blocking agents can directly activate mast cells through MRGPRX2 without IgE-mediated sensitization. These reactions are dose-dependent and not reproducible by skin-prick testing, which detects only IgE-mediated sensitivity.

Acute and Chronic Urticaria: Classification and Clinical Features

Classification by Duration and Etiology

Urticaria is classified by duration into acute (less than 6 weeks) and chronic (6 weeks or longer). Acute urticaria is the most common form, affecting approximately 15 to 25 percent of individuals at least once in their lifetime. In the majority of cases, the cause is identifiable: viral infections (particularly upper respiratory tract infections in children), drug reactions (NSAIDs, antibiotics, opioids), food allergens (nuts, shellfish, egg, milk), insect stings, and contact allergens. The wheals of acute urticaria are transient (individual lesions lasting less than 24 hours), migratory (appearing and resolving in different locations), intensely pruritic, and leave no residual mark upon resolution — this evanescent quality is the defining clinical feature that distinguishes urticaria from other erythematous conditions. Angioedema (deep dermal and subcutaneous swelling, most commonly of the lips, eyelids, tongue, and genitalia) accompanies urticaria in approximately 40 percent of cases and may occur in isolation.

Chronic Urticaria: Clinical Burden and Evaluation

Chronic urticaria, defined by the persistence of wheals on most days of the week for 6 weeks or more, affects approximately 0.5 to 1 percent of the population and imposes a disease burden comparable to coronary artery disease when measured by quality-of-life instruments. The Urticaria Activity Score (UAS7) quantifies disease severity over 7 days by summing daily wheal count (0-3) and itch intensity (0-3) scores, yielding a range of 0 to 42. The Urticaria Control Test (UCT) provides a patient-reported outcome measure of disease control. Routine laboratory evaluation of chronic urticaria should be limited to a complete blood count with differential (screening for eosinophilia, which raises the possibility of urticarial vasculitis or parasitic infection), erythrocyte sedimentation rate or C-reactive protein (elevated in urticarial vasculitis), and thyroid function tests with anti-thyroid antibodies (autoimmune thyroid disease is associated with chronic urticaria in approximately 10 to 25 percent of patients). Extensive allergy testing, food elimination diets, and screening for infections or malignancy are not recommended in the routine evaluation of chronic urticaria unless the clinical history suggests a specific trigger, because the vast majority of chronic urticaria is spontaneous (no identifiable external cause) and the diagnostic yield of unfocused testing is extremely low.

Chronic Spontaneous Urticaria: Autoimmune Mechanisms and Biomarkers

Autoimmune Pathogenesis

Chronic spontaneous urticaria (CSU) is now understood to be an autoimmune disease in a substantial proportion of patients. Two autoimmune mechanisms have been characterized. Type I autoimmune CSU involves IgE autoantibodies directed against self-antigens (including thyroid peroxidase, IL-24, and other autoantigens), which bind to FcepsilonRI on mast cells and are cross-linked by the corresponding autoantigen, triggering degranulation through the same mechanism as allergen-induced urticaria. This subtype is associated with elevated total IgE and responds well to omalizumab (which reduces free IgE and downregulates FcepsilonRI expression). Type IIb autoimmune CSU involves IgG autoantibodies directed against FcepsilonRI itself or against IgE, which directly cross-link and activate the receptor. This subtype is associated with a positive basophil histamine release assay (BHRA) and autologous serum skin test (ASST), lower total IgE levels, a higher rate of concomitant autoimmune disease (particularly thyroid autoimmunity), and a poorer response to omalizumab — because the pathogenic mechanism bypasses IgE. The distinction between type I and type IIb autoimmune CSU has implications for treatment selection and prognosis and is an area of active clinical research.

Biomarkers and Clinical Phenotyping

The clinical phenotyping of CSU is increasingly guided by biomarkers that predict disease course and treatment response. Total serum IgE is the most accessible predictor of omalizumab response: patients with higher baseline IgE tend to respond more rapidly and completely, while patients with low IgE (particularly those with positive ASST) are more likely to be partial or non-responders to omalizumab. Basophil markers — including basophil CD63 expression (a degranulation marker assessed by flow cytometry) and the BHRA — identify patients with functional autoantibodies. D-dimer and prothrombin fragment 1+2 are elevated in a subset of CSU patients and correlate with disease severity, reflecting activation of the extrinsic coagulation cascade and thrombin-mediated mast cell activation through protease-activated receptors. Blood eosinophil count and eosinophil cationic protein may identify patients with eosinophilic CSU who respond to eosinophil-targeted therapies. The integration of these biomarkers into a precision-medicine framework for CSU is evolving, with the goal of matching individual patients to the therapy most likely to achieve complete urticaria control.

Natural History, Prognosis, and Quality of Life Impact

The natural history of chronic spontaneous urticaria is characterized by eventual spontaneous remission in the majority of patients, though the time course is highly variable and unpredictable at the individual level. Population-based studies indicate that approximately 30 to 50 percent of patients achieve complete remission within 1 year, 50 to 70 percent within 3 years, and 80 to 90 percent within 5 years. However, a substantial minority (10 to 20 percent) experience disease lasting a decade or longer, and recurrence after apparent remission occurs in approximately 20 to 30 percent of cases, necessitating ongoing follow-up even after clinical resolution. Predictors of prolonged disease duration include severe baseline disease activity (UAS7 greater than 28), concomitant angioedema, positive autologous serum skin test (indicating type IIb autoimmune CSU), concomitant inducible urticaria, the presence of autoimmune comorbidities (particularly thyroid autoimmunity), and elevated baseline inflammatory markers (CRP, D-dimer). The impact of CSU on quality of life is substantial and frequently underestimated by clinicians who view urticaria as a cosmetically bothersome but medically benign condition: patients report sleep disruption from nocturnal pruritus, impaired work productivity, social withdrawal due to visible lesions and unpredictable flares, and psychological distress including clinically significant anxiety and depression at rates two to three times higher than the general population. The Dermatology Life Quality Index (DLQI) scores in CSU are comparable to those reported in severe psoriasis and atopic dermatitis, and CSU has been shown to impair overall health utility to a degree comparable to ischemic heart disease when measured by generic preference-based instruments. Disease monitoring should incorporate both physician-assessed activity measures (UAS7) and patient-reported outcome measures (Urticaria Control Test, DLQI, Chronic Urticaria Quality of Life Questionnaire) at regular intervals to guide treatment escalation or de-escalation decisions. The target of therapy is complete symptom control (UAS7 of 0 and UCT of 16), not merely partial improvement, and this treat-to-target approach — analogous to the treat-to-target paradigm in rheumatology and cardiology — drives the stepwise escalation algorithm.

Physical Urticarias and Inducible Urticarias

Classification and Pathophysiology

Inducible urticarias are forms of chronic urticaria triggered by specific physical or environmental stimuli. They account for approximately 15 to 25 percent of chronic urticaria cases and may coexist with chronic spontaneous urticaria. Symptomatic dermographism (the most common inducible urticaria) produces linear wheals at sites of skin stroking or friction within 2 to 5 minutes, persisting for 30 to 60 minutes. Cold urticaria is triggered by cold exposure (cold air, cold water, cold objects) and presents with wheals at sites of cold contact; it carries a risk of systemic anaphylaxis with extensive cold exposure (cold water immersion, swimming), making patient education about water safety essential. Cholinergic urticaria is triggered by a rise in core body temperature (exercise, hot baths, emotional stress) and produces distinctive small (2 to 4 mm), monomorphic wheals surrounded by prominent erythematous flares. Delayed pressure urticaria produces deep, painful, swollen plaques (rather than superficial wheals) 4 to 6 hours after sustained pressure (tight clothing, sitting on hard surfaces, carrying heavy bags), and it responds poorly to antihistamines because the mediators involved are predominantly leukotrienes and prostaglandins rather than histamine. Solar urticaria, aquagenic urticaria, vibratory urticaria, and contact heat urticaria are rarer variants, each defined by their specific trigger.

Diagnostic Provocation Testing

Diagnosis of inducible urticaria requires standardized provocation testing that reproduces the trigger under controlled conditions. Dermographism is confirmed by stroking the skin with a standardized dermographometer (calibrated to a pressure of 36 g/mm2) and observing the wheal response at 10 minutes. Cold urticaria is confirmed by applying an ice cube or TempTest (a standardized Peltier element device that delivers precise temperature stimuli) to the forearm for 5 minutes and observing the wheal response upon rewarming. Cholinergic urticaria is confirmed by exercise provocation testing (typically a treadmill protocol to raise core body temperature by 1 degree Celsius) or by a methacholine skin test. Delayed pressure urticaria is confirmed by applying a weight (approximately 7 kg) over the shoulder or thigh for 15 minutes and assessing for swelling at 6 hours. These provocation tests not only confirm the diagnosis but establish the stimulation threshold, which guides counseling about trigger avoidance and can be repeated to monitor treatment response.

Special Populations: Pediatric, Geriatric, and Pregnancy Considerations

Urticaria in pediatric patients is overwhelmingly acute and infection-triggered: viral upper respiratory tract infections (rhinovirus, adenovirus, enterovirus) account for the majority of episodes, and the condition is self-limited in most children, resolving within days to weeks without specific therapy beyond supportive antihistamines. Chronic urticaria in children is less common than in adults (estimated prevalence 0.1 to 0.3 percent) but follows similar pathophysiologic mechanisms and autoimmune associations. The stepwise treatment algorithm applies with age-appropriate dose adjustments: second-generation antihistamines (cetirizine, loratadine, fexofenadine) are first-line in children and may be updosed following the same fourfold protocol used in adults. Omalizumab is approved for CSU in patients aged 12 years and older and has been used off-label in younger children with refractory disease, with safety data from case series supporting its tolerability in the pediatric population. The evaluation of chronic urticaria in children should include screening for infection-related triggers (including Helicobacter pylori in endemic regions) and parasitic infection where epidemiologically relevant, as these treatable causes are proportionally more common in pediatric CSU than in adult CSU. In elderly patients, the differential diagnosis of urticaria-like eruptions must be broadened to include the pre-bullous phase of bullous pemphigoid, urticarial vasculitis with systemic implications, and drug-induced urticaria from polypharmacy, and the threshold for skin biopsy should be substantially lower than in younger patients.

Urticaria in pregnancy requires careful attention to drug safety and a balanced approach to maternal symptom control and fetal risk minimization. Second-generation antihistamines (cetirizine and loratadine) have the strongest safety data in pregnancy, with extensive post-marketing surveillance and registry data showing no increased risk of major congenital malformations, and are the preferred first-line agents. First-generation antihistamines should be avoided due to sedation, anticholinergic effects, and more limited safety documentation. Omalizumab has accumulated reassuring safety data from pregnancy registries (the EXPECT study enrolled over 250 pregnancies with omalizumab exposure), showing no increased risk of major congenital malformations, preterm birth, or small-for-gestational-age infants, though it remains reserved for refractory disease in which the maternal benefit clearly outweighs the theoretical risk. Systemic corticosteroids should be minimized during pregnancy due to the risks of gestational diabetes, hypertension, premature rupture of membranes, and cleft palate with first-trimester exposure. Cyclosporine is generally avoided in pregnancy. For inducible urticarias during pregnancy, trigger avoidance is the primary strategy, supplemented by pregnancy-safe antihistamines as needed.

Urticarial Vasculitis and Urticaria-Like Conditions

Urticarial Vasculitis

Urticarial vasculitis is a clinicopathologic entity defined by urticarial lesions that, on biopsy, demonstrate leukocytoclastic vasculitis rather than the simple perivascular edema of ordinary urticaria. Clinical features that distinguish urticarial vasculitis from common urticaria include lesions that persist in the same location for more than 24 hours (ordinary urticarial wheals are transient), lesions that are painful or burning rather than purely pruritic, lesions that resolve with residual purpura or hemosiderin staining (ordinary wheals resolve without trace), and systemic symptoms (arthralgias, fever, malaise, abdominal pain, renal involvement). Urticarial vasculitis is classified by complement levels into normocomplementemic (typically milder, limited cutaneous disease) and hypocomplementemic forms. Hypocomplementemic urticarial vasculitis syndrome (HUVS) is a serious systemic disease associated with anti-C1q antibodies, low C3 and C4, angioedema, obstructive lung disease, nephritis, and ocular inflammation, and it overlaps clinically with systemic lupus erythematosus. Biopsy is mandatory when urticarial vasculitis is suspected; histopathology shows neutrophilic infiltration of vessel walls with fibrinoid necrosis, nuclear dust (leukocytoclasia), and erythrocyte extravasation, distinguishing it from the perivascular edema and eosinophilic infiltrate of ordinary urticaria. Management of urticarial vasculitis is directed by severity: mild disease may respond to antihistamines, colchicine, or dapsone, while severe or hypocomplementemic disease requires systemic immunosuppression (corticosteroids, mycophenolate mofetil, rituximab).

Differential Diagnosis of Urticaria-Like Eruptions

Several conditions produce urticaria-like eruptions that require differentiation from true urticaria. Urticarial drug eruptions (particularly from ACE inhibitors, which cause bradykinin-mediated angioedema without wheals) must be distinguished from allergic urticaria because the management differs (drug withdrawal rather than antihistamines). The pre-bullous phase of bullous pemphigoid may present as urticarial plaques (intensely pruritic, edematous, erythematous plaques) before bullae develop, and this urticated pemphigoid phase can persist for weeks or months, leading to misdiagnosis as chronic urticaria — direct immunofluorescence of a perilesional biopsy showing linear C3 and IgG deposition at the basement membrane zone resolves the diagnosis. Sweet syndrome (acute febrile neutrophilic dermatosis) produces tender, edematous, erythematous plaques that may resemble urticaria but are accompanied by fever, neutrophilia, and a dense dermal neutrophilic infiltrate on biopsy without vasculitis. Schnitzler syndrome is a rare autoinflammatory disorder defined by chronic urticaria and monoclonal IgM (or occasionally IgG) gammopathy, accompanied by intermittent fever, arthralgias, bone pain, lymphadenopathy, and markedly elevated inflammatory markers; it requires treatment with IL-1 receptor antagonist (anakinra) rather than antihistamines. Recognizing these urticaria mimickers prevents diagnostic delay and inappropriate long-term antihistamine therapy for conditions that require fundamentally different treatment.

THE CUTANEOUS MIMICKER RECOGNITION ATLAS — Chronic Spontaneous Urticaria versus Urticarial Bullous Pemphigoid

The Clinical Pattern: Chronic spontaneous urticaria presents as recurrent transient wheals (individual lesions lasting less than 24 hours, migratory, leaving no residual mark) with intense pruritus, occurring most days for 6 weeks or more, in the absence of an identifiable external trigger. The wheals are superficial, well-circumscribed, erythematous, and edematous, and the surrounding skin is normal between episodes.

The Mimicker: The pre-bullous (urticarial) phase of bullous pemphigoid presents as intensely pruritic, erythematous, edematous plaques that closely resemble urticarial wheals. However, unlike true urticaria, these plaques persist in the same location for days, are often accompanied by eczematous or excoriated features, and may show peripheral eosinophilia on CBC. The urticarial phase may precede the development of tense bullae by weeks to months, and in some elderly patients, bullae never develop (non-bullous pemphigoid), making the diagnosis particularly elusive.

Trap Logic: Anchoring bias is the cognitive trap. The clinician anchors on the initial pattern (pruritic erythematous plaques = urticaria), initiates antihistamine therapy, and does not reassess the diagnosis when the patient returns with persistent, fixed lesions and incomplete response to treatment. In elderly patients, the anchoring is reinforced by the assumption that new-onset urticaria in an older adult is unremarkable, when in fact new-onset urticaria-like eruptions in patients over 60 should specifically prompt consideration of bullous pemphigoid.

The Decision Anchor: The discriminating features are **lesion persistence beyond 24 hours at the same site, peripheral eosinophilia, and direct immunofluorescence showing linear IgG and C3 at the basement membrane zone**. Ordinary urticarial wheals are evanescent (less than 24 hours per individual wheal); pemphigoid plaques are persistent. The definitive test is a perilesional skin biopsy for direct immunofluorescence and serum anti-BP180/BP230 antibodies (ELISA). In any patient over 60 with urticaria-like eruptions that do not resolve with standard antihistamine therapy, obtain DIF biopsy before escalating urticaria-directed treatment.

Illustrative Clinical Scenario: Persistent Urticaria-Like Eruption in an Elderly Patient

A 74-year-old woman presents with a 3-month history of intensely pruritic, erythematous, edematous plaques on the trunk and proximal extremities. She has been treated with cetirizine 10 mg daily by her primary care physician with minimal improvement, and a subsequent trial of hydroxyzine 25 mg at bedtime provided only marginal additional relief. She reports that the lesions seem to persist in the same locations for several days before slowly fading, and new lesions continue to appear at adjacent sites. She has no history of atopy, denies any new medications within the preceding 6 months, and reports no recent infections or known allergen exposures. Physical examination reveals widespread erythematous, edematous, urticaria-like plaques on the trunk, proximal upper and lower extremities, and inner thighs, some with overlying excoriations from scratching. No frank bullae or vesicles are visible. A complete blood count reveals a peripheral eosinophil count of 1.8 × 10^9/L (markedly elevated above the normal range of 0.1 to 0.5 × 10^9/L), and the erythrocyte sedimentation rate is 38 mm/hour. The initial clinical impression is chronic spontaneous urticaria, and the treatment plan is to updose cetirizine to 20 mg twice daily per the stepwise algorithm. However, the combination of several atypical features — older age at onset (new-onset CSU after age 60 is uncommon and warrants broadened differential diagnosis), lesion persistence beyond 24 hours at the same anatomical site (true urticarial wheals resolve within 24 hours and migrate), incomplete response to H1-antihistamine therapy, and marked peripheral eosinophilia — triggers diagnostic reassessment. A 4 mm punch biopsy of lesional skin shows a superficial perivascular and interstitial eosinophilic infiltrate with focal vacuolar interface change at the dermoepidermal junction. A perilesional biopsy submitted for direct immunofluorescence reveals linear IgG and C3 deposition along the basement membrane zone, the hallmark immunopathologic finding of bullous pemphigoid. Serum anti-BP180 (NC16A domain) antibodies are strongly positive by ELISA. The diagnosis is revised to pre-bullous (urticarial) bullous pemphigoid, a well-recognized clinical phenotype in which the urticarial phase precedes the development of tense bullae by weeks to months — or in some elderly patients, frank bullae never develop (non-bullous pemphigoid). Management is transitioned from antihistamines to superpotent topical corticosteroid (clobetasol propionate 0.05% cream applied to active lesions twice daily) and oral doxycycline as a steroid-sparing agent, with resolution of the eruption over 8 weeks and normalization of eosinophil count. This scenario illustrates the diagnostic importance of reassessing the urticaria diagnosis when the clinical pattern deviates from expectation: fixed-site persistence, antihistamine refractoriness, late age at onset, and peripheral eosinophilia are the four anchors that should prompt DIF biopsy before escalating urticaria-directed therapy.

Erythema Multiforme, Erythema Nodosum, and Reactive Erythemas

Erythema Multiforme

Erythema multiforme (EM) is an acute, self-limited, immune-mediated reaction pattern that produces targetoid (target-shaped) lesions with a characteristic three-zone morphology: a central dusky or vesicular zone, an inner pale edematous ring, and an outer erythematous ring. The distribution favors the acral sites (dorsal hands, palms, soles, elbows, knees) and face, and mucosal involvement (oral, genital, ocular) occurs in the more severe form (EM major). The most common trigger is herpes simplex virus (HSV) infection, which accounts for the majority of recurrent EM cases: HSV DNA has been detected in EM lesional skin by polymerase chain reaction, and the immune response is directed against HSV antigens expressed in keratinocytes. Mycoplasma pneumoniae is the second most common infectious trigger, particularly in children and adolescents, and is more likely to cause mucosal-predominant disease. EM is now understood as pathogenetically distinct from Stevens-Johnson syndrome (SJS) and toxic epidermal necrolysis (TEN): EM is infection-driven (predominantly HSV and Mycoplasma), acral-predominant, self-limited, and recurrent, while SJS/TEN is drug-driven, trunk-predominant, potentially life-threatening, and does not recur unless re-exposed to the causative drug. This distinction has direct clinical implications: recurrent EM is managed with antiviral prophylaxis (suppressive acyclovir or valacyclovir), whereas SJS/TEN management centers on immediate withdrawal of the causative drug.

Erythema Nodosum and Panniculitis

Erythema nodosum (EN) is the most common clinicopathologic pattern of panniculitis (inflammation of subcutaneous fat). It presents as bilateral, tender, warm, erythematous nodules on the anterior shins, typically in women aged 20 to 40 years. The nodules resolve over 3 to 6 weeks without ulceration, scarring, or atrophy, evolving through bruise-like color changes (erythematous to violaceous to yellow-green, a sequence termed erythema contusiformis). Histopathology shows a septal panniculitis with Miescher radial granulomas (small, well-defined histiocytic aggregates arranged radially around a central cleft within the septa), without vasculitis. EN is a reactive condition with a broad differential of underlying causes: infections (streptococcal pharyngitis is the most common trigger, followed by tuberculosis, coccidioidomycosis, histoplasmosis, and Yersinia enterocolitica), medications (oral contraceptives, sulfonamides), sarcoidosis (EN is part of Lofgren syndrome: bilateral hilar lymphadenopathy, EN, fever, and polyarthralgia), inflammatory bowel disease (EN correlates with intestinal disease activity in Crohn disease more reliably than in ulcerative colitis), and pregnancy. The diagnostic workup includes throat culture or anti-streptolysin O titer, chest radiograph (screening for sarcoidosis and tuberculosis), complete blood count, and ESR/CRP. Treatment is symptomatic (rest, leg elevation, NSAIDs, potassium iodide) and directed at the underlying cause.

Other Reactive Erythemas

Several additional reactive erythemas are encountered in clinical dermatology. Erythema annulare centrifugum (EAC) presents as annular or arciform erythematous plaques with a trailing scale at the inner edge of the advancing border (the pathognomonic trailing scale), expanding centrifugally over weeks. It is usually idiopathic but may be associated with infections (dermatophytosis, Candida), malignancy, or medications. Erythema gyratum repens, a rare paraneoplastic dermatosis, produces rapidly advancing (approximately 1 cm per day), concentric, wood-grain-patterned erythematous bands with fine trailing scale, most commonly associated with underlying bronchogenic carcinoma. Erythema marginatum is the characteristic cutaneous manifestation of acute rheumatic fever, presenting as transient, migratory, non-pruritic, erythematous rings and arcs on the trunk and proximal extremities that wax and wane over hours and are included among the Jones criteria for rheumatic fever diagnosis. Erythema chronicum migrans is the expanding erythematous annular plaque at the site of an Ixodes tick bite that signals early Lyme disease (Borrelia burgdorferi infection), and its recognition is one of the most consequential clinical diagnoses in dermatology because it allows treatment with antibiotics (doxycycline, amoxicillin) before the disseminated complications of Lyme disease develop.

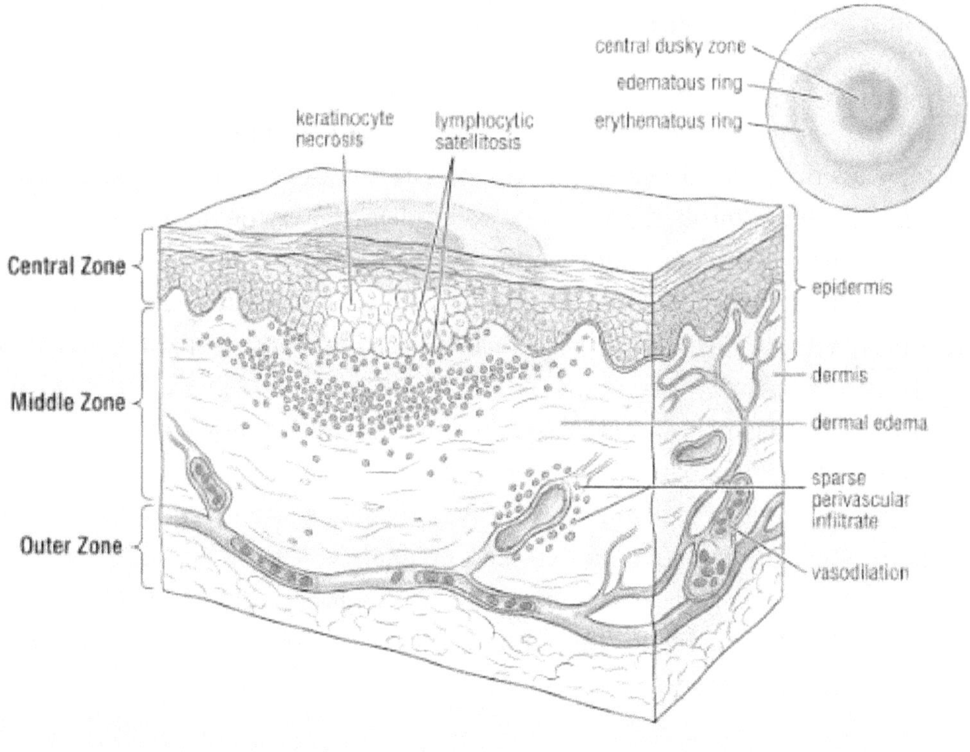

Evidence-Based Management of Urticaria

Stepwise Pharmacotherapy

The current international guidelines (EAACI/GA2LEN/EuroGuiDerm/APAAACI) recommend a stepwise approach to chronic urticaria management. Step 1 is a standard-dose second-generation H1-antihistamine (cetirizine, loratadine, fexofenadine, desloratadine, levocetirizine, bilastine, rupatadine). If symptoms persist after 2 to 4 weeks, Step 2 is updosing the same second-generation antihistamine up to four times the standard dose — a critical step that many clinicians skip prematurely, moving to add-on therapy before maximizing antihistamine dosing. If symptoms persist at fourfold dosing for 2 to 4 weeks, Step 3 is the addition of omalizumab (anti-IgE monoclonal antibody) to the updosed antihistamine. Omalizumab has demonstrated consistent efficacy in randomized controlled trials, with approximately 70 to 80 percent of patients achieving meaningful improvement (UAS7 reduction of 50 percent or greater) and 30 to 40 percent achieving complete urticaria control. It works by binding free IgE, reducing FcepsilonRI expression on mast cells and basophils, and in autoimmune CSU, potentially disrupting autoantibody-mediated mast cell activation. Step 4, reserved for omalizumab-refractory cases, is cyclosporine added to the antihistamine, though its use is limited by nephrotoxicity, hypertension, and the requirement for laboratory monitoring.

Emerging Therapies and Antihistamine Principles

Several emerging therapies target novel pathways in chronic urticaria. Anti-IgE agents with enhanced potency (ligelizumab), Bruton tyrosine kinase (BTK) inhibitors (remibrutinib, which blocks the FcepsilonRI signaling cascade upstream of mast cell degranulation), and anti-TSLP/anti-IL-4R agents are in advanced clinical development and may expand the therapeutic armamentarium for antihistamine- and omalizumab-refractory disease. First-generation (sedating) antihistamines (diphenhydramine, hydroxyzine, chlorpheniramine) should not be used as first-line therapy for chronic urticaria: their anticholinergic side effects, sedation, psychomotor impairment, and short half-lives make them inferior to second-generation agents, and their sedative properties do not add clinical benefit for urticaria management beyond what second-generation agents provide. Systemic corticosteroids may be used for short rescue courses (3 to 7 days) in acute flares of chronic urticaria or severe acute urticaria with angioedema but must never be used as maintenance therapy due to the cumulative toxicity of chronic corticosteroid exposure. Leukotriene receptor antagonists (montelukast) may provide modest additional benefit as add-on therapy in patients with concomitant NSAID-exacerbated urticaria or aspirin-sensitive urticaria but are not recommended as monotherapy and are not part of the current stepwise algorithm.

CAUTION: Updosing second-generation antihistamines to four times the standard dose (Step 2 of the international guideline algorithm) is safe, evidence-based, and achieves additional urticaria control in approximately 60 to 75 percent of patients who fail standard dosing. This step should not be skipped. Moving directly from standard-dose antihistamines to omalizumab or cyclosporine without trialing updosed antihistamines denies the patient a well-tolerated, effective intervention and adds unnecessary cost and complexity.

EVIDENCE: The ASTERIA I, ASTERIA II, and GLACIAL randomized controlled trials established the efficacy and safety of omalizumab 300 mg subcutaneously every 4 weeks in chronic spontaneous urticaria refractory to H1-antihistamines at both standard and updosed levels. Approximately 35 to 44 percent of patients achieved complete response (UAS7 of 0) at 12 weeks, with onset of benefit typically at 4 to 8 weeks. Relapse after discontinuation was common, with symptoms returning in the majority of patients within 8 to 10 weeks of stopping, supporting ongoing treatment for the duration of active disease followed by reassessment attempts at intervals of 6 to 12 months.

Treatment Step	Intervention	Duration Before Escalation	Expected Response Rate
Step 1	Second-generation H1-antihistamine (standard dose)	2-4 weeks	Approximately 50%
Step 2	Updose same antihistamine to 4x standard dose	2-4 weeks	Additional 60-75% of Step 1 non-responders
Step 3	Add omalizumab (anti-IgE) to updosed antihistamine	6 months (assess response at 3-6 months)	70-80% meaningful improvement
Step 4	Add cyclosporine to antihistamine (omalizumab-refractory)	Variable, limited by toxicity	60-70% improvement, limited by side effects

Angioedema: Classification and Emergency Management

Angioedema accompanies urticaria in approximately 40 percent of cases (histaminergic angioedema) and may also occur in isolation without wheals. The critical clinical distinction is between histamine-mediated angioedema (which accompanies urticaria, responds to antihistamines and epinephrine, and involves mast cell degranulation) and bradykinin-mediated angioedema (which does NOT accompany urticaria, does NOT respond to antihistamines or epinephrine, and involves the kallikrein-kinin system). Bradykinin-mediated angioedema includes hereditary angioedema (HAE, caused by C1-inhibitor deficiency or dysfunction — types I and II — or by gain-of-function mutations in factor XII, plasminogen, angiopoietin-1, kininogen-1, or myoferlin in HAE with normal C1-inhibitor) and ACE inhibitor-induced angioedema (caused by reduced bradykinin degradation due to pharmacologic inhibition of angiotensin-converting enzyme, which also degrades bradykinin). The distinction is clinically urgent because bradykinin-mediated angioedema involving the upper airway is a life-threatening emergency that does not respond to the standard anaphylaxis protocol (epinephrine, antihistamines, corticosteroids). HAE acute attacks are treated with on-demand therapies: C1-inhibitor concentrate (plasma-derived or recombinant), icatibant (bradykinin B2 receptor antagonist), or ecallantide (kallikrein inhibitor). Long-term prophylaxis for HAE includes subcutaneous C1-inhibitor replacement, lanadelumab (anti-kallikrein monoclonal antibody), and berotralstat (oral kallikrein inhibitor). ACE inhibitor-induced angioedema is managed by permanent drug discontinuation; angiotensin receptor blockers may be substituted, as true cross-reactivity is rare (estimated at less than 2 percent). Any patient presenting with angioedema without urticaria — particularly with a family history of angioedema, recurrent episodes without an allergic trigger, or onset after starting an ACE inhibitor — requires evaluation for bradykinin-mediated angioedema with serum C4 (low in HAE types I and II even between attacks, serving as an effective screening test), C1-inhibitor antigenic level, and C1-inhibitor functional activity.

Patient Education and Long-Term Self-Management

Patient education is integral to chronic urticaria management and directly improves treatment adherence and outcomes. Patients should understand that CSU is not an allergy (extensive allergen testing and elimination diets are not indicated in the absence of a clear clinical history of allergen-triggered symptoms), that the condition is autoimmune in a substantial proportion of cases, and that spontaneous remission is the expected long-term outcome for most patients — typically within 2 to 5 years — though the timeline cannot be predicted for any individual. Counseling should address the importance of adherence to daily (not as-needed) antihistamine therapy, the safety and evidence-based rationale for updosing to four times the standard dose (a concept that many patients and some clinicians find counterintuitive), and the mechanism of action and expected response timeline for omalizumab (onset of benefit typically within 4 to 12 weeks, with full effect assessed at 6 months). For inducible urticarias, trigger-specific education is essential: patients with cold urticaria must be counseled about the risk of systemic anaphylaxis with cold water immersion (swimming in cold water, jumping into lakes or pools), and aquatic activities should be accompanied by a companion who is aware of the risk, with injectable epinephrine available on scene. Patients with delayed pressure urticaria benefit from practical modifications such as padded seats, cushioned bag straps, and avoidance of prolonged standing or sitting on hard surfaces. Written action plans that outline the stepwise escalation protocol, indications for emergency evaluation (airway angioedema, anaphylaxis symptoms including respiratory distress, hypotension, and loss of consciousness), and expected disease trajectory improve patient engagement, reduce anxiety, and decrease unnecessary emergency department visits for manageable flares.

THE CUTANEOUS MIMICKER RECOGNITION ATLAS — Erythema Multiforme versus Stevens-Johnson Syndrome

---

The Clinical Pattern: Erythema multiforme presents as acute-onset, well-defined target lesions (three-zone morphology: central dusky or vesicular zone, edematous pale ring, outer erythematous ring) distributed predominantly on the acral surfaces (dorsal hands, palms, soles, elbows, knees). It is typically triggered by herpes simplex virus or Mycoplasma pneumoniae infection, is self-limited, and recurs in association with HSV reactivation.

The Mimicker: Stevens-Johnson syndrome (SJS) produces dusky erythematous macules, atypical flat target lesions (two-zone, without a raised palpable border), and epidermal detachment affecting less than 10 percent of body surface area (or 10 to 30 percent for SJS/TEN overlap, or greater than 30 percent for TEN). Distribution is trunk-predominant. Mucosal involvement (oral, ocular, genital) is typically more severe than in EM major. The trigger is almost always a medication (sulfonamides, allopurinol, aromatic anticonvulsants, NSAIDs, antibiotics), and the condition is not recurrent unless re-exposed to the causative drug.

Trap Logic: Conflation of EM and SJS as a single spectrum is the cognitive trap. Historically, EM, SJS, and TEN were taught as points on a severity continuum (EM minor → EM major → SJS → TEN). This outdated model leads clinicians to assume that severe EM will progress to SJS, or that SJS is simply EM with mucosal involvement. In reality, EM and SJS are pathogenetically distinct entities (infection-driven vs. drug-driven) with different prognoses, treatment strategies, and recurrence patterns. Conflating them delays drug withdrawal in SJS (because the clinician is managing EM) or leads to unnecessary drug withdrawal in EM (because the clinician fears SJS progression).

The Decision Anchor: The discriminating features are **lesion morphology (raised three-zone targets in EM vs. flat two-zone atypical targets or purpuric macules in SJS), distribution (acral in EM vs. truncal in SJS), and trigger (infection, especially HSV, in EM vs. drug in SJS)**. Recurrence with HSV reactivation clinches EM. Onset 1 to 3 weeks after starting a new medication clinches SJS. When in doubt, biopsy shows satellite cell necrosis of keratinocytes in both, but the clinical context — acral targets after a cold sore (EM) versus truncal dusky macules after starting allopurinol (SJS) — provides the distinction.

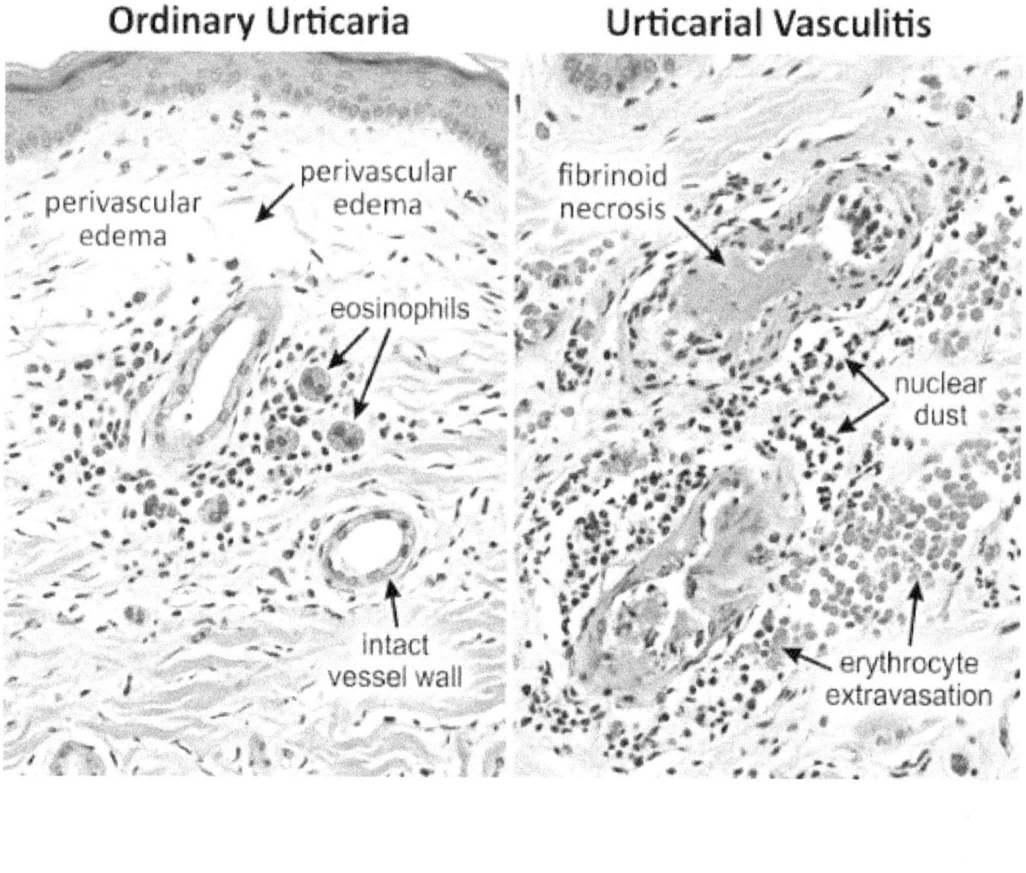

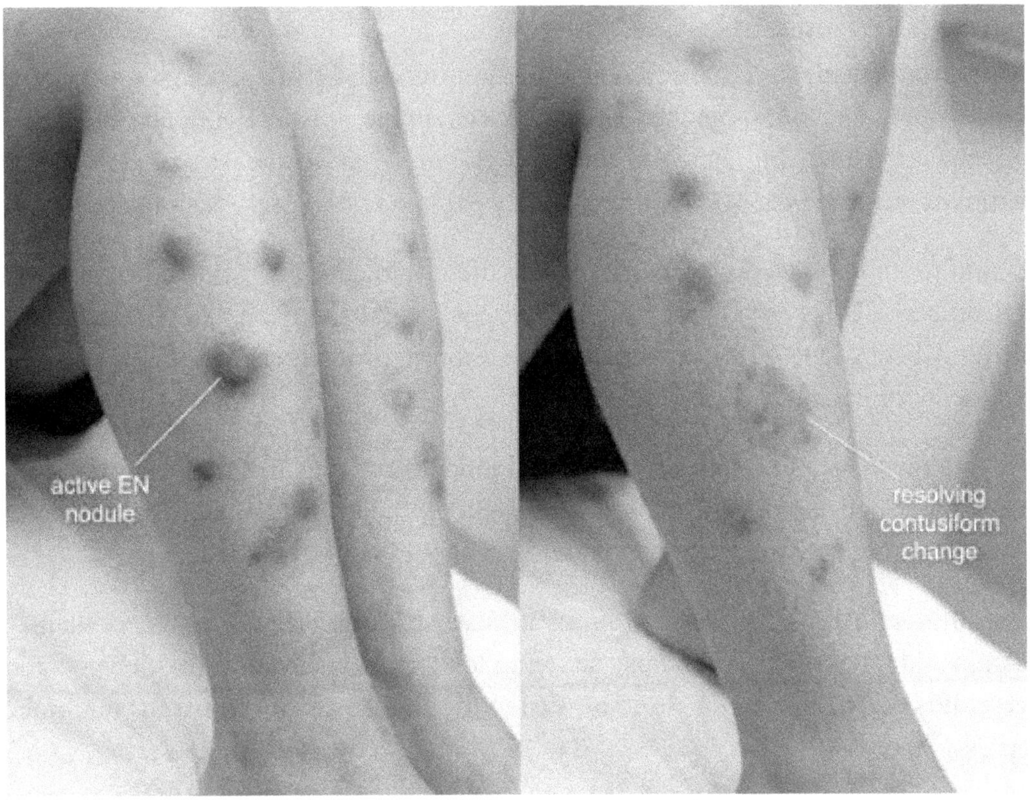

THE CUTANEOUS MIMICKER RECOGNITION ATLAS — Urticarial and Erythematous Diagnostic Arcs

Chronic Spontaneous Urticaria vs. Urticarial Bullous Pemphigoid: The discriminating features are lesion persistence beyond 24 hours at the same site, peripheral eosinophilia, and direct immunofluorescence showing linear IgG and C3 at the basement membrane zone. Urticarial wheals are evanescent; pemphigoid plaques are persistent. Biopsy with DIF is mandatory in any patient over 60 with urticaria-like eruptions refractory to antihistamines. Cognitive trap: anchoring bias on the urticaria diagnosis in elderly patients.

Erythema Multiforme vs. Stevens-Johnson Syndrome: The discriminating features are lesion morphology (raised three-zone targets in EM vs. flat two-zone atypical targets in SJS), distribution (acral vs. truncal), and trigger (infection/HSV in EM vs. drug in SJS). EM and SJS are pathogenetically distinct entities, not points on a severity spectrum. Recurrence with HSV reactivation clinches EM; onset after a new medication clinches SJS. Cognitive trap: conflation of EM and SJS as a single spectrum.

Summary and Key Concepts

Urticaria results from cutaneous mast cell degranulation through IgE-dependent, complement-mediated, MRGPRX2-mediated, and autoimmune pathways. Histamine is the dominant mediator (producing wheals, erythema, pruritus), but lipid mediators, cytokines, and proteases sustain the inflammatory response. Serum tryptase and the MRGPRX2 pathway explain non-allergic pseudoallergic drug reactions.

Chronic urticaria (duration 6 weeks or longer) is classified into chronic spontaneous urticaria (CSU) and inducible urticarias. CSU has two autoimmune subtypes: type I (anti-self IgE, omalizumab-responsive) and type IIb (anti-FcepsilonRI IgG, omalizumab-resistant). Biomarkers (total IgE, ASST, BHRA, D-dimer) guide phenotyping and treatment selection.

Stepwise urticaria management follows international guidelines: Step 1 standard-dose second-generation antihistamine, Step 2 updose to four times standard, Step 3 add omalizumab, Step 4 add cyclosporine. Updosing (Step 2) is a critical evidence-based step that should not be skipped.

Urticarial vasculitis is distinguished from ordinary urticaria by lesions persisting more than 24 hours, pain rather than itch, residual purpura, and biopsy showing leukocytoclastic vasculitis. Hypocomplementemic urticarial vasculitis syndrome is a serious systemic disease with anti-C1q antibodies requiring immunosuppression.

Erythema multiforme and Stevens-Johnson syndrome are pathogenetically distinct: EM is infection-driven (HSV, Mycoplasma), acral, self-limited, and recurrent; SJS is drug-driven (sulfonamides, allopurinol, anticonvulsants), truncal, potentially life-threatening, and not recurrent unless re-exposed. Erythema nodosum is a septal panniculitis most commonly triggered by streptococcal infection and sarcoidosis.

CHAPTER 6: LICHENOID AND INTERFACE DERMATOSES

Learning Objectives

1. Describe the immunopathogenesis of lichen planus, including the role of CD8+ cytotoxic T cell-mediated attack on basal keratinocytes and the mechanisms of apoptosis at the dermoepidermal junction.
2. Recognize the clinical variants of lichen planus — classic cutaneous, oral, hypertrophic, follicular, and nail — and their distinctive presentations across Fitzpatrick skin types.
3. Distinguish lichenoid drug eruptions from idiopathic lichen planus using clinical, temporal, and histopathologic features, and identify the most common causative agents.
4. Explain the histopathologic hallmarks of interface dermatitis and classify the major interface patterns (vacuolar versus lichenoid) with their clinical disease correlates.
5. Apply evidence-based management strategies for lichenoid dermatoses, including topical, systemic, and procedural approaches for cutaneous and mucosal disease, and understand the risk of malignant transformation in oral lichen planus.

Lichen Planus: Pathogenesis, Clinical Variants, and Oral Disease

Immunopathogenesis and the CD8+ T Cell Attack on Basal Keratinocytes

Lichen planus (LP) is a chronic, immune-mediated inflammatory dermatosis driven by CD8+ cytotoxic T lymphocytes that target basal keratinocytes at the dermoepidermal junction. The pathogenetic cascade begins with the aberrant expression or unmasking of autoantigens on basal keratinocytes — the precise antigen remains unidentified, but candidates include modified self-peptides presented by MHC class I molecules on the keratinocyte surface. Langerhans cells and plasmacytoid dendritic cells process and present these antigens to CD8+ T cells, which infiltrate the basal layer and release perforin and granzyme B, inducing keratinocyte apoptosis through the Fas-FasL pathway and the perforin-granzyme pathway. The apoptotic keratinocytes become Civatte bodies (colloid bodies) — eosinophilic, round, hyaline structures that are the histopathologic hallmark of interface dermatitis in LP. Simultaneously, CXCL9, CXCL10, and CXCL11 recruit additional CXCR3+ T cells to the site, creating a self-amplifying inflammatory loop. The basal layer damage disrupts melanocyte function and releases melanin into the upper dermis, where it is phagocytosed by melanophages — this dermal melanin incontinence is responsible for the violaceous color of LP lesions and for the post-inflammatory hyperpigmentation that persists after the inflammation resolves, a feature particularly prominent in individuals with Fitzpatrick IV–VI skin. TNF-alpha and IFN-gamma produced by the infiltrating T cells upregulate adhesion molecules and perpetuate the inflammatory cascade.

Hepatitis C Association and Screening

Hepatitis C virus (HCV) infection has a well-established epidemiologic and pathogenetic association with lichen planus, particularly oral lichen planus. Meta-analyses demonstrate that HCV infection is significantly more prevalent in LP patients than in the general population (odds ratio approximately 4 to 5), and the geographic distribution of the association is strongest in Mediterranean and East Asian populations. The proposed mechanism involves HCV replication within hepatocytes and lymphocytes, which triggers a cross-reactive cytotoxic T cell response against HCV epitopes expressed on or cross-presented by keratinocytes — the same CD8+ T cell-mediated interface attack that characterizes idiopathic LP. Successful antiviral treatment of HCV (with direct-acting antiviral agents) has been shown to improve or resolve LP in some patients, providing further evidence for a causal relationship. Current guidelines recommend screening for HCV infection (serum anti-HCV antibody followed by HCV RNA confirmation if positive) in all patients presenting with new-onset lichen planus, particularly those with oral LP, oral plus cutaneous LP, or erosive LP. Additionally, liver function tests should be obtained at baseline, both for HCV screening and because systemic therapies used in LP management (methotrexate, acitretin) require hepatic monitoring.

Classic Cutaneous Lichen Planus: The Five Ps and Morphologic Features

Classic cutaneous LP is characterized by the five Ps: pruritic, polygonal, planar (flat-topped), purple (violaceous) papules and plaques. The distribution favors the flexural surfaces of the wrists, forearms, lower legs (particularly the ankles), and the sacral region. Individual papules are typically 2 to 10 mm, well-demarcated, and flat-topped, with a characteristic violaceous to lilac hue in lighter skin (Fitzpatrick I–III) or a hyperpigmented, dark brown to slate-gray color in darker skin (Fitzpatrick IV–VI). The surface of LP papules displays Wickham striae — fine, white, reticular (lace-like) lines visible to the naked eye or with dermoscopy — which represent areas of irregular hypergranulosis (thickened granular layer) overlying the wedge-shaped dermal inflammatory infiltrate. Wickham striae are a critical diagnostic feature: their presence on dermoscopy distinguishes LP from other violaceous papular eruptions and is particularly useful in pigmented skin where the violaceous color is obscured. The Koebner phenomenon (isomorphic response) is common in LP: new lesions develop at sites of trauma, scratching, or surgical scars, and its presence helps confirm the diagnosis. LP may present in a generalized distribution (widespread papules on the trunk and extremities) or in a localized pattern (limited to one or two anatomic sites). Generalized LP tends to be more symptomatic, with intense pruritus that significantly impairs quality of life.

Clinical Variants: Hypertrophic, Atrophic, Vesiculobullous, and Annular

Several morphologic variants of cutaneous LP are recognized, each with distinct clinical behavior. Hypertrophic LP (lichen planus verrucosus) presents as thick, hyperkeratotic, verrucous plaques on the anterior shins and ankles — the most pruritic variant and the most resistant to treatment, often persisting for years and carrying a small but real risk of squamous cell carcinoma arising within long-standing lesions (particularly on the lower extremities). Atrophic LP produces thinned, atrophic plaques with a violaceous hue, typically on the lower legs, and may represent resolved hypertrophic LP or primary atrophic disease. Vesiculobullous LP develops when the intensity of basal cell damage at the dermoepidermal junction produces subepidermal clefting (Max-Joseph spaces) sufficient to form vesicles or bullae, most commonly on the lower extremities and feet; it must be distinguished from bullous pemphigoid arising in LP (LP-BP overlap), which shows linear immunoglobulin and complement deposition at the basement membrane zone on direct immunofluorescence. Annular LP presents as ring-shaped plaques with raised, violaceous borders and a central clearing or hyperpigmentation, most commonly on the glans penis (where it may be the sole manifestation of LP) and the trunk. Actinic LP (LP subtropicus) is a photodistributed variant occurring on sun-exposed sites (face, dorsal forearms, V of neck) in individuals from the Middle East, South Asia, North Africa, and East Africa, and may mimic discoid lupus erythematosus in distribution and morphology.

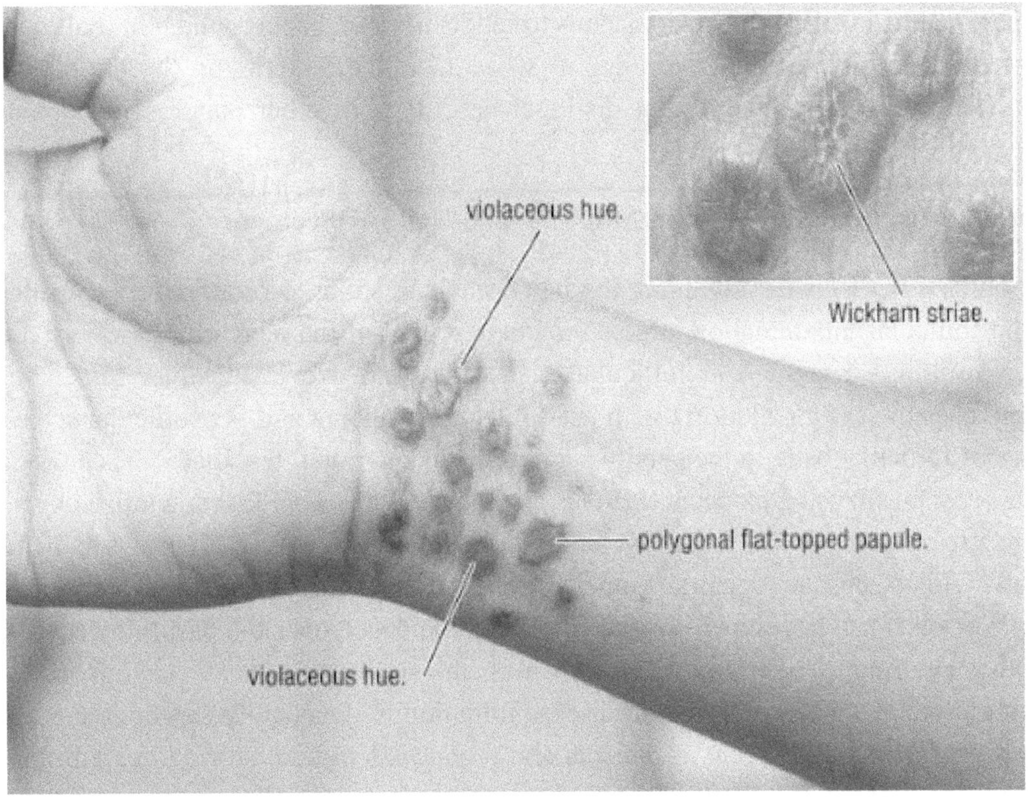

Oral Lichen Planus: Reticular, Erosive, and Atrophic Forms

Oral lichen planus (OLP) affects approximately 50 to 70 percent of patients with cutaneous LP and may be the sole manifestation of disease in up to 25 percent of cases. OLP occurs most commonly on the buccal mucosa (bilaterally), tongue, and gingiva, and presents in three principal clinical forms. Reticular OLP (the most common form) produces asymptomatic, bilateral, white, lace-like Wickham striae on the buccal mucosa — the classic presentation is pathognomonic and often incidentally discovered during dental examination. Erosive (ulcerative) OLP produces painful, well-demarcated erosions and ulcerations with a fibrinous base, surrounded by a peripheral rim of white striae, most commonly on the buccal mucosa, tongue, and gingiva. Erosive OLP causes significant morbidity: burning pain exacerbated by spicy, acidic, or hot foods impairs nutrition and quality of life, and chronic erosive OLP carries a malignant transformation risk estimated at 0.5 to 2 percent over 5 to 10 years, mandating clinical surveillance and biopsy of any area that develops induration, verrucous change, or a non-healing ulcer. Atrophic (erythematous) OLP presents as areas of mucosal thinning and erythema, often on the attached gingiva (desquamative gingivitis), and may be mistaken for chronic gingivitis. Desquamative gingivitis is not specific to OLP — it also occurs in mucous membrane pemphigoid and pemphigus vulgaris — and requires biopsy with direct immunofluorescence for definitive differential diagnosis. Genital lichen planus (vulvar and penile LP) produces painful erosions, scarring, and architectural distortion that can cause urinary and sexual dysfunction, and requires multidisciplinary management.

CLINICAL PEARL: Wickham striae — the fine, white, reticular lines on the surface of lichen planus papules — are best visualized with dermoscopy, which reveals white crossing lines (corresponding to areas of hypergranulosis) overlying a violaceous to reddish-brown background. On oral mucosal lesions, Wickham striae are visible to the naked eye as white lace-like patterns on the buccal mucosa. Their presence is a key diagnostic feature that distinguishes LP from other papulosquamous and interface dermatoses.

Lichen Planopilaris, Frontal Fibrosing Alopecia, and Nail Involvement

Lichen planopilaris (LPP) is LP involving the hair follicle, leading to progressive, scarring (cicatricial) alopecia. The follicular inflammation targets the bulge region of the hair follicle, where follicular stem cells reside, resulting in permanent follicular destruction and irreversible hair loss. Clinically, LPP presents as patches of scarring alopecia with perifollicular erythema and perifollicular scale at the active margins, loss of follicular ostia in the central scarred zone, and a pull test that yields anagen hairs at the active border. Frontal fibrosing alopecia (FFA) is a clinical variant of LPP characterized by a progressive, symmetric recession of the frontal and temporal hairline, often with loss of eyebrows and body hair. FFA predominantly affects postmenopausal women (though cases in men and premenopausal women are increasingly reported) and has shown a markedly rising incidence over the past two decades, raising the hypothesis that environmental triggers (sunscreen chemical filters such as benzophenone-3, leave-on facial skincare products) may contribute to disease initiation in genetically susceptible individuals. Nail LP affects approximately 10 percent of patients and produces longitudinal ridging, nail thinning, dorsal pterygium (adhesion of the proximal nail fold to the nail bed, which is pathognomonic for LP), twenty-nail dystrophy (trachyonychia), and in severe cases, permanent nail loss. Early treatment is essential because nail matrix scarring is irreversible.

Lichenoid Drug Eruptions and Lichenoid Keratoses

Pathogenesis and Causative Agents

Lichenoid drug eruptions (LDE) are drug-induced inflammatory reactions that mimic lichen planus both clinically and histopathologically. The pathogenesis involves drug-specific T cell activation: the offending drug or its metabolite acts as a hapten, binding to keratinocyte proteins and altering their antigenicity, which triggers a CD8+ T cell-mediated cytotoxic response against the modified basal keratinocytes — the same effector mechanism as idiopathic LP. The latency period between drug initiation and eruption onset is typically weeks to months (commonly 2 to 12 months), reflecting the time required for sensitization, and this prolonged latency often makes the causal association difficult to recognize. The most commonly implicated drug classes include antihypertensives (ACE inhibitors, thiazide diuretics, beta-blockers, calcium channel blockers), antimalarials (hydroxychloroquine, chloroquine — important because these drugs are also used to treat discoid lupus, which is in the differential diagnosis of LDE), gold compounds, penicillamine, NSAIDs, proton pump inhibitors, TNF-alpha inhibitors, and checkpoint inhibitor immunotherapy drugs (pembrolizumab, nivolumab, ipilimumab — a growing cause of LDE as immunotherapy use expands). Hepatitis C virus infection is a well-established trigger of lichen planus and should be screened for in all patients presenting with new-onset LP, particularly those with oral LP or oral plus cutaneous disease.

Clinical and Histopathologic Distinction From Idiopathic Lichen Planus

Several clinical features help distinguish LDE from idiopathic LP, though considerable overlap exists. LDE lesions tend to be larger, more psoriasiform (with greater scale), and more widely distributed than idiopathic LP. LDE more commonly involves the trunk and may be photodistributed (favoring sun-exposed sites), whereas idiopathic LP favors flexural wrists, ankles, and oral mucosa. LDE less commonly displays Wickham striae than idiopathic LP. Oral involvement is less common in LDE, though it occurs. Resolution after drug withdrawal (which may take weeks to months given the prolonged immunologic memory) supports the diagnosis of LDE, whereas idiopathic LP follows an independent clinical course. Histopathologically, LDE shares the interface dermatitis pattern with idiopathic LP (band-like lymphocytic infiltrate obscuring the dermoepidermal junction, Civatte bodies, pigment incontinence) but is more likely to show eosinophils within the infiltrate, focal parakeratosis (rather than the wedge-shaped hypergranulosis of LP), perivascular extension of the inflammatory infiltrate deeper into the dermis, and cytoid bodies at all levels of the epidermis rather than confined to the basal layer. None of these histopathologic features is individually diagnostic, but the overall pattern — eosinophils + deeper perivascular inflammation + parakeratosis in a lichenoid interface reaction — should raise suspicion for a drug-related etiology and prompt a thorough medication history.

KEY POINT: Checkpoint inhibitor immunotherapy (anti-PD-1, anti-PD-L1, anti-CTLA-4) is an increasingly common cause of lichenoid drug eruptions, affecting 5 to 20 percent of treated patients. The eruption may occur weeks to months after starting therapy and can be severe, involving the oral mucosa and mimicking erosive lichen planus. Importantly, the development of a lichenoid immune-related adverse event may correlate with antitumor response, and management aims to control the cutaneous disease without necessarily discontinuing the immunotherapy unless the eruption is severe or refractory.

Benign Lichenoid Keratosis

Benign lichenoid keratosis (BLK), also known as lichen planus-like keratosis, is a common, solitary lesion that represents an immunologic regression reaction within a pre-existing solar lentigo, seborrheic keratosis, or large cell acanthoma. It presents as a solitary, erythematous to violaceous, scaly papule or plaque, typically on the trunk or upper extremities of middle-aged and older adults, and clinically mimics basal cell carcinoma, squamous cell carcinoma in situ (Bowen disease), or superficial spreading melanoma. Dermoscopy of BLK shows a structureless gray to blue-gray pattern or granular structures corresponding to dermal melanophages, which overlaps with the dermoscopic features of melanoma and frequently prompts biopsy. Histopathology shows a lichenoid interface reaction (band-like lymphocytic infiltrate at the dermoepidermal junction with Civatte bodies) superimposed on the features of the underlying benign lesion. BLK is entirely benign and requires no treatment beyond diagnostic biopsy, but its importance lies in its role as a clinical mimicker: it is one of the most common lesions biopsied to rule out melanoma or non-melanoma skin cancer.

Interface Dermatitis: Mechanisms and Histopathologic Patterns

Definition and Pathophysiology of Interface Dermatitis

Interface dermatitis is a histopathologic reaction pattern defined by lymphocyte-mediated damage to the basal layer of the epidermis at the dermoepidermal junction (the interface zone). This damage produces keratinocyte apoptosis (Civatte bodies), basal cell vacuolization, basement membrane zone disruption, and melanin incontinence (release of melanin from damaged melanocytes into the upper dermis, where it is engulfed by dermal melanophages). Interface dermatitis is not a single disease but a reaction pattern shared by a broad group of inflammatory dermatoses and systemic diseases. The common pathogenetic denominator is cytotoxic T cell-mediated or antibody-mediated attack on basal keratinocytes, driven by autoantigens (in lichen planus, lupus erythematosus), drug-modified antigens (in lichenoid drug eruptions), viral antigens (in viral exanthems), or minor histocompatibility antigens (in graft-versus-host disease). Understanding interface dermatitis as a reaction pattern rather than a diagnosis is clinically important because the histopathologic finding of interface change narrows the differential but does not specify the etiology — the diagnosis requires integration of the biopsy findings with the clinical presentation, distribution, and history.

Vacuolar Interface Pattern Versus Lichenoid Interface Pattern

Interface dermatitis is subclassified into two principal histopathologic patterns based on the density and distribution of the inflammatory infiltrate, and each pattern is associated with a distinct group of clinical diseases. The vacuolar (cell-poor) interface pattern is characterized by sparse lymphocytic infiltrate at the dermoepidermal junction with prominent basal cell vacuolization, scattered apoptotic keratinocytes, and minimal inflammatory obscuring of the junction. This pattern is seen in erythema multiforme, lupus erythematosus (particularly subacute cutaneous lupus and acute cutaneous lupus), dermatomyositis, acute graft-versus-host disease, fixed drug eruption, and viral exanthems. The lichenoid (cell-rich) interface pattern is characterized by a dense, band-like lymphocytic infiltrate that hugs and obscures the dermoepidermal junction, with extensive basal cell damage, sawtooth-pattern rete ridge irregularity, and prominent Civatte body formation. This pattern is the histopathologic hallmark of lichen planus, lichenoid drug eruptions, chronic graft-versus-host disease (lichenoid phase), and lichen sclerosus (early stage). The distinction between vacuolar and lichenoid interface patterns has direct clinical implications: a vacuolar pattern on biopsy prompts serologic evaluation for lupus erythematosus and dermatomyositis (ANA, anti-dsDNA, anti-Ro/SSA, anti-La/SSB, creatine kinase, aldolase), while a lichenoid pattern prompts evaluation for drug-related etiology and hepatitis C screening.

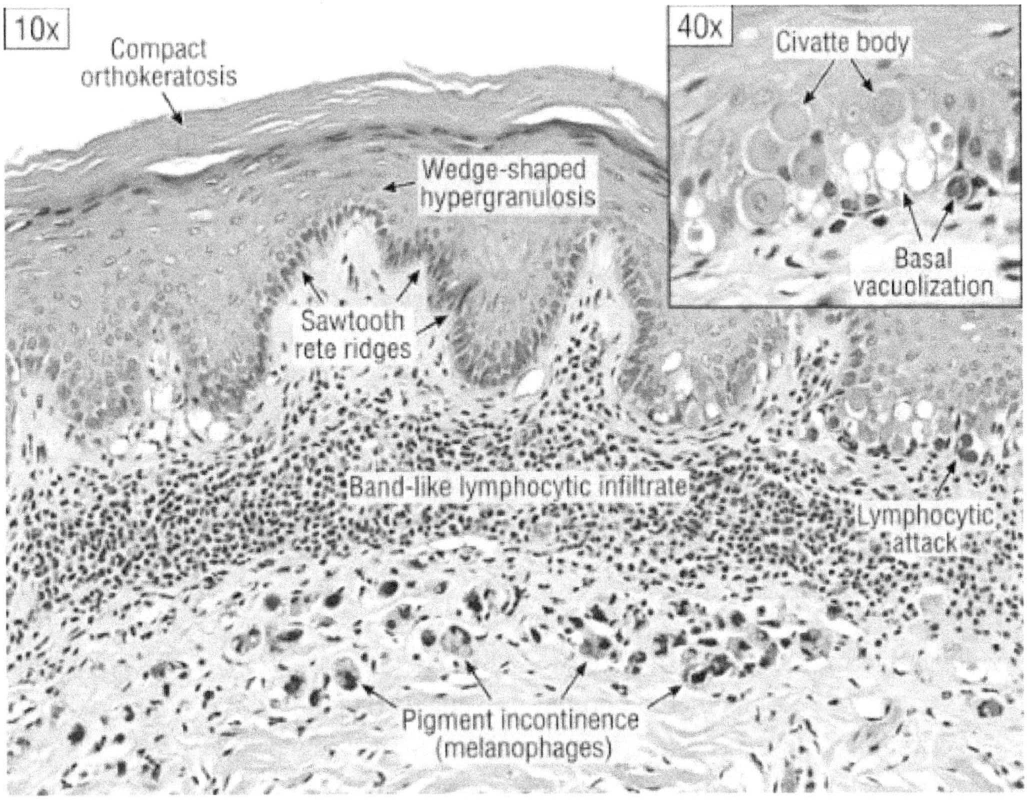

Clinical Correlates and Diagnostic Integration

The clinician uses the interface dermatitis classification as a diagnostic framework. When a biopsy reports interface dermatitis, the next question is which subtype — vacuolar or lichenoid — because this determines the clinical differential. A vacuolar interface pattern on the face of a young woman with photosensitivity and arthralgias raises lupus erythematosus (order ANA, anti-dsDNA). A vacuolar interface pattern on the proximal extremities with heliotrope eyelid discoloration raises dermatomyositis (order myositis-specific antibodies, muscle enzymes). A lichenoid interface pattern on the wrists of a patient with oral white striae is lichen planus. A lichenoid interface pattern in a patient who started a new medication 3 months ago is a lichenoid drug eruption. Direct immunofluorescence (DIF) further refines the diagnosis: LP shows shaggy fibrinogen deposition at the basement membrane zone and scattered IgM-positive Civatte bodies (neither is specific), lupus shows granular IgG, IgM, and C3 deposition at the basement membrane zone (the lupus band test), and pemphigus and pemphigoid show distinct patterns that distinguish them from interface dermatitis. The integration of histopathology, DIF, clinical distribution, and clinical history transforms the nonspecific finding of interface dermatitis into a specific diagnosis.

Interface Pattern	Histopathologic Features	Clinical Disease Associations
Vacuolar (cell-poor)	Sparse infiltrate, prominent basal vacuolization, scattered apoptotic keratinocytes, dermal edema	Lupus erythematosus, dermatomyositis, erythema multiforme, acute GVHD, fixed drug eruption, viral exanthems
Lichenoid (cell-rich)	Dense band-like infiltrate obscuring DEJ, extensive Civatte bodies, sawtooth rete ridges, hypergranulosis, pigment incontinence	Lichen planus, lichenoid drug eruption, chronic GVHD, lichen sclerosus (early)
Mixed vacuolar-lichenoid	Features of both patterns at different biopsy levels or sites	LP-lupus overlap, drug reactions with mixed features, pityriasis lichenoides

THE CUTANEOUS MIMICKER RECOGNITION ATLAS — Lichen Planus versus Lichenoid Drug Eruption

The Clinical Pattern: Idiopathic lichen planus presents as pruritic, polygonal, flat-topped, violaceous papules and plaques favoring the flexural wrists, ankles, and sacral region, with Wickham striae visible on dermoscopy, frequently accompanied by oral involvement (reticular white striae on the buccal mucosa bilaterally). The eruption may be generalized or localized, with Koebner phenomenon at sites of trauma. Nail involvement (longitudinal ridging, dorsal pterygium) and scalp involvement (lichen planopilaris) may coexist.

The Mimicker: Lichenoid drug eruptions closely mimic idiopathic LP — violaceous papules and plaques with similar morphology — but tend to be larger and more psoriasiform, more widely distributed (trunk predominance rather than flexural wrist/ankle predilection), more commonly photodistributed, and less likely to display Wickham striae. Oral involvement is less frequent than in idiopathic LP. The eruption develops weeks to months after starting the causative medication (ACE inhibitors, thiazides, beta-blockers, antimalarials, checkpoint inhibitors, NSAIDs, proton pump inhibitors), and the prolonged latency obscures the drug-disease relationship.

Trap Logic: Latency bias is the cognitive trap. The 2- to 12-month latency between drug initiation and eruption onset means that the clinician does not temporally associate the eruption with the drug — the medication was started long before the skin disease appeared, so it is not considered a suspect. This is compounded by **familiarity bias**: LP is a common diagnosis, and once the clinical pattern is recognized as lichenoid, the clinician anchors on idiopathic LP without reviewing the medication list for recent additions. The result is ongoing exposure to the causative drug and failure to resolve a treatable cause.

The Decision Anchor: The discriminating approach is a **thorough medication history with specific attention to drugs started within the preceding 12 months**, correlated with the clinical features (trunk-predominant or photodistributed, psoriasiform morphology, absence of Wickham striae). On biopsy, eosinophils in the infiltrate, parakeratosis, and deeper perivascular extension favor LDE over idiopathic LP. The definitive test is clinical: resolution after withdrawal of the suspected drug (which may take 2 to 6 months) confirms the diagnosis. In any patient presenting with new-onset lichenoid eruption, a complete medication review is mandatory before accepting the diagnosis of idiopathic LP.

Lichen Nitidus, Lichen Striatus, and Other Lichenoid Conditions

Lichen Nitidus

Lichen nitidus is a chronic, usually asymptomatic dermatosis of unknown etiology characterized by tiny (1 to 2 mm), skin-colored to slightly hypopigmented, flat-topped, shiny papules. The papules typically cluster on the trunk, genitalia, upper extremities, and abdomen. In darker skin (Fitzpatrick IV–VI), the papules may appear hypopigmented and can be confused with pityriasis alba or vitiligo. Histopathology is distinctive and diagnostic: a well-circumscribed, ball-and-claw granulomatous infiltrate (lymphocytes, histiocytes, and giant cells) within an expanded dermal papilla, flanked by elongated rete ridges that appear to clutch the infiltrate, with overlying thinned epidermis and focal parakeratosis. The condition is self-limited in most patients (resolving spontaneously over months to years), and treatment is generally unnecessary. In symptomatic or cosmetically bothersome cases, topical corticosteroids, topical calcineurin inhibitors, or narrow-band UVB phototherapy may provide partial relief.

Lichen Striatus

Lichen striatus is an acquired, self-limited, linear inflammatory dermatosis that follows the lines of Blaschko — embryologic migration pathways of keratinocyte clones that are distinct from dermatomes and neurovascular distributions. It presents as a unilateral, linear band of small, flat-topped, skin-colored to slightly erythematous papules extending along a limb (most commonly) or the trunk, developing over days to weeks and resolving spontaneously within 6 to 24 months. The condition most commonly affects children aged 5 to 15 years and is usually asymptomatic, though mild pruritus may occur. Histopathology shows a lichenoid and spongiotic interface dermatitis with exocytosis of lymphocytes and focal necrosis of keratinocytes along the dermoepidermal junction. The pathogenesis is believed to involve an immune response against a mosaically distributed keratinocyte clone carrying a somatic mutation along a Blaschko line — the same concept that underlies inflammatory linear verrucous epidermal nevus (ILVEN), with which lichen striatus must be differentiated. No treatment is required beyond reassurance, though post-inflammatory hypopigmentation may persist after the inflammation resolves (particularly in darker skin types) and should be anticipated in counseling.

Lichen Aureus and Pigmented Purpuric Dermatoses

Lichen aureus is a variant of pigmented purpuric dermatosis (capillaritis) that presents as a solitary or localized, golden-brown to russet-colored patch, most commonly on the lower extremities. It is classified among the pigmented purpuric dermatoses (PPD) — a group of chronic, benign capillaritides that include Schamberg disease (progressive pigmentary dermatosis), Majocchi disease (purpura annularis telangiectodes), Gougerot-Blum syndrome (pigmented purpuric lichenoid dermatitis), and Doucas-Kapetanakis (eczematoid purpura). All PPD variants share a histopathologic pattern of perivascular lymphocytic infiltrate with erythrocyte extravasation, hemosiderin deposition, and endothelial swelling in the superficial dermal capillaries — a capillaritis pattern. What distinguishes lichen aureus from the other PPD variants is the dense, band-like (lichenoid) lymphocytic infiltrate in the superficial dermis, which gives it a lichenoid histopathologic appearance. Clinically, PPD is important because of the differential diagnosis it raises: the petechial and purpuric lesions can mimic cutaneous vasculitis (particularly hypersensitivity vasculitis), drug-induced purpura, mycosis fungoides (patch-stage cutaneous T-cell lymphoma), and stasis dermatitis. Biopsy distinguishes PPD from vasculitis (no fibrinoid necrosis or vessel wall destruction) and from mycosis fungoides (no epidermotropism or atypical lymphocytes on immunohistochemistry).

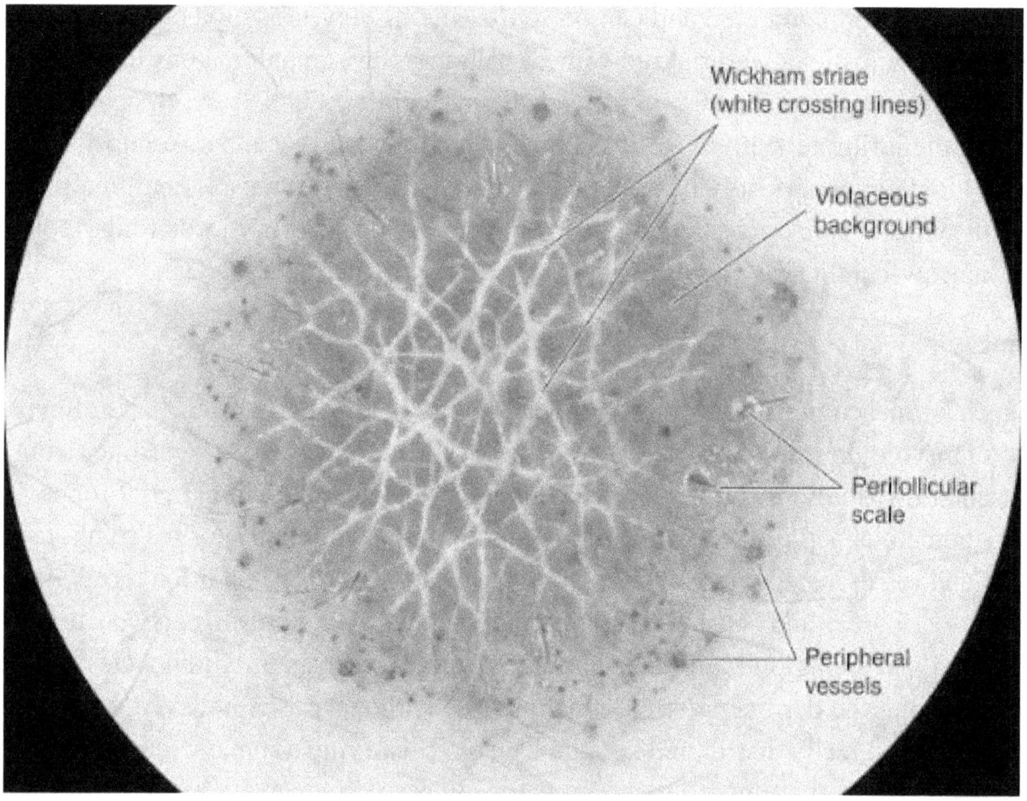

Differential Diagnosis of Lichenoid Eruptions

The differential diagnosis of lichenoid papules and plaques extends beyond LP and LDE to include several conditions that share the morphology of flat-topped, violaceous lesions. Secondary syphilis (the great mimicker) can produce widespread, copper-colored, flat-topped papules that closely resemble LP — the distribution (palms and soles involvement is a critical distinguishing feature of syphilis), oral mucous patches, condylomata lata, and serologic testing (RPR/VDRL, FTA-ABS) differentiate syphilis from LP. Pityriasis rosea presents as a herald patch followed by a Christmas tree distribution of oval, salmon-colored papules with collarette scaling — the collarette scale (scaling at the periphery of the lesion) and the long-axis alignment along skin tension lines distinguish pityriasis rosea from LP. Guttate psoriasis produces small, scattered, erythematous, scaly papules that may overlap morphologically with LP, but the silvery micaceous scale of psoriasis, the Auspitz sign (pinpoint bleeding upon scale removal), and the predilection for the trunk and proximal extremities differentiate it. Chronic graft-versus-host disease (lichenoid phase) produces lichenoid papules and plaques indistinguishable from LP in bone marrow transplant recipients — the clinical context and timing after transplant confirm the diagnosis.

Management of Lichenoid Dermatoses

Topical Therapies: Corticosteroids and Calcineurin Inhibitors

Topical corticosteroids are the first-line treatment for cutaneous LP. For lesions on the trunk and extremities, superpotent topical corticosteroids (clobetasol propionate 0.05%) are applied under occlusion for 2 to 4 weeks, followed by a taper to mid-potency agents. For flexural, facial, and genital LP, mid-potency corticosteroids (triamcinolone acetonide 0.1%) or topical calcineurin inhibitors (tacrolimus 0.1% ointment, pimecrolimus 1% cream) are preferred to minimize the risk of corticosteroid-induced skin atrophy. Topical calcineurin inhibitors are particularly valuable for oral and genital LP, where they provide effective anti-inflammatory therapy without the mucosal atrophy risk of prolonged topical corticosteroids. For hypertrophic LP, intralesional corticosteroid injection (triamcinolone acetonide, concentration per institutional protocol, injected into the plaque at 4- to 6-week intervals) is often necessary because topical agents fail to penetrate the thickened, hyperkeratotic surface. Topical retinoids (tretinoin 0.05% cream) may be used as adjunctive therapy for hypertrophic LP to reduce hyperkeratosis and improve penetration of topical corticosteroids.

Systemic Therapies: Retinoids, Immunosuppressants, and Targeted Agents

Systemic therapy is reserved for widespread cutaneous LP, severe erosive oral LP, or LP refractory to topical treatment. Systemic corticosteroids (oral prednisone, initial dose per weight-based protocol, tapered over 4 to 8 weeks) provide rapid control of widespread or acutely symptomatic LP but are limited by relapse upon discontinuation and cumulative toxicity with prolonged use. Acitretin (systemic retinoid) is effective for widespread cutaneous LP and hypertrophic LP, acting through normalization of keratinization and reduction of T cell-mediated inflammation; it is teratogenic and requires pregnancy prevention counseling and monitoring. Methotrexate (oral, low-dose weekly regimen) has demonstrated efficacy in case series and small trials for widespread cutaneous LP and erosive OLP, with monitoring for hepatotoxicity and myelosuppression. Mycophenolate mofetil is used as a steroid-sparing agent for severe erosive oral LP and vulvovaginal LP. For lichen planopilaris and frontal fibrosing alopecia, oral hydroxychloroquine is considered first-line systemic therapy based on moderate evidence from retrospective studies, with the goal of halting disease progression (hair regrowth is uncommon because follicular scarring is irreversible). Doxycycline has shown efficacy in some LPP/FFA patients as an alternative to hydroxychloroquine. Rituximab and JAK inhibitors (tofacitinib, baricitinib) have been reported as effective in refractory LP in case reports and small series, representing emerging options for difficult cases.

CAUTION: Erosive oral lichen planus carries a malignant transformation risk estimated at 0.5 to 2 percent over 5 to 10 years, with squamous cell carcinoma developing in chronically eroded or atrophic areas. All patients with erosive OLP require regular clinical surveillance (every 6 to 12 months), and any area that develops induration, verrucous change, rapid growth, or a non-healing ulcer must be biopsied to exclude dysplasia or squamous cell carcinoma. This surveillance obligation continues indefinitely, even if the LP enters clinical remission.

EVIDENCE: A systematic review of treatment outcomes in frontal fibrosing alopecia found that hydroxychloroquine stabilized or improved hairline recession in approximately 55 to 70 percent of patients in retrospective cohorts, making it the most commonly used and best-studied systemic agent for FFA. The treatment effect is primarily stabilization (halting further recession) rather than regrowth, because follicular scarring is irreversible. Combination with topical minoxidil may provide additional benefit for cosmetic density in preserved follicles. Treatment duration is typically 12 to 24 months, with monitoring for retinal toxicity per ophthalmologic screening guidelines.

Management of Oral Lichen Planus

The management of oral LP is stratified by clinical subtype. Reticular OLP is typically asymptomatic and requires no treatment beyond monitoring. Erosive and atrophic OLP require active management because of their symptomatic burden and malignant transformation risk. First-line treatment is a superpotent topical corticosteroid (clobetasol propionate 0.05% in a mucosal adhesive base such as Orabase or applied with a custom oral tray) or topical tacrolimus (0.1% ointment applied to erosive areas twice daily). Intralesional corticosteroid injection is used for localized, refractory erosions. For severe erosive OLP unresponsive to topical therapy, systemic options include short courses of oral corticosteroids for acute flares, followed by steroid-sparing agents (mycophenolate mofetil, methotrexate, or azathioprine) for maintenance. Good oral hygiene and the avoidance of irritants (alcohol-containing mouthwashes, sharp dental restorations, poorly fitting dentures) are essential adjuncts. Dental amalgam restorations should be evaluated as a potential cause of oral lichenoid contact reactions (clinically indistinguishable from OLP, but localized to areas in direct contact with amalgam), and patch testing to dental metals may be warranted in selected cases.

Prognosis and Natural History

The natural history of cutaneous LP is favorable: the majority of cases resolve spontaneously within 1 to 2 years, though relapse occurs in approximately 15 to 20 percent of patients. Post-inflammatory hyperpigmentation may persist for months to years after the inflammation resolves, particularly in Fitzpatrick IV–VI skin, and can be more distressing to the patient than the LP itself. Hypertrophic LP follows a more protracted course, often persisting for years and requiring sustained treatment. Oral LP tends to be chronic and relapsing, with the erosive form showing a more persistent course and requiring long-term management. Lichen planopilaris and frontal fibrosing alopecia cause irreversible scarring alopecia, and the goal of treatment is stabilization (preventing further hair loss) rather than regrowth. Nail LP may cause permanent nail destruction if treatment is delayed, but early systemic therapy can halt progression. The overall prognosis of LP is good for cutaneous disease; the key long-term concerns are post-inflammatory pigmentary change, scarring from follicular and nail variants, and the small but real malignant transformation risk in erosive oral LP requiring ongoing surveillance.

Illustrative Clinical Scenario: New-Onset Lichenoid Eruption on a Background of Recent Medication Change

A 58-year-old man with hypertension and type 2 diabetes presents with a 2-month history of a widespread, pruritic eruption on the trunk and extremities. His primary care physician diagnosed eczema and prescribed triamcinolone acetonide 0.1% cream, which provided minimal improvement. On dermatologic examination, the eruption consists of flat-topped, violaceous to dusky-brown papules and thin plaques, predominantly on the trunk, upper back, and proximal extremities, with extension to the forearms. The distribution is widespread and includes sun-exposed sites. Wickham striae are not clearly visible on clinical examination or dermoscopy. The oral mucosa is uninvolved. The clinical impression is a lichenoid eruption, and the differential includes idiopathic lichen planus versus lichenoid drug eruption. A careful medication history reveals that lisinopril (ACE inhibitor) was added to his antihypertensive regimen 4 months ago — a latency of 2 months between drug initiation and eruption onset. A 4 mm punch biopsy shows a band-like lymphocytic infiltrate at the dermoepidermal junction with Civatte bodies, focal parakeratosis, and scattered eosinophils within the infiltrate. Hepatitis C serology is negative. The histopathologic findings (eosinophils, parakeratosis in a lichenoid interface reaction) and the clinical features (trunk-predominant distribution, photodistributed extension, absence of Wickham striae, no oral involvement) favor a lichenoid drug eruption over idiopathic LP. Lisinopril is discontinued and replaced with losartan. The eruption begins to improve after 6 weeks and clears completely over 4 months, leaving post-inflammatory hyperpigmentation that gradually fades over the subsequent year. This case illustrates the importance of a complete medication review — with attention to drugs started within the preceding 12 months — in every new presentation of a lichenoid eruption, and the histopathologic clues (eosinophils, parakeratosis) that tilt the diagnosis toward drug-related etiology.

THE CUTANEOUS MIMICKER RECOGNITION ATLAS — Erosive Oral Lichen Planus versus Oral Squamous Cell Carcinoma

The Clinical Pattern: Erosive oral lichen planus presents as chronic, painful, well-demarcated erosions with a fibrinous base and a peripheral rim of white reticular striae (Wickham striae), typically on the buccal mucosa bilaterally and the tongue. The erosions wax and wane over months to years, are exacerbated by spicy or acidic foods, and respond partially to topical corticosteroids or calcineurin inhibitors. The surrounding mucosa shows the characteristic white lace-like striae of reticular OLP.

The Mimicker: Oral squamous cell carcinoma (OSCC) arising within chronic erosive OLP presents as a non-healing ulcer, an area of induration within a previously flat erosion, verrucous or exophytic change, or a rapidly enlarging erosion that no longer responds to topical therapy. OSCC may develop at the periphery of a chronic erosive OLP site, and its early features can be subtle — a slightly indurated border, a deeper ulcer bed, or a change in the pain character (from burning to deep, constant pain) — making it difficult to detect against the background of chronic erosive disease.

Trap Logic: Surveillance fatigue and attribution bias are the cognitive traps. Patients with long-standing erosive OLP have chronic ulcers that wax and wane as a normal part of their disease. The clinician — and the patient — become habituated to the presence of oral erosions and attribute new changes to the underlying OLP rather than recognizing a malignant transformation event. The low absolute risk (0.5 to 2 percent over 5 to 10 years) reinforces complacency: the transformation is rare enough that many surveillance visits are normal, which erodes vigilance over time.

The Decision Anchor: The discriminating features are **induration (hardness on palpation that was not present before), verrucous change (raised, rough, warty surface developing within a flat erosion), fixation to underlying structures, failure to respond to adequate topical therapy when it previously responded, and a change in pain quality from burning to deep or constant**. Any of these findings in a patient with erosive OLP mandates incisional biopsy of the suspicious area. Biopsy specimens should be taken from the border of the lesion (not the ulcer center, which shows only necrosis) and should include adjacent clinically involved mucosa for comparison. The surveillance interval for erosive OLP is every 6 to 12 months, with clinical photography to document the baseline pattern against which new changes can be detected.

THE CUTANEOUS MIMICKER RECOGNITION ATLAS — Lichenoid Diagnostic Arcs

Lichen Planus vs. Lichenoid Drug Eruption: The discriminating approach is a thorough medication history with specific attention to drugs started within the preceding 12 months. Clinical features favoring LDE include trunk-predominant or photodistributed pattern, psoriasiform morphology, absence of Wickham striae, and less frequent oral involvement. On biopsy, eosinophils, parakeratosis, and deeper perivascular extension favor LDE. Definitive confirmation is clinical resolution after drug withdrawal (2 to 6 months). Cognitive trap: latency bias — the 2- to 12-month drug-to-eruption interval obscures the causal association.

Erosive Oral Lichen Planus vs. Oral Squamous Cell Carcinoma: The discriminating features are induration, verrucous change, fixation, failure to respond to previously effective topical therapy, and a change in pain quality. Any of these findings in erosive OLP mandates incisional biopsy. The malignant transformation risk is 0.5 to 2 percent over 5 to 10 years. Cognitive trap: surveillance fatigue and attribution bias — clinicians habituated to chronic oral erosions attribute new changes to the underlying OLP rather than recognizing transformation.

Summary and Key Concepts

Lichen planus is driven by CD8+ cytotoxic T lymphocytes targeting basal keratinocytes through perforin-granzyme and Fas-FasL pathways, producing the hallmark interface dermatitis with Civatte bodies, sawtooth rete ridges, and wedge-shaped hypergranulosis. The violaceous color and post-inflammatory hyperpigmentation result from melanin incontinence following basal cell destruction.

Classic cutaneous LP is defined by the five Ps (pruritic, polygonal, planar, purple papules) with Wickham striae — white reticular lines visible on dermoscopy corresponding to hypergranulosis. Variants include hypertrophic, atrophic, vesiculobullous, annular, and actinic forms, each with distinct clinical behavior and prognosis.

Oral lichen planus affects 50 to 70 percent of LP patients and presents as reticular (asymptomatic white striae), erosive (painful ulcerations with malignant transformation risk of 0.5 to 2 percent), or atrophic (desquamative gingivitis) forms. Erosive OLP requires lifelong surveillance for squamous cell carcinoma development.

Interface dermatitis is classified into vacuolar (cell-poor, seen in lupus, dermatomyositis, EM, acute GVHD) and lichenoid (cell-rich, seen in LP, LDE, chronic GVHD) patterns. The histopathologic subtype narrows the clinical differential and directs the diagnostic workup.

Management of LP is stratified by site and severity: topical corticosteroids and calcineurin inhibitors for localized disease, systemic retinoids or immunosuppressants for widespread or refractory disease, and hydroxychloroquine for lichen planopilaris and frontal fibrosing alopecia. Lichenoid drug eruptions are managed by identification and withdrawal of the causative medication.

CHAPTER 7: AUTOIMMUNE BLISTERING DISEASES

Learning Objectives

1. Explain the immunopathogenesis of pemphigus vulgaris and pemphigus foliaceus, including the roles of anti-desmoglein 1 and anti-desmoglein 3 autoantibodies in determining clinical phenotype.
2. Distinguish the clinical, histopathologic, and immunofluorescence features of bullous pemphigoid from pemphigus vulgaris and apply the desmoglein compensation theory to predict mucosal versus cutaneous involvement.
3. Recognize the clinical presentations of linear IgA bullous dermatosis, epidermolysis bullosa acquisita, and dermatitis herpetiformis and their respective diagnostic immunofluorescence patterns.
4. Interpret direct and indirect immunofluorescence findings and serologic markers (anti-desmoglein, anti-BP180, anti-BP230 antibodies) to classify autoimmune blistering diseases.
5. Apply evidence-based management strategies for autoimmune blistering diseases, including rituximab as first-line therapy for pemphigus and corticosteroid-sparing approaches for bullous pemphigoid.

Pemphigus Vulgaris and Pemphigus Foliaceus

Immunopathogenesis and the Desmoglein Compensation Theory

Pemphigus vulgaris (PV) and pemphigus foliaceus (PF) are autoimmune blistering diseases caused by IgG autoantibodies directed against desmogleins, transmembrane glycoproteins of the cadherin superfamily that form the adhesive core of desmosomes — the intercellular junctions responsible for keratinocyte-to-keratinocyte adhesion. In PV, autoantibodies target desmoglein 3 (Dsg3), with or without concurrent anti-desmoglein 1 (Dsg1) antibodies. In PF, autoantibodies target Dsg1 exclusively. The desmoglein compensation theory explains the clinical phenotypes: Dsg3 is the dominant desmosomal cadherin in the mucous membranes (oral, pharyngeal, esophageal, genital), and Dsg1 predominates in the superficial epidermis (granular and cornified layers). In mucosal epithelium, Dsg3 is expressed throughout the full thickness, so anti-Dsg3 antibodies alone (mucosal-dominant PV) cause loss of cell adhesion (acantholysis) in the mucosa but not the skin, because cutaneous Dsg1 compensates for the loss of Dsg3 in the deep epidermis. When anti-Dsg1 antibodies are also present (mucocutaneous PV), both mucosal and cutaneous blistering occurs because compensation is lost at all levels. In PF, anti-Dsg1 antibodies cause acantholysis only in the superficial epidermis (where Dsg1 is the dominant adhesion molecule and Dsg3 is absent or sparse), producing superficial, fragile blisters that rupture easily and present as crusted erosions rather than intact blisters.

Clinical Presentation of Pemphigus Vulgaris

PV is the most common form of pemphigus (incidence approximately 1 to 5 per million per year, with higher rates in Ashkenazi Jewish and Mediterranean populations). The disease typically presents in the fifth and sixth decades of life. Oral mucosal involvement is often the initial manifestation, preceding cutaneous disease by weeks to months: painful, irregularly shaped erosions on the buccal mucosa, palate, pharynx, and gingiva that fail to heal. The oral erosions are often misdiagnosed as aphthous stomatitis, oral candidiasis, or herpes simplex — the key distinguishing feature is that pemphigus erosions are persistent, widespread, and do not respond to antifungal or antiviral therapy. Cutaneous PV presents as flaccid blisters (easily ruptured, leaving painful erosions with a moist, denuded base) on otherwise normal-appearing or slightly erythematous skin. The Nikolsky sign (lateral pressure on uninvolved perilesional skin produces epidermal detachment and a new blister or erosion) is positive in active PV and reflects the subclinical loss of keratinocyte adhesion beyond the visible lesion. The Asboe-Hansen sign (direct pressure on an intact blister causes lateral extension of the blister) is also positive. Lesions favor the scalp, face, chest, axillae, and groin. Without treatment, PV follows a progressive course with increasing body surface involvement and significant morbidity from pain, secondary infection, fluid and protein loss, and nutritional impairment due to oral erosions.

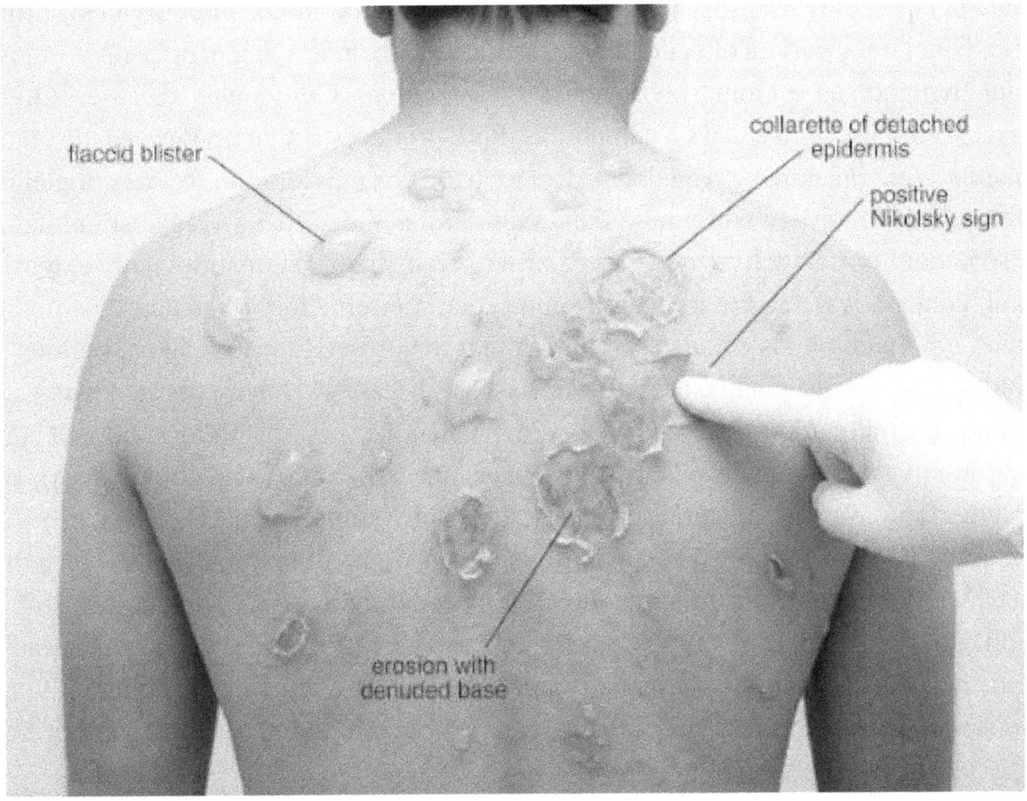

Clinical Presentation of Pemphigus Foliaceus

PF presents as superficial, fragile blisters that rupture almost immediately, producing crusted, scaly erosions on an erythematous base. Intact blisters are rarely seen because the superficial plane of acantholysis (within the granular layer) produces blisters too thin to survive mechanical stress. The distribution is seborrheic — scalp, face (malar region, producing a butterfly distribution that mimics lupus erythematosus), upper chest, and upper back — reflecting the anatomic regions where Dsg1 expression is highest. Oral mucosal involvement does NOT occur in PF (because the mucosa is protected by Dsg3 compensation), and this is the critical clinical distinction from PV. Fogo selvagem (endemic pemphigus foliaceus) is a variant of PF occurring in rural areas of Brazil and other South American regions, linked to an environmental trigger (possibly sand fly bites from Simuliidae), with an identical autoantibody profile (anti-Dsg1) but an epidemiologic pattern suggesting an infectious or environmental cofactor in genetically susceptible populations. Drug-induced pemphigus (triggered by thiol-containing drugs such as penicillamine and captopril, or by non-thiol drugs such as ACE inhibitors and some antibiotics) most commonly presents as a PF-like phenotype with anti-Dsg1 antibodies.

Paraneoplastic Pemphigus

Paraneoplastic pemphigus (PNP), also termed paraneoplastic autoimmune multiorgan syndrome (PAMS), is a distinct and often fatal variant of pemphigus associated with underlying neoplasms — most commonly non-Hodgkin lymphoma, chronic lymphocytic leukemia, Castleman disease, thymoma, and retroperitoneal sarcomas. Unlike classic pemphigus, PNP produces autoantibodies against multiple plakin family proteins (envoplakin, periplakin, desmoplakin) in addition to desmogleins, and the immunopathogenesis involves both humoral and cell-mediated cytotoxicity against epithelial cells. The clinical presentation is distinctive: severe, painful, hemorrhagic stomatitis with extensive mucosal erosions (oral, conjunctival, nasopharyngeal, genital) that are refractory to standard pemphigus therapy, combined with a polymorphous cutaneous eruption that may resemble pemphigus, bullous pemphigoid, erythema multiforme, lichen planus, or graft-versus-host disease — often simultaneously. This clinical polymorphism is the hallmark of PNP and a key diagnostic clue. Histopathology shows a combination of suprabasal acantholysis (pemphigus pattern) AND interface dermatitis (lichenoid pattern), a dual pattern not seen in other autoimmune blistering diseases. DIF shows intercellular IgG (as in PV) plus linear complement at the BMZ. The most specific serologic test is indirect immunofluorescence on rat bladder epithelium, which detects anti-plakin antibodies. Pulmonary involvement (bronchiolitis obliterans) is a feared complication that occurs in approximately 30 percent of PNP cases and is the leading cause of death. Treatment requires aggressive immunosuppression AND treatment of the underlying neoplasm; Castleman disease, when resectable, may produce complete remission of PNP after tumor excision.

Histopathology and Diagnostic Confirmation

The histopathologic hallmark of PV is suprabasal acantholysis: loss of intercellular adhesion just above the basal cell layer produces a cleft above the basal keratinocytes, which remain attached to the basement membrane like a row of tombstones (the tombstone pattern). The suprabasal cleft contains acantholytic keratinocytes — rounded, detached keratinocytes with condensed cytoplasm and hyperchromatic nuclei. In PF, acantholysis occurs in the superficial epidermis (within the granular layer), producing a subcorneal or intragranular cleft. Direct immunofluorescence (DIF) of perilesional skin in both PV and PF shows intercellular (chicken-wire or fishnet pattern) IgG and C3 deposition throughout the epidermis, reflecting autoantibody binding to desmosomal antigens on the keratinocyte surface. Serum anti-desmoglein antibodies are measured by ELISA: anti-Dsg3 is specific for PV (mucosal-dominant PV shows anti-Dsg3 alone, mucocutaneous PV shows both anti-Dsg3 and anti-Dsg1), and anti-Dsg1 alone is specific for PF. Antibody titers correlate with disease activity and are used to monitor treatment response and predict relapse.

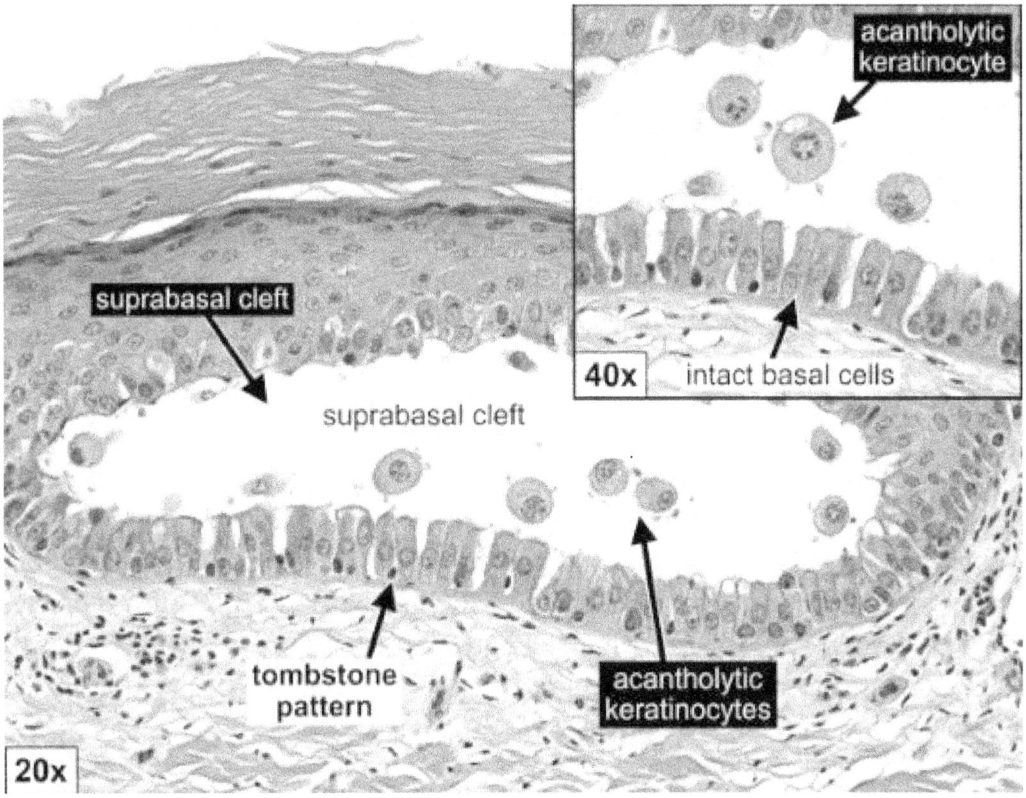

Bullous Pemphigoid and Mucous Membrane Pemphigoid

Immunopathogenesis of Bullous Pemphigoid

Bullous pemphigoid (BP) is the most common autoimmune blistering disease (incidence approximately 7 to 43 per million per year, increasing with age). It is caused by IgG autoantibodies directed against two hemidesmosomal antigens at the basement membrane zone: BP180 (type XVII collagen, also called BPAG2) and BP230 (BPAG1). BP180 is a transmembrane protein whose extracellular domain (the

NC16A domain is the immunodominant epitope) spans the lamina lucida and anchors the basal keratinocyte to the underlying lamina densa. Anti-BP180 antibodies bind to the NC16A domain, activate the classical complement pathway (C3, C5a), recruit neutrophils and eosinophils to the basement membrane zone, and trigger protease release (neutrophil elastase, matrix metalloproteinases) that cleaves the lamina lucida and produces subepidermal blistering. The subepidermal plane of cleavage — below the basal keratinocytes, at the level of the lamina lucida — produces tense blisters (because the full-thickness epidermis forms the blister roof), in contrast to the flaccid blisters of pemphigus (where only a portion of the epidermis forms the blister roof). Anti-BP180 antibody levels (measured by ELISA) correlate with disease activity and are used to monitor treatment response.

Clinical Presentation and Pre-Bullous Phase

BP predominantly affects elderly patients (mean age at onset 75 to 80 years), and its incidence has increased markedly over the past two decades, in part due to aging populations and in part due to drug-induced BP (dipeptidyl peptidase-4 inhibitors/gliptins, used in type 2 diabetes, are the most commonly implicated drug class). The classic presentation is tense, dome-shaped blisters on an erythematous or urticarial base, distributed on the trunk, proximal extremities, and flexural areas. The blisters are thick-walled and may persist intact for days before rupturing, in contrast to the fragile, immediately rupturing blisters of pemphigus. However, the pre-bullous phase of BP — which may precede frank blistering by weeks to months — is the most diagnostically challenging presentation: it presents as urticarial plaques, eczematous patches, or prurigo-like papules and excoriations without visible blisters, closely mimicking eczema, urticaria, drug eruption, or scabies. This pre-bullous phase is particularly treacherous in elderly patients, in whom pruritus may be attributed to xerosis or senile pruritus, and the correct diagnosis is delayed until blisters finally appear. The Nikolsky sign is typically negative in BP (the epidermis is intact and adherent above the subepidermal blister), which helps distinguish it from pemphigus.

CLINICAL PEARL: Dipeptidyl peptidase-4 (DPP-4) inhibitors (gliptins: sitagliptin, vildagliptin, linagliptin, saxagliptin) are an increasingly recognized cause of drug-induced bullous pemphigoid, with the eruption typically developing months to years after drug initiation. The clinical presentation is indistinguishable from idiopathic BP, and the diagnosis is confirmed by DIF. Drug withdrawal alone may be sufficient for mild cases; severe cases require the same immunosuppressive management as idiopathic BP. DPP-4 inhibitor-associated BP should be considered in every diabetic patient presenting with a new blistering eruption.

Pemphigoid Gestationis

Pemphigoid gestationis (PG, formerly herpes gestationis) is a rare autoimmune subepidermal blistering disease that occurs during pregnancy, typically in the second or third trimester, or in the immediate postpartum period. PG shares the same immunopathogenesis as BP — IgG autoantibodies against the NC16A domain of BP180 activate complement at the basement membrane zone, producing subepidermal blistering — but the antigenic trigger is thought to be aberrant expression of MHC class II molecules in the placenta, which presents BP180 (expressed in placental trophoblast and amniotic epithelium) to maternal T cells. The clinical presentation begins as intensely pruritic urticarial papules and plaques, often starting periumbilically and spreading to the trunk and extremities, followed by the development of tense vesicles and bullae on an erythematous base. PG may flare at delivery and recur with subsequent pregnancies (often earlier and more severely) and with oral contraceptive use. The fetal impact includes a small risk of prematurity and small-for-gestational-age neonates. Transient neonatal blistering occurs in approximately 5 to 10 percent of cases due to passive transplacental transfer of maternal anti-BP180 antibodies, resolving spontaneously as maternal antibodies are cleared. Management depends on severity: mild PG responds to potent topical corticosteroids and oral antihistamines, while severe PG requires systemic corticosteroids (prednisone, managed in collaboration with obstetrics). DIF shows linear C3 (with or without IgG) at the basement membrane zone — complement is the dominant finding, distinguishing PG from polymorphic eruption of pregnancy and other gestational dermatoses.

Mucous Membrane Pemphigoid

Mucous membrane pemphigoid (MMP, formerly cicatricial pemphigoid) is a group of autoimmune subepidermal blistering diseases that predominantly affect the mucous membranes and produce scarring. The target antigens overlap with those of BP (BP180, BP230) but also include laminin-332, integrin alpha-6/beta-4, and type VII collagen, and the specific antigen determines the clinical phenotype and prognosis. Oral involvement (desquamative gingivitis, erosions of the buccal mucosa and palate) is the most common site. Ocular involvement is the most feared complication: conjunctival inflammation leads to symblepharon (adhesion of the palpebral and bulbar conjunctiva), ankyloblepharon, entropion with trichiasis, corneal scarring, and potentially irreversible blindness if untreated. Anti-laminin-332 MMP carries a possible paraneoplastic association and warrants malignancy screening. Management of MMP is guided by the involved sites and the risk of scarring: low-risk MMP (oral only) may be managed with topical corticosteroids and dapsone, while high-risk MMP (ocular, laryngeal, esophageal, or genital involvement) requires systemic immunosuppression (rituximab, cyclophosphamide, or mycophenolate mofetil) with ophthalmologic co-management.

Linear IgA Bullous Dermatosis and Epidermolysis Bullosa Acquisita

Linear IgA Bullous Dermatosis

Linear IgA bullous dermatosis (LAD) is an autoimmune blistering disease defined by linear IgA deposition at the basement membrane zone on direct immunofluorescence — the diagnostic hallmark that distinguishes it from BP (which shows linear IgG and C3) and dermatitis herpetiformis (which shows granular IgA at the dermal papillae). The autoantibodies target multiple antigens within the basement membrane zone, most commonly the cleaved ectodomain of BP180 (97 kDa LAD-1 antigen) and type VII collagen. LAD presents as tense vesicles and blisters, often arranged in an annular or rosette configuration (the string of pearls or cluster of jewels sign), distributed on the trunk, extremities, buttocks, and face. In children (the childhood form is also known as chronic bullous disease of childhood), the presentation favors the perioral and perineal areas with large, tense bullae. Drug-induced LAD is common and most frequently caused by vancomycin (the strongest drug association in any autoimmune blistering disease), and less commonly by NSAIDs, lithium, diclofenac, amiodarone, and trimethoprim-sulfamethoxazole.

Drug-induced LAD typically resolves within weeks of drug withdrawal. Dapsone is the first-line treatment for idiopathic LAD, with monitoring for methemoglobinemia and hemolytic anemia (particularly in patients with glucose-6-phosphate dehydrogenase deficiency, which must be tested before dapsone initiation).

Epidermolysis Bullosa Acquisita

Epidermolysis bullosa acquisita (EBA) is an autoimmune blistering disease caused by IgG autoantibodies against type VII collagen, the major structural component of anchoring fibrils that tether the lamina densa to the papillary dermis. Loss of anchoring fibril function produces subepidermal blistering at a level below the lamina densa (the deepest level of any autoimmune blistering disease), resulting in a mechanobullous phenotype: skin fragility, trauma-induced blisters on the dorsal hands, knuckles, elbows, knees, and feet, healing with scarring and milia formation (small, white, keratin-filled cysts within scars). This mechanobullous presentation closely mimics hereditary epidermolysis bullosa and porphyria cutanea tarda. An inflammatory variant of EBA mimics bullous pemphigoid (widespread tense blisters on an erythematous base), and diagnostic differentiation requires specialized techniques. DIF shows linear IgG and C3 at the basement membrane zone (indistinguishable from BP on standard DIF). Salt-split skin immunofluorescence, which cleaves the skin at the lamina lucida, localizes the antibody to the dermal side (floor) of the split in EBA (because type VII collagen is below the lamina lucida) versus the epidermal side (roof) in BP (because BP180 is above the lamina lucida). Anti-type VII collagen ELISA confirms the diagnosis. EBA is one of the most treatment-resistant autoimmune blistering diseases; options include dapsone, colchicine, rituximab, and intravenous immunoglobulin.

Complications and Differential Diagnosis of EBA

The scarring sequelae of EBA distinguish it from most other autoimmune blistering diseases and are the primary source of long-term morbidity. Repeated blistering and erosion on the dorsal hands and fingers leads to digital scarring, flexion contractures, and pseudosyndactyly (fusion of digits by scar tissue) that mimics recessive dystrophic epidermolysis bullosa. Nail dystrophy and eventual nail loss are common. Scarring alopecia occurs when the scalp is involved. Esophageal involvement produces dysphagia and stricture formation, and ocular involvement (in the inflammatory variant) can cause symblepharon and visual impairment, paralleling the complications of mucous membrane pemphigoid. The differential diagnosis of the mechanobullous variant includes porphyria cutanea tarda (which also produces skin fragility, blisters, and milia on the dorsal hands — distinguished by urine porphyrin analysis and the absence of autoantibodies on DIF), hereditary dystrophic epidermolysis bullosa (distinguished by age of onset and family history), and bullous systemic lupus erythematosus (which shares anti-type VII collagen antibodies and responds to dapsone but occurs in the context of active SLE with positive ANA and anti-dsDNA). EBA has a recognized association with inflammatory bowel disease, particularly Crohn disease, and screening for gastrointestinal symptoms is warranted.

Dermatitis Herpetiformis and Gluten-Sensitive Enteropathy

Pathogenesis and Gluten-Driven Autoimmunity

Dermatitis herpetiformis (DH) is the cutaneous manifestation of celiac disease (gluten-sensitive enteropathy), driven by IgA autoantibodies against epidermal transglutaminase (eTG), a close homolog of tissue transglutaminase (tTG), the primary autoantigen in celiac disease. The pathogenetic sequence begins in the gut: ingestion of gluten (gliadin peptides from wheat, barley, and rye) triggers a T cell-mediated immune response in the small intestinal mucosa in genetically susceptible individuals (HLA-DQ2 or HLA-DQ8), producing anti-tTG IgA antibodies. These IgA antibodies cross-react with eTG in the dermal papillae of the skin, where they deposit as granular IgA aggregates and activate complement, recruit neutrophils, and produce the characteristic neutrophilic microabscesses at the tips of the dermal papillae that lead to subepidermal vesicle formation. Virtually all DH patients have underlying celiac disease on small intestinal biopsy (villous atrophy, crypt hyperplasia, increased intraepithelial lymphocytes), though the majority are clinically asymptomatic or have only subclinical gastrointestinal symptoms — the skin disease is their presenting manifestation.

Clinical Presentation and Diagnostic Features

DH presents as intensely pruritic, grouped (herpetiform) vesicles and papulovesicles on the extensor surfaces: elbows, knees, buttocks, posterior scalp, and upper back. The distribution is symmetric. The vesicles are extremely pruritic and are often excoriated before clinical examination, so the presenting findings may be excoriations, crusted papules, and post-inflammatory hyperpigmentation rather than intact vesicles — a diagnostic challenge that leads to delay in diagnosis (average delay from symptom onset to diagnosis is approximately 1 to 2 years). DH must be distinguished from linear IgA bullous dermatosis, scabies (which shares the intensely pruritic papulovesicular eruption on extensor surfaces and buttocks), and dermatitis artefacta. The diagnostic gold standard is DIF of uninvolved perilesional skin, which shows granular IgA deposition at the tips of dermal papillae — the pathognomonic finding. Serum anti-tTG IgA and anti-eTG IgA antibodies support the diagnosis and can be used for monitoring. Small intestinal biopsy is recommended to confirm celiac disease and assess the degree of enteropathy, which has implications for lymphoma risk and nutritional management.

Management: Gluten-Free Diet and Dapsone

The definitive treatment of DH is a strict, lifelong gluten-free diet (GFD), which addresses both the cutaneous and the gastrointestinal components of the disease. The GFD eliminates the antigenic trigger (gliadin peptides), reduces anti-tTG and anti-eTG antibody production, and clears the granular IgA deposits from the dermal papillae — though the skin response to GFD is slow, typically requiring 6 to 24 months for complete resolution, because existing IgA deposits are cleared gradually. Dapsone provides rapid symptomatic relief (improvement within 24 to 72 hours), acting by inhibiting neutrophil chemotaxis and neutrophil-mediated tissue damage at the dermal papillae. Dapsone is used as initial therapy to control symptoms while the GFD takes effect, with the goal of tapering and discontinuing dapsone once the GFD achieves full disease control. Glucose-6-phosphate dehydrogenase activity must be measured before dapsone initiation because dapsone causes dose-dependent hemolysis that is exacerbated in G6PD deficiency, potentially causing severe, life-threatening hemolytic anemia. Regular monitoring of complete blood count and reticulocyte count is required during dapsone therapy. Patients with DH carry a small but increased lifetime risk of non-Hodgkin lymphoma (particularly enteropathy-associated T-cell lymphoma), and adherence to a strict GFD reduces this risk.

KEY POINT: Dapsone produces dramatic improvement in dermatitis herpetiformis within 24 to 72 hours — a therapeutic response so rapid and specific that it has diagnostic value: if a suspected DH eruption does not respond promptly to dapsone, the diagnosis should be reconsidered. However, dapsone controls only the skin disease; it does not treat the underlying celiac enteropathy. The gluten-free diet is the definitive treatment that addresses both skin and gut, and dapsone should be viewed as a bridge therapy, not as a substitute for the GFD.

Long-Term Complications and Screening

The long-term complications of DH are driven primarily by the underlying celiac disease rather than the skin disease itself. Patients with DH carry an increased lifetime risk of enteropathy-associated T-cell lymphoma (EATL) and other non-Hodgkin lymphomas, with the risk correlating with duration and degree of gluten exposure — strict adherence to a gluten-free diet reduces this lymphoma risk substantially. Nutritional deficiencies are common in patients with undiagnosed or poorly controlled celiac disease, including iron deficiency anemia (due to malabsorption in the proximal duodenum), folate deficiency, vitamin D deficiency (with resultant osteopenia and osteoporosis), vitamin B12 deficiency, and zinc deficiency. Bone mineral density screening with DEXA scan is recommended at diagnosis. Additional autoimmune comorbidities occur at increased frequency in DH and celiac disease, including type 1 diabetes mellitus, autoimmune thyroid disease (Hashimoto thyroiditis, Graves disease), Sjogren syndrome, and autoimmune hepatitis. First-degree relatives of DH patients carry a 10 to 15 percent risk of celiac disease and should be offered serologic screening with anti-tTG IgA.

Diagnostic Approach: Direct and Indirect Immunofluorescence

Direct Immunofluorescence: Technique and Interpretation

Direct immunofluorescence (DIF) is the single most important diagnostic test in autoimmune blistering diseases. It detects in vivo-bound immunoglobulins (IgG, IgA, IgM) and complement (C3) in the patient's tissue using fluorescein-labeled anti-human antibodies. The biopsy for DIF must be taken from perilesional, clinically uninvolved skin (not from a blister or erosion, which shows nonspecific findings due to tissue damage) and submitted in Michel transport medium or frozen immediately (not in formalin, which destroys immunoglobulins). The DIF pattern determines the diagnosis: intercellular (chicken-wire) IgG and C3 throughout the epidermis indicates pemphigus (PV or PF). Linear IgG and C3 at the basement membrane zone indicates BP, EBA, or MMP (further distinction requires salt-split skin or serologic testing). Linear IgA at the basement membrane zone indicates LAD. Granular IgA at the dermal papillae indicates dermatitis herpetiformis. The lupus band test shows granular IgG, IgM, IgA, and C3 at the basement membrane zone in a full-house pattern. DIF is positive in approximately 90 to 95 percent of autoimmune blistering diseases when the biopsy is properly obtained and processed, making it the gold standard for diagnosis.

Indirect Immunofluorescence and Serologic Testing

Indirect immunofluorescence (IIF) detects circulating autoantibodies in the patient's serum by applying the serum to a substrate tissue (monkey esophagus for pemphigus, salt-split human skin for subepidermal blistering diseases) and detecting bound antibody with fluorescein-labeled anti-human IgG. IIF on monkey esophagus shows an intercellular pattern in pemphigus. IIF on salt-split skin shows antibody binding to the epidermal side (roof) in BP and LAD, and to the dermal side (floor) in EBA and anti-laminin-332 MMP — this localization is diagnostically critical because standard DIF cannot distinguish BP from EBA (both show linear IgG at the BMZ). ELISA testing for specific autoantibodies provides the highest diagnostic specificity: anti-Dsg1 and anti-Dsg3 for pemphigus (with antibody profiles predicting clinical phenotype per the desmoglein compensation theory), anti-BP180 (NC16A) and anti-BP230 for BP, anti-type VII collagen for EBA, and anti-endomysial/anti-tTG IgA for DH. Antibody titers correlate with disease activity in pemphigus and BP and are used to guide treatment adjustments: a rising titer may predict clinical relapse before symptoms appear, allowing preemptive treatment escalation.

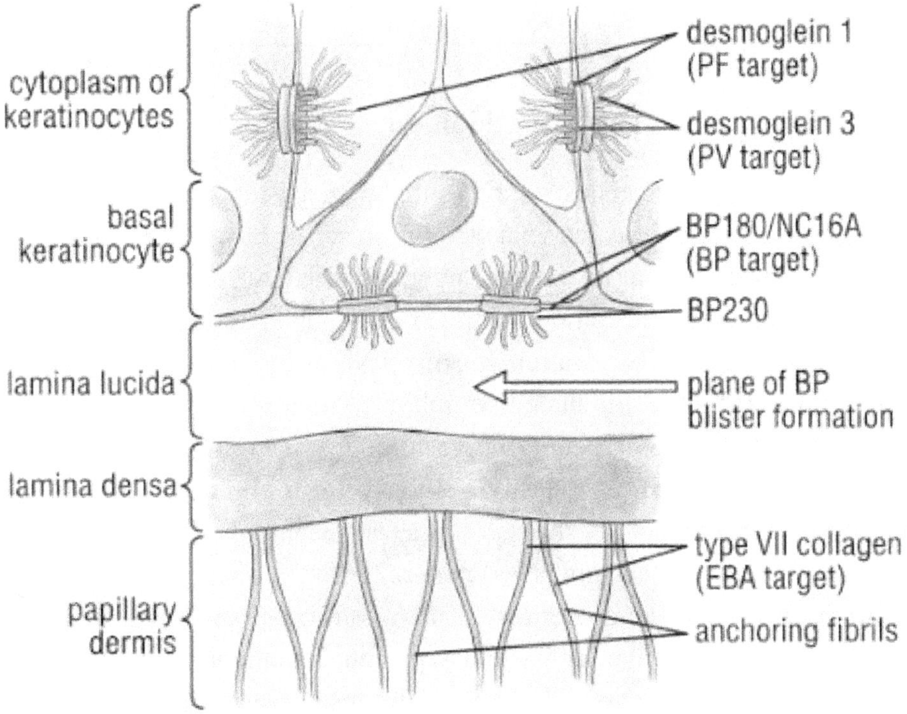

Disease	DIF Pattern	DIF Location	Key Serology
Pemphigus vulgaris	Intercellular (chicken-wire) IgG, C3	Epidermis (intercellular spaces)	Anti-Dsg3 ± anti-Dsg1 (ELISA)
Pemphigus foliaceus	Intercellular (chicken-wire) IgG, C3	Epidermis (intercellular spaces)	Anti-Dsg1 only (ELISA)
Bullous pemphigoid	Linear IgG, C3	Basement membrane zone (roof on salt-split)	Anti-BP180 NC16A, anti-BP230 (ELISA)
Epidermolysis bullosa acquisita	Linear IgG, C3	BMZ (floor on salt-split)	Anti-type VII collagen (ELISA)
Linear IgA bullous dermatosis	Linear IgA	Basement membrane zone	Anti-LAD-1 (97 kDa BP180 fragment)
Dermatitis herpetiformis	Granular IgA	Dermal papillae tips	Anti-tTG IgA, anti-eTG IgA
Mucous membrane pemphigoid	Linear IgG, IgA, C3	BMZ (variable roof/floor on salt-split)	Anti-BP180, anti-laminin-332

Clinical Case: Persistent Oral Erosions in a Middle-Aged Woman

A 52-year-old woman of Mediterranean descent presented with a 4-month history of painful oral erosions that had failed to respond to fluconazole and valacyclovir prescribed by her dentist. Examination revealed widespread, irregularly shaped erosions on the buccal mucosa bilaterally, the hard palate, and the posterior pharynx. Two flaccid blisters were present on the upper chest, and gentle lateral pressure on perilesional skin produced immediate epidermal separation (positive Nikolsky sign). No intact tense blisters were present. The initial clinical differential included pemphigus vulgaris, erosive oral lichen planus, mucous membrane pemphigoid, and chronic herpetic gingivostomatitis. Two biopsies were obtained: a lesional biopsy for H&E histopathology and a perilesional biopsy from clinically uninvolved skin in Michel transport medium for DIF. Histopathology showed suprabasal acantholysis with intact basal keratinocytes attached to the basement membrane in a tombstone pattern. DIF demonstrated intercellular (chicken-wire) IgG and C3 deposition throughout the epidermis. ELISA confirmed anti-Dsg3 antibodies at a high titer with anti-Dsg1 antibodies also positive, consistent with mucocutaneous pemphigus vulgaris. She was started on rituximab (first-line) with a short course of low-dose prednisone for initial disease control. At 6 months, her oral erosions had healed completely, cutaneous blistering had ceased, and anti-Dsg3 titers had declined by 80 percent. Prednisone was tapered and discontinued. This case illustrates the importance of pursuing immunopathologic workup — DIF and serology — in any patient with persistent oral erosions that fail to respond to antimicrobial therapy, rather than relying on clinical diagnosis alone.

EVIDENCE: The RITUX 3 randomized controlled trial (Joly et al., 2017) established rituximab as first-line therapy for moderate-to-severe pemphigus. Patients randomized to rituximab plus low-dose prednisone achieved complete remission off therapy in 89% at 24 months, versus 34% with prednisone alone. The rituximab group also experienced fewer corticosteroid-related adverse events and required a significantly lower cumulative prednisone dose. These findings transformed the treatment paradigm and are reflected in current international consensus guidelines recommending rituximab as first-line therapy over high-dose systemic corticosteroids.

THE CUTANEOUS MIMICKER RECOGNITION ATLAS — Pemphigus Vulgaris versus Bullous Pemphigoid

The Clinical Pattern: Pemphigus vulgaris presents as flaccid blisters on non-inflamed skin that rupture easily, leaving painful, slow-healing erosions with a moist base and peripheral collarette of detached epidermis. Oral mucosal erosions are typically the first manifestation, preceding cutaneous disease by weeks to months. The Nikolsky sign is positive. The clinical pattern is flaccid blisters, persistent erosions, mucosal involvement, and a positive Nikolsky sign.

The Mimicker: Bullous pemphigoid presents as tense, dome-shaped blisters on an erythematous or urticarial base, typically in elderly patients. The blisters are thick-walled and may persist intact for days. Oral involvement is less common (10 to 30 percent of cases) and less severe than in PV. The Nikolsky sign is typically negative. The pre-bullous phase may present as urticarial plaques or prurigo-like lesions without visible blisters, mimicking eczema or chronic urticaria for weeks before blisters develop.

Trap Logic: Age-driven diagnostic anchoring is the cognitive trap. Because BP is far more common than PV in elderly patients, clinicians may assume that any new blistering eruption in an older patient is BP without performing the immunopathologic workup. Conversely, when oral erosions are the presenting feature, they may be dismissed as aphthous stomatitis or denture-related trauma, delaying the diagnosis of PV until widespread cutaneous blistering develops. The more subtle trap is misinterpreting the pre-bullous phase of BP as eczema or urticaria and treating with topical steroids — which may partially suppress blistering and further delay diagnosis.

The Decision Anchor: The discriminating features are **blister tension (flaccid in PV, tense in BP), Nikolsky sign (positive in PV, negative in BP), mucosal involvement (early and prominent in PV, uncommon and mild in BP), and histopathologic level of cleavage (suprabasal in PV, subepidermal in BP)**. DIF is the definitive discriminator: intercellular IgG in PV versus linear IgG at the BMZ in BP. Serology confirms: anti-Dsg3/Dsg1 in PV, anti-BP180/BP230 in BP. Both a lesional biopsy for H&E and a perilesional biopsy for DIF should be obtained in every new blistering eruption.

Evidence-Based Management of Autoimmune Blistering Diseases

Pemphigus: Rituximab as First-Line Therapy

The management of pemphigus has been transformed by the RITUX 3 trial, which demonstrated that rituximab (anti-CD20 monoclonal antibody) as first-line therapy, combined with short-course low-dose prednisone, achieved complete remission off therapy in 89 percent of patients at 24 months — compared to 34 percent with prednisone alone. Based on this and subsequent confirmatory studies, rituximab is now recommended as first-line therapy for moderate-to-severe pemphigus in international consensus guidelines. The mechanism of action involves depletion of CD20+ B cells (which are the precursors of the plasma cells that produce pathogenic anti-desmoglein antibodies), leading to a gradual decline in autoantibody titers and clinical remission over weeks to months. The standard dosing protocol is two infusions of rituximab (per institutional protocol) separated by 2 weeks, with low-dose prednisone for initial disease control while rituximab takes effect (onset of benefit typically at 4 to 12 weeks). Maintenance infusions at 6 and 12 months may be given to consolidate remission. Before the rituximab era, pemphigus management relied on high-dose systemic corticosteroids (with their substantial cumulative toxicity) combined with conventional steroid-sparing immunosuppressants (mycophenolate mofetil, azathioprine) — these agents remain important for patients who cannot receive rituximab or who relapse after rituximab therapy.

Bullous Pemphigoid: Corticosteroid-Sparing Strategies

The management of BP aims to control blistering while minimizing corticosteroid exposure, which is particularly important given the elderly age of the typical patient and the excess mortality associated with systemic corticosteroid use in this population. A landmark randomized controlled trial demonstrated that superpotent topical corticosteroid (clobetasol propionate 0.05% cream applied to the entire body surface twice daily, including uninvolved skin) was as effective as systemic prednisone for moderate-to-severe BP and was associated with significantly lower mortality and fewer serious adverse events. Topical corticosteroid therapy is therefore preferred as initial treatment for localized to moderate-severity BP. For widespread or rapidly progressive BP, systemic corticosteroids (oral prednisone, dose per weight-based protocol, tapered over 4 to 6 months) may be necessary. Doxycycline has been shown in the BLISTER trial to be non-inferior to oral prednisolone for BP at 6 weeks with a superior long-term safety profile, making it an attractive steroid-sparing option for mild-to-moderate disease. Dapsone, methotrexate, mycophenolate mofetil, and azathioprine are additional steroid-sparing agents used in BP. Rituximab is reserved for refractory BP and has shown efficacy in case series. For all patients with BP, DPP-4 inhibitors and other potentially causative medications should be reviewed and discontinued if appropriate.

CAUTION: Systemic corticosteroid use in elderly patients with bullous pemphigoid carries significant excess mortality — predominantly from infectious complications (sepsis, pneumonia), metabolic derangements (hyperglycemia, adrenal suppression), cardiovascular events, and osteoporotic fractures. The mortality difference between topical and systemic corticosteroid regimens in BP was a key finding of the French randomized trial. Use the minimum effective corticosteroid dose, taper as rapidly as disease control allows, and use steroid-sparing agents early.

Monitoring, Relapse Prevention, and Prognosis

Disease monitoring in autoimmune blistering diseases relies on the combination of clinical assessment (lesion count, healing rate, mucosal examination), autoantibody titers (anti-Dsg for pemphigus, anti-BP180 for BP), and patient-reported outcomes. In pemphigus, the Pemphigus Disease Area Index (PDAI) quantifies disease activity. Serial anti-Dsg3 and anti-Dsg1 titers guide treatment decisions: a rising titer during corticosteroid taper predicts clinical relapse and may warrant preemptive treatment intensification before new blisters appear. Complete remission off therapy (no new lesions for at least 2 months while off all systemic therapy) is the treatment goal in pemphigus. In BP, anti-BP180 titers may predict relapse but are less consistently correlated with clinical activity than anti-desmoglein titers in pemphigus. Relapse after successful treatment occurs in approximately 30 to 50 percent of PV patients and 20 to 30 percent of BP patients, typically within the first 2 years after treatment discontinuation. The prognosis of pemphigus has improved dramatically with rituximab: mortality has declined from 75 percent in the pre-corticosteroid era to 5 to 10 percent in the current era. BP carries a 1-year mortality of approximately 20 to 40 percent in elderly patients, driven primarily by comorbidities and treatment-related complications rather than the disease itself.

Patient Education and Counseling

Patient education is essential in the management of autoimmune blistering diseases, which are chronic conditions requiring prolonged immunosuppressive therapy and lifestyle modification. Patients with pemphigus should understand that rituximab-based treatment typically requires 4 to 12 weeks to produce clinical improvement, and that short-term corticosteroids provide a bridge during this interval. They should be educated about signs of infection (the primary risk of immunosuppression and a leading cause of morbidity), the importance of wound care for open erosions, and the need for nutritional support when oral involvement impairs eating. Vaccination status should be reviewed and updated before rituximab initiation, as live vaccines are contraindicated during B-cell depletion. Patients with BP should be counseled about the importance of medication adherence during taper (premature corticosteroid discontinuation is a common cause of relapse), fall prevention (given the elderly population and corticosteroid-related osteoporosis), and recognition of new blistering that warrants prompt medical evaluation. Patients with DH require comprehensive dietary counseling from a dietitian experienced in celiac disease, because a strict gluten-free diet is both the definitive treatment for the skin disease and the primary means of preventing long-term gastrointestinal complications, nutritional deficiencies, and lymphoma. Hidden sources of gluten in medications, supplements, and processed foods should be identified. All patients should be informed that autoimmune blistering diseases are manageable chronic conditions and that current therapies — particularly rituximab for pemphigus — have transformed the prognosis from a historically fatal disease to one in which complete remission is achievable.

THE CUTANEOUS MIMICKER RECOGNITION ATLAS — Dermatitis Herpetiformis versus Linear IgA Bullous Dermatosis

The Clinical Pattern: Dermatitis herpetiformis presents as intensely pruritic, grouped (herpetiform) vesicles and papulovesicles symmetrically distributed on the extensor surfaces — elbows, knees, buttocks, posterior scalp, and upper back. Vesicles are often excoriated before examination, leaving crusted papules and excoriations. The patient has underlying celiac disease (confirmed by small intestinal biopsy), and serologic markers of celiac disease (anti-tTG IgA, anti-eTG IgA) are positive.

The Mimicker: Linear IgA bullous dermatosis presents as tense vesicles and blisters, often in an annular or rosette configuration (the string of pearls sign), distributed on the trunk, extremities, buttocks, and perioral/perineal areas. It may be drug-induced (vancomycin is the most common trigger) or idiopathic. Unlike DH, LAD is not associated with celiac disease, anti-tTG/anti-eTG antibodies are negative, and small intestinal biopsy is normal. The clinical morphology can overlap with DH, particularly when both present as vesicles on the buttocks and proximal extremities.

Trap Logic: Pattern matching to the vesicular eruption without immunopathologic confirmation is the cognitive trap. Both DH and LAD present as pruritic vesiculobullous eruptions, and their clinical distributions partially overlap. The clinician may diagnose DH based on clinical appearance and prescribe dapsone (which treats both diseases symptomatically) without obtaining the DIF biopsy that distinguishes them — granular IgA at dermal papillae (DH) versus linear IgA at the BMZ (LAD). This matters because DH requires a lifelong GFD and celiac disease surveillance, while LAD does not — and drug-induced LAD resolves with drug withdrawal.

The Decision Anchor: The discriminating test is **DIF of perilesional uninvolved skin: granular IgA at the dermal papillae indicates DH; linear IgA at the basement membrane zone indicates LAD**. This single test is definitive. Supporting evidence: anti-tTG and anti-eTG antibodies are positive in DH and negative in LAD; small intestinal biopsy shows villous atrophy in DH and is normal in LAD; a clear temporal association with vancomycin or another causative drug supports drug-induced LAD. DIF biopsy must be obtained in every vesiculobullous eruption before initiating dapsone therapy.

THE CUTANEOUS MIMICKER RECOGNITION ATLAS — Autoimmune Blistering Diagnostic Arcs

Pemphigus Vulgaris vs. Bullous Pemphigoid: The discriminating features are blister tension (flaccid in PV, tense in BP), Nikolsky sign (positive in PV, negative in BP), mucosal involvement (early and prominent in PV, uncommon in BP), and DIF pattern (intercellular IgG in PV versus linear IgG at the BMZ in BP). Histopathology shows suprabasal acantholysis in PV and subepidermal cleft with eosinophils in BP. Cognitive trap: age-driven anchoring on BP in elderly patients without immunopathologic workup; dismissal of oral erosions as aphthous stomatitis.

Dermatitis Herpetiformis vs. Linear IgA Bullous Dermatosis: The discriminating test is DIF: granular IgA at dermal papillae (DH) versus linear IgA at the BMZ (LAD). DH requires lifelong GFD and celiac disease surveillance; LAD does not. Drug-induced LAD (vancomycin) resolves with drug withdrawal.

Anti-tTG IgA is positive in DH, negative in LAD. Cognitive trap: treating both with dapsone without DIF confirmation, which misses the need for GFD in DH and drug withdrawal in LAD.

Summary and Key Concepts

Pemphigus vulgaris and pemphigus foliaceus are caused by IgG autoantibodies against desmogleins (Dsg3 and Dsg1), producing intraepidermal acantholysis. The desmoglein compensation theory explains phenotype: anti-Dsg3 alone causes mucosal-dominant PV; anti-Dsg3 plus anti-Dsg1 causes mucocutaneous PV; anti-Dsg1 alone causes PF (superficial blisters, no mucosal involvement). Rituximab is now first-line therapy for moderate-to-severe pemphigus.

Bullous pemphigoid is the most common autoimmune blistering disease, caused by anti-BP180 and anti-BP230 antibodies producing subepidermal (tense) blisters. The pre-bullous phase mimics eczema, urticaria, or prurigo. Superpotent topical corticosteroid is preferred over systemic prednisone for initial treatment due to lower mortality in elderly patients.

Linear IgA bullous dermatosis is defined by linear IgA on DIF and may be drug-induced (vancomycin). Epidermolysis bullosa acquisita targets type VII collagen (anchoring fibrils) and produces mechanobullous fragility with scarring. Salt-split skin localizes antibodies to dermal floor (EBA) versus epidermal roof (BP).

Dermatitis herpetiformis is the cutaneous manifestation of celiac disease, with granular IgA at dermal papillae on DIF. Dapsone provides rapid symptom control, but the gluten-free diet is the definitive treatment addressing both skin and gut disease. DH patients require celiac disease surveillance and carry an increased lymphoma risk.

DIF of perilesional uninvolved skin is the single most important diagnostic test in autoimmune blistering diseases. The DIF pattern (intercellular vs. linear IgG vs. linear IgA vs. granular IgA) and salt-split skin localization (roof vs. floor) classify the disease and direct serologic testing and management.

CHAPTER 8: GRANULOMATOUS AND DEPOSITIONAL SKIN DISEASES

Learning Objectives

1. Describe the immunopathogenesis of granuloma formation in the skin, distinguishing sarcoidal (naked) granulomas from palisading, suppurative, and foreign body granulomatous patterns and their diagnostic implications.
2. Recognize the protean cutaneous manifestations of sarcoidosis and correlate skin findings with systemic organ involvement, including the prognostic significance of specific morphologic subtypes.
3. Differentiate granuloma annulare from necrobiosis lipoidica, annular elastolytic giant cell granuloma, and other palisading granulomatous dermatoses based on clinical, histopathologic, and dermoscopic features.
4. Apply a systematic diagnostic approach to cutaneous depositional disorders, including amyloidosis, mucinoses, xanthomas, and calcinosis, correlating skin findings with underlying metabolic and systemic diseases.
5. Identify the clinical and histopathologic features that distinguish foreign body granulomas and infectious granulomatous diseases from non-infectious granulomatous dermatoses.

Sarcoidosis: Cutaneous Manifestations and Systemic Correlation

Pathogenesis of Granuloma Formation

Sarcoidosis is a systemic granulomatous disease of unknown etiology characterized by the formation of non-caseating (naked) epithelioid granulomas in affected organs. The immunopathogenesis involves an exaggerated Th1/Th17 cell-mediated immune response to an unidentified antigen (proposed candidates include mycobacterial antigens, Propionibacterium acnes, and environmental inorganic particles) in genetically susceptible individuals. The granuloma consists of a compact core of epithelioid histiocytes and multinucleated giant cells (Langhans and foreign body types), surrounded by a sparse rim of lymphocytes — hence the term naked granuloma, reflecting the relative paucity of the surrounding lymphocytic infiltrate compared to the dense lymphocytic cuff of infectious granulomas. Asteroid bodies (stellate cytoplasmic inclusions within giant cells) and Schaumann bodies (laminated calcified inclusions) are characteristic but not pathognomonic. The granulomatous inflammation is driven by local secretion of TNF-alpha, IFN-gamma, and IL-12 by activated macrophages and T cells, creating a self-perpetuating inflammatory loop that sustains granuloma formation even in the absence of identifiable organisms. Genetic susceptibility is linked to HLA alleles (HLA-DRB1*03 associated with acute, self-limited disease; HLA-DRB1*15 associated with chronic, progressive disease) and polymorphisms in genes regulating innate immunity and TNF-alpha production.

Epidemiology and Special Populations

Sarcoidosis has a worldwide distribution with a peak incidence in the third and fourth decades of life and a slight female predominance. Incidence and prevalence vary markedly by ethnicity and geography: in the United States, sarcoidosis is three to four times more common in African Americans than in white Americans (age-adjusted annual incidence approximately 35 per 100,000 versus 11 per 100,000), and African American patients tend to have more severe, chronic, multiorgan disease with higher rates of pulmonary fibrosis, cardiac involvement, and extrapulmonary complications. Scandinavian populations have a relatively high incidence of sarcoidosis but tend toward acute, self-limited disease (Lofgren syndrome is particularly common in Scandinavian women). Pediatric sarcoidosis presents differently by age: children under 5 years old (early-onset sarcoidosis) typically present with a triad of skin rash, uveitis, and arthritis without pulmonary involvement (this constellation overlaps with Blau syndrome, a monogenic autoinflammatory granulomatous disease caused by NOD2 mutations that must be excluded), while older children present with the adult pattern of bilateral hilar lymphadenopathy and pulmonary disease. In pregnancy, sarcoidosis generally improves during the second and third trimesters (due to physiologic immunosuppression and elevated endogenous cortisol) and may flare postpartum, requiring close monitoring during the postpartum period.

Cutaneous Morphologic Subtypes

Cutaneous involvement occurs in approximately 25 to 35 percent of sarcoidosis patients and may be the presenting manifestation. The protean morphology of cutaneous sarcoidosis is one of its defining diagnostic challenges — sarcoidosis is a great imitator of the skin. Specific cutaneous lesions (containing sarcoidal granulomas on histopathology) include papular sarcoidosis (the most common morphology: red-brown to violaceous papules, 2 to 5 mm, typically on the face, periorbital skin, and nares), plaque sarcoidosis (indurated, annular or discoid plaques, often on the trunk, extremities, and buttocks), nodular sarcoidosis (subcutaneous nodules mimicking lipomas or cysts), lupus pernio (violaceous, indurated plaques on the nose, cheeks, ears, and fingers — the morphology most strongly associated with chronic, fibrotic pulmonary sarcoidosis and upper airway involvement), and scar sarcoidosis (infiltration and reactivation of old scars, tattoos, or sites of prior trauma). Less common presentations include ichthyosiform, psoriasiform, verrucous, ulcerative, hypopigmented (particularly in patients with deeply pigmented skin, where hypopigmented macules and patches may be the dominant finding), and erythrodermic sarcoidosis. Non-specific cutaneous findings include erythema nodosum (which, in the context of bilateral hilar lymphadenopathy and polyarthralgia, constitutes Lofgren syndrome — an acute, self-limited form of sarcoidosis with an excellent prognosis).

Systemic Correlation and Diagnostic Workup

The diagnostic evaluation of suspected cutaneous sarcoidosis begins with a skin biopsy demonstrating non-caseating granulomas, followed by special stains (Ziehl-Neelsen, GMS, PAS) and tissue culture to exclude infectious etiologies (mycobacteria, fungi), which is obligatory because infectious granulomatous diseases are histopathologically similar and require fundamentally different treatment. Once sarcoidosis is confirmed, systemic staging is essential because cutaneous disease correlates with specific patterns of organ involvement. The baseline workup includes pulmonary function tests with diffusing capacity (DLCO), chest imaging (chest radiograph for Scadding staging; high-resolution CT if abnormal), serum angiotensin-converting enzyme (ACE, elevated in approximately 60% of cases but neither sensitive nor specific), complete blood count (lymphopenia is common), comprehensive metabolic panel (hypercalcemia from granuloma-derived 1,25-dihydroxyvitamin D production), liver function tests, urinalysis, electrocardiogram, and ophthalmologic examination (uveitis occurs in 25 to 50 percent of sarcoidosis patients). Lupus pernio specifically warrants evaluation for upper airway involvement (nasal, laryngeal, sinonasal) and chronic pulmonary fibrosis. Serum ACE levels may be followed as a marker of granuloma burden during treatment but should not be used alone for treatment decisions because the correlation with clinical activity is imperfect.

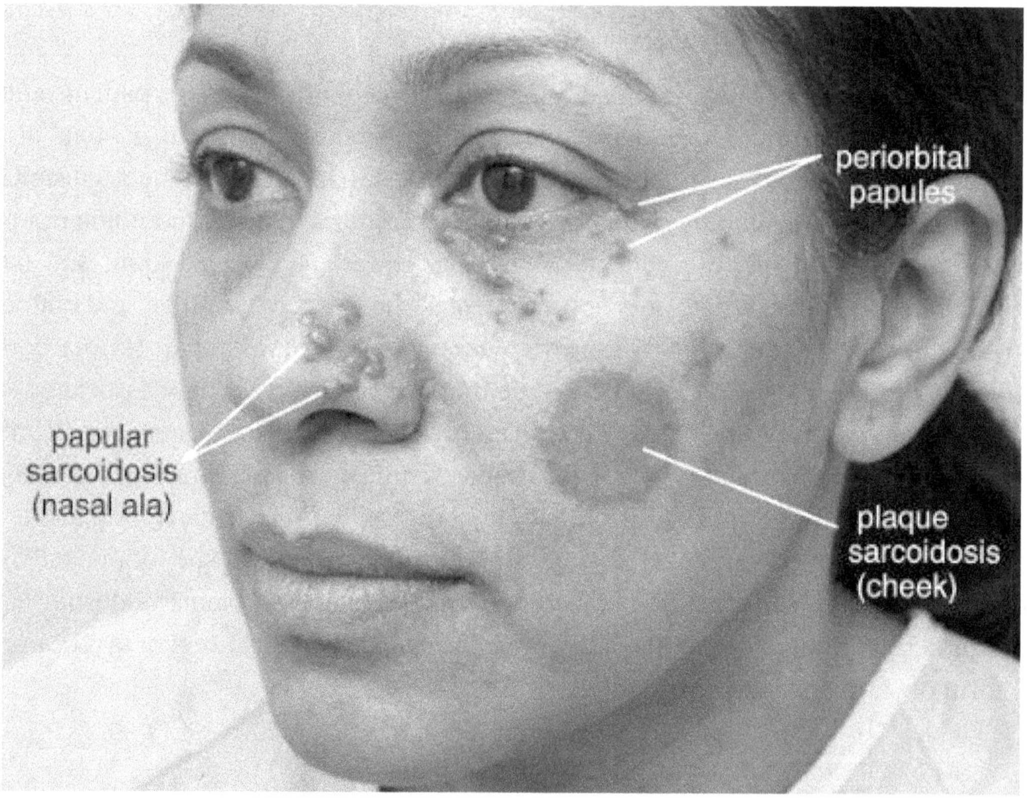

CLINICAL PEARL: Diascopy (pressing a glass slide against the skin) is a simple bedside test that aids in the clinical recognition of granulomatous dermatoses. In sarcoidosis, diascopy reveals an apple-jelly (brownish-yellow, translucent) color within the papules and plaques, reflecting the underlying granulomatous infiltrate. This finding, while not specific to sarcoidosis (it is also positive in lupus vulgaris and other granulomatous conditions), helps distinguish granulomatous lesions from non-granulomatous inflammatory dermatoses and should prompt a biopsy.

Granuloma Annulare and Necrobiosis Lipoidica

Granuloma Annulare: Clinical Variants and Pathogenesis

Granuloma annulare (GA) is a common, benign, self-limited granulomatous dermatosis characterized by palisading granulomas surrounding foci of altered collagen (necrobiosis) and mucin deposition in the dermis. The pathogenesis is incompletely understood but is thought to involve a Th1 cell-mediated immune response to an unknown trigger, with macrophage-derived matrix metalloproteinases degrading collagen and fibroblasts producing excess mucin. The classic localized variant (the most common, accounting for approximately 75 percent of cases) presents as flesh-colored to erythematous, annular plaques with a raised, beaded border and a flat or slightly depressed center, distributed on the dorsal hands and feet, elbows, and knees. The central clearing occurs because granulomatous inflammation resolves in the center while advancing peripherally. Subcutaneous (deep) GA presents as firm, painless, skin-colored nodules on the lower extremities, scalp, and hands — most common in children, where it may be confused with rheumatoid nodules. Generalized GA (disseminated, with numerous papules and plaques widely distributed on the trunk and extremities) is the variant most frequently associated with systemic disease, particularly diabetes mellitus, though the strength of this association has been debated and large epidemiologic studies have produced conflicting results. Perforating GA presents as umbilicated papules that extrude necrobiotic material through the epidermis, usually on the dorsal hands and fingers. The histopathologic hallmark of all GA variants is a palisading granuloma: histiocytes arranged in a palisade around a central zone of degenerated collagen and mucin (demonstrated by Alcian blue or colloidal iron staining). The dermis between granulomas shows increased interstitial mucin.

Necrobiosis Lipoidica: Clinical Features and Diabetic Association

Necrobiosis lipoidica (NL) is a chronic granulomatous dermatosis strongly associated with diabetes mellitus (approximately 65 percent of NL patients have diabetes, and an additional 10 to 15 percent have impaired glucose tolerance). The pathogenesis involves diabetic microangiopathy, immune complex-mediated vasculitis, and granulomatous inflammation around areas of collagen degeneration. The classic presentation is one or more well-demarcated, oval to irregular plaques on the bilateral pretibial areas (shins), with a characteristic evolution: early lesions are erythematous papules or plaques that evolve into waxy, yellow-brown, atrophic plaques with prominent telangiectasias and a violaceous, raised, active border. The center of established lesions becomes markedly atrophic, with the underlying vasculature visible through the thinned, transparent skin. Ulceration occurs in approximately 15 to 35 percent of cases, typically following minor trauma, and the ulcers are slow to heal due to the underlying microangiopathy and granulomatous inflammation. NL is distinguished from GA by its strong diabetic association, pretibial predilection, atrophic (rather than firm) center, visible telangiectasias, and ulceration tendency. Histopathologically, NL shows layered (tier-cake) granulomatous inflammation extending through the full thickness of the dermis and into the subcutis, with horizontal palisading granulomas alternating with zones of degenerated collagen — a layered pattern that distinguishes it from the focal, discrete granulomas of GA. Plasma cells and obliterative vasculopathy are characteristic of NL but not GA.

Complications, Prognosis, and Long-Term Monitoring of Necrobiosis Lipoidica

The long-term prognosis of NL is characterized by chronicity and recurrence: spontaneous resolution occurs in fewer than 20 percent of cases, and the majority of patients have persistent lesions over years to decades. Ulceration is the most significant complication, occurring in approximately one-third of patients, and the resulting wounds are notoriously slow to heal because the underlying granulomatous inflammation and microangiopathy impair normal wound repair. Secondary bacterial infection of ulcerated NL is common and may produce cellulitis, osteomyelitis (particularly over the tibial surface), or sepsis in diabetic patients with impaired immunity. Squamous cell carcinoma arising within longstanding ulcerated NL has been reported in rare cases, warranting biopsy of any non-healing ulcer that changes character. Patients with NL and concurrent diabetes mellitus require ongoing monitoring of glycemic control, peripheral neuropathy assessment (which compounds the risk of unrecognized wound progression), and vascular status evaluation. The cosmetic impact of NL is substantial — the yellow-brown, atrophic, scarred plaques on the anterior shins cause significant psychosocial distress, particularly in younger patients, and this aspect of disease burden should be addressed in management discussions.

Differential Diagnosis and Management of Palisading Granulomatous Dermatoses

The differential diagnosis of annular granulomatous lesions includes GA, NL, annular elastolytic giant cell granuloma (AEGCG, which presents as annular plaques on sun-exposed skin with elastolysis and multinucleated giant cells on histopathology), rheumatoid nodules (in patients with rheumatoid arthritis), and, importantly, tinea corporis — misdiagnosis of GA as tinea is common because both present as annular lesions with central clearing on the extremities, and a KOH preparation should be performed when clinical doubt exists. Sarcoidosis may also present as annular plaques. Management of localized GA is conservative because the majority of lesions resolve spontaneously within 2 years. For symptomatic or cosmetically bothersome lesions, potent topical or intralesional corticosteroids are first-line. For generalized GA, phototherapy (narrowband UVB or PUVA), dapsone, hydroxychloroquine, and TNF-alpha inhibitors have been used with variable success, though evidence is limited to case series and small trials. Management of NL is challenging: strict glycemic control does not reliably improve the skin disease, but it reduces the risk of progression and ulceration. Topical and intralesional corticosteroids suppress the active inflammatory border; calcineurin inhibitors (tacrolimus ointment) may be used as steroid-sparing alternatives; and compression therapy assists wound healing in ulcerated lesions.

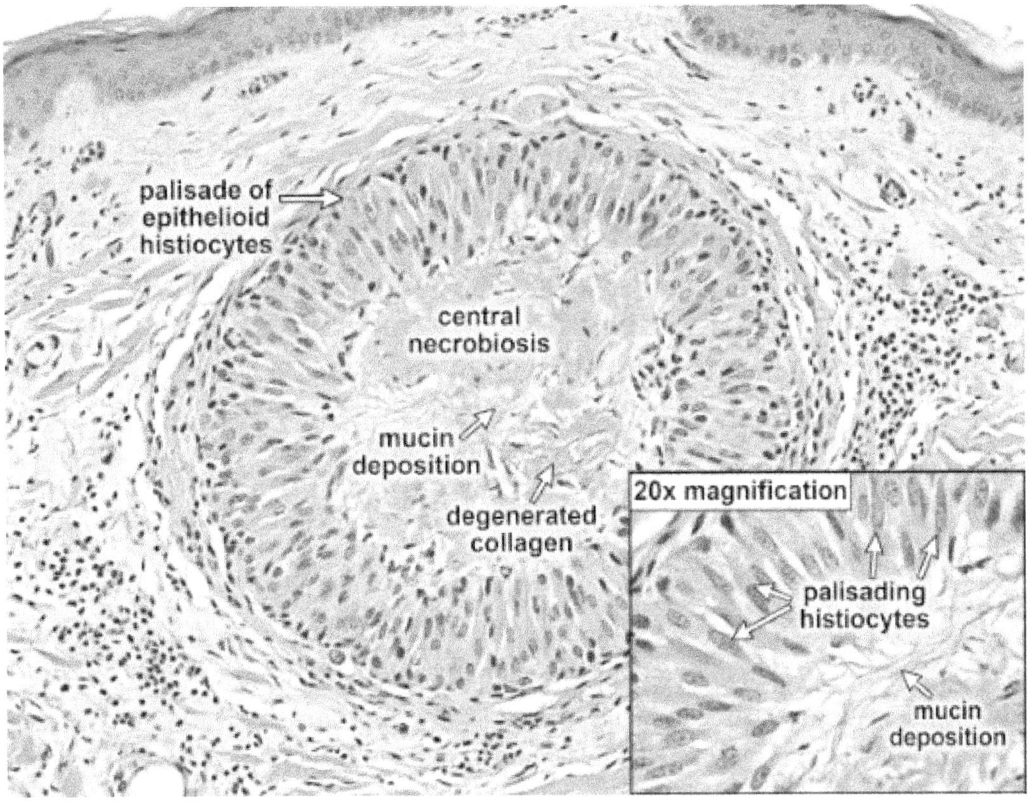

Foreign Body Granulomas and Infectious Granulomatous Diseases

Foreign Body Granulomas

Foreign body granulomas develop when the immune system encounters exogenous material that cannot be degraded by macrophage enzymatic machinery, triggering persistent granulomatous inflammation around the indigestible particle. Common causes include silica (from occupational exposure or road rash), talc (from surgical glove powder or intravenous drug use with crushed tablets), suture material, implanted medical devices, and cosmetic injectable fillers (silicone, hyaluronic acid, polymethylmethacrylate, calcium hydroxylapatite). Tattoo granulomas occur when pigment particles (particularly red pigment containing mercury sulfide, and more recently organic azo dyes) provoke an immune response — the granulomatous reaction may develop years after tattoo placement. The histopathology of foreign body granulomas shows multinucleated foreign body-type giant cells (with randomly scattered nuclei, unlike the peripheral ring of nuclei in Langhans giant cells) engulfing or surrounding the foreign material, which may be identifiable under polarized light (birefringent materials such as silica, talc, suture). The clinical presentation is firm, non-tender nodules or plaques at the site of foreign material introduction, and the temporal relationship to the inciting event (surgery, injection, tattoo, trauma) is the critical diagnostic clue.

Cutaneous Tuberculosis and Atypical Mycobacterial Infections

Cutaneous tuberculosis results from Mycobacterium tuberculosis infection of the skin, with clinical phenotype determined by the route of infection and the host immune status. Lupus vulgaris is the most common form in immunocompetent individuals in endemic regions: a chronic, progressive, red-brown plaque (classically on the face) with an apple-jelly appearance on diascopy, showing well-formed caseating granulomas on histopathology. Scrofuloderma develops by direct extension from an underlying tuberculous lymph node or bone, producing draining sinuses and ulcers. Tuberculosis verrucosa cutis (warty tuberculosis) is an exogenous inoculation form in previously sensitized individuals, presenting as a verrucous plaque on the hands or feet. Atypical (non-tuberculous) mycobacterial skin infections are increasingly common, particularly Mycobacterium marinum (fish tank granuloma: a nodular or sporotrichoid eruption on the hand or arm following aquarium or fish exposure), Mycobacterium chelonae and M. abscessus (rapidly growing mycobacteria causing post-procedural infections, injection site abscesses, and disseminated cutaneous disease in immunosuppressed patients), and Mycobacterium leprae (leprosy/Hansen disease, with its spectrum from tuberculoid to lepromatous forms). Tissue culture and molecular identification (PCR) are essential for species identification and antimicrobial susceptibility testing.

Deep Fungal Infections and Other Infectious Granulomas

Deep (systemic) fungal infections produce granulomatous inflammation in the skin and are particularly important in immunosuppressed patients and in endemic regions. Sporotrichosis (Sporothrix schenckii, acquired through plant-thorn or soil inoculation) classically presents as a lymphocutaneous pattern: an initial nodule at the inoculation site followed by a chain of nodules ascending along the lymphatic drainage (sporotrichoid spread). Histoplasmosis (Histoplasma capsulatum) and blastomycosis (Blastomyces dermatitidis) produce cutaneous lesions in the context of disseminated disease (papules, nodules, verrucous plaques, or ulcers) with granulomatous histopathology showing organisms identifiable on GMS or PAS staining. Coccidioidomycosis (Coccidioides immitis) produces granulomatous nodules, plaques, and abscesses; erythema nodosum in coccidioidomycosis, as in sarcoidosis, is a reactive (non-infectious) process indicating robust cell-mediated immunity. Leishmaniasis, a protozoal infection transmitted by sandfly bite, produces granulomatous papules, nodules, and ulcers at the bite site. The histopathologic approach to all infectious granulomas requires special stains (GMS, PAS for fungi; Ziehl-Neelsen, Fite for mycobacteria; Giemsa for Leishmania amastigotes), tissue culture, and increasingly molecular diagnostics. The key principle is that no granuloma should be assumed to be non-infectious without appropriate staining and culture — sarcoidosis remains a diagnosis of exclusion.

Amyloidosis, Mucinoses, and Cutaneous Depositional Disorders

Cutaneous Amyloidosis: Primary, Macular, and Systemic Forms

Cutaneous amyloidosis results from the deposition of amyloid — misfolded, insoluble fibrillar proteins arranged in a beta-pleated sheet configuration — in the skin. Primary cutaneous amyloidosis (localized to the skin without systemic involvement) has two main forms. Macular amyloidosis presents as rippled, hyperpigmented patches on the upper back (classically in the interscapular region), often intensely pruritic and associated with chronic rubbing or scratching (notalgia paresthetica is a recognized predisposing factor). The amyloid is derived from degenerated keratinocyte-derived keratin (amyloid K). Lichen amyloidosis presents as discrete, firm, pruritic, hyperkeratotic papules on the shins and extensor extremities, often arranged in a rippled or corrugated pattern. Nodular amyloidosis presents as waxy, smooth nodules or plaques, most commonly on the legs, trunk, or genitalia, with the amyloid derived from immunoglobulin light chains (amyloid AL) produced locally by dermal plasma cells — because the amyloid is AL-type, nodular amyloidosis carries a small risk (approximately 7 to 10 percent over follow-up) of progression to systemic AL amyloidosis, and long-term monitoring with serum free light chains and urine protein electrophoresis is recommended. Systemic AL amyloidosis (primary systemic amyloidosis, associated with plasma cell dyscrasias and multiple myeloma) produces characteristic cutaneous findings including periorbital purpura (raccoon eyes — the earliest and most specific skin finding), waxy papules and plaques (particularly on the eyelids, nasolabial folds, and perioral skin), macroglossia, pinch purpura (purpura at sites of minor trauma), and bullous lesions. Histopathologically, amyloid deposits appear as amorphous, eosinophilic material in the papillary dermis (in macular and lichen forms) or throughout the dermis and subcutis (in nodular and systemic forms), showing apple-green birefringence under polarized light after Congo red staining — the definitive histochemical test for amyloid.

Cutaneous Mucinoses

Cutaneous mucinoses are disorders characterized by excessive dermal mucin deposition (glycosaminoglycans, predominantly hyaluronic acid and dermatan sulfate, produced by fibroblasts). Pretibial myxedema (thyroid dermopathy) presents as flesh-colored to yellowish, non-pitting, indurated plaques on the pretibial areas and dorsal feet in patients with Graves disease — it is almost always associated with concurrent or preceding Graves ophthalmopathy and high levels of thyroid-stimulating immunoglobulins, which stimulate fibroblast glycosaminoglycan production via the TSH receptor expressed on dermal fibroblasts. Scleromyxedema (papular mucinosis) presents as a generalized eruption of firm, waxy, closely spaced papules (lichenoid papular mucinosis) on the face, neck, forearms, and hands, with diffuse skin thickening that produces a leonine facies and limited joint mobility. It is associated with an IgG lambda monoclonal gammopathy and carries a risk of internal organ involvement (neurologic, cardiac, pulmonary). Reticular erythematous mucinosis (REM syndrome) presents as reticular erythematous plaques on the central chest and back. Scleredema (scleredema adultorum of Buschke) presents as diffuse, symmetric, non-pitting induration of the upper back, neck, and shoulders, and is associated with diabetes mellitus (the most common association in adults), streptococcal infection, or monoclonal gammopathy.

Diagnostic Approach to Depositional Disorders

The diagnostic approach to cutaneous depositional disorders relies on the integration of clinical presentation, histopathology with appropriate special stains, and directed laboratory evaluation for associated systemic diseases. Congo red staining with polarized microscopy is the gold standard for amyloid detection. Alcian blue and colloidal iron staining at pH 2.5 identifies mucin deposition (distinguishing mucinoses from other dermal depositional processes). For suspected systemic amyloidosis, the workup includes serum and urine protein electrophoresis with immunofixation, serum free light chain assay, cardiac evaluation (echocardiography, NT-proBNP, cardiac MRI), renal function assessment, and often fat pad aspiration biopsy or bone marrow biopsy for tissue confirmation. For mucinoses, thyroid function tests (Graves disease for pretibial myxedema), serum protein electrophoresis (monoclonal gammopathy for scleromyxedema), and hemoglobin A1c (diabetes for scleredema) are directed by the clinical pattern. The key clinical question in any depositional disorder is whether the deposition is localized (a primary cutaneous process with generally favorable prognosis) or represents cutaneous involvement by a systemic disease (requiring multidisciplinary management and ongoing surveillance).

THE CUTANEOUS MIMICKER RECOGNITION ATLAS — Granuloma Annulare versus Tinea Corporis

The Clinical Pattern: Granuloma annulare presents as flesh-colored to erythematous, annular plaques with a raised, beaded border composed of firm, non-scaly papules and a flat or slightly depressed center. The surface is smooth and non-scaly. Lesions favor the dorsal hands, feet, elbows, and knees. The patient is often asymptomatic. The annular configuration with firm papular border and absent scaling is the clinical signature.

The Mimicker: Tinea corporis presents as annular, erythematous, scaly plaques with an active, raised, scaly border and central clearing. The key distinguishing feature is the presence of scale along the advancing border, which contains fungal hyphae identifiable on KOH preparation. Tinea may produce pruritus and a more inflammatory appearance. The annular shape with central clearing mimics GA closely when surface texture is not carefully assessed.

Trap Logic: Visual pattern matching to the annular shape without examining surface texture is the cognitive trap. Both conditions present as annular lesions with central clearing on the extremities, and clinicians may diagnose tinea based on morphology alone and prescribe antifungals — or, conversely, assume GA and withhold antifungals from a patient with actual tinea. The failure point is omitting the KOH preparation and the tactile examination: GA is firm and non-scaly (smooth surface), while tinea has a fine, adherent scale at the active border.

The Decision Anchor: The discriminating feature is **surface scale: tinea corporis has a scaly advancing border (KOH-positive); granuloma annulare is smooth and non-scaly (KOH-negative)**. Perform a KOH preparation on every annular lesion before assigning a diagnosis. If KOH is negative and the clinical suspicion for GA remains, a punch biopsy showing palisading granulomas with mucin confirms the diagnosis.

Xanthomas, Calcification Disorders, and Metabolic Deposition

Xanthomas: Classification and Lipid Correlation

Xanthomas are localized collections of lipid-laden macrophages (foam cells) in the skin and tendons, serving as cutaneous markers of underlying lipid metabolism disorders. The clinical morphology of xanthomas directly correlates with the specific lipoprotein abnormality. Eruptive xanthomas (crops of small, 1 to 4 mm, yellowish papules with an erythematous halo on the buttocks, shoulders, and extensor extremities, appearing rapidly over days to weeks) signal severe hypertriglyceridemia (triglycerides typically exceeding 1,000 mg/dL, approximately 11.3 mmol/L) and carry a risk of pancreatitis requiring urgent lipid-lowering therapy. Tuberous xanthomas (firm, yellowish nodules on the elbows, knees, and buttocks) and tendinous xanthomas (subcutaneous nodules within tendons, classically the Achilles tendon and extensor tendons of the hands) are associated with familial hypercholesterolemia (elevated LDL cholesterol due to LDL receptor mutations), indicating very high cardiovascular risk. Xanthelasma palpebrarum (soft, yellowish plaques on the medial eyelids) is the most common xanthoma; approximately 50 percent of patients with xanthelasma have normal lipid levels, but it is an independent cardiovascular risk marker regardless of lipid status. Plane xanthomas (flat, yellowish patches in the palmar creases — xanthoma striatum palmare — or generalized plane xanthomas) are associated with dysbetalipoproteinemia (type III) and, in the case of generalized plane xanthomas, with monoclonal gammopathy or multiple myeloma. A fasting lipid panel is mandatory for every patient presenting with any xanthoma type.

Calcinosis Cutis and Calciphylaxis

Calcinosis cutis is the deposition of calcium salts (calcium phosphate, hydroxyapatite) in the skin and subcutaneous tissue. The classification is based on pathogenesis: dystrophic calcification (the most common type, occurring in damaged or inflamed tissue with normal serum calcium and phosphate — seen in dermatomyositis, systemic sclerosis/CREST syndrome, panniculitis, and at sites of prior trauma or injection), metastatic calcification (deposition in normal tissue due to elevated calcium-phosphate product — seen in chronic kidney disease, hyperparathyroidism, hypervitaminosis D, and milk-alkali syndrome), idiopathic calcification (in the absence of tissue damage or metabolic abnormality — includes idiopathic scrotal calcinosis and subepidermal calcified nodule), and iatrogenic calcification (at sites of intravenous calcium gluconate or calcium chloride extravasation). Clinical presentation varies from firm, white or skin-colored papules and nodules to large, stony-hard subcutaneous plaques, sometimes with ulceration and extrusion of chalky white material. Calciphylaxis (calcific uremic arteriolopathy) is a distinct and life-threatening entity: mural calcification of small dermal and subcutaneous arterioles leading to thrombosis, ischemia, and necrosis, presenting as exquisitely painful, violaceous, reticulated (livedo) patches that rapidly evolve into necrotic eschars, most commonly on the thighs, abdomen, and buttocks of patients with end-stage renal disease on dialysis. Calciphylaxis carries a mortality rate of 60 to 80 percent, primarily from sepsis in the necrotic wounds. Management includes sodium thiosulfate (which chelates calcium and has anti-oxidant properties), wound care, and optimization of calcium-phosphate metabolism (discontinue calcium-based phosphate binders and vitamin D supplements, consider cinacalcet for secondary hyperparathyroidism). Non-uremic calciphylaxis, though rarer, occurs in patients with primary hyperparathyroidism, malignancy, warfarin use, or obesity.

Pathogenesis of Calciphylaxis (Calcific Uremic Arteriolopathy)

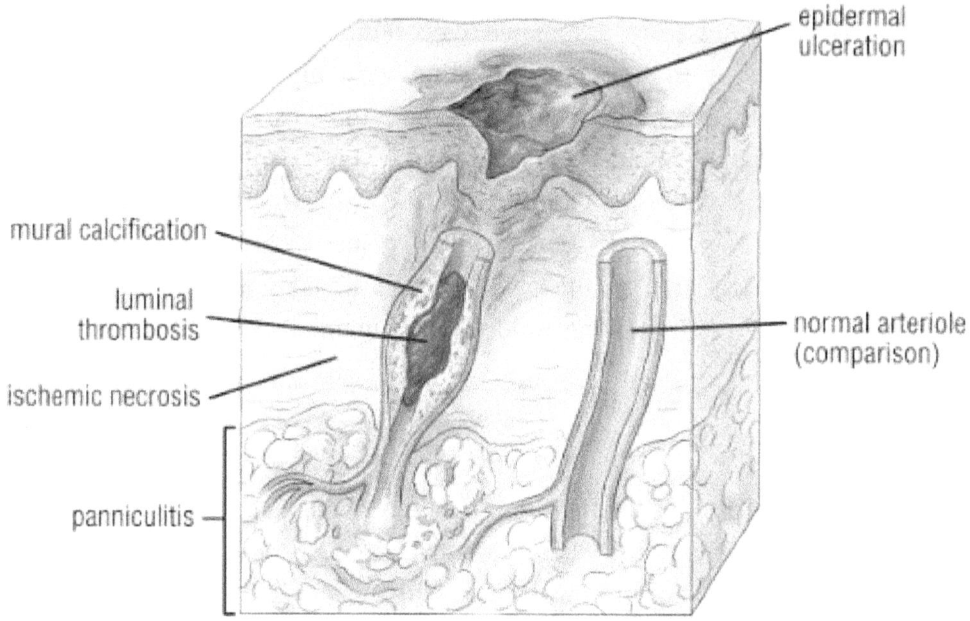

Clinical Case: Papular Eruption on the Face of a Young Woman

A 32-year-old African American woman presented with a 3-month history of asymptomatic, red-brown papules on her face, progressively increasing in number. She had also noticed mild dry cough and bilateral ankle swelling over the same period. Examination revealed approximately 20 firm, 2 to 5 mm, red-brown papules on the nasal ala, periorbital skin, and cheeks, with a few similar lesions on the nape of the neck. Diascopy showed apple-jelly discoloration. The clinical differential included cutaneous sarcoidosis, granulomatous rosacea, lupus vulgaris, foreign body granulomas, and secondary syphilis. A punch biopsy showed well-formed, non-caseating epithelioid granulomas with sparse peripheral lymphocytes (naked granulomas), multinucleated giant cells, and no necrosis. Special stains for acid-fast bacilli and fungi were negative, and tissue culture was sterile. These findings were consistent with cutaneous sarcoidosis. Systemic workup revealed bilateral hilar lymphadenopathy on chest radiograph (Scadding stage II), mildly reduced DLCO, elevated serum ACE, and hypercalcemia. Ophthalmologic examination detected asymptomatic anterior uveitis. She was started on oral corticosteroid therapy (prednisone, per weight-based protocol) with steroid-sparing transition to methotrexate, producing resolution of cutaneous papules and improvement in pulmonary function over 6 months. This case illustrates the importance of systemic staging in every patient diagnosed with cutaneous sarcoidosis, because subclinical organ involvement (pulmonary, ocular, cardiac) is common and may require treatment independently of the skin disease.

EVIDENCE: Infliximab (anti-TNF-alpha monoclonal antibody) has demonstrated efficacy in refractory cutaneous sarcoidosis in multiple case series and small trials, with particular benefit in lupus pernio and disfiguring nodular disease that has not responded to methotrexate or hydroxychloroquine. TNF-alpha is the central cytokine driving granuloma formation and maintenance in sarcoidosis, and its blockade disrupts the self-perpetuating inflammatory loop. Adalimumab has also shown efficacy. Paradoxically, TNF-alpha inhibitors used for other indications (rheumatoid arthritis, inflammatory bowel disease) have been reported to cause drug-induced sarcoidosis, predominantly etanercept — a finding attributed to the different mechanisms of action among TNF-alpha inhibitors.

CAUTION: Calciphylaxis (calcific uremic arteriolopathy) is a dermatologic emergency. The characteristic presentation — exquisitely painful, reticulated violaceous patches progressing to necrotic eschars on the thighs or abdomen of a dialysis patient — demands immediate recognition because delayed treatment increases mortality. A skin biopsy (punch or incisional, avoiding the necrotic center) showing arteriolar mural calcification with thrombosis confirms the diagnosis. Do not debride aggressively — surgical debridement of calciphylaxis wounds can extend the necrosis. Initiate sodium thiosulfate, optimize phosphate control, and pursue multidisciplinary management with nephrology, wound care, and pain management.

Metabolic Deposition and Gout

Gouty tophi are deposits of monosodium urate crystals in the skin and periarticular soft tissues, occurring in patients with chronic hyperuricemia and gout. Tophi present as firm, whitish-yellow nodules within or beneath the skin, classically on the ears (helix), olecranon bursae, fingers, toes, and Achilles tendons. The overlying skin may ulcerate, extruding a chalky, white, paste-like material composed of urate crystals. Histopathology shows amorphous, pale, eosinophilic deposits surrounded by a foreign body giant cell reaction — the crystals are dissolved during formalin fixation and appear as negative birefringent, needle-shaped crystals under compensated polarized light on fresh tissue or aspirated material. Ochronosis is a rare depositional disorder caused by accumulation of homogentisic acid in connective tissues (including the skin, cartilage, and sclera) in patients with alkaptonuria, an autosomal recessive deficiency of homogentisic acid oxidase. Cutaneous ochronosis presents as blue-black discoloration, particularly in the ear cartilage, nasal tip, and sclera. Exogenous ochronosis, produced by chronic topical hydroquinone use, is more common and presents as blue-black papules and hyperpigmentation in the treated areas — the paradoxical darkening produced by a bleaching agent, caused by dermal deposition of hydroquinone-derived oxidized polymers that resemble homogentisic acid histochemically.

Cardiovascular Risk Stratification and Screening

Because xanthomas are the visible cutaneous manifestation of an underlying lipid disorder — and because the specific xanthoma morphology predicts the lipoprotein abnormality and associated cardiovascular risk — every patient presenting with any xanthoma type requires a comprehensive cardiovascular risk assessment beyond the fasting lipid panel. Patients with tendinous xanthomas should be evaluated for familial hypercholesterolemia using validated clinical scoring systems (Dutch Lipid Clinic Network criteria, Simon Broome register criteria) and referred for genetic testing (LDL receptor, apolipoprotein B, PCSK9 mutations) because cascade screening of first-degree relatives identifies additional affected individuals who require early, aggressive lipid-lowering therapy to prevent premature cardiovascular events. The presence of xanthelasma, even in patients with normal lipid levels, is associated with an increased risk of myocardial infarction, ischemic heart disease, and cardiovascular death, and these patients benefit from global cardiovascular risk assessment (Framingham Risk Score, SCORE, or equivalent) with appropriate preventive interventions. For patients with eruptive xanthomas and severe hypertriglyceridemia, the immediate priority is pancreatitis prevention through urgent triglyceride-lowering therapy (fibrates, omega-3 fatty acids, dietary fat restriction, management of secondary causes including uncontrolled diabetes, hypothyroidism, and alcohol), followed by cardiovascular risk stratification once triglycerides are controlled.

Depositional Disorder	Deposited Material	Classic Cutaneous Presentation	Associated Systemic Disease	Diagnostic Test
Macular/lichen amyloidosis	Amyloid K (keratin-derived)	Rippled hyperpigmented patches (macular) or hyperkeratotic papules (lichen) — upper back, shins	None (primary cutaneous)	Congo red with apple-green birefringence
Systemic AL amyloidosis	Amyloid AL (light chain)	Periorbital purpura, waxy papules, macroglossia, pinch purpura	Plasma cell dyscrasia, multiple myeloma	Congo red; serum free light chains; SPEP/UPEP
Pretibial myxedema	Mucin (glycosaminoglycans)	Flesh-colored, non-pitting, indurated plaques on pretibial areas	Graves disease (with ophthalmopathy)	Alcian blue staining; thyroid function tests
Scleromyxedema	Mucin + fibrosis	Widespread waxy papules, skin thickening, leonine facies	IgG lambda monoclonal gammopathy	Alcian blue; SPEP with immunofixation
Xanthoma (eruptive)	Lipid (foam cells)	Crops of yellowish papules with erythematous halo — buttocks, shoulders	Severe hypertriglyceridemia (>1,000 mg/dL)	Fasting lipid panel

Xanthoma (tendinous)	Lipid (foam cells)	Subcutaneous nodules in Achilles and extensor tendons	Familial hypercholesterolemia	Fasting lipid panel; LDL receptor genetics
Calcinosis cutis (dystrophic)	Calcium phosphate	Firm white papules/nodules at sites of tissue damage	Dermatomyositis, systemic sclerosis, CREST	Radiograph; serum calcium/phosphate (normal)
Calciphylaxis	Arteriolar calcium + thrombus	Painful reticulated livedo → necrotic eschars — thighs, abdomen	End-stage renal disease on dialysis	Biopsy: arteriolar mural calcification + thrombosis
Gouty tophi	Monosodium urate crystals	Firm whitish-yellow nodules — ears, olecranon, fingers, toes	Chronic hyperuricemia, gout	Polarized light: negatively birefringent needle crystals

THE CUTANEOUS MIMICKER RECOGNITION ATLAS — Necrobiosis Lipoidica versus Granuloma Annulare

The Clinical Pattern: Necrobiosis lipoidica presents as well-demarcated, oval to irregular plaques on the bilateral pretibial areas with a characteristic progression: early erythematous papules evolve into waxy, yellow-brown, atrophic plaques with prominent telangiectasias visible through the thinned, transparent skin. The center is depressed and atrophic, and the border is violaceous and raised (active). Ulceration occurs in 15 to 35 percent of cases. The patient frequently has diabetes mellitus or impaired glucose tolerance.

The Mimicker: Granuloma annulare presents as flesh-colored to erythematous, annular plaques with a firm, beaded border and a flat or slightly depressed center — but the center is not atrophic, telangiectatic, or transparent. The surface is smooth and non-scaly. GA favors the dorsal hands and feet, elbows, and knees (less commonly the pretibial area). GA is not reliably associated with diabetes mellitus, the skin is firm rather than atrophic, and ulceration does not occur.

Trap Logic: Premature diagnostic closure based on annular morphology and pretibial location is the cognitive trap. When an annular plaque appears on the shin of a diabetic patient, both NL and GA are in the differential, and clinicians may assign the diagnosis based on the diabetic history alone (favoring NL) without assessing the qualitative features of the plaque center. The failure point is not examining whether the center is atrophic with telangiectasias (NL) or firm and non-atrophic (GA), because this single observation separates the two diagnoses at the bedside.

The Decision Anchor: The discriminating feature is **the quality of the plaque center: NL has an atrophic, transparent center with visible telangiectasias and a risk of ulceration; GA has a firm, non-atrophic center without telangiectasias and does not ulcerate**. Histopathology confirms: NL shows layered (tier-cake) granulomatous inflammation with plasma cells and obliterative vasculopathy extending through the full dermis; GA shows focal palisading granulomas with central mucin, confined to the superficial and mid-dermis. Biopsy is definitive when the clinical distinction is unclear.

Patient Education and Counseling

Patient education in granulomatous and depositional skin diseases varies by condition but centers on the relationship between the skin finding and the underlying systemic disease. Patients with cutaneous sarcoidosis should understand that the skin disease, while often the most visible manifestation, may indicate organ involvement elsewhere — and that ongoing systemic monitoring is necessary even when skin lesions improve. They should be counseled about sun protection (sarcoidosis lesions may be photosensitive or exacerbated by UV exposure) and vitamin D supplementation should be managed carefully because sarcoid granulomas produce 1,25-dihydroxyvitamin D, which can exacerbate hypercalcemia. Patients with NL require wound prevention counseling (avoiding leg trauma, wearing protective shin guards during activities), recognition of early ulceration requiring prompt medical evaluation, and understanding that glycemic control alone does not resolve the skin disease. Patients with xanthomas should be counseled that the skin lesions themselves are markers of an underlying lipid disorder that carries cardiovascular risk, and that adherence to lipid-lowering therapy and lifestyle modification addresses both the skin lesions and the cardiovascular risk — eruptive xanthomas resolve rapidly with effective triglyceride lowering, while tendinous xanthomas regress slowly over years of sustained LDL cholesterol reduction.

KEY POINT: Every xanthoma requires a fasting lipid panel because the xanthoma morphology predicts the underlying lipoprotein abnormality and determines cardiovascular risk. Eruptive xanthomas signal severe hypertriglyceridemia with pancreatitis risk (urgent treatment). Tendinous xanthomas signal familial hypercholesterolemia with very high cardiovascular risk (aggressive statin therapy and possible PCSK9 inhibitors). Xanthelasma is an independent cardiovascular risk marker even when lipid levels are normal. Palmar crease xanthomas are nearly pathognomonic for dysbetalipoproteinemia (type III hyperlipoproteinemia).

THE CUTANEOUS MIMICKER RECOGNITION ATLAS — Granulomatous and Depositional Diagnostic Arcs

---

Granuloma Annulare vs. Tinea Corporis: The discriminating feature is surface scale: tinea has a scaly advancing border (KOH-positive) while GA is smooth and non-scaly (KOH-negative). Always perform KOH preparation on annular lesions before assigning a diagnosis. Cognitive trap: visual pattern matching to the annular shape without examining surface texture or performing KOH preparation.

Necrobiosis Lipoidica vs. Granuloma Annulare: The discriminating feature is the quality of the plaque center: NL has an atrophic, transparent center with visible telangiectasias and ulceration risk; GA has a firm, non-atrophic center without telangiectasias. Histopathology confirms: layered (tier-cake) full-dermal granulomas with plasma cells and vasculopathy in NL versus focal palisading granulomas with mucin in GA. Cognitive trap: premature diagnostic closure based on annular morphology and pretibial location without assessing the plaque center.

Summary and Key Concepts

Sarcoidosis produces non-caseating (naked) epithelioid granulomas driven by Th1/Th17 immunity against an unidentified antigen. Cutaneous sarcoidosis manifests as papular, plaque, nodular, lupus pernio, scar, and other morphologic subtypes. Lupus pernio predicts chronic fibrotic pulmonary disease. Special stains and tissue culture to exclude infectious granulomas are mandatory before diagnosing sarcoidosis.

Granuloma annulare is characterized by palisading granulomas surrounding necrobiotic collagen and mucin. Localized GA is self-limited; generalized GA has a debated association with diabetes mellitus. Necrobiosis lipoidica is strongly associated with diabetes and produces atrophic, telangiectatic pretibial plaques that may ulcerate, distinguished from GA by the atrophic transparent center and full-dermal layered histopathology.

Foreign body granulomas develop around indigestible exogenous material identifiable on polarized light microscopy. Infectious granulomas (tuberculosis, atypical mycobacteria, deep fungal infections) require special stains, tissue culture, and molecular diagnostics for pathogen identification. No granuloma should be assumed non-infectious without appropriate workup.

Cutaneous amyloidosis (macular, lichen, nodular forms) is diagnosed by Congo red staining with apple-green birefringence. Nodular amyloidosis carries a risk of progression to systemic AL amyloidosis. Mucinoses (pretibial myxedema, scleromyxedema, scleredema) correlate with thyroid disease, monoclonal gammopathy, and diabetes mellitus, respectively.

Xanthomas are cutaneous markers of lipoprotein abnormalities — eruptive xanthomas signal severe hypertriglyceridemia with pancreatitis risk; tendinous xanthomas signal familial hypercholesterolemia with high cardiovascular risk. Calciphylaxis is a dermatologic emergency in dialysis patients requiring urgent sodium thiosulfate and multidisciplinary management.

CHAPTER 9: BACTERIAL SKIN INFECTIONS

Learning Objectives

1. Classify bacterial skin infections by depth and severity, from superficial pyodermas (impetigo, ecthyma) through deep soft tissue infections (cellulitis, necrotizing fasciitis), and select appropriate empiric antimicrobial therapy.
2. Recognize the clinical features and common mimickers of cellulitis and erysipelas, applying validated diagnostic criteria to distinguish true cellulitis from conditions that account for its misdiagnosis in up to 30 percent of cases.
3. Identify necrotizing soft tissue infections as a surgical emergency, applying the clinical features that distinguish necrotizing fasciitis from uncomplicated cellulitis and understanding that delay in surgical debridement increases mortality.
4. Distinguish staphylococcal scalded skin syndrome from toxic epidermal necrolysis based on the level of epidermal cleavage and the clinical context, and apply appropriate management for each.
5. Apply antibiotic stewardship principles in dermatology, selecting targeted narrow-spectrum agents when possible, limiting unnecessary antibiotic courses for inflammatory conditions, and recognizing the dermatologic consequences of antimicrobial resistance.

Impetigo, Ecthyma, and Superficial Pyodermas

Pathogenesis and Classification

Impetigo is the most common bacterial skin infection, predominantly affecting children, caused by Staphylococcus aureus (the dominant pathogen in most geographic regions) or Streptococcus pyogenes (group A Streptococcus, GAS), or both. The infection develops when bacteria colonize the skin surface and penetrate the stratum corneum through minor breaks in the epidermal barrier — abrasions, insect bites, eczematous skin, or macerated skin in intertriginous areas. Two clinical forms are recognized: non-bullous impetigo (the more common form, approximately 70 percent of cases) begins as erythematous macules that rapidly evolve into vesicles and pustules that rupture, leaving the pathognomonic honey-colored (golden-yellow) crusted erosions on an erythematous base, most commonly on the face (perioral, perinasal) and extremities. Bullous impetigo (approximately 30 percent of cases, caused exclusively by phage group II S. aureus producing exfoliative toxins A and B) presents as superficial, flaccid, thin-walled bullae containing clear yellow fluid on otherwise normal skin, primarily on the trunk and intertriginous areas in neonates and young children. The exfoliative toxins cleave desmoglein 1 in the granular layer of the epidermis, producing the same superficial plane of cleavage as pemphigus foliaceus — the toxin-mediated mechanism of bullous impetigo is the localized form of the same pathologic process that produces staphylococcal scalded skin syndrome when the toxin enters the systemic circulation.

Ecthyma and Differential Diagnosis

Ecthyma is a deeper form of pyoderma that extends through the epidermis into the superficial dermis, producing punched-out ulcers with thick, adherent, grey-brown crusts surrounded by a violaceous border, most commonly on the lower extremities. It typically follows untreated impetigo or develops de novo in immunocompromised patients or those with poor hygiene. Ecthyma gangrenosum, by contrast, is a distinct entity caused by Pseudomonas aeruginosa bacteremia (or other gram-negative organisms), presenting as hemorrhagic bullae that rapidly evolve into necrotic eschars with surrounding erythema — a cutaneous sign of disseminated Pseudomonas infection that requires urgent blood cultures and anti-pseudomonal antibiotic therapy. The differential diagnosis of impetigo includes herpes simplex (grouped vesicles on an erythematous base, distinguishable by Tzanck smear and viral PCR), contact dermatitis (pruritic vesicles with a geometric distribution suggesting external exposure), dermatophytosis (annular, scaly plaques, KOH-positive), and pemphigus foliaceus (which shares the superficial plane of cleavage but presents in adults with persistent, widespread erosions and positive DIF).

Management of Superficial Pyodermas

For localized non-bullous impetigo (fewer than five lesions, limited area), topical antibiotics are first-line: mupirocin 2% ointment or retapamulin 1% ointment applied three times daily for 5 days. For widespread impetigo, bullous impetigo, ecthyma, or impetigo failing topical therapy, systemic antibiotics are indicated — first-generation cephalosporins (cephalexin) or anti-staphylococcal penicillins (dicloxacillin) cover both S. aureus and GAS; in areas with high methicillin-resistant S. aureus (MRSA) prevalence, trimethoprim-sulfamethoxazole or clindamycin provides coverage, though clindamycin also covers GAS while TMP-SMX does not reliably cover streptococci. Wound care (gentle debridement of crusts with warm compresses, hand hygiene, avoidance of sharing towels and personal items) is an important adjunct. Post-streptococcal glomerulonephritis (PSGN) is a recognized complication of streptococcal impetigo (nephritogenic strains of GAS, primarily affecting children), developing 1 to 3 weeks after the skin infection; antibiotic treatment of the skin infection does not prevent PSGN (unlike treatment of streptococcal pharyngitis, which prevents rheumatic fever), but treatment reduces transmission of nephritogenic strains.

Cellulitis and Erysipelas: Diagnosis, Mimickers, and Management

Clinical Presentation and Distinction Between Cellulitis and Erysipelas

Cellulitis is an acute bacterial infection of the deep dermis and subcutaneous fat presenting as a rapidly expanding area of erythema, warmth, swelling, and tenderness, most commonly on the lower extremities. The borders of cellulitis are poorly defined (because the infection spreads through the deep dermal and subcutaneous tissue, where the advancing edge is not visible through the overlying skin). Erysipelas is a more superficial infection involving the upper dermis and superficial lymphatics, distinguished from cellulitis by its sharply demarcated, raised borders (reflecting the superficial plane of infection) and its predilection for the face and lower extremities. Erysipelas is almost always caused by GAS, whereas cellulitis is caused by GAS and S. aureus (including MRSA in appropriate epidemiologic contexts). Risk factors for lower extremity cellulitis include lymphedema, chronic venous insufficiency, prior cellulitis (which damages lymphatic drainage and predisposes to recurrence), tinea pedis (which provides a portal of entry), obesity, and leg edema from any cause. Systemic signs (fever, tachycardia, leukocytosis) accompany both conditions but are more pronounced in erysipelas.

Cellulitis Mimickers and Diagnostic Challenges

Cellulitis is misdiagnosed in approximately 30 percent of cases, and the conditions that mimic cellulitis (pseudocellulitis) account for a substantial proportion of unnecessary hospital admissions and antibiotic courses. The most common cellulitis mimickers include stasis dermatitis (bilateral, symmetrical erythema and edema of the lower legs with chronic venous insufficiency findings — hemosiderin staining, varicose veins, lipodermatosclerosis — that is often treated as recurrent bilateral cellulitis despite the fact that bilateral cellulitis is rare), contact dermatitis (pruritic erythema with vesicles in a geometric distribution), deep venous thrombosis (unilateral leg swelling and erythema, differentiated by Doppler ultrasonography), erythema migrans of early Lyme disease (expanding erythematous patch with central clearing and tick exposure history), gout and acute crystalline arthropathy (periarticular erythema and swelling over a joint), lipodermatosclerosis (acute phase with tender, indurated, erythematous plaque on the medial lower leg), and inflammatory breast carcinoma (mimicking breast cellulitis). The ALT-70 score (a clinical prediction tool based on asymmetric involvement, leukocytosis, tachycardia, and age over 70) has been validated to help distinguish true cellulitis from its mimickers, though clinical judgment remains paramount.

CLINICAL PEARL: Bilateral lower extremity cellulitis is exceptionally rare because cellulitis is a unilateral infection entering through a breach in the skin barrier. When both legs are red, warm, swollen, and tender, the diagnosis is almost always stasis dermatitis, not cellulitis. Stasis dermatitis is treated with compression, emollients, and topical corticosteroids — not antibiotics. Recognizing this pattern prevents unnecessary antibiotic exposure and addresses the actual underlying pathology.

Clinical Case: Recurrent Bilateral Leg Erythema

A 68-year-old woman with a history of obesity, bilateral varicose veins, and chronic lower extremity edema presented to the emergency department for the fourth time in 6 months with bilateral lower leg erythema. Each prior visit resulted in a diagnosis of cellulitis and a 10-day course of cephalexin, with perceived improvement. On examination, both lower legs showed symmetric, poorly demarcated erythema extending from the ankles to mid-calf, with pitting edema, prominent varicose veins, brownish hemosiderin staining around the medial malleoli, mild scaling, and lipodermatosclerosis (inverted champagne-bottle narrowing of the distal leg). No warmth differential between involved and uninvolved skin was noted. Temperature was 36.8°C, and white blood cell count was normal. There were no portals of entry — interdigital spaces were intact without tinea pedis. The bilateral, symmetric, chronic nature of the erythema, the absence of systemic signs, the hemosiderin deposition, and the lipodermatosclerosis were all consistent with bilateral chronic stasis dermatitis, not cellulitis. The prior perceived antibiotic responses reflected the natural fluctuation of stasis dermatitis (which worsens with prolonged standing and improves with rest and elevation — which typically coincides with the antibiotic course). She was started on compression therapy (graduated compression stockings, 30 to 40 mmHg), mid-potency topical corticosteroid for the acute eczematous component, and emollients, with complete resolution of erythema at 4-week follow-up and no further emergency department visits for cellulitis over the subsequent year. This case illustrates how stasis dermatitis is one of the most commonly misdiagnosed conditions in emergency and urgent care settings, and how the pattern of bilateral, chronic, symmetric erythema with signs of venous insufficiency should trigger reassessment of the cellulitis diagnosis.

Evidence-Based Management

Empiric antibiotic therapy for non-purulent cellulitis (no abscess or purulent drainage) should cover beta-hemolytic streptococci and methicillin-susceptible S. aureus: oral cephalexin or dicloxacillin for outpatient management; intravenous cefazolin or nafcillin for patients requiring hospitalization. For purulent cellulitis (associated with abscess or purulent drainage, where MRSA is the likely pathogen), incision and drainage is the primary intervention for abscesses, with oral TMP-SMX or doxycycline for surrounding cellulitis. Duration of therapy is typically 5 to 7 days, extended to 10 to 14 days for slow-resolving infections. Patients with recurrent cellulitis (two or more episodes per year) benefit from prophylactic low-dose penicillin or erythromycin, concurrent treatment of tinea pedis and interdigital maceration (which eliminates the bacterial portal of entry), and management of lymphedema and chronic venous insufficiency.

Folliculitis, Furuncles, Carbuncles, and Abscesses

Pathogenesis and Clinical Spectrum

Folliculitis, furuncles, carbuncles, and cutaneous abscesses represent a spectrum of follicular and perifollicular infections of increasing depth and severity. Superficial folliculitis (Bockhart impetigo) presents as small, dome-shaped pustules at the follicular ostia, each pierced by a hair, most commonly on the scalp, extremities, buttocks, and areas of friction or occlusion. The dominant pathogen is S. aureus. Hot tub folliculitis (caused by Pseudomonas aeruginosa) produces pruritic follicular papules and pustules on areas covered by the bathing suit, developing 8 to 48 hours after exposure to contaminated water. Gram-negative folliculitis (caused by Klebsiella, Enterobacter, or Proteus) occurs in patients on long-term oral antibiotic therapy for acne. Pityrosporum folliculitis (Malassezia folliculitis) presents as pruritic, monomorphous follicular papules and pustules on the trunk, often misdiagnosed as acne — the monomorphous appearance, truncal distribution, pruritus, and failure to respond to standard acne therapy are clinical clues.

Furuncles, Carbuncles, and Abscess Management

A furuncle (boil) is a deep follicular infection extending into the surrounding dermis and subcutis, presenting as a tender, erythematous, fluctuant nodule with a central pustule or necrotic plug. Furuncles most commonly develop on hair-bearing areas subject to friction and moisture: the neck, axillae, groin, buttocks, and inner thighs. Community-associated MRSA (CA-MRSA) is the most common cause of skin abscesses and furuncles in the United States, and the USA300 strain (carrying the Panton-Valentine leukocidin virulence factor) predominates. A carbuncle is a coalescence of multiple furuncles forming a deep, multiloculated abscess with multiple draining sinuses, typically on the posterior neck or upper back. Management of skin abscesses follows a size-stratified approach: incision and drainage alone is adequate for most uncomplicated abscesses (less than 5 cm), because randomized trials have demonstrated that antibiotics provide only modest additional benefit when adequate drainage is performed. For abscesses larger than 5 cm, abscesses associated with surrounding cellulitis, immunosuppressed patients, or patients with systemic signs, adjunctive antibiotics (TMP-SMX or doxycycline for empiric MRSA coverage) are recommended alongside incision and drainage.

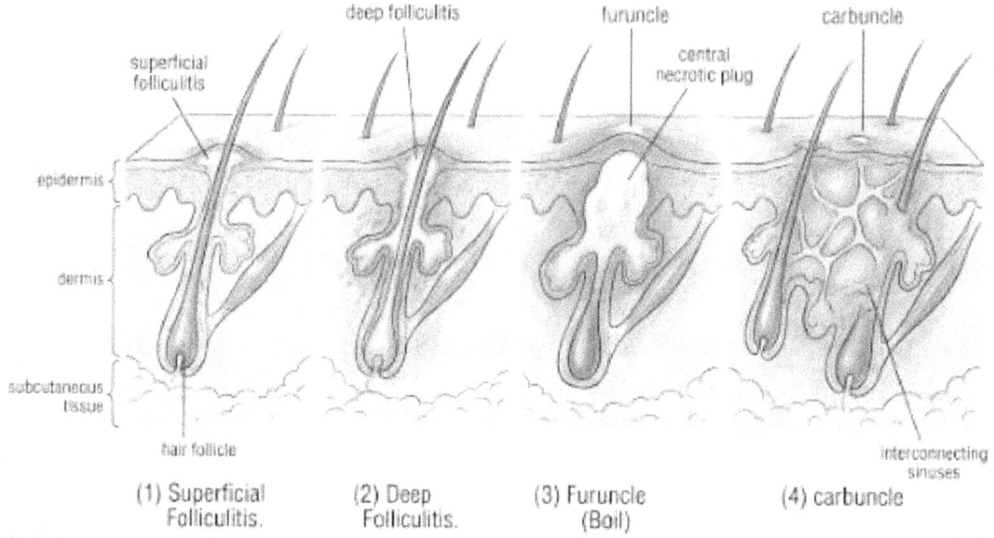

Necrotizing Soft Tissue Infections: Early Recognition and Surgical Emergency

Classification and Microbiology

Necrotizing soft tissue infections (NSTIs) are rapidly progressive, life-threatening infections of the skin, subcutaneous tissue, and fascia (and sometimes muscle) characterized by tissue necrosis, systemic toxicity, and high mortality (20 to 40 percent despite optimal management). NSTIs are classified by microbiology: Type I (polymicrobial, involving mixed aerobic and anaerobic organisms — the most common type, typically occurring in patients with diabetes, peripheral vascular disease, or following abdominal or perineal surgery) and Type II (monomicrobial, caused by GAS alone or in combination with S. aureus — the classic streptococcal necrotizing fasciitis, which can occur in young, otherwise healthy individuals). Fournier gangrene is a type I NSTI of the perineum and genital area, representing a surgical emergency. The tissue destruction in NSTIs is driven by a combination of bacterial toxin production (streptococcal pyrogenic exotoxins act as superantigens triggering massive cytokine release), thrombosis of nutrient vessels in the subcutaneous tissue (producing ischemia and anaerobic conditions that favor bacterial proliferation), and liquefactive necrosis of fascia and fat.

Clinical Recognition and the Diagnostic Window

The central clinical challenge in NSTIs is early recognition, because the skin findings may be deceptively mild in the early stages while the fascial necrosis spreads rapidly in the deep tissue planes. Early NSTI may present as a cellulitis-like picture — erythema, swelling, warmth, tenderness — but several features should raise suspicion for NSTI over uncomplicated cellulitis: pain disproportionate to the clinical findings (the hallmark early sign — the patient describes excruciating pain while the skin looks only mildly erythematous), rapid progression over hours (cellulitis typically evolves over days), systemic toxicity (high fever, tachycardia, hypotension, altered mental status) early in the course, and failure to respond to appropriate intravenous antibiotics within 24 to 48 hours. Late findings include crepitus (gas in the subcutaneous tissue, indicating anaerobic infection), hemorrhagic bullae, grey-purple or dusky skin discoloration (reflecting underlying tissue necrosis and thrombosis), cutaneous anesthesia (due to destruction of cutaneous nerves), and frank gangrene. The LRINEC (Laboratory Risk Indicator for Necrotizing Fasciitis) score uses laboratory values (CRP, white blood cell count, hemoglobin, sodium, creatinine, glucose) to stratify risk, though its sensitivity is imperfect and clinical suspicion must override a low score.

CAUTION: Pain disproportionate to the visible skin findings is the earliest and most important clinical clue to necrotizing fasciitis. A patient with severe, escalating pain over an area that appears only mildly erythematous should be treated as a surgical emergency until proven otherwise. The definitive diagnosis is made in the operating room (dishwater-grey necrotic fascia that separates easily from the underlying muscle with blunt dissection, absence of bleeding from the necrotic tissue). Imaging (CT showing fascial thickening and gas) may support the diagnosis but must not delay surgical exploration when clinical suspicion is high.

Complications and Long-Term Sequelae

Survivors of NSTIs face significant long-term morbidity. The extensive tissue loss from debridement frequently requires complex reconstructive procedures (split-thickness skin grafts, rotational flaps, free tissue transfer) and prolonged wound care. Functional impairment — including limb contractures, chronic pain, sensory deficits, and amputation — is common, particularly when NSTIs involve the extremities or perineum. Fournier gangrene survivors may require colostomy, urinary diversion, and genital reconstruction. Psychological sequelae are pervasive: post-traumatic stress disorder, depression, body image disturbance, and chronic pain syndromes are reported in the majority of NSTI survivors and warrant formal psychiatric and psychological support as part of the multidisciplinary rehabilitation program. Long-term surveillance for secondary complications including chronic osteomyelitis (if debridement extended to bone), heterotopic ossification, and wound-related squamous cell carcinoma (Marjolin ulcer in chronic non-healing wounds) is recommended.

Surgical and Medical Management

Aggressive surgical debridement of all necrotic tissue is the cornerstone of NSTI management — every hour of delay in surgical intervention increases mortality. Debridement is continued until only viable, bleeding tissue remains, and re-exploration at 24 to 48 hours is standard because necrosis often extends beyond the initial debridement margins. Empiric broad-spectrum antibiotic therapy covering gram-positive organisms (including MRSA), gram-negative organisms, and anaerobes is initiated immediately (vancomycin or linezolid plus a carbapenem or piperacillin-tazobactam, with the addition of clindamycin for its anti-toxin properties — clindamycin inhibits bacterial protein synthesis and suppresses the production of streptococcal and staphylococcal exotoxins). Intravenous immunoglobulin (IVIG) may be considered as adjunctive therapy in streptococcal toxic shock syndrome. Hemodynamic resuscitation, intensive care monitoring, and nutritional support are essential. Reconstructive surgery (skin grafting, flap closure) is performed after the infection is controlled and the wound bed is clean.

Staphylococcal Scalded Skin Syndrome and Toxic Shock Syndrome

Staphylococcal Scalded Skin Syndrome

Staphylococcal scalded skin syndrome (SSSS) is a toxin-mediated disease caused by exfoliative toxins (ET-A and ET-B) produced by S. aureus phage group II at a distant infection site (conjunctivitis, otitis media, nasopharyngeal colonization, umbilical stump infection in neonates). The exfoliative toxins are serine proteases that cleave desmoglein 1 specifically in the granular layer of the epidermis, producing generalized superficial epidermal separation — the same molecular target as in bullous impetigo and pemphigus foliaceus, but in SSSS the toxin enters the systemic circulation and causes widespread rather than localized cleavage. SSSS predominantly affects neonates and children under 5 years (who lack anti-exfoliative toxin antibodies and have immature renal clearance of the toxin). The clinical presentation begins with diffuse, tender erythema (the scalded appearance), followed by formation of flaccid blisters and large sheets of superficial epidermal detachment with a positive Nikolsky sign. The blistering is superficial (within the epidermis), so the exposed surface is moist and glistening but does not show the deeper, grey, necrotic wound base seen in toxic epidermal necrolysis (TEN). Perioral radial fissuring and crusting are characteristic. SSSS in adults is rare and occurs almost exclusively in patients with renal insufficiency (impaired toxin clearance) or immunosuppression.

Toxic Shock Syndrome

Toxic shock syndrome (TSS) is a superantigen-mediated multisystem disease caused by S. aureus (toxic shock syndrome toxin-1, TSST-1) or GAS (streptococcal pyrogenic exotoxins). Staphylococcal TSS presents with abrupt onset of high fever, diffuse macular erythroderma (sunburn-like rash), hypotension, and multiorgan involvement (diarrhea, myalgias, confusion, renal and hepatic dysfunction), followed by characteristic desquamation (full-thickness peeling) of the palms and soles 1 to 2 weeks after onset. Originally associated with superabsorbent tampon use (menstrual TSS), staphylococcal TSS now occurs equally in non-menstrual settings — wound infections, surgical sites, nasal packing, and soft tissue abscesses. Streptococcal TSS is associated with invasive GAS infections (necrotizing fasciitis, bacteremia) and carries a higher mortality rate (30 to 70 percent) than staphylococcal TSS (less than 5 percent with treatment). Management includes hemodynamic resuscitation, source control (removal of tampons, foreign bodies, or debridement of infected wounds), anti-staphylococcal antibiotics (nafcillin or vancomycin) with clindamycin (to suppress toxin production), and IVIG for refractory cases.

THE CUTANEOUS MIMICKER RECOGNITION ATLAS — Staphylococcal Scalded Skin Syndrome versus Toxic Epidermal Necrolysis

---

The Clinical Pattern: Staphylococcal scalded skin syndrome presents in neonates and young children with diffuse, tender erythema followed by superficial epidermal separation and flaccid blistering. The Nikolsky sign is positive. The exposed surface is moist and glistening without grey necrosis. Perioral radial fissuring is characteristic. Mucous membranes are spared. The biopsy site (or a frozen section of the blister roof) shows a superficial, subcorneal/intragranular plane of cleavage within the epidermis.

The Mimicker: Toxic epidermal necrolysis presents in adults (most commonly) with widespread erythema followed by full-thickness epidermal necrosis and sheet-like detachment. The Nikolsky sign is positive. The exposed wound surface is deeper, grey-purple, and weeping, resembling a full-thickness burn. Mucous membrane involvement (oral, ocular, genital) is present in over 90 percent of cases. TEN is drug-induced (sulfonamides, anticonvulsants, allopurinol, NSAIDs, antibiotics) in most cases. Biopsy shows full-thickness epidermal necrosis with subepidermal cleavage at the dermoepidermal junction.

Trap Logic: Assuming drug-induced TEN in any patient with widespread epidermal detachment, without considering SSSS based on age and biopsy is the cognitive trap. In a child under 5 with diffuse erythema and superficial peeling, SSSS is far more likely than TEN, and the management is fundamentally different — SSSS is treated with anti-staphylococcal antibiotics (not drug withdrawal), and the prognosis is excellent with mortality under 5 percent. In adults, SSSS is rare but occurs in renal failure patients and must still be considered. The reverse trap is assuming SSSS in an adolescent or adult who actually has TEN, delaying drug withdrawal and supportive care.

The Decision Anchor: The discriminating test is the **level of epidermal cleavage: SSSS cleaves within the granular layer (superficial, subcorneal — the blister roof contains the full epidermis below the granular layer); TEN cleaves at the dermoepidermal junction (full-thickness — the blister roof is the entire necrotic epidermis)**. A frozen section of the blister roof provides the answer within minutes and guides immediate management. Clinical clues: SSSS spares mucous membranes and occurs in children; TEN involves mucous membranes and is drug-induced. Both are dermatologic emergencies, but their treatments differ fundamentally.

Mycobacterial Skin Infections: Tuberculosis Cutis, Nontuberculous Mycobacteria, and Leprosy

Cutaneous Tuberculosis

Cutaneous tuberculosis encompasses a spectrum of clinical presentations determined by the route of infection and the host immune response. Lupus vulgaris is the most common form in immunocompetent patients, presenting as a slowly progressive, red-brown plaque on the head and neck with apple-jelly nodules on diascopy, showing well-formed caseating granulomas on histopathology; untreated, it may cause extensive disfigurement over years. Scrofuloderma presents as bluish-red nodules that break down into draining sinuses and undermined ulcers overlying infected lymph nodes (cervical, axillary) or bones, representing direct extension from deep tuberculous foci. Warty tuberculosis (tuberculosis verrucosa cutis) presents as a verrucous plaque on the hand or foot following exogenous inoculation in previously sensitized individuals. The tuberculid reactions (papulonecrotic tuberculid, erythema induratum/Bazin disease) are hypersensitivity reactions to M. tuberculosis antigens in patients with strong immunity, and the skin lesions are paucibacillary or culture-negative. Diagnosis relies on clinical presentation, histopathology (caseating granulomas), tissue culture (gold standard but slow — 4 to 8 weeks), and PCR for M. tuberculosis DNA. Treatment follows standard multidrug anti-tuberculosis regimens.

EVIDENCE: A landmark randomized controlled trial (Talan et al., 2016, NEJM) demonstrated that trimethoprim-sulfamethoxazole combined with incision and drainage of skin abscesses significantly increased cure rates compared with incision and drainage plus placebo (80.5% vs. 73.6%), with the benefit most pronounced for abscesses larger than 5 cm and those with surrounding cellulitis. This trial provided the evidence base for the current recommendation to add systemic antibiotics for larger abscesses while confirming that incision and drainage alone remains adequate for smaller, uncomplicated abscesses.

Nontuberculous Mycobacteria and Leprosy

Nontuberculous mycobacteria (NTM) produce a range of cutaneous infections. M. marinum (fish tank granuloma) presents as a solitary papulonodule at the inoculation site (hand, finger) following aquarium or marine exposure, sometimes with proximal lymphatic spread in a sporotrichoid pattern. M. chelonae and M. abscessus (rapidly growing mycobacteria) cause post-procedural wound infections, injection site abscesses, and disseminated cutaneous disease in immunosuppressed patients. M. ulcerans causes Buruli ulcer, an indolent, undermined ulcer with necrotic edges found in tropical and subtropical regions. Leprosy (Hansen disease, caused by M. leprae) presents along a clinical spectrum determined by the host immune response: tuberculoid leprosy (strong cell-mediated immunity) produces well-defined, hypopigmented, anesthetic patches with thickened peripheral nerves, while lepromatous leprosy (poor cell-mediated immunity) produces diffuse infiltration, nodules (lepromas), leonine facies, and widespread nerve involvement. Histoid leprosy presents as firm, dome-shaped nodules containing spindle-shaped bacillary-laden macrophages. Slit-skin smear with Ziehl-Neelsen staining and histopathology with Fite staining provide diagnostic confirmation. Multidrug therapy (dapsone, rifampicin, and clofazimine) is the standard treatment per WHO guidelines.

Leprosy Reactions and Their Management

Leprosy reactions are acute immunologic events that cause sudden worsening of clinical disease and are the primary cause of nerve damage and disability in leprosy. Type 1 reactions (reversal reactions) occur in borderline leprosy when a shift toward the tuberculoid pole produces a sudden increase in cell-mediated immunity: existing skin lesions become acutely inflamed, erythematous, and edematous, and peripheral nerves develop acute neuritis with pain, tenderness, and motor and sensory loss. If untreated, reversal reactions produce irreversible nerve damage within hours to days. Systemic corticosteroids (prednisone, tapered over months) are the cornerstone of type 1 reaction management. Type 2 reactions (erythema nodosum leprosum, ENL) occur in lepromatous and borderline-lepromatous leprosy and are mediated by immune complex deposition: crops of tender, erythematous nodules appear on the trunk and extremities, accompanied by fever, arthralgia, iridocyclitis, and orchitis. Thalidomide is the most effective treatment for ENL but is strictly contraindicated in women of childbearing potential due to teratogenicity; corticosteroids and clofazimine are alternatives. Both reaction types can occur before, during, or after completion of multidrug therapy — patients and clinicians must be aware that completed treatment does not eliminate the risk of reactions, and monitoring must continue for at least 2 years after treatment completion.

Sexually Transmitted Bacterial Infections With Cutaneous Manifestations: Syphilis and Gonorrhea

Syphilis: Protean Cutaneous Manifestations

Syphilis (caused by Treponema pallidum) is re-emerging globally and produces protean cutaneous manifestations across its clinical stages. Primary syphilis presents as the chancre: a painless, indurated, clean-based ulcer at the site of inoculation (genitalia, anus, oral mucosa), developing 10 to 90 days after exposure, with nontender regional lymphadenopathy. The chancre heals spontaneously in 3 to 6 weeks regardless of treatment. Secondary syphilis develops 6 to 8 weeks later with a widespread symmetric rash — the great imitator — that may present as copper-colored macules and papules (the classic roseola syphilitica), papulosquamous plaques mimicking psoriasis or pityriasis rosea, annular plaques, moth-eaten alopecia (patchy, irregular hair loss on the scalp), mucous patches (painless, greyish-white erosions on oral or genital mucosa), and condylomata lata (moist, flat-topped, grey-white plaques in intertriginous areas, highly infectious). The palms and soles are characteristically involved in secondary syphilis — palmoplantar involvement in a generalized rash should always prompt syphilis testing. Serologic diagnosis uses a two-step algorithm: nontreponemal screening tests (RPR or VDRL, which correlate with disease activity) confirmed by treponemal-specific tests (FTA-ABS or TP-PA). Treatment of primary and secondary syphilis is intramuscular benzathine penicillin G, a single dose for primary and secondary stages.

Disseminated Gonococcal Infection

Disseminated gonococcal infection (DGI) is the most common systemic complication of Neisseria gonorrhoeae infection, occurring in 0.5 to 3 percent of untreated mucosal gonococcal infections. The classic presentation includes the dermatitis-arthritis syndrome: scattered, few (typically fewer than 30), hemorrhagic pustules or papulopustules on an erythematous base, often with a grey necrotic center, distributed on the distal extremities (fingers, hands, wrists, feet); polyarthralgias or migratory polyarthritis; and tenosynovitis (particularly of the wrists and hands). The skin lesions are vasculitic in nature and contain N. gonorrhoeae DNA (detectable by PCR) even when cultures are negative. DGI must be distinguished from acute meningococcemia (which also presents with purpuric skin lesions but is more rapidly fulminant), infective endocarditis (Janeway lesions, Osler nodes), and reactive arthritis. Diagnosis is confirmed by nucleic acid amplification testing (NAAT) from mucosal sites (pharynx, urethra, cervix, rectum) and blood or joint fluid culture. Treatment is intravenous ceftriaxone (to cover penicillin- and fluoroquinolone-resistant strains) with concurrent treatment for chlamydial coinfection.

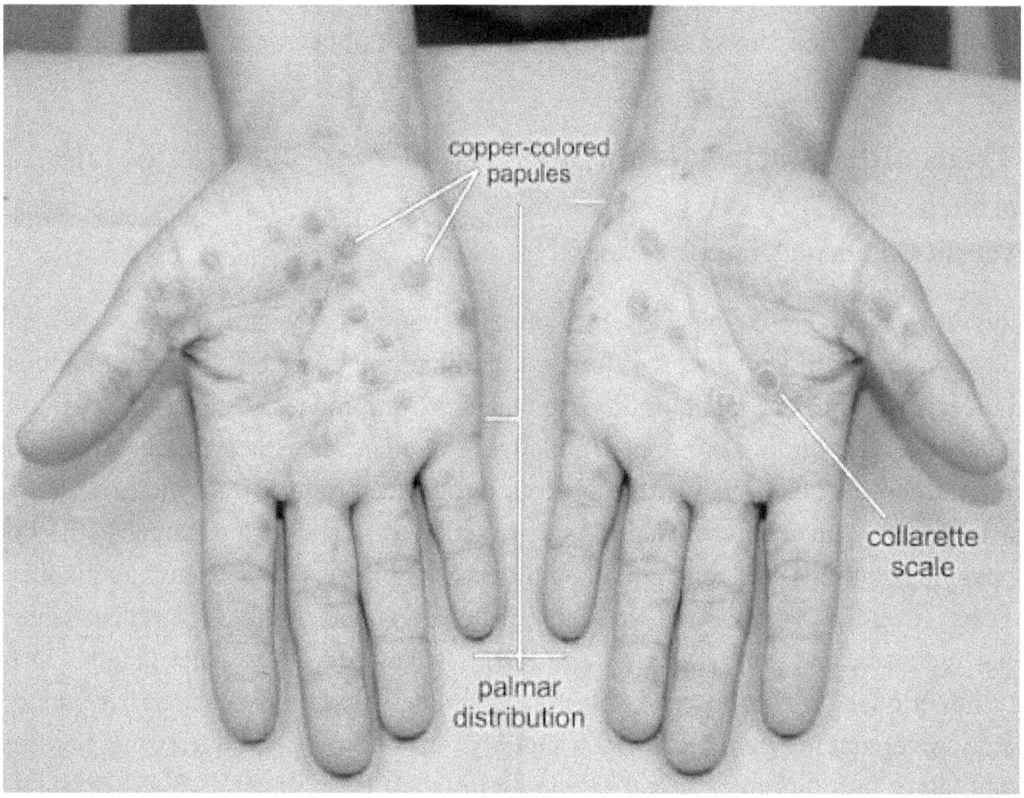

Patient Education and Screening

Patient education regarding sexually transmitted infections with cutaneous manifestations is an integral component of dermatologic management. Patients diagnosed with syphilis must be counseled about the mandatory reporting of syphilis to public health authorities, the necessity of partner notification and treatment (to interrupt transmission chains), and the importance of completing serologic follow-up after treatment (RPR or VDRL titers should decline fourfold within 6 to 12 months of adequate treatment for primary or secondary syphilis; failure to decline suggests treatment failure or reinfection). HIV testing should be offered to every patient diagnosed with syphilis or gonococcal infection, because these infections are markers of high-risk sexual behavior and because syphilis-HIV coinfection alters the natural history and management of both diseases. Screening for concurrent infections (chlamydia, hepatitis B, hepatitis C) is standard of care. Patients should be educated about condom use for prevention, the window periods of serologic testing, and the importance of early treatment to prevent complications — neurosyphilis, cardiovascular syphilis, and congenital syphilis in pregnant women are all preventable with timely penicillin therapy.

Antibiotic Stewardship in Dermatology

Principles and Dermatologic-Specific Concerns

Antibiotic stewardship in dermatology addresses the outsized contribution of dermatologic prescribing to overall antibiotic consumption — dermatologists prescribe antibiotics at higher rates per visit than any other outpatient specialty, primarily for acne vulgaris. Prolonged courses of oral antibiotics (tetracyclines, macrolides) for acne contribute to antimicrobial resistance in Cutibacterium acnes (previously Propionibacterium acnes), S. aureus, and GAS, with potential downstream effects on resistance patterns in non-dermatologic infections. Stewardship principles relevant to dermatology include using topical rather than systemic antibiotics when appropriate (for localized impetigo, mild folliculitis), limiting antibiotic duration to the shortest effective course (5 to 7 days for uncomplicated cellulitis, not 14 days), avoiding antibiotics for inflammatory conditions that do not require them (stasis dermatitis misdiagnosed as cellulitis, sterile inflammatory abscesses), and using non-antibiotic alternatives for acne (benzoyl peroxide, retinoids, hormonal therapy, isotretinoin) rather than chronic antibiotic courses. When oral antibiotics are necessary for acne, the course should be limited to 3 months and combined with topical benzoyl peroxide (which reduces resistance selection by killing bacteria through oxidative stress rather than a resistance-susceptible mechanism).

MRSA Decolonization and Prevention of Recurrent Skin Infections

For patients with recurrent S. aureus skin infections (furunculosis, recurrent abscesses), decolonization protocols reduce recurrence rates. The standard decolonization regimen includes nasal mupirocin ointment (applied to the anterior nares twice daily for 5 days), chlorhexidine or dilute bleach baths (one-quarter cup of household bleach in a full bathtub, soaking for 15 minutes twice weekly), and environmental decontamination (washing linens and towels in hot water, not sharing personal items). Household decolonization (treating all household members simultaneously) is more effective than treating the index patient alone, because household transmission of MRSA is a major driver of recurrence. Systemic decolonization with oral antibiotics (rifampin plus TMP-SMX or doxycycline) is reserved for cases failing topical decolonization.

THE CUTANEOUS MIMICKER RECOGNITION ATLAS — Cellulitis versus Stasis Dermatitis

The Clinical Pattern: Cellulitis presents as a unilateral area of erythema, warmth, swelling, and tenderness on the lower extremity, often with a portal of entry (interdigital tinea pedis, wound, or ulcer). Systemic signs (fever, leukocytosis) are typically present. The erythema has poorly defined borders and progresses over 24 to 72 hours. Lymphangitic streaking (red streaks extending proximally from the infection) or regional lymphadenopathy supports the diagnosis.

The Mimicker: Stasis dermatitis presents as bilateral erythema, scaling, edema, and hyperpigmentation of the lower extremities in the setting of chronic venous insufficiency. Hemosiderin staining (brown discoloration), varicose veins, and lipodermatosclerosis (inverted champagne-bottle deformity of the leg) are present. The erythema is chronic and relatively stable rather than acutely progressive. Fever and leukocytosis are absent. Pruritus is a prominent symptom (cellulitis is painful, not typically pruritic).

Trap Logic: Treating bilateral leg erythema as recurrent cellulitis without recognizing the chronic, symmetric pattern of venous disease is the cognitive trap. Patients with chronic venous insufficiency may present repeatedly to emergency departments with bilateral lower extremity erythema diagnosed as cellulitis and treated with antibiotics, leading to unnecessary antibiotic exposure, potential adverse effects, and failure to treat the underlying venous disease. The trap is reinforced when the patient reports improvement after each antibiotic course — which reflects the natural fluctuation of stasis dermatitis rather than genuine infection clearance.

The Decision Anchor: The discriminating features are **laterality (cellulitis is unilateral; bilateral leg erythema is almost always stasis dermatitis, not cellulitis), chronicity (cellulitis is acute and progressive over hours to days; stasis dermatitis is chronic and stable), signs of chronic venous insufficiency (hemosiderin staining, varicose veins, lipodermatosclerosis), and systemic signs (present in cellulitis, absent in stasis dermatitis)**. If both legs are red in a patient with varicose veins and hemosiderin staining, the diagnosis is stasis dermatitis — treat the venous disease, not the infection that is not there.

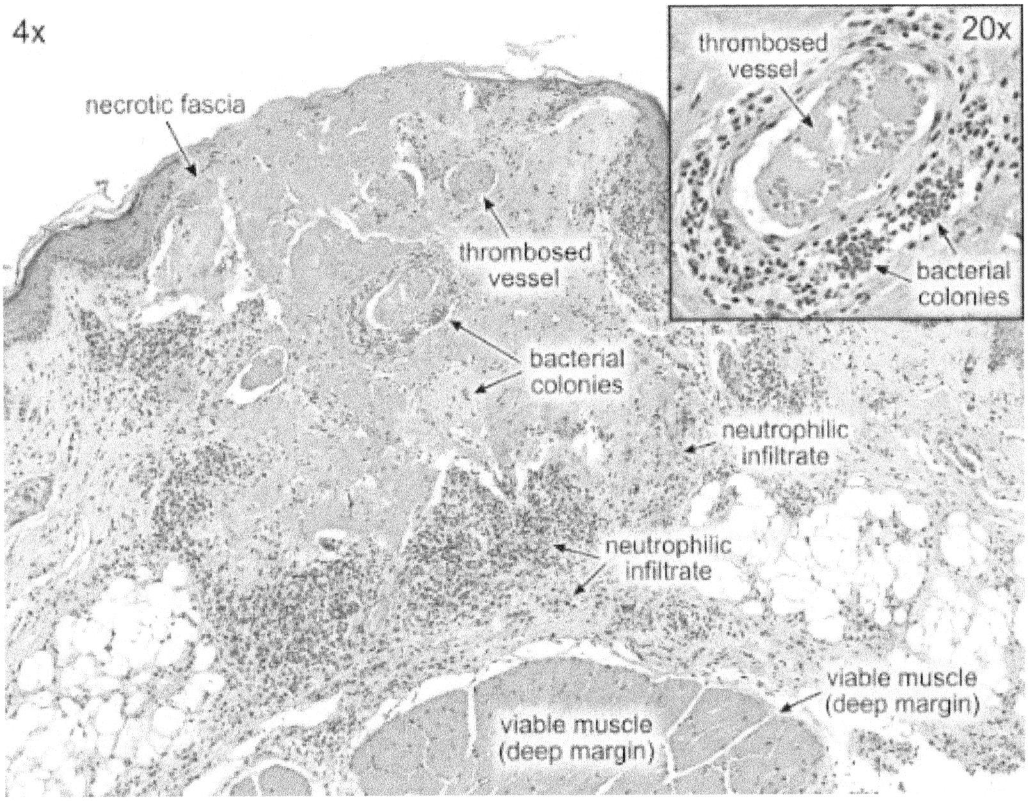

THE CUTANEOUS MIMICKER RECOGNITION ATLAS — Bacterial Infection Diagnostic Arcs

SSSS vs. Toxic Epidermal Necrolysis: The discriminating test is the level of epidermal cleavage: SSSS cleaves within the granular layer (superficial, subcorneal) while TEN cleaves at the dermoepidermal junction (full-thickness epidermal necrosis). A frozen section of the blister roof provides the answer within minutes. Clinical clues: SSSS spares mucous membranes and occurs predominantly in children; TEN involves mucous membranes and is drug-induced. Cognitive trap: assuming drug-induced TEN in any patient with widespread epidermal detachment without considering SSSS based on age and biopsy.

Cellulitis vs. Stasis Dermatitis: The discriminating features are laterality (cellulitis is unilateral; bilateral erythema is almost always stasis dermatitis), chronicity (acute progressive vs. chronic stable), signs of chronic venous insufficiency (hemosiderin staining, varicose veins), and systemic signs (present in cellulitis, absent in stasis dermatitis). Cognitive trap: treating bilateral leg erythema as recurrent cellulitis without recognizing the chronic symmetric pattern of venous disease.

Summary and Key Concepts

Impetigo is the most common bacterial skin infection, presenting as honey-colored crusted erosions (non-bullous) or superficial flaccid bullae (bullous, toxin-mediated). Bullous impetigo and SSSS share the same molecular target (desmoglein 1 cleavage by exfoliative toxins) but differ in whether the toxin acts locally or systemically. Ecthyma gangrenosum is a distinct Pseudomonas-associated entity requiring urgent systemic therapy.

Cellulitis is misdiagnosed in approximately 30 percent of cases. Bilateral lower extremity erythema is almost always stasis dermatitis, not cellulitis. The ALT-70 score and clinical features (unilaterality, portal of entry, systemic signs) help distinguish true cellulitis from its mimickers and prevent unnecessary antibiotic exposure.

Necrotizing soft tissue infections are surgical emergencies in which pain disproportionate to clinical findings is the earliest and most important clue. Every hour of delay in surgical debridement increases mortality. Empiric therapy includes broad-spectrum antibiotics with clindamycin for toxin suppression.

SSSS and TEN are distinguished by the level of epidermal cleavage: superficial (granular layer) in SSSS versus full-thickness (dermoepidermal junction) in TEN. A frozen section of the blister roof provides the answer within minutes. SSSS spares mucous membranes and occurs in children; TEN involves mucous membranes and is drug-induced.

Syphilis is the great imitator — secondary syphilis produces protean cutaneous manifestations. Palmoplantar involvement in a generalized rash should always prompt syphilis testing. Antibiotic stewardship in dermatology addresses the specialty's high prescribing rates, emphasizing topical alternatives, short courses, and non-antibiotic acne treatments.

CHAPTER 10: VIRAL SKIN INFECTIONS

Learning Objectives

1. Classify cutaneous viral infections by pathogen family and clinical presentation, distinguishing verrucae, condylomata, herpetic vesicles, varicella-zoster eruptions, poxvirus lesions, and viral exanthems by their morphologic and distributional features.
2. Apply the clinical and dermoscopic features that distinguish verrucae from other papillomatous lesions and identify high-risk HPV-associated lesions requiring surveillance for dysplasia and malignant transformation.
3. Recognize the clinical spectrum of herpes simplex and varicella-zoster virus infections, including atypical presentations in immunocompromised patients, and apply evidence-based antiviral strategies for treatment and prevention.
4. Identify the characteristic features of childhood viral exanthems and distinguish them from drug eruptions, bacterial infections, and other causes of generalized rash in pediatric patients.
5. Recognize HIV-associated dermatoses as potential markers of immunosuppression severity and apply the dermatologic findings that should prompt HIV testing in undiagnosed patients.

Human Papillomavirus: Verrucae, Condylomata, and Oncogenic Associations

Virology and Oncogenic Risk Stratification

Human papillomaviruses (HPVs) are a family of over 200 genotypes of small, non-enveloped, double-stranded DNA viruses with tropism for cutaneous and mucosal epithelium. HPV infects basal keratinocytes through microabrasions in the epithelial surface, and the virus persists in the basal layer where it hijacks the host cell replication machinery through the viral oncoproteins E6 and E7. HPV types are classified by oncogenic potential: low-risk types (HPV 6, 11) cause benign anogenital warts (condylomata acuminata) and respiratory papillomatosis but carry minimal malignant potential. High-risk types (HPV 16, 18, 31, 33, 45, and others) are causally linked to cervical, anal, penile, vulvar, vaginal, and oropharyngeal squamous cell carcinoma. Cutaneous HPV types (HPV 1, 2, 3, 4, 27, 57) cause common warts (verrucae vulgaris), plantar warts (verrucae plantaris), and flat warts (verrucae plana) — these types have low oncogenic potential except in immunosuppressed patients, where HPV 5 and 8 (epidermodysplasia verruciformis-associated types) can drive cutaneous squamous cell carcinoma in sun-exposed areas. The HPV vaccine (9-valent: HPV 6, 11, 16, 18, 31, 33, 45, 52, 58) prevents infection with the most important low-risk and high-risk types and has dramatically reduced the incidence of anogenital warts and HPV-associated dysplasia in vaccinated populations.

Epidemiology and Prevention

Cutaneous warts are among the most common dermatologic conditions, affecting an estimated 7 to 12 percent of the general population, with peak prevalence in school-aged children and young adults. Anogenital HPV is the most prevalent sexually transmitted infection worldwide, with an estimated lifetime acquisition risk exceeding 80 percent in sexually active individuals. The epidemiologic landscape has shifted substantially since the introduction of HPV vaccination: countries with high vaccine coverage have reported reductions of 60 to 90 percent in anogenital wart incidence among vaccinated cohorts, and emerging data demonstrate declining rates of cervical high-grade dysplasia and cervical cancer in vaccinated populations. Current guidelines recommend routine HPV vaccination beginning at age 9 to 12 years, with catch-up vaccination through age 26 and shared clinical decision-making for ages 27 to 45. Immunosuppressed patients — organ transplant recipients, HIV-infected individuals, and patients on chronic immunosuppressive therapy — carry markedly elevated risks of HPV persistence, treatment-resistant warts, and HPV-driven malignancies, necessitating enhanced surveillance with annual skin examinations and mucosal screening.

Clinical Presentation of Verrucae and Condylomata

Common warts (verrucae vulgaris, predominantly HPV 2 and 4) present as firm, dome-shaped, skin-colored to grey-brown papules with a rough, verrucous surface and characteristic thrombosed capillaries (black dots) visible within the wart. They favor the dorsal hands, fingers, and periungual skin, and spread by autoinoculation. Plantar warts (verrucae plantaris, HPV 1) present as endophytic, painful, hyperkeratotic plaques on the plantar surface of the foot, with black dots visible on paring (distinguishing them from calluses, which lack thrombosed capillaries and show a preserved dermatoglyphic pattern). Mosaic warts are coalescent clusters of superficial plantar warts. Flat warts (verrucae plana, HPV 3, 10) present as multiple small, 2 to 4 mm, flat-topped, skin-colored to slightly pigmented papules on the face, dorsal hands, and shins, often spreading in a linear pattern along scratch lines (Koebner phenomenon). Condylomata acuminata (anogenital warts, HPV 6, 11) present as soft, flesh-colored to pink, pedunculated papillomas in the anogenital region. Bowenoid papulosis (HPV 16) presents as pigmented papules on the genitalia that histologically show full-thickness keratinocyte dysplasia (Bowen disease pattern) — this is a high-risk HPV-driven in situ carcinoma that warrants close surveillance and treatment.

Dermoscopic Features and Differential Diagnosis

Dermoscopy enhances the clinical diagnosis of verrucae and helps distinguish them from other papillomatous or hyperkeratotic lesions. Common warts show a pattern of thrombosed vessels (appearing as red-to-black globules or dots arranged in clusters) against a white-to-yellow background of hyperkeratosis. Plantar warts show the same thrombosed vessel pattern plus loss of the normal dermatoglyphic lines across the lesion (whereas calluses preserve dermatoglyphics). Flat warts show a subtle pattern of tiny red dots in a regular arrangement. The differential diagnosis of verrucae includes seborrheic keratoses (stuck-on appearance, brain-like fissures on dermoscopy), squamous cell carcinoma (particularly for longstanding, solitary, or rapidly changing verrucous lesions — biopsy is indicated), amelanotic melanoma (which may mimic a verrucous papule on the foot), and corns/calluses (preserved dermatoglyphics, no thrombosed capillaries). Management options include destructive therapies (cryotherapy with liquid nitrogen, salicylic acid, electrosurgery, laser ablation), immunologic approaches (imiquimod, contact immunotherapy with squaric acid dibutylester), and intralesional therapies (bleomycin, Candida antigen injection), with selection based on wart location, size, patient age, and immune status.

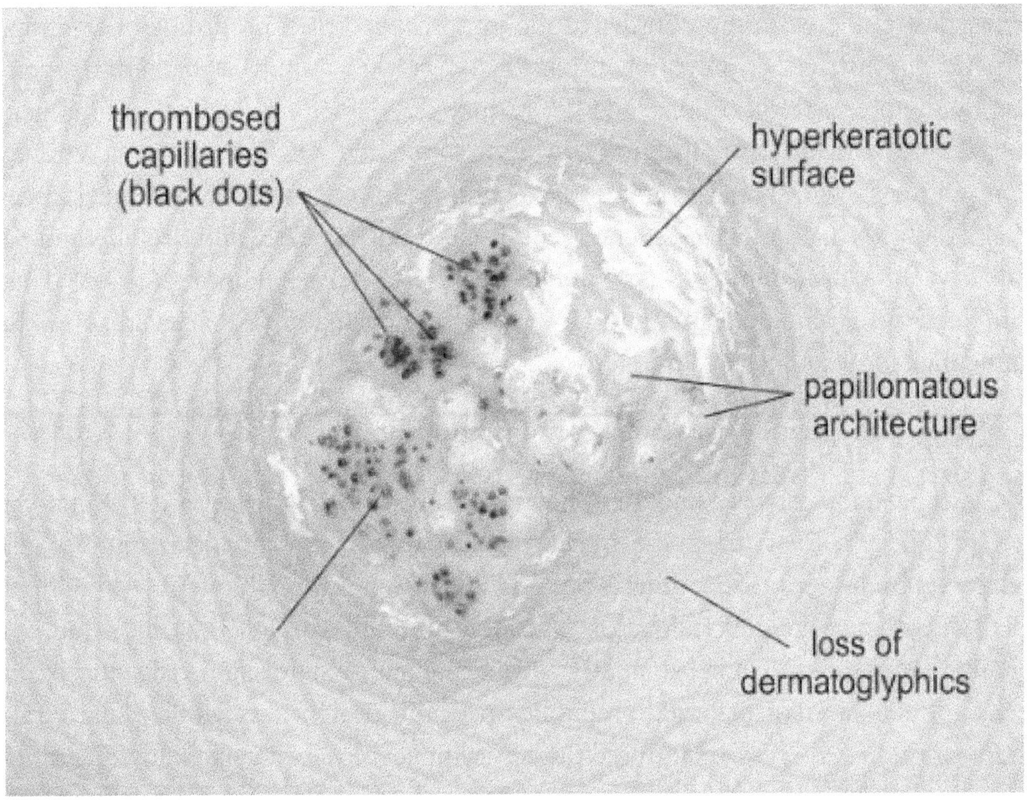

Herpes Simplex Virus: Orofacial, Genital, and Disseminated Infections

Virology, Latency, and Reactivation

Herpes simplex virus types 1 and 2 (HSV-1, HSV-2) are neurotropic alpha-herpesviruses that establish lifelong latency in sensory ganglia after primary infection. HSV-1 classically causes orofacial herpes (herpes labialis) with latency in the trigeminal ganglion, while HSV-2 classically causes genital herpes with latency in the sacral ganglia — though cross-infection is common and HSV-1 is now the leading cause of new genital herpes in young adults in many countries. Primary infection occurs through direct contact with infected secretions or skin and may be asymptomatic (the majority of HSV acquisitions) or symptomatic (primary herpetic gingivostomatitis in children, primary genital herpes in adolescents and adults). The virus infects epithelial cells, producing intraepidermal vesicles through ballooning degeneration and reticular degeneration of keratinocytes, then travels via retrograde axonal transport to the sensory ganglion where it establishes latency in neuronal cell bodies. Periodic reactivation produces anterograde viral transport back to the skin, causing recurrent vesicular eruptions at or near the site of original infection.

Clinical Presentations and Complications

Primary herpetic gingivostomatitis presents in children as multiple painful vesicles and erosions on the oral mucosa, lips, and perioral skin, accompanied by fever, malaise, and cervical lymphadenopathy. Primary genital herpes presents as painful, grouped vesicles on an erythematous base on the genitalia, perineum, or perianal skin, progressing to shallow, painful ulcers; dysuria, inguinal lymphadenopathy, and systemic symptoms are common in primary episodes. Recurrent herpes labialis (cold sores) presents as grouped vesicles on the vermillion border of the lip, preceded by a prodrome of tingling, burning, or itching. Herpetic whitlow (HSV infection of the distal finger) mimics a bacterial paronychia but is distinguished by the presence of vesicles and the history of contact with oral or genital herpes. Eczema herpeticum (Kaposi varicelliform eruption) is a disseminated HSV infection complicating atopic dermatitis, presenting as widespread monomorphous punched-out erosions and vesicles superimposed on eczematous skin — a dermatologic emergency requiring urgent systemic antiviral therapy because of the risk of viremia, systemic dissemination, and rarely encephalitis. Neonatal herpes (acquired during passage through an infected birth canal or, less commonly, in utero or postnatally) is a severe, often fatal infection requiring immediate intravenous acyclovir.

Special Populations: Pregnancy, Neonates, and Immunosuppression

Genital HSV in pregnancy carries critical implications for neonatal transmission. Primary genital HSV acquired near the time of delivery poses the highest transmission risk (30 to 50 percent) because the mother lacks protective antibodies, viral shedding is prolonged, and viral titers are high — cesarean delivery is recommended when active genital lesions or a positive viral culture are present at the onset of labor. Recurrent genital herpes carries a substantially lower neonatal transmission risk (approximately 1 to 3 percent) because transplacental maternal antibodies partially protect the neonate and viral shedding is shorter with lower titers. Suppressive antiviral therapy with acyclovir or valacyclovir starting at 36 weeks of gestation reduces the risk of clinical recurrence at delivery and lowers cesarean delivery rates. Neonatal herpes manifests in three patterns: skin-eyes-mouth disease (the mildest form, with vesicles on the skin, keratoconjunctivitis, and oral ulcers), central nervous system disease (encephalitis with seizures and lethargy), and disseminated disease (multi-organ involvement with hepatitis, pneumonitis, and disseminated intravascular coagulation, carrying the highest mortality). In immunocompromised patients, HSV produces chronic, non-healing ulcerations (lasting more than one month — an AIDS-defining condition), verrucous or hypertrophic HSV lesions that mimic squamous cell carcinoma, and acyclovir-resistant infection requiring foscarnet or cidofovir.

KEY POINT: Eczema herpeticum is a dermatologic emergency. The clinical clue is the sudden appearance of monomorphous, punched-out erosions and vesicles disseminated across eczematous skin — the monomorphous quality distinguishes eczema herpeticum from an exacerbation of atopic dermatitis (which produces polymorphous lesions). Immediate systemic acyclovir or valacyclovir is required. Tzanck smear (showing multinucleated giant cells) provides rapid bedside confirmation, and viral PCR is definitive.

Varicella-Zoster Virus: Primary Varicella, Herpes Zoster, and Postherpetic Neuralgia

Primary Varicella (Chickenpox)

Primary varicella (chickenpox) is caused by primary infection with varicella-zoster virus (VZV), a neurotropic alpha-herpesvirus that, like HSV, establishes lifelong latency in sensory ganglia. The classic presentation is a generalized, pruritic vesicular eruption that evolves through stages: erythematous macules → papules → vesicles (described as dewdrops on a rose petal because of the superficial, clear vesicle on an erythematous base) → pustules → crusting. The hallmark feature is lesions in different stages of evolution simultaneously (unlike smallpox, where lesions are all in the same stage), and the distribution is centripetal (concentrated on the trunk, spreading peripherally). Varicella is highly contagious via respiratory droplets and direct contact with vesicle fluid. Complications include secondary bacterial superinfection (the most common complication), varicella pneumonia (more severe in adults, smokers, and pregnant women), encephalitis (cerebellar ataxia in children, diffuse encephalitis in adults), and congenital varicella syndrome (limb hypoplasia, skin scarring, microcephaly) when maternal infection occurs in the first 20 weeks of pregnancy.

Herpes Zoster (Shingles) and Postherpetic Neuralgia

Herpes zoster (shingles) results from reactivation of latent VZV in a sensory ganglion, producing a unilateral, dermatomal vesicular eruption accompanied by pain. The eruption follows the dermatome of the affected sensory ganglion (thoracic dermatomes are most common, followed by the ophthalmic division of the trigeminal nerve) and does not cross the midline. The rash progresses through the same stages as varicella (papule → vesicle → pustule → crust) over 7 to 10 days. A prodrome of dermatomal pain, burning, or dysesthesia precedes the rash by 1 to 5 days, and this prodromal pain phase — before any visible rash — is a diagnostic pitfall because it may mimic myocardial infarction, cholecystitis, renal colic, or radiculopathy depending on the dermatome involved. Herpes zoster ophthalmicus (HZO) involves the ophthalmic division of the trigeminal nerve and carries a risk of keratitis, uveitis, and vision loss — the Hutchinson sign (vesicles on the tip of the nose, indicating nasociliary nerve involvement) predicts ocular complications and requires urgent ophthalmologic referral. Postherpetic neuralgia (PHN) — persistent dermatomal pain lasting more than 90 days after the acute rash — is the most common chronic complication, occurring in 10 to 18 percent of herpes zoster patients overall and in up to 30 percent of patients over age 60. The recombinant adjuvanted zoster vaccine (RZV) reduces the incidence of herpes zoster by over 90 percent and the incidence of PHN by over 85 percent in adults over 50.

Complications, Prognosis, and Zoster in Special Populations

Beyond postherpetic neuralgia, herpes zoster produces several serious complications that influence prognosis and management urgency. Zoster oticus (Ramsay Hunt syndrome) results from VZV reactivation in the geniculate ganglion and presents with the triad of ipsilateral facial nerve palsy, vesicles in the external ear canal or on the auricle, and sensorineural hearing loss — complete facial nerve recovery occurs in only approximately 50 percent of cases, making early antiviral therapy critical. Motor zoster

(zoster paresis) occurs when the virus extends from the sensory ganglion to involve the anterior horn cells or motor nerve roots, producing segmental motor weakness in the corresponding myotome. Disseminated zoster (more than 20 vesicles outside the primary and adjacent dermatomes) occurs in immunocompromised patients and carries a risk of visceral involvement including pneumonitis, hepatitis, and encephalitis. Herpes zoster in a patient under 50 years of age — particularly recurrent or multidermatomal zoster — should prompt HIV testing, because VZV reactivation at an unusually young age is a recognized early marker of immunosuppression. In pregnancy, maternal varicella in the first 20 weeks carries a 1 to 2 percent risk of congenital varicella syndrome, while maternal varicella within 5 days before to 2 days after delivery can cause severe neonatal varicella requiring varicella-zoster immune globulin (VZIG) for the neonate.

CLINICAL PEARL: The Hutchinson sign — vesicles on the tip or side of the nose — indicates involvement of the nasociliary branch of the ophthalmic division of the trigeminal nerve and strongly predicts ocular complications (keratitis, uveitis, acute retinal necrosis) in herpes zoster ophthalmicus. Any patient with herpes zoster ophthalmicus should receive urgent ophthalmologic consultation regardless of whether the Hutchinson sign is present, because ocular involvement can occur without this sign in approximately one-third of cases.

CAUTION: Herpes zoster in a patient younger than 50 — especially if recurrent, multidermatomal, or disseminated — should prompt HIV testing. VZV reactivation at an atypically young age is a recognized early clinical marker of immunosuppression, often preceding other manifestations of HIV disease. Similarly, any patient with disseminated zoster (defined as more than 20 vesicles outside the primary and immediately adjacent dermatomes) requires evaluation for underlying immunodeficiency, hematologic malignancy, or iatrogenic immunosuppression.

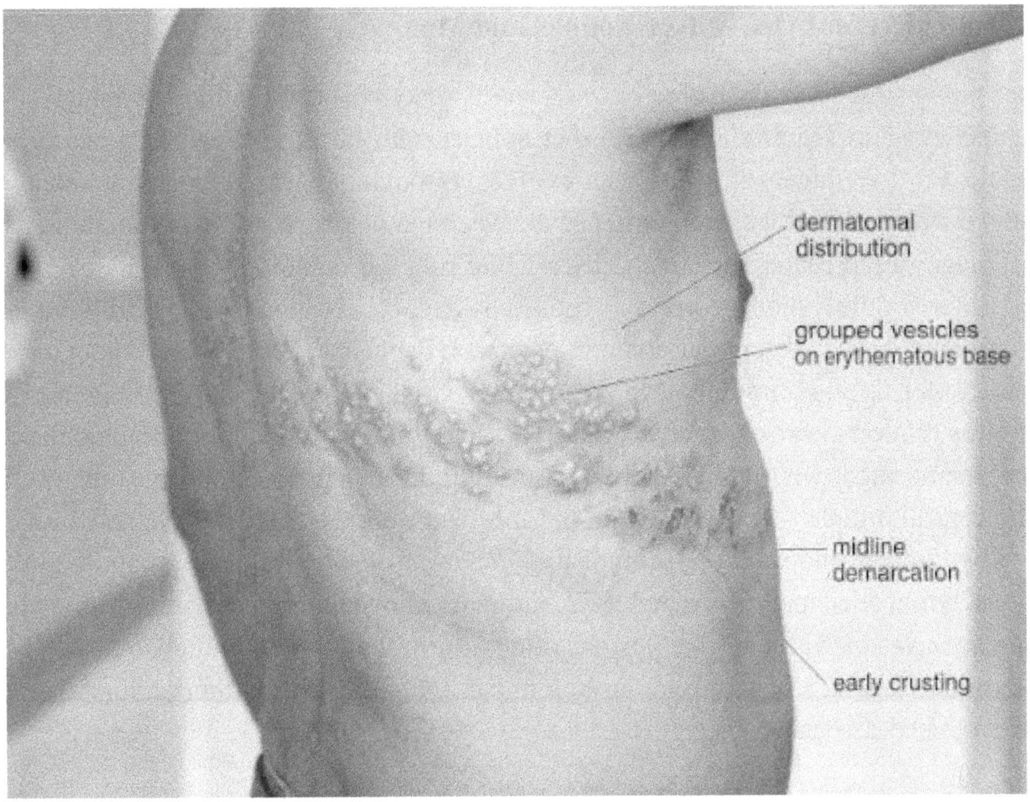

EVIDENCE: The Shingrix (recombinant adjuvanted zoster vaccine, RZV) pivotal trials demonstrated greater than 97 percent efficacy against herpes zoster in adults aged 50 and older and greater than 91 percent efficacy in adults aged 70 and older, with sustained protection exceeding 85 percent at 4 years post-vaccination. Efficacy against postherpetic neuralgia was 91 percent in adults aged 50 and older. RZV is recommended for all immunocompetent adults aged 50 and older and for immunocompromised adults aged 19 and older, replacing the previously used live attenuated zoster vaccine.

Molluscum Contagiosum and Poxvirus Infections

Molluscum Contagiosum

Molluscum contagiosum is caused by the molluscum contagiosum virus (MCV), a large, double-stranded DNA poxvirus with exclusive tropism for human keratinocytes. It presents as discrete, firm, dome-shaped, flesh-colored to pearly papules (2 to 5 mm) with a characteristic central umbilication (dimple or dell) from which a waxy, white core (the molluscum body) can be expressed. The central umbilication is the pathognomonic clinical feature and is best seen with magnification or dermoscopy. In children (the most commonly affected population), lesions occur on the face, trunk, extremities, and axillae, and spread by autoinoculation, direct skin-to-skin contact, and fomite transmission (shared towels, pool toys). In adults, molluscum is typically sexually transmitted when it presents in the genital and inguinal region. In HIV-infected patients with advanced immunosuppression (CD4 count below 200 cells/mm3), molluscum can become widespread with hundreds of large, treatment-resistant lesions — extensive molluscum in an adult should prompt HIV testing. The molluscum dermatitis (a surrounding eczematous ring around individual lesions) represents a host immune response to the virus and often heralds spontaneous resolution.

Other Poxvirus Infections: Orf, Milker Nodule, and Mpox

Several other poxviruses produce distinctive cutaneous infections. Orf (ecthyma contagiosum) is caused by the parapoxvirus and acquired through direct contact with infected sheep or goats. It presents as a solitary nodule on the finger or hand that evolves through six characteristic clinical stages over approximately 6 weeks: maculopapular, target, acute weeping, regenerative, papillomatous, and regressive — the target stage (a red center surrounded by a white ring surrounded by a red halo) is diagnostically distinctive. Milker nodule (pseudocowpox) is caused by a closely related parapoxvirus and acquired from infected cow udders, producing similar nodular lesions on the hands. Both resolve spontaneously without treatment and confer lasting immunity. Mpox (formerly monkeypox) is caused by the monkeypox virus, an orthopoxvirus related to variola and vaccinia. The 2022 global outbreak highlighted the dermatologic presentation: deep-seated, well-circumscribed, firm, umbilicated papules and pustules — often with a characteristic central dimple — distributed on the face, extremities, palms, soles, and anogenital region, accompanied by lymphadenopathy (a distinguishing feature from varicella and smallpox, which typically lack prominent lymphadenopathy). In the 2022 outbreak, anogenital and perioral lesions predominated among men who have sex with men, and lesions often occurred at sites of sexual contact. Tecovirimat, an anti-orthopoxvirus agent, has been used under emergency authorization for severe or immunocompromised-associated mpox.

Differential Diagnosis and Management of Molluscum

The differential diagnosis of molluscum includes verrucae (rough surface, thrombosed capillaries on dermoscopy), basal cell carcinoma (pearly papule with telangiectasias in adults, usually solitary), cryptococcosis (umbilicated papules in immunocompromised patients — a life-threatening disseminated fungal infection that mimics molluscum morphologically), and histoplasmosis (similar umbilicated papules in HIV-infected patients). In immunocompromised patients, every new umbilicated papule warrants biopsy to exclude disseminated opportunistic infections. Treatment of molluscum in immunocompetent children is often expectant (spontaneous resolution typically occurs within 6 to 18 months), but active treatment may be warranted for widespread lesions, lesions in cosmetically sensitive areas, or to prevent autoinoculation and transmission. Treatment options include physical destruction (curettage, cryotherapy), topical agents (cantharidin, tretinoin, imiquimod, potassium hydroxide), and intralesional cidofovir for immunocompromised patients with extensive disease.

Viral Exanthems: Measles, Rubella, Erythema Infectiosum, Roseola, and Hand-Foot-Mouth Disease

Classic Childhood Exanthems

Viral exanthems are generalized skin rashes caused by systemic viral infections, and they represent some of the most common causes of rash in children. Measles (rubeola, caused by the measles virus, a paramyxovirus) presents with a prodrome of fever, cough, coryza, conjunctivitis (the three Cs), and Koplik spots (bluish-white papules on an erythematous base on the buccal mucosa opposite the premolars — pathognomonic, appearing 1 to 2 days before the rash), followed by a maculopapular rash starting on the face and spreading cephalocaudally over 3 to 4 days. Complications include pneumonia, encephalitis, and subacute sclerosing panencephalitis. Rubella (German measles) presents with a milder maculopapular rash (also cephalocaudal spread), prominent posterior cervical and postauricular lymphadenopathy, and arthralgia (particularly in adult women). Congenital rubella syndrome (cardiac defects, cataracts, deafness) is the feared consequence of maternal infection in the first trimester. Erythema infectiosum (fifth disease, caused by parvovirus B19) presents with the slapped cheek rash (bilateral facial erythema sparing the nose) followed by a reticular, lace-like erythema on the trunk and extremities. Parvovirus B19 causes transient aplastic crisis in patients with hemolytic anemias (sickle cell disease, hereditary spherocytosis) and hydrops fetalis in pregnant women.

Roseola, Hand-Foot-Mouth Disease, and Exanthem Differential Diagnosis

Roseola infantum (exanthem subitum, caused by HHV-6, less commonly HHV-7) follows a characteristic sequence: 3 to 5 days of high fever (often exceeding 40 degrees Celsius), followed by defervescence and the simultaneous appearance of a diffuse, blanchable, maculopapular rash on the trunk spreading to the extremities. The rash appears as the fever breaks — the diagnostic clue is the temporal sequence of fever followed by rash, not concurrent with it. HHV-6 primary infection is the most common cause of febrile seizures in infants. Hand-foot-mouth disease (caused by coxsackievirus A16, enterovirus 71) presents as vesicles and erosions on the oral mucosa (herpangina pattern) accompanied by oval vesicles on the palms, soles, and sometimes the buttocks and knees — the acral vesicular distribution in a febrile child is diagnostically distinctive. Enterovirus 71-associated HFMD carries a risk of neurologic complications including brainstem encephalitis. The differential diagnosis of viral exanthems includes drug eruptions (which lack the viral prodrome and specific clinical sequences), Kawasaki disease (which shares the erythematous rash, conjunctivitis, and fever but includes strawberry tongue, palmoplantar erythema with desquamation, and coronary artery aneurysm risk), and scarlet fever (sandpaper-like rash with Pastia lines and pharyngitis caused by GAS).

Viral Exanthem	Causative Agent	Pathognomonic Feature	Rash Morphology and Distribution	Key Complications
Measles (Rubeola)	Paramyxovirus	Koplik spots on buccal mucosa	Maculopapular; cephalocaudal spread, face to trunk to extremities	Pneumonia, encephalitis, SSPE
Rubella (German Measles)	Togavirus (Rubivirus)	Posterior cervical and postauricular lymphadenopathy	Fine maculopapular; cephalocaudal, milder than measles	Congenital rubella syndrome (first trimester)

Erythema Infectiosum (Fifth Disease)	Parvovirus B19	Slapped cheek bilateral facial erythema	Reticular, lace-like erythema on trunk and extremities	Aplastic crisis (hemolytic anemias), hydrops fetalis
Roseola Infantum (Sixth Disease)	HHV-6 (HHV-7)	Fever then rash sequence (rash appears as fever breaks)	Diffuse blanchable maculopapular; trunk to extremities	Febrile seizures
Hand-Foot-Mouth Disease	Coxsackievirus A16, EV71	Oral vesicles plus acral papulovesicles (palms, soles)	Oval vesicles on palms, soles, buttocks; oral erosions	Brainstem encephalitis (EV71)

HIV-Associated Dermatoses

Dermatologic Markers of Immunosuppression

Cutaneous disease occurs in over 90 percent of HIV-infected patients during the course of their illness, and specific dermatologic findings correlate with the degree of immunosuppression, making the skin a window into immune status. Early HIV infection (CD4 count above 500 cells/mm3) is associated with acute retroviral syndrome (morbilliform exanthem, oral ulcers, pharyngitis, lymphadenopathy within 2 to 4 weeks of infection), seborrheic dermatitis (often the earliest cutaneous manifestation of HIV, with widespread, severe seborrheic dermatitis on the face, scalp, and chest in a young adult without prior history), oral hairy leukoplakia (corrugated white plaques on the lateral tongue caused by Epstein-Barr virus, virtually pathognomonic for HIV infection), and herpes zoster in a patient under 50 (which should prompt HIV testing). Moderate immunosuppression (CD4 200 to 500 cells/mm3) is associated with worsening of pre-existing dermatoses (psoriasis, atopic dermatitis), eosinophilic folliculitis (intensely pruritic follicular papules on the face, trunk, and proximal extremities), and increasingly recalcitrant molluscum contagiosum. Severe immunosuppression (CD4 below 200 cells/mm3) is associated with disseminated opportunistic infections — cryptococcosis (umbilicated papules mimicking molluscum), histoplasmosis, disseminated herpes simplex (chronic non-healing ulcers), cytomegalovirus (perineal ulcers), Kaposi sarcoma (violaceous patches, plaques, and nodules caused by HHV-8), bacillary angiomatosis (vascular papules and nodules caused by Bartonella, resembling pyogenic granulomas or KS), and extensive HPV-associated condylomata and dysplasia.

Dermatologic Clues Prompting HIV Testing

Several dermatologic presentations should prompt clinicians to offer HIV testing when the patient's status is unknown: severe or treatment-resistant seborrheic dermatitis in a young adult, herpes zoster in a patient under 50, oral hairy leukoplakia, extensive molluscum contagiosum in an adult, unexplained eosinophilic folliculitis, chronic non-healing herpes simplex ulcer (lasting more than 1 month), new-onset Kaposi sarcoma, and widespread condylomata acuminata or anal dysplasia. Pruritic papular eruption (PPE), a severely pruritic, symmetrical papular eruption on the trunk and extremities, is one of the most common dermatoses in HIV-infected patients in resource-limited settings and often prompts the initial HIV diagnosis. Antiretroviral therapy (ART) produces immune reconstitution inflammatory syndrome (IRIS) in approximately 10 to 25 percent of patients initiating ART with low CD4 counts — the paradoxical worsening of pre-existing infections (herpes zoster flare, new KS lesions, tuberculosis worsening) or the unmasking of previously subclinical infections, occurring within the first 2 to 8 weeks of ART as the recovering immune system mounts an exuberant inflammatory response.

THE CUTANEOUS MIMICKER RECOGNITION ATLAS — Herpes Zoster versus Contact Dermatitis

The Clinical Pattern: Herpes zoster presents as grouped vesicles on erythematous bases arranged in a unilateral, band-like distribution following a single dermatome from the posterior midline around the trunk, without crossing the midline. A prodrome of dermatomal pain or burning precedes the rash by 1 to 5 days. The vesicles evolve through vesicle-pustule-crust stages over 7 to 10 days. The patient is typically over 50 years old or immunocompromised.

The Mimicker: Allergic contact dermatitis may present as a unilateral, linear or grouped vesicular eruption that can mimic the dermatomal distribution of herpes zoster — particularly poison ivy/oak dermatitis, which produces linear streaks of vesicles on erythematous, edematous skin in the distribution of plant contact. Contact dermatitis is intensely pruritic (zoster is predominantly painful), lacks a pain prodrome, is not dermatomal (its distribution follows the pattern of external contact, which may cross dermatomes and the midline), and shows spongiotic dermatitis rather than viral cytopathic effect on histopathology.

Trap Logic: Diagnosing contact dermatitis based on vesicles and assuming the distribution is explained by external exposure, without considering dermatomal anatomy is the cognitive trap. When linear vesicles appear on the trunk, the clinician may attribute them to a contactant (plant exposure, clothing, occupational chemical) without recognizing the dermatomal pattern. The reverse trap occurs when a true contact dermatitis (which can be unilateral and band-like on the trunk) is treated as herpes zoster with antivirals. The failure point is not assessing the symptom quality: herpes zoster is painful with a prodrome; contact dermatitis is pruritic without a prodrome.

The Decision Anchor: The discriminating features are **symptom quality (pain and prodrome in zoster versus pruritus without prodrome in contact dermatitis), dermatomal versus contactant distribution (zoster follows a single dermatome and does not cross the midline; contact dermatitis follows the pattern of external exposure and may cross dermatomes and the midline), and Tzanck smear or viral PCR (positive for multinucleated giant cells and VZV DNA in zoster, negative in contact dermatitis)**. Perform a Tzanck smear when in doubt — it provides rapid bedside confirmation.

Evidence-Based Antiviral Therapeutics

Systemic Antiviral Agents

The nucleoside analogue antivirals — acyclovir, valacyclovir, and famciclovir — are the cornerstone of herpesvirus management. These agents are phosphorylated by viral thymidine kinase (TK) to their active triphosphate form, which inhibits viral DNA polymerase and terminates viral DNA chain elongation. Viral TK selectivity makes these drugs highly specific for virus-infected cells with minimal toxicity to uninfected host cells. Valacyclovir (the L-valine ester prodrug of acyclovir) has three to five times greater oral bioavailability than acyclovir and allows less frequent dosing. For primary genital herpes, valacyclovir or acyclovir for 7 to 10 days reduces symptom duration and viral shedding. For recurrent genital herpes, episodic therapy (initiated within 24 hours of prodrome) shortens episodes by 1 to 2 days, and suppressive therapy (daily valacyclovir) reduces recurrence frequency by 70 to 80 percent and reduces asymptomatic viral shedding by approximately 50 percent. For herpes zoster, antiviral therapy (valacyclovir, famciclovir, or acyclovir, initiated within 72 hours of rash onset) accelerates healing, reduces acute pain, and may reduce the risk and duration of PHN. Intravenous acyclovir is required for disseminated HSV, eczema herpeticum, HSV encephalitis, neonatal herpes, and varicella or zoster in severely immunocompromised patients.

Topical Antivirals and Emerging Therapies

Topical antiviral agents have limited efficacy compared to systemic therapy but play a role in mild, localized disease. Topical acyclovir and penciclovir cream may modestly shorten the duration of herpes labialis episodes when applied early in the prodromal phase, but they do not prevent recurrences and are inferior to systemic therapy for all indications. Cidofovir (a nucleotide analogue that does not require viral TK for activation) is used topically and intravenously for acyclovir-resistant HSV and CMV infections in immunocompromised patients — resistance to acyclovir develops through mutations in the viral TK gene and occurs almost exclusively in immunosuppressed patients receiving prolonged antiviral therapy. Foscarnet (a pyrophosphate analogue that directly inhibits viral DNA polymerase) is the primary alternative for acyclovir-resistant herpes infections. For HPV, cidofovir injection and topical sinecatechins (green tea polyphenols) are options for recalcitrant genital warts; the systemic immunologic agents (imiquimod, 5-fluorouracil) work through immune stimulation rather than direct antiviral activity. Tecovirimat (an anti-orthopoxvirus agent originally developed for smallpox) has been deployed for mpox in select cases with severe or immunocompromised-associated disease.

Patient Education and Counseling

Patient education is integral to the management of chronic and recurrent viral infections. For genital herpes, counseling should address the natural history of HSV infection (lifelong latency with periodic reactivation, which tends to decrease in frequency over years), the distinction between symptomatic and asymptomatic viral shedding (asymptomatic shedding accounts for the majority of HSV transmissions), the role of suppressive therapy in reducing transmission to uninfected partners, and the importance of disclosure to sexual partners. Condom use reduces but does not eliminate transmission risk because HSV can be shed from areas not covered by condoms. For herpes zoster, patients should understand that the rash is contagious to VZV-naive individuals (who would develop varicella, not zoster) until all lesions have crusted, and that postherpetic neuralgia may require multimodal pain management including gabapentinoids, tricyclic antidepressants, and topical lidocaine or capsaicin. For HPV, patient counseling should include discussion of the high lifetime prevalence of infection, the difference between low-risk and high-risk types, the availability and importance of vaccination even after prior infection (vaccination protects against types not yet acquired), and the need for continued screening per guidelines.

THE CUTANEOUS MIMICKER RECOGNITION ATLAS — Molluscum Contagiosum versus Disseminated Cryptococcosis

The Clinical Pattern: Molluscum contagiosum presents as multiple discrete, flesh-colored to pearly, dome-shaped papules (2 to 5 mm) with a characteristic central umbilication. In immunocompetent children, lesions are scattered on the face, trunk, and extremities. The surrounding skin is normal unless a molluscum dermatitis (eczematous halo) is present. The patient is otherwise well without systemic symptoms.

The Mimicker: Disseminated cryptococcosis (caused by Cryptococcus neoformans in severely immunocompromised patients, particularly those with AIDS and CD4 counts below 100 cells/mm3) presents as multiple, dome-shaped, umbilicated papules that are morphologically identical to molluscum contagiosum. The papules may be flesh-colored, translucent, or hemorrhagic. The patient is systemically ill with fever, headache (meningeal involvement), and malaise.

Trap Logic: Assuming molluscum in an immunosuppressed patient with multiple umbilicated papules without performing a biopsy is the cognitive trap. In an HIV-positive patient with advanced immunosuppression, the morphologic overlap between molluscum and disseminated cryptococcosis (and histoplasmosis, which also produces umbilicated papules) is near-total. Treating the lesions as molluscum delays the diagnosis of a life-threatening disseminated fungal infection that requires urgent systemic antifungal therapy. The clue is the clinical context: an immunosuppressed patient who appears systemically ill requires biopsy of umbilicated papules to exclude opportunistic infection.

The Decision Anchor: The discriminating test is **skin biopsy with histopathology and special stains: molluscum shows large, eosinophilic intracytoplasmic inclusion bodies (Henderson-Patterson bodies/molluscum bodies) in the epidermis; cryptococcosis shows encapsulated yeast organisms with a clear halo (representing the polysaccharide capsule) in the dermis, positive on GMS, PAS, and mucicarmine staining**. In any immunocompromised patient with umbilicated papules, biopsy before assuming molluscum. Serum and CSF cryptococcal antigen testing should be sent simultaneously to evaluate for disseminated disease and meningitis.

Clinical Case: Recurrent Oral Erosions in an Immunocompromised Patient

A 42-year-old man with recently diagnosed HIV infection (CD4 count 85 cells/mm3, not yet on antiretroviral therapy) presents with a 3-week history of painful, non-healing ulcers on the lower lip and chin. He reports that similar but smaller lesions had occurred intermittently over the prior year, each resolving within 1 to 2 weeks, but the current episode has been progressive and unresponsive to over-the-counter lip balm and topical antibiotics. On examination, there are multiple shallow, well-demarcated ulcers with scalloped borders on the lower lip vermillion and adjacent skin, some coalescing into a large, crusted plaque on the chin. Scattered umbilicated papules are noted on the forehead and neck.

The clinical differential includes chronic HSV infection (the leading consideration given the HIV status and duration exceeding 1 month), squamous cell carcinoma (verrucous or ulcerated), and deep fungal infection. Tzanck smear from an ulcer edge shows multinucleated giant cells with molding (Cowdry type A inclusions), and HSV PCR confirms HSV-1. The umbilicated papules on the forehead and neck are biopsied: histopathology shows intracytoplasmic molluscum bodies, confirming molluscum contagiosum — biopsy was appropriate to exclude disseminated cryptococcosis given the profound immunosuppression. The chronic HSV ulcer (lasting more than 1 month) meets criteria for an AIDS-defining condition. Treatment is initiated with intravenous acyclovir given the extensive disease and immunosuppression, with transition to oral valacyclovir for long-term suppression. Antiretroviral therapy is initiated with careful monitoring for immune reconstitution inflammatory syndrome. This case illustrates two principles: first, HSV in immunocompromised patients produces atypical, chronic, non-healing ulcerations rather than the classic grouped vesicles seen in immunocompetent hosts; second, umbilicated papules in severely immunosuppressed patients require histopathologic confirmation to exclude life-threatening mimickers.

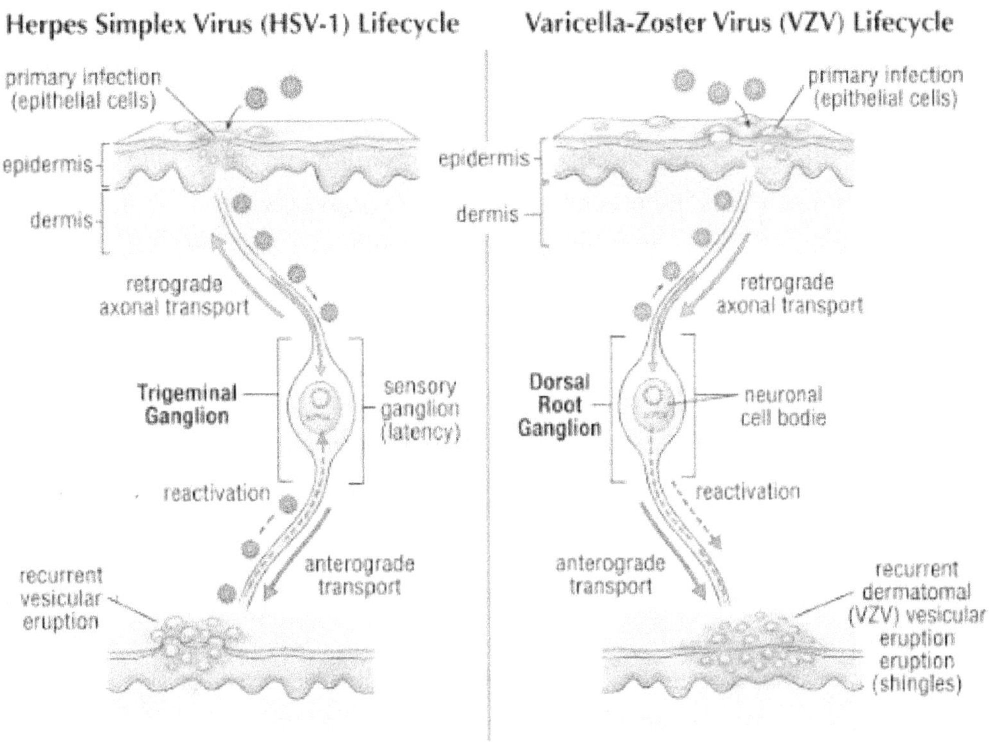

THE CUTANEOUS MIMICKER RECOGNITION ATLAS — Viral Infection Diagnostic Arcs

Herpes Zoster vs. Contact Dermatitis: The discriminating features are symptom quality (pain and prodrome in zoster versus pruritus without prodrome in contact dermatitis) and distribution (dermatomal without midline crossing in zoster versus contactant pattern that may cross dermatomes and the midline in contact dermatitis). Tzanck smear or VZV PCR confirms the diagnosis. Cognitive trap: attributing unilateral vesicles to external contactant exposure without recognizing the dermatomal anatomy.

Molluscum Contagiosum vs. Disseminated Cryptococcosis: The discriminating test is skin biopsy: molluscum shows intracytoplasmic Henderson-Patterson bodies; cryptococcosis shows encapsulated yeast with a clear capsular halo on mucicarmine staining. In any immunocompromised patient with umbilicated papules, biopsy before assuming molluscum — disseminated cryptococcosis is morphologically identical and is life-threatening if missed.

Summary and Key Concepts

HPV infection is stratified by oncogenic risk: low-risk types (6, 11) cause benign condylomata; high-risk types (16, 18) cause anogenital and oropharyngeal carcinoma. Dermoscopy aids verruca diagnosis by revealing thrombosed capillaries and loss of dermatoglyphics. The 9-valent HPV vaccine prevents the most important oncogenic and condyloma-causing types, with vaccination recommended beginning at age 9 to 12 years.

HSV-1 and HSV-2 establish lifelong latency in sensory ganglia with periodic reactivation. Eczema herpeticum is a dermatologic emergency (disseminated HSV on eczematous skin) requiring urgent systemic acyclovir. In pregnancy, primary genital HSV near delivery carries 30 to 50 percent neonatal transmission risk, warranting cesarean delivery and suppressive antiviral therapy from 36 weeks of gestation.

Herpes zoster follows a unilateral dermatomal distribution without crossing the midline. The Hutchinson sign predicts ocular complications in herpes zoster ophthalmicus. Postherpetic neuralgia occurs in up to 30 percent of patients over 60. The recombinant zoster vaccine reduces herpes zoster incidence by over 90 percent and is recommended for adults aged 50 and older and immunocompromised adults aged 19 and older.

Classic childhood exanthems each have a characteristic clinical sequence: measles (Koplik spots then cephalocaudal maculopapular rash), fifth disease (slapped cheek then reticular rash), roseola (high fever then rash), hand-foot-mouth disease (oral vesicles plus acral papulovesicles). Kawasaki disease and drug eruptions are key differential diagnoses.

HIV-associated dermatoses correlate with immunosuppression severity. Severe seborrheic dermatitis, oral hairy leukoplakia, herpes zoster in patients under 50, and extensive adult molluscum should prompt HIV testing. In immunocompromised patients, umbilicated papules require biopsy to exclude disseminated cryptococcosis or histoplasmosis — morphologic overlap is near-total.

CHAPTER 11: FUNGAL AND YEAST INFECTIONS OF THE SKIN

Learning Objectives

1. Classify cutaneous fungal infections by causative organism — dermatophytes, yeasts (Candida, Malassezia), dimorphic fungi, and subcutaneous mycoses — and correlate each with its characteristic clinical presentation, anatomic predilection, and diagnostic approach.
2. Apply the clinical, dermoscopic, and mycologic features that distinguish dermatophyte infections from their common mimickers, including nummular eczema, psoriasis, and erythema annulare centrifugum.
3. Recognize the cutaneous manifestations of systemic (endemic) mycoses as potential markers of disseminated infection requiring urgent systemic antifungal therapy, and correlate skin findings with the patient's geographic and immunologic risk profile.
4. Select appropriate topical and systemic antifungal agents based on the infection's causative organism, anatomic site, severity, and the patient's comorbidities, and monitor for adverse effects of prolonged systemic antifungal therapy.

Dermatophytosis: Tinea Corporis, Cruris, Pedis, Capitis, Unguium, and Faciei

Mycology and Pathophysiology

Dermatophytes are keratinophilic fungi that infect the stratum corneum, hair, and nails — tissues rich in keratin, which serves as their primary nutrient source. Three genera cause the vast majority of human dermatophytosis: Trichophyton (the most common genus worldwide, including T. rubrum, T. tonsurans, and T. interdigitale), Microsporum (M. canis, M. audouinii), and Epidermophyton (E. floccosum). Dermatophytes are classified by ecological reservoir: anthropophilic species (adapted to humans, causing milder but more chronic infections — T. rubrum, T. tonsurans), zoophilic species (animal reservoirs, causing more inflammatory infections — M. canis from cats and dogs, T. verrucosum from cattle), and geophilic species (soil reservoir — M. gypseum). Infection occurs through direct contact with infected individuals, animals, fomites, or soil. The dermatophyte invades the stratum corneum and grows centrifugally, producing the characteristic annular morphology with an active, advancing, raised border (where fungal hyphae are most concentrated and the host inflammatory response is most vigorous) and a relatively clear center (where the infection has been partially controlled by the immune response).

Epidemiology and Risk Factors

Dermatophytosis is among the most prevalent infectious diseases globally, affecting an estimated 20 to 25 percent of the world's population. T. rubrum is the most common causative species worldwide, responsible for the majority of tinea corporis, cruris, pedis, and unguium cases. Tinea capitis epidemiology varies by region: T. tonsurans predominates in the United States, the United Kingdom, and parts of Africa, while M. canis is more common in continental Europe, the Mediterranean, and parts of South America. Risk factors for dermatophytosis include warm and humid environments (occlusive footwear, athletic activities, tropical climates), diabetes mellitus (particularly for onychomycosis and chronic tinea pedis), peripheral vascular disease, immunosuppression (corticosteroid therapy, HIV infection, organ transplant), and shared communal facilities (swimming pools, gymnasium locker rooms, military barracks). The increasing prevalence of terbinafine-resistant T. indotineae (formerly T. mentagrophytes genotype VIII) — first reported in South Asia and now spreading globally — has introduced antifungal resistance as an emerging challenge in dermatophyte management, presenting as extensive, treatment-resistant dermatophytosis requiring susceptibility-guided therapy.

Clinical Presentations by Anatomic Site

Tinea corporis (ringworm of the body) presents as annular or arciform erythematous plaques with a raised, scaly, advancing border and central clearing — the classic ringworm morphology. Lesions are often pruritic and may be single or multiple. Tinea cruris (jock itch) involves the inguinal folds and inner thighs, presenting as bilateral erythematous plaques with a raised, scaly border extending from the inguinal crease — characteristically sparing the scrotum (unlike candidal intertrigo, which involves the scrotum). Tinea pedis (athlete's foot) has three clinical patterns: interdigital (maceration and scaling in the web spaces, particularly the fourth interdigital space), moccasin (diffuse hyperkeratosis and fine scaling of the entire sole, heel, and lateral foot — the most chronic and treatment-resistant pattern, caused predominantly by T. rubrum), and vesiculobullous (inflammatory vesicles and bullae on the instep). Tinea capitis (scalp ringworm) is predominantly a disease of prepubertal children and presents as patches of alopecia with scaling, broken hair shafts, and varying degrees of inflammation depending on the causative species — the severe inflammatory form (kerion) presents as a boggy, tender, purulent nodule or plaque that is an exuberant host immune response to the fungus and should not be misdiagnosed as a bacterial abscess requiring incision and drainage.

Tinea unguium (dermatophyte onychomycosis) is the most common cause of onychomycosis and presents in several clinical patterns: distal and lateral subungual onychomycosis (DLSO — the most common, with subungual hyperkeratosis, onycholysis, and yellow-white discoloration beginning at the distal nail), proximal subungual onychomycosis (PSO — white discoloration beginning at the proximal nail fold, considered a marker of immunosuppression when seen in younger patients), white superficial onychomycosis (WSO — chalky white patches on the dorsal nail plate), and total dystrophic onychomycosis (complete nail destruction). Tinea faciei (face) and tinea manuum (hand, characteristically unilateral — the two feet, one hand syndrome with bilateral tinea pedis plus unilateral tinea manuum) complete the spectrum. Majocchi granuloma (nodular granulomatous perifolliculitis) occurs when dermatophytes invade hair follicles and extend into the dermis, producing deep inflammatory nodules — this is seen most commonly in women shaving the lower legs and in immunosuppressed patients.

Dermatophyte Infection	Anatomic Site	Classic Morphology	Key Diagnostic Clue	First-Line Treatment
Tinea corporis	Trunk, extremities	Annular plaque, raised scaly border, central clearing	KOH: septate branching hyphae from border	Topical terbinafine or azole
Tinea cruris	Inguinal folds, inner thighs	Bilateral erythematous plaques, scrotum spared	Scrotal sparing (candida involves scrotum)	Topical terbinafine or azole
Tinea pedis (moccasin)	Sole, heel, lateral foot	Diffuse hyperkeratosis, fine scaling, chronic	Bilateral chronic plantar scaling	Oral terbinafine (topical often insufficient)
Tinea capitis	Scalp (children)	Alopecia, scaling, broken hairs; kerion if inflammatory	Comma hairs and corkscrew hairs on trichoscopy	Oral griseofulvin or terbinafine (systemic required)
Tinea unguium (DLSO)	Nails	Subungual hyperkeratosis, onycholysis, yellow discoloration	PSO pattern suggests immunosuppress ion	Oral terbinafine 12–16 weeks
Tinea manuum	Palm (usually unilateral)	Unilateral palmar hyperkeratosis	Two feet, one hand syndrome	Oral terbinafine

Diagnostic Workup and KOH Examination

The gold standard for diagnosing dermatophytosis is direct microscopy with potassium hydroxide (KOH) preparation. Scales are collected from the active, advancing border of the lesion (where hyphae are most abundant), placed on a glass slide with 10 to 20 percent KOH solution, gently heated to dissolve keratin, and examined under light microscopy for septate, branching hyphae. The sensitivity of KOH preparation ranges from 40 to 70 percent and is operator-dependent. Fungal culture on Sabouraud dextrose agar or dermatophyte test medium (DTM) identifies the species and is useful when species identification changes management (e.g., tinea capitis, where the causative species determines treatment duration and public health measures). Wood lamp examination produces bright green fluorescence with Microsporum infections (M. canis, M. audouinii) due to pteridine metabolites in infected hair, but does not fluoresce with Trichophyton species — a negative Wood lamp does not exclude dermatophytosis. Dermoscopy of tinea capitis shows comma hairs (short, C-shaped broken hairs), corkscrew hairs, zigzag hairs, and Morse code hairs, which are highly specific for tinea capitis and help distinguish it from alopecia areata (exclamation point hairs, yellow dots) and trichotillomania (broken hairs at varying lengths, flame hairs).

CLINICAL PEARL: The two feet, one hand pattern — bilateral tinea pedis with unilateral tinea manuum — is a classic presentation of T. rubrum dermatophytosis. When a patient presents with one scaly, hyperkeratotic palm and bilateral moccasin-type scaling of the feet, think dermatophyte infection and perform KOH preparation from the active border of the palm lesion. The unilateral hand involvement is explained by autoinoculation from the foot (typically the dominant hand, which scratches the pruritic foot).

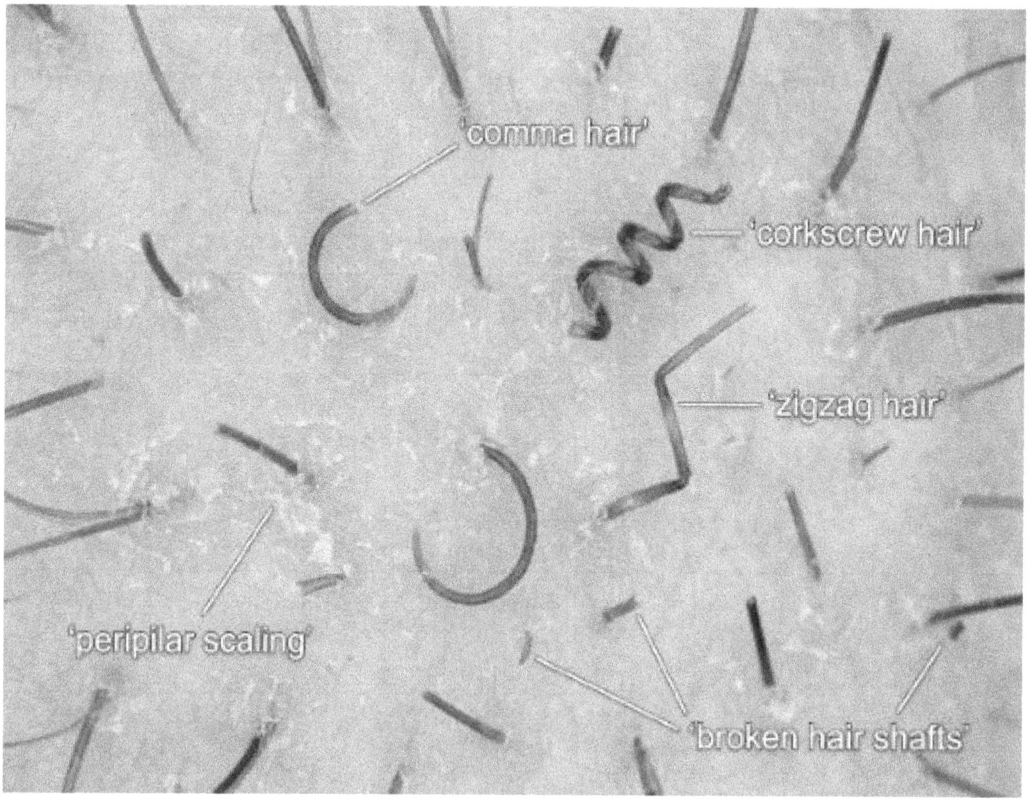

Candidiasis: Mucocutaneous, Intertriginous, and Invasive Forms

Pathogenesis and Risk Factors

Candida species (predominantly C. albicans, with increasing prevalence of non-albicans species including C. glabrata, C. tropicalis, C. parapsilosis, and C. auris) are commensal yeasts that inhabit the gastrointestinal tract, oral cavity, and vaginal mucosa. Candida transitions from commensal to pathogen when host defenses are compromised — predisposing factors include moisture and occlusion (intertriginous skin), disruption of the cutaneous barrier (maceration, dentures), alteration of the normal bacterial flora (broad-spectrum antibiotics), endocrine dysfunction (diabetes mellitus, Cushing syndrome), immunosuppression (HIV/AIDS, chemotherapy, organ transplant), and extremes of age (neonates, elderly). The virulence of C. albicans derives from its ability to switch between yeast (blastospore) and hyphal (filamentous) forms — the hyphal form is invasive and produces tissue-penetrating enzymes (secreted aspartyl proteinases, phospholipases) that enable mucosal and cutaneous invasion.

Clinical Presentations

Oropharyngeal candidiasis (thrush) presents as creamy white, curd-like plaques on the buccal mucosa, palate, and tongue that can be scraped off to reveal an erythematous, sometimes bleeding base. Angular cheilitis (perleche) presents as erythematous, fissured patches at the oral commissures, often with satellite papules. Candidal intertrigo occurs in skin folds (axillary, inframammary, inguinal, intergluteal, pannicular folds) presenting as beefy red, macerated, well-demarcated erythematous plaques with characteristic satellite pustules — the satellite pustules (small papules and pustules extending beyond the main plaque border) are the pathognomonic clinical clue distinguishing candidal intertrigo from dermatophyte infection (which lacks satellites) and inverse psoriasis (which is well-demarcated, glazed, and shiny without satellites). Vulvovaginal candidiasis presents with thick, white, cottage cheese-like vaginal discharge, vulvar erythema, pruritus, and dysuria. Candidal balanitis (erythematous papules and plaques on the glans penis) and candidal paronychia (chronic, boggy swelling of the proximal nail fold, often with loss of the cuticle) are additional recognized presentations. Chronic mucocutaneous candidiasis (CMC) is a group of rare primary immunodeficiency syndromes (often STAT1 gain-of-function or AIRE deficiency) characterized by persistent, recalcitrant Candida infection of the skin, nails, and mucous membranes beginning in early childhood.

Diagnostic Approach and Differential Diagnosis

The diagnosis of cutaneous candidiasis is primarily clinical, supported by KOH preparation and culture when confirmation is needed. KOH preparation from the edge of a candidal lesion shows pseudohyphae (elongated yeast cells connected end-to-end in chains) and budding yeast cells — this distinguishes Candida from dermatophytes (which show true septate hyphae) and Malassezia (which shows the spaghetti and meatballs pattern). Culture on Sabouraud dextrose agar confirms the species and is particularly important when azole resistance is suspected (C. glabrata, C. auris). The differential diagnosis of candidal intertrigo includes inverse psoriasis (well-demarcated, glazed, shiny plaques in skin folds without satellite pustules), dermatophyte intertrigo (scaly border without satellites, scrotal sparing in the groin), erythrasma (coral-red fluorescence under Wood lamp, caused by Corynebacterium minutissimum), and irritant or allergic contact dermatitis. Recurrent vulvovaginal candidiasis (defined as four or more episodes per year) warrants investigation for predisposing factors including uncontrolled diabetes mellitus, immunosuppression, and antibiotic overuse, and may benefit from prolonged suppressive fluconazole therapy.

Congenital and Neonatal Candidiasis

Congenital cutaneous candidiasis results from ascending intrauterine infection and presents at birth or within the first 24 hours of life as a widespread erythematous papulopustular eruption covering the trunk, extremities, palms, and soles, often with desquamation. In premature infants, this can progress to systemic candidemia with significant mortality. Neonatal candidiasis (acquired during passage through a colonized birth canal) typically presents after the first week of life as oral thrush, candidal diaper dermatitis, or a combination. Candidal diaper dermatitis is distinguished from irritant diaper dermatitis by its involvement of the inguinal folds (irritant dermatitis typically spares the folds), beefy red erythema, and satellite pustules.

Malassezia-Associated Conditions: Pityriasis Versicolor, Malassezia Folliculitis, and Seborrheic Dermatitis

Malassezia Biology and Pathogenesis

Malassezia species are lipophilic yeasts that are part of the normal cutaneous flora, particularly in sebum-rich areas (scalp, face, upper trunk). The genus includes multiple species (M. globosa, M. restricta, M. sympodialis, M. furfur) that require exogenous lipids for growth, which is why they colonize sebaceous areas. Malassezia contributes to cutaneous disease through multiple mechanisms: direct infection of the stratum corneum (pityriasis versicolor), follicular occlusion and inflammation (Malassezia folliculitis), and inflammatory lipid metabolism that triggers an immune response (seborrheic dermatitis, where Malassezia metabolizes sebum triglycerides into unsaturated fatty acids — particularly oleic acid — that irritate the epidermis and drive inflammation in genetically susceptible individuals).

Clinical Presentations and Diagnostic Features

Pityriasis versicolor (tinea versicolor) presents as multiple, well-demarcated, oval macules and thin plaques with fine, powdery scale on the trunk, upper arms, and neck. The name versicolor reflects the variable pigmentation: lesions appear hypopigmented on dark skin (because the fungus produces azelaic acid, which inhibits melanocyte tyrosinase) and hyperpigmented (tan, pink, or brown) on fair skin. The distribution pattern — multiple oval macules on the upper trunk and proximal arms — is characteristic and often described as a rain-drop pattern. KOH preparation shows the diagnostic spaghetti and meatballs pattern (short, thick hyphae interspersed with round yeast cells in clusters). Malassezia folliculitis presents as monomorphous, pruritic, follicular papules and pustules on the upper trunk, shoulders, and upper arms — the monomorphous quality and the distribution distinguish it from acne vulgaris (which produces a mix of comedones, papules, pustules, and nodules on the face, chest, and back) and bacterial folliculitis. Malassezia folliculitis commonly occurs in young adults in hot, humid climates, after antibiotic use, and in immunosuppressed patients. Seborrheic dermatitis presents as erythematous patches and plaques with greasy, yellowish scale in sebaceous areas — the nasolabial folds, eyebrows, glabella, scalp (dandruff), external ear canals, and presternal chest.

Management and Recurrence Prevention

Pityriasis versicolor is treated with topical azole or selenium sulfide-based agents for localized disease (ketoconazole cream or shampoo, selenium sulfide 2.5 percent lotion applied as a body wash) and oral fluconazole or itraconazole for widespread or recurrent disease. Patients should be counseled that the pigmentary changes (particularly hypopigmentation) persist for weeks to months after successful eradication of the fungus — the slow return of normal pigmentation reflects the time required for melanocyte recovery and re-pigmentation, and does not indicate treatment failure. Recurrence rates for pityriasis versicolor exceed 60 percent within one year because the causative Malassezia is a normal skin commensal that cannot be permanently eradicated, and re-colonization in warm, humid conditions is inevitable. Prophylactic strategies include monthly pulse dosing of oral fluconazole or application of ketoconazole shampoo as a body wash once to twice weekly. Seborrheic dermatitis management combines topical antifungals (ketoconazole shampoo or cream) with low-potency topical corticosteroids for flares, and topical calcineurin inhibitors (pimecrolimus, tacrolimus) for steroid-sparing maintenance on facial skin.

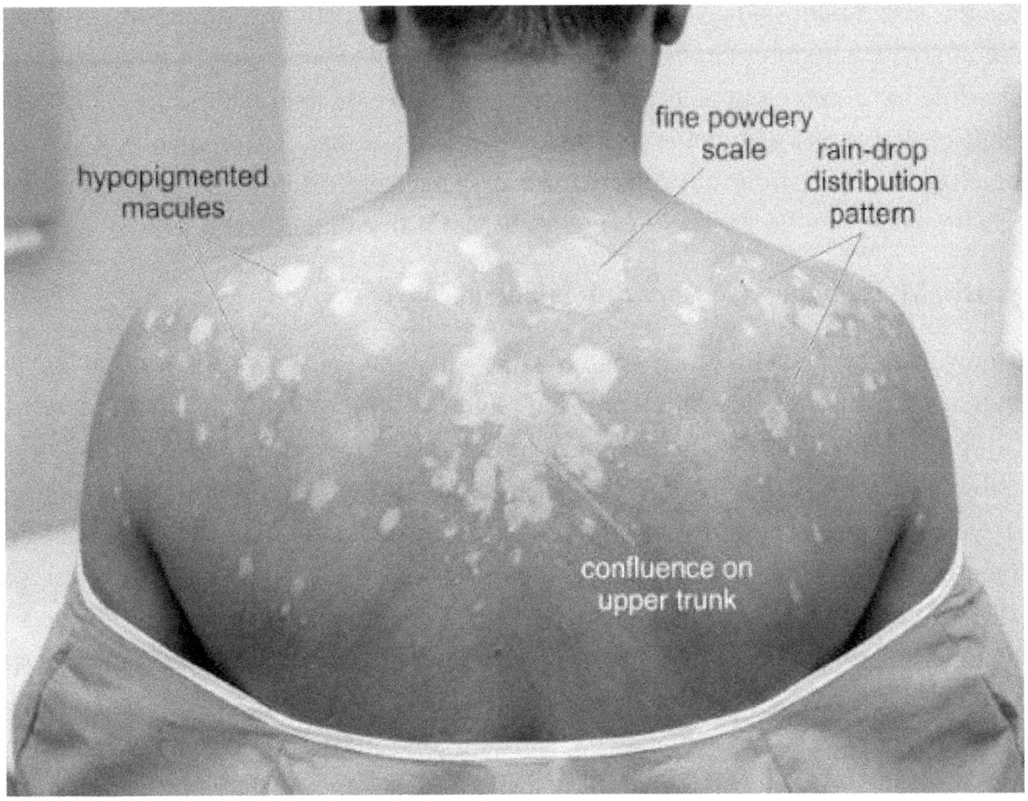

Deep Fungal Infections: Sporotrichosis, Chromomycosis, Mycetoma, and Subcutaneous Mycoses

Sporotrichosis

Sporotrichosis is caused by the dimorphic fungus Sporothrix schenckii (and related species in the S. schenckii complex), which inhabits soil, decaying vegetation, sphagnum moss, and rose thorns. The classic clinical presentation is lymphocutaneous sporotrichosis: after inoculation through a thorn prick, splinter, or animal scratch (cat scratch is an increasingly recognized vector, particularly in South America), a painless papule or nodule develops at the inoculation site, followed by the appearance of additional nodules in a linear, ascending pattern along the draining lymphatic vessels (lymphangitic spread). This linear, sporotrichoid nodular pattern — a chain of nodules along a lymphatic — is the pathognomonic clinical signature and narrows the differential to sporotrichosis, atypical mycobacterial infection (M. marinum, which produces an identical sporotrichoid pattern in patients with aquatic exposure), nocardiosis, leishmaniasis, and tularemia. Fixed cutaneous sporotrichosis (a single nodule or plaque without lymphangitic spread) occurs in endemic areas in individuals with partial immunity. Disseminated and osteoarticular sporotrichosis occur in immunocompromised patients and require prolonged systemic antifungal therapy with amphotericin B followed by itraconazole. Treatment of lymphocutaneous disease is oral itraconazole for 3 to 6 months; the traditional alternative of saturated solution of potassium iodide (SSKI) remains effective and affordable in resource-limited settings. Histopathology shows suppurative and granulomatous inflammation, but organisms are sparse and often difficult to identify on H&E — culture on Sabouraud agar at 25 degrees Celsius is the definitive diagnostic test.

Chromomycosis, Mycetoma, and Other Subcutaneous Mycoses

Chromoblastomycosis (chromomycosis) is a chronic subcutaneous mycosis caused by dematiaceous (dark-pigmented) fungi (Fonsecaea pedrosoi, Cladophialophora carrionii, Phialophora verrucosa) and is endemic in tropical and subtropical regions, predominantly affecting barefoot agricultural workers. It presents as slowly progressive, verrucous plaques and nodules — often on the lower extremity — that evolve over years to decades into cauliflower-like, verrucous masses. Histopathology shows the pathognomonic muriform cells (sclerotic bodies, copper pennies) — thick-walled, brown, septate fungal cells in the dermis visible on H&E without special stains. Treatment is prolonged (months to years) with itraconazole or terbinafine, often combined with cryotherapy or surgical excision for small lesions. Mycetoma (Madura foot) is a chronic, destructive subcutaneous infection caused by either fungi (eumycetoma — Madurella mycetomatis, Scedosporium apiospermum) or bacteria (actinomycetoma — Nocardia, Actinomadura, Streptomyces). The clinical triad is a subcutaneous mass, draining sinuses, and grains (compacted colonies of the causative organism) discharged from the sinuses — grain color helps distinguish eumycetoma (black grains in Madurella) from actinomycetoma (white to yellow grains), which is therapeutically important because actinomycetoma responds to antibiotics while eumycetoma requires antifungals and often surgical excision. Lobomycosis (lacaziosis, caused by Lacazia loboi) produces slowly progressive keloid-like nodules on the ears, extremities, and trunk in patients from the Amazon basin.

Systemic Mycoses With Cutaneous Dissemination: Histoplasmosis, Coccidioidomycosis, Blastomycosis, and Cryptococcosis

Endemic Mycoses: Geographic Distribution and Pathogenesis

The endemic (dimorphic) fungi — Histoplasma capsulatum, Coccidioides immitis/posadasii, Blastomyces dermatitidis, and Talaromyces (Penicillium) marneffei — exist as molds in the environment and convert to yeast (or spherules, in the case of Coccidioides) at body temperature after inhalation of spores. Primary infection is pulmonary, and cutaneous involvement typically indicates disseminated disease, particularly in immunocompromised patients. Geographic distribution is a critical diagnostic clue: histoplasmosis is endemic in the Ohio and Mississippi River valleys (bat and bird guano in caves), coccidioidomycosis in the southwestern US and northern Mexico (San Joaquin Valley fever), blastomycosis in the Great Lakes region and Ohio/Mississippi River valleys, and talaromycosis in Southeast Asia (a defining opportunistic infection in HIV-positive patients in that region).

Cutaneous Manifestations and Diagnostic Approach

Disseminated histoplasmosis produces polymorphous skin lesions including papules, nodules, plaques, and ulcers — notably, umbilicated papules morphologically identical to molluscum contagiosum, which is the key mimicker in immunocompromised patients. Oral ulcers (painful, indurated ulcers on the tongue, palate, or pharynx) are the most common mucosal finding. Disseminated coccidioidomycosis produces papules, nodules, verrucous plaques, abscesses, and draining sinuses; erythema nodosum and erythema multiforme are immunologic skin reactions that occur during primary coccidioidal infection and are associated with a favorable prognosis (they indicate a robust immune response). Blastomycosis produces distinctive verrucous plaques and nodules (often on the face, nose, and extremities) with raised, crusted borders and central healing — these verrucous lesions are frequently misdiagnosed as squamous cell carcinoma, and biopsy with histopathology (showing broad-based budding yeast, 8 to 15 micrometers in diameter, with a thick refractile cell wall) is diagnostic. Cryptococcosis (C. neoformans, C. gattii) produces umbilicated papules, cellulitis-like plaques, and nodules, particularly in immunocompromised patients — the umbilicated papules that mimic molluscum are the cutaneous presentation that should prompt urgent workup for disseminated disease including cryptococcal meningitis.

Special Populations and Immunocompromised Hosts

The clinical behavior of endemic mycoses is profoundly influenced by the patient's immune status. In immunocompetent individuals, primary infection with endemic fungi is often asymptomatic or self-limited (pulmonary granulomas, erythema nodosum in coccidioidomycosis), and cutaneous dissemination is rare. In immunocompromised patients — particularly those with HIV/AIDS (CD4 count below 150 cells/mm3), organ transplant recipients on immunosuppressive therapy, and patients receiving biologic agents (anti-TNF therapy) — primary infection may fail to contain the organism, leading to progressive disseminated disease with skin involvement as a sentinel marker. The dermatologist who recognizes cutaneous histoplasmosis umbilicated papules, blastomycosis verrucous plaques, or cryptococcosis cellulitis in an immunocompromised patient may be the first clinician to diagnose a life-threatening disseminated infection. Biopsy of suspicious lesions with tissue culture and histopathologic examination using GMS and PAS stains is essential — serologic testing (Histoplasma urinary antigen, cryptococcal serum antigen) provides complementary diagnostic data but should not delay tissue diagnosis.

CAUTION: Verrucous or ulcerated skin lesions in a patient from an endemic fungal region — particularly if immunocompromised — should prompt biopsy with fungal culture and histopathologic examination with special stains (GMS, PAS) rather than empiric antibiotics or observation. Blastomycosis verrucous plaques are frequently misdiagnosed as squamous cell carcinoma, and disseminated histoplasmosis umbilicated papules are misidentified as molluscum contagiosum, delaying life-saving antifungal therapy.

THE CUTANEOUS MIMICKER RECOGNITION ATLAS — Tinea Corporis versus Nummular Eczema

The Clinical Pattern: Tinea corporis presents as an annular or arciform plaque with a raised, scaly, advancing border and central clearing — the classic ringworm morphology. The border is the most active zone (where fungal hyphae are concentrated), and KOH preparation from the advancing edge reveals septate, branching hyphae. Lesions may be single or few, are usually asymmetric, and are frequently pruritic. The annular shape, advancing scaly border, and central clearing are the defining clinical triad.

The Mimicker: Nummular eczema (discoid eczema) presents as round or coin-shaped (nummular), erythematous, scaly plaques that closely mimic the annular morphology of tinea corporis. However, nummular eczema plaques are typically uniformly scaly across the entire plaque (without the distinct border-versus-center differential of tinea), are often weepy or crusted in the acute phase, tend to be multiple and bilateral on the extensor surfaces of the extremities, and lack an advancing border with central clearing. Nummular eczema responds to topical corticosteroids; tinea corporis worsens with topical corticosteroids (tinea incognito).

Trap Logic: Treating a round, scaly plaque with topical corticosteroids without performing KOH preparation is the cognitive trap. When a clinician sees a round, pruritic, scaly lesion and assumes eczema, application of topical corticosteroids suppresses the inflammatory border of tinea, partially clearing the scale and redness while allowing the fungus to spread — producing tinea incognito (a modified dermatophyte infection with atypical morphology that is even harder to diagnose). The reverse trap occurs when nummular eczema is treated with prolonged antifungals based on its annular shape, without response, before recognizing it as eczema.

The Decision Anchor: The discriminating test is **KOH preparation from the active border: septate, branching hyphae confirm dermatophyte infection; a negative KOH (ideally confirmed with fungal culture) supports eczema**. The clinical clue is the border: tinea has a raised, scaly, advancing border with relative central clearing (the border is more active than the center); nummular eczema is uniformly involved across the entire plaque without a distinct advancing border. When in doubt, scrape before you treat — KOH takes 5 minutes and prevents tinea incognito.

Antifungal Therapeutics: Topical and Systemic Agents

Topical Antifungal Agents

Topical antifungals are first-line for superficial, localized dermatophyte infections (tinea corporis, cruris, pedis — interdigital and vesiculobullous patterns) and for pityriasis versicolor. The azole class (clotrimazole, miconazole, ketoconazole, econazole, luliconazole, efinaconazole) inhibits lanosterol 14-alpha-demethylase (CYP51), blocking ergosterol synthesis and disrupting the fungal cell membrane. Allylamines (terbinafine, naftifine, butenafine) inhibit squalene epoxidase, an earlier step in ergosterol synthesis, and are fungicidal against dermatophytes (compared to the primarily fungistatic azoles), making them preferred for dermatophyte infections. Ciclopirox olamine works through iron chelation and disruption of fungal mitochondrial electron transport. Topical nystatin is effective only against Candida (not dermatophytes) and is used for oral thrush (nystatin oral suspension) and cutaneous candidiasis.

Systemic Antifungal Agents and Monitoring

Systemic antifungals are required for dermatophyte infections that are extensive, involve hair (tinea capitis — systemic therapy is always required because topical agents do not penetrate the hair follicle), involve nails (onychomycosis), or fail topical therapy. Terbinafine (an allylamine) is the preferred systemic agent for dermatophyte infections due to its fungicidal activity, keratin affinity (it concentrates in the stratum corneum, hair, and nail plate and persists for weeks after discontinuation), and favorable efficacy profile. For tinea capitis, oral terbinafine or griseofulvin (which has historically been the standard of care) for 4 to 8 weeks is the treatment — griseofulvin is more effective against Microsporum species while terbinafine is more effective against Trichophyton. For onychomycosis, terbinafine for 12 weeks (fingernails) or 12 to 16 weeks (toenails) achieves mycologic cure rates of 70 to 80 percent. Itraconazole (a triazole) is an alternative for onychomycosis and is the drug of choice for sporotrichosis (itraconazole for 3 to 6 months), chromomycosis, and the endemic mycoses. Fluconazole is the preferred agent for Candida infections (oropharyngeal, esophageal, vulvovaginal) and for cryptococcal maintenance therapy. Amphotericin B (which binds directly to ergosterol, creating pores in the fungal cell membrane) remains the gold standard for life-threatening systemic mycoses including disseminated histoplasmosis, coccidioidomycosis, blastomycosis, and cryptococcal meningitis — the lipid formulations (liposomal amphotericin B) have substantially reduced nephrotoxicity compared to conventional amphotericin B deoxycholate.

EVIDENCE: A systematic review and meta-analysis comparing oral terbinafine with griseofulvin for tinea capitis in children found that terbinafine demonstrated higher complete cure rates for Trichophyton infections (relative risk 1.47), while griseofulvin showed superiority for Microsporum infections. This species-dependent efficacy difference has led to the recommendation that species identification (via culture) should guide systemic antifungal selection for tinea capitis, rather than empiric therapy with a single agent. Duration of therapy is also species-dependent: Trichophyton requires 4 weeks of terbinafine, while Microsporum requires 8 to 12 weeks of griseofulvin (confirm doses against current formulary).

Drug Interactions, Safety Monitoring, and Patient Counseling

Systemic antifungal therapy requires attention to drug interactions and hepatotoxicity monitoring. Terbinafine is associated with rare hepatotoxicity (confirm against current formulary); baseline and periodic liver function testing is recommended for courses exceeding 4 weeks. Terbinafine inhibits CYP2D6 and may increase levels of drugs metabolized by this enzyme. The azole antifungals (itraconazole, fluconazole, voriconazole, posaconazole) are potent CYP3A4 inhibitors with extensive drug interaction potential — concurrent use with statins, calcineurin inhibitors, certain anticoagulants, and benzodiazepines requires dose adjustment or avoidance. Itraconazole has negative inotropic effects and is contraindicated in heart failure. Voriconazole causes visual disturbances (photopsia) in approximately 30 percent of patients, photosensitivity (long-term use increases cutaneous squamous cell carcinoma risk in transplant patients), and periostitis. Griseofulvin is a CYP3A4 inducer that reduces the efficacy of oral contraceptives and warfarin. The emerging threat of C. auris — a multidrug-resistant Candida species with high rates of resistance to fluconazole, variable susceptibility to echinocandins, and occasional resistance to amphotericin B — has necessitated updated antifungal stewardship protocols in healthcare settings. Patient counseling should address the prolonged treatment courses required for onychomycosis (3 to 4 months of oral therapy, with visible nail improvement taking 9 to 12 months as the healthy nail grows out), the importance of adherence to prevent relapse, and the need for concurrent environmental measures (treating shoes with antifungal powder, avoiding shared bathing facilities, keeping intertriginous areas dry) to reduce reinfection risk. For tinea capitis, counseling should include the importance of treating all household contacts who may be asymptomatic carriers (particularly in T. tonsurans outbreaks), the use of antifungal shampoo (ketoconazole or selenium sulfide) as an adjunct to reduce spore shedding and transmission, and reassurance that the child can return to school once systemic therapy has been initiated. For recurrent dermatophytosis, patients should be counseled on environmental risk reduction — drying intertriginous areas thoroughly after bathing, wearing moisture-wicking fabrics during exercise, treating athletic footwear with antifungal powder, avoiding walking barefoot in communal showers and locker rooms, and not sharing towels, combs, or hats (particularly relevant for tinea capitis prevention in children).

KEY POINT: For Malassezia folliculitis, the diagnostic clue is the monomorphous quality of the follicular papules and pustules — all lesions look the same, unlike acne vulgaris which produces a polymorphous mix of comedones, papules, pustules, and nodules. Malassezia folliculitis worsens with antibiotics (which further suppress competing bacterial flora and allow Malassezia overgrowth) and responds to topical or systemic antifungals, making the distinction from acne therapeutically critical.

THE CUTANEOUS MIMICKER RECOGNITION ATLAS — Pityriasis Versicolor versus Vitiligo

---

The Clinical Pattern: Pityriasis versicolor presents as multiple, well-demarcated, oval macules and thin plaques with fine, powdery scale on the upper trunk, shoulders, and neck. Lesions are hypopigmented on darker skin and tan-to-brown on lighter skin. The distribution is upper trunk-predominant, and the lesions have a subtle but palpable fine scale best appreciated by gently stretching the skin (the evoked scale sign). KOH preparation shows the spaghetti and meatballs pattern (short hyphae and round yeast clusters).

The Mimicker: Vitiligo presents as well-demarcated, depigmented (not merely hypopigmented) macules and patches that are completely devoid of melanin — they appear chalky white under room light and fluoresce bright white under Wood lamp examination (enhanced contrast). Vitiligo patches have NO scale, no palpable texture change, and a smooth surface. The distribution may involve the upper trunk but also favors acral sites (hands, feet, periocular, perioral) and areas of friction or trauma (Koebner phenomenon). Vitiligo is an autoimmune destruction of melanocytes; pityriasis versicolor is a superficial fungal infection that inhibits melanin transfer.

Trap Logic: Diagnosing vitiligo in a patient with hypopigmented macules on the trunk without performing KOH preparation or Wood lamp examination is the cognitive trap. The light spots of pityriasis versicolor may be casually labeled vitiligo, leading to unnecessary autoimmune workup and missing a treatable fungal infection. The reverse trap — treating depigmented vitiligo patches with antifungals because they are on the trunk — delays appropriate therapy. The failure point is not distinguishing hypopigmentation (partial melanin reduction, as in pityriasis versicolor) from depigmentation (complete melanin loss, as in vitiligo).

The Decision Anchor: The discriminating features are **pigment quality (hypopigmented in pityriasis versicolor versus depigmented/chalk-white in vitiligo), surface texture (fine powdery scale in pityriasis versicolor versus smooth, non-scaly surface in vitiligo), Wood lamp (pityriasis versicolor shows yellow-green fluorescence and subtle enhancement; vitiligo shows bright chalk-white fluorescence due to complete melanin absence), and KOH preparation (positive spaghetti and meatballs in pityriasis versicolor; negative in vitiligo)**. The evoked scale sign (stretching the skin to reveal fine scale) is a quick bedside test that favors pityriasis versicolor.

Clinical Case: Pruritic Follicular Papules Unresponsive to Antibiotics

A 24-year-old woman presents with a 4-month history of pruritic, monomorphous papules and pustules on the upper back, chest, and shoulders. She has been treated with two courses of oral antibiotics (doxycycline, then minocycline) for presumed acne with no improvement — in fact, the eruption has worsened during antibiotic therapy. She lives in a hot, humid climate and exercises daily. On examination, there are numerous uniform, 2 to 3 mm, follicular papules and pustules distributed symmetrically on the upper trunk and proximal arms. Comedones are absent. The face is relatively spared.

The key diagnostic clues are the monomorphous follicular morphology (all papules and pustules are the same size and shape, without the polymorphous comedone-papule-pustule-nodule mix of acne vulgaris), the worsening with antibiotic therapy (which suppresses competing bacterial flora and allows Malassezia overgrowth), the hot and humid climate exposure, and the distribution pattern favoring the upper trunk over the face. KOH preparation of pustule contents shows round yeast cells consistent with Malassezia, confirming Malassezia folliculitis. Treatment is initiated with oral fluconazole (confirm dose against current formulary) combined with ketoconazole shampoo as a body wash. Antibiotics are discontinued. At 4-week follow-up, the eruption has cleared substantially. Maintenance therapy with twice-weekly ketoconazole shampoo body wash is recommended to prevent recurrence. This case illustrates the clinical and therapeutic consequences of misdiagnosing Malassezia folliculitis as bacterial acne: the monomorphous quality, the trunk-predominant distribution, and the paradoxical worsening with antibiotics are the three red flags that should prompt fungal evaluation rather than escalation of antibiotic therapy.

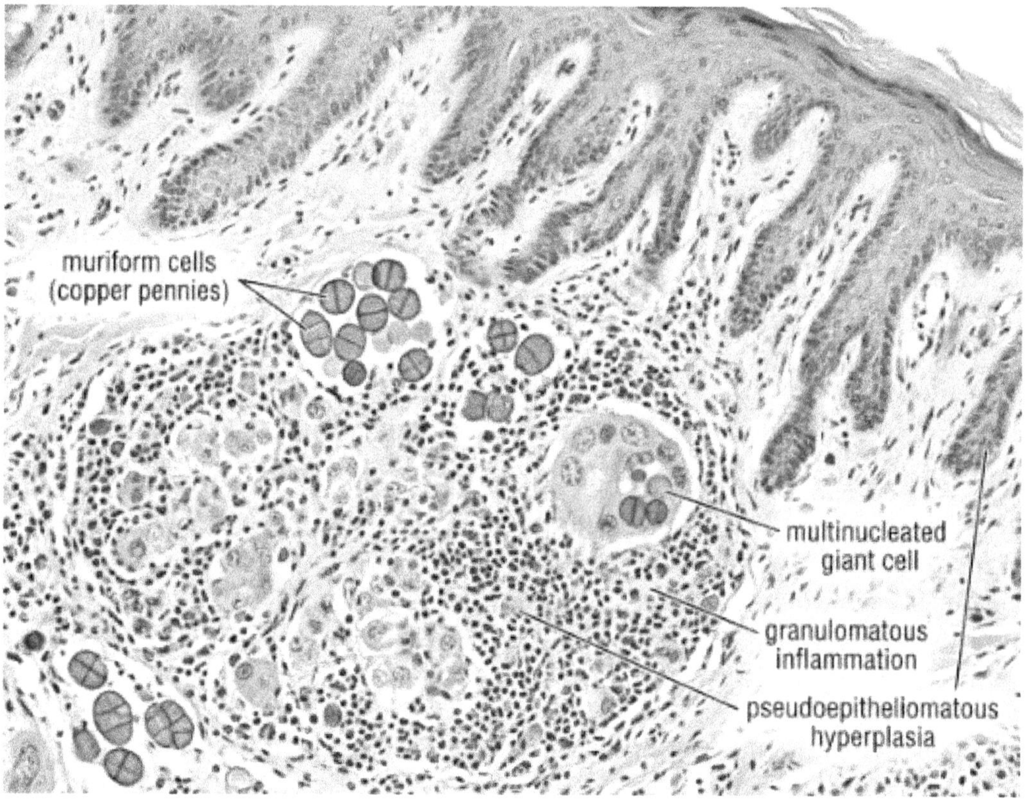

Tinea Corporis vs. Nummular Eczema: The discriminating test is KOH preparation from the active border: septate, branching hyphae confirm dermatophyte infection. The clinical clue is the border morphology — tinea has a raised, advancing border with central clearing, while nummular eczema is uniformly scaly across the entire plaque without a distinct advancing edge. Treating a round plaque with topical corticosteroids without performing KOH creates tinea incognito — a modified dermatophyte infection with atypical morphology.

Pityriasis Versicolor vs. Vitiligo: The discriminating features are pigment quality (hypopigmented versus depigmented), surface texture (fine powdery scale versus smooth), Wood lamp pattern (yellow-green fluorescence versus bright chalk-white), and KOH preparation (spaghetti and meatballs pattern versus negative). The evoked scale sign — stretching the skin to reveal fine scale — is a rapid bedside test favoring pityriasis versicolor over vitiligo.

Summary and Key Concepts

Dermatophytes are keratinophilic fungi classified by genus (Trichophyton, Microsporum, Epidermophyton) and ecological reservoir (anthropophilic, zoophilic, geophilic). KOH preparation from the active border is the gold standard for diagnosis. The two feet, one hand pattern is classic for T. rubrum, and tinea capitis always requires systemic antifungal therapy because topical agents cannot penetrate the hair follicle.

Candidal intertrigo is distinguished from dermatophyte infection by the presence of satellite pustules and involvement of the scrotum (which dermatophytes characteristically spare). Chronic mucocutaneous candidiasis results from primary immunodeficiency syndromes (STAT1 gain-of-function, AIRE deficiency) and presents with persistent, recalcitrant Candida infection from early childhood.

Pityriasis versicolor produces hypopigmented (dark skin) or hyperpigmented (light skin) macules with fine scale and the diagnostic spaghetti and meatballs KOH pattern. Malassezia folliculitis is distinguished from acne by its monomorphous follicular papules, trunk-predominant distribution, absence of comedones, and worsening with antibiotics.

Subcutaneous mycoses produce characteristic clinical patterns: sporotrichosis causes lymphocutaneous nodular spread along lymphatics, chromoblastomycosis shows muriform cells on histopathology, and mycetoma presents with the triad of subcutaneous mass, draining sinuses, and grains.

Endemic dimorphic fungi cause cutaneous lesions through hematogenous dissemination from primary pulmonary infection. Blastomycosis verrucous plaques mimic squamous cell carcinoma, histoplasmosis umbilicated papules mimic molluscum, and all require biopsy with special stains for diagnosis. Systemic therapy selection is guided by organism, severity, and immune status.

CHAPTER 12: PARASITIC, ARTHROPOD, AND INFESTATIONAL SKIN DISEASES

Learning Objectives

1. Recognize the clinical features and dermoscopic findings of scabies infestation, including classic, crusted, and nodular variants, and apply evidence-based treatment strategies for affected patients and their close contacts.
2. Distinguish the three forms of pediculosis by anatomic site, clinical presentation, and epidemiologic context, and identify the public health implications of body lice as vectors for epidemic typhus, trench fever, and relapsing fever.
3. Identify arthropod bite and sting reactions by their morphologic patterns, and correlate clinical findings with the causative arthropod for targeted management and prevention.
4. Recognize the cutaneous manifestations of tropical and travel-associated parasitic infections — cutaneous larva migrans, leishmaniasis, onchocerciasis, and filariasis — and apply the geographic and exposure history that distinguishes these from their clinical mimickers.

Scabies: Classic, Crusted, and Nodular Variants

Epidemiology and Risk Factors

Scabies is one of the most common dermatologic conditions worldwide, with an estimated global prevalence of 100 to 200 million people at any given time. The highest burden falls on tropical and subtropical regions with overcrowded living conditions: Pacific Island nations report prevalence rates exceeding 25 percent in children, and community-level prevalence in parts of sub-Saharan Africa, Southeast Asia, and Indigenous Australian communities reaches 30 to 50 percent in pediatric populations. In high-income countries, scabies occurs in cyclical outbreaks within institutional settings — nursing homes, prisons, daycare centers, and homeless shelters — and in household clusters linked to prolonged skin-to-skin contact. Risk factors include crowding, poverty, lack of access to regular laundering, immunosuppression (HIV/AIDS, organ transplant recipients, systemic corticosteroid use), and neurologic conditions that impair the itch-scratch reflex (dementia, spinal cord injury). The elderly institutionalized population is at highest risk for crusted scabies because of age-related immune senescence compounded by comorbid immunosuppression. Scabies transmission is not related to personal hygiene — the mite is equally capable of infesting clean and unwashed skin, and the persistent social stigma associated with scabies remains a barrier to timely diagnosis and treatment in many communities.

Etiology and Pathophysiology

Scabies is caused by the obligate human ectoparasite Sarcoptes scabiei var. hominis, a microscopic mite (0.3 to 0.4 mm) that burrows into the stratum corneum to lay eggs. The female mite excavates a serpentine burrow 1 to 10 mm long in the superficial epidermis, depositing 2 to 3 eggs per day over her 4 to 6 week lifespan. The characteristic pruritus of scabies is not caused by the mite itself but by a delayed type IV hypersensitivity reaction to mite proteins, fecal pellets (scybala), and egg antigens — this immunologic mechanism explains why pruritus in primary infestation takes 4 to 6 weeks to develop (the time required for sensitization), while reinfestation produces pruritus within 24 to 48 hours in a previously sensitized individual. Transmission occurs through prolonged, direct skin-to-skin contact (15 to 20 minutes minimum), which is why scabies spreads readily within households, between sexual partners, and in institutional settings (nursing homes, prisons, military barracks, refugee camps). Fomite transmission (bedding, clothing) is uncommon in classic scabies (the mite survives only 48 to 72 hours off the host) but is a major transmission route in crusted scabies, where mite burden is massively elevated.

Clinical Presentation and Dermoscopic Features

Classic scabies presents as intensely pruritic papules, vesicles, and excoriations in a characteristic distribution: interdigital web spaces of the hands, wrists (flexor surface), axillary folds, periareolar skin in women, periumbilical area, belt line, genitalia (penile papules and nodules are highly characteristic), buttocks, and the medial feet. The face and scalp are characteristically spared in adults but are commonly involved in infants. The pathognomonic clinical finding is the burrow — a thin, grey, slightly elevated, serpentine line representing the mite's tunnel — best seen in the interdigital web spaces and on the wrists. Dermoscopy greatly enhances burrow detection: the delta-wing jet sign (a dark, triangular structure at the leading end of the burrow, representing the mite's anterior body and legs) is pathognomonic for scabies and visible with a standard dermatoscope. The contrail sign (the trailing burrow behind the mite, resembling a jet contrail) completes the dermoscopic picture. Scabies pruritus is characteristically worse at night (the mite is more active in warm environments), and the generalized pruritus often extends beyond the sites of actual mite colonization due to the systemic nature of the hypersensitivity response.

Crusted (Norwegian) Scabies and Nodular Scabies

Crusted scabies (formerly Norwegian scabies) is a hyperinfestation variant occurring in immunocompromised patients (HIV/AIDS, organ transplant recipients, those receiving immunosuppressive therapy), elderly institutionalized individuals, and patients with neurologic conditions that impair the itch-scratch reflex. While classic scabies involves 10 to 15 mites on the entire body, crusted scabies harbors millions of mites, producing thick, hyperkeratotic, crusted plaques on the hands, feet, elbows, and scalp that resemble psoriasis — the failure to recognize this psoriasis-mimicking presentation as scabies leads to delayed diagnosis and sustained transmission in institutional settings, because each crusted patient sheds millions of mites into the environment. Crusted scabies requires combination therapy (topical permethrin plus oral ivermectin) and intensive environmental decontamination. Nodular scabies presents as persistent, intensely pruritic, red-brown nodules (5 to 20 mm) on the genitalia, axillae, and groin that may persist for weeks to months after successful mite eradication — these nodules represent a persistent granulomatous hypersensitivity reaction to retained mite antigens and respond to potent topical corticosteroids or intralesional corticosteroid injection.

Complications and Special Populations

Secondary bacterial infection (impetiginization) of scabies lesions by Streptococcus pyogenes and Staphylococcus aureus is the most common complication and, in resource-limited settings where scabies is endemic, represents a major driver of post-streptococcal glomerulonephritis and rheumatic heart disease — the World Health Organization has designated scabies as a neglected tropical disease in part because of this downstream burden of secondary bacterial sequelae. In infants and young children, scabies often presents atypically: the distribution includes the palms, soles, face, and scalp (sites spared in adults), vesicles and pustules may predominate, and the clinical picture may mimic atopic dermatitis, impetigo, or even Langerhans cell histiocytosis. In elderly patients, scabies may present as generalized itch with minimal visible skin findings (scabies of the clean), making diagnosis difficult without a high index of suspicion and dermoscopic examination.

CLINICAL PEARL: In any patient presenting with generalized pruritus worse at night — particularly when household contacts or sexual partners are also pruritic — consider scabies regardless of the initial clinical impression. The delta-wing jet sign on dermoscopy is pathognomonic and can be identified in under 30 seconds with a standard dermatoscope. In institutional settings, a single case of crusted scabies can cause a facility-wide outbreak because the massive mite burden produces environmental contamination far exceeding that of classic scabies.

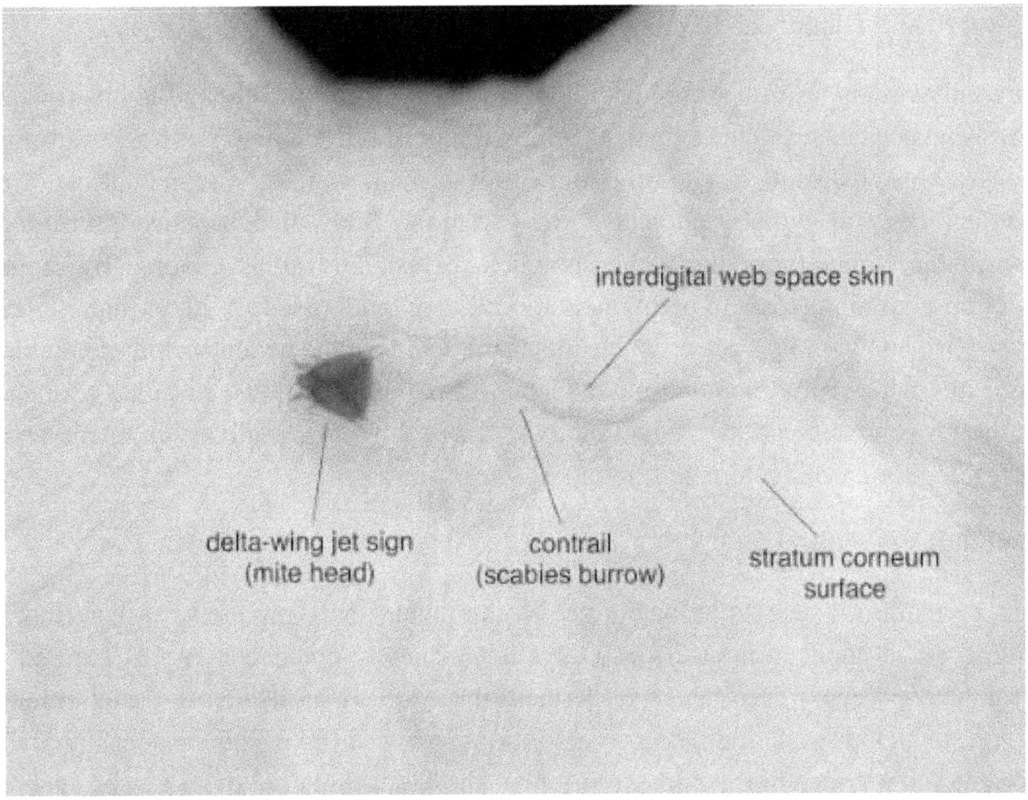

Pediculosis: Head Lice, Body Lice, and Pubic Lice

Biology and Epidemiology

Human lice are obligate ectoparasites that feed on human blood and are classified by anatomic site: Pediculus humanus capitis (head louse), Pediculus humanus corporis (body louse), and Pthirus pubis (pubic louse, crab louse). Head lice are the most common form, with an estimated 6 to 12 million infestations per year among children aged 3 to 11 in the United States alone. Head lice spread through direct head-to-head contact and occasionally through shared personal items (combs, hats, pillows); they do not transmit systemic infections. Body lice live and lay eggs (nits) in the seams of clothing (not on the body itself) and crawl onto the skin to feed; they are associated with conditions of crowding, poverty, and limited access to laundry facilities (homelessness, refugee settings, military deployment). Body lice are medically significant because they are vectors for three serious systemic infections: epidemic typhus (Rickettsia prowazekii), trench fever (Bartonella quintana), and louse-borne relapsing fever (Borrelia recurrentis). Pubic lice infest the coarse hair of the genital region and are transmitted primarily through sexual contact; their prevalence has declined substantially with the increasing practice of genital hair removal.

Clinical Features and Diagnosis

Head lice present as scalp pruritus (often occipital and postauricular), with visible nits (oval, grey-white, 0.8 mm egg casings cemented to the hair shaft within 6 mm of the scalp — nits further from the scalp are typically non-viable) and adult lice (1 to 3 mm, grey-brown, visible with magnification). Secondary excoriations and cervical lymphadenopathy are common. Body lice produce pruritic papules and excoriations on the trunk (particularly the shoulders, waist, and areas covered by clothing) with a characteristic post-inflammatory hyperpigmentation (vagabond disease) in chronic infestation. The diagnosis is confirmed by finding lice or viable nits in the seams of the patient's clothing. Pubic lice present as genital pruritus with visible lice and nits attached to pubic hair shafts; maculae ceruleae (blue-grey macules on the lower abdomen, thighs, and buttocks, caused by louse salivary pigment deposited in the skin during feeding) are a characteristic finding.

Management and Prevention

For head lice, permethrin 1 percent lotion applied to damp hair for 10 minutes and then rinsed is first-line therapy, with a repeat application at 7 to 10 days to kill newly hatched nymphs (permethrin does not reliably kill unhatched eggs). Resistance to permethrin is well documented in many communities, and second-line agents include malathion 0.5 percent lotion, spinosad 0.9 percent suspension, benzyl alcohol 5 percent lotion, and ivermectin 0.5 percent lotion — the latter three are ovicidal and may not require a repeat application. Oral ivermectin (two doses, 7 days apart) is effective for resistant cases. Wet combing with a fine-toothed nit comb every 3 to 4 days for 2 weeks is a non-chemical alternative. School-based no-nit policies (which exclude children until all nits are removed) are not recommended by the American Academy of Pediatrics because they lead to unnecessary school absence and stigma without reducing transmission rates. For body lice, treatment is primarily environmental: laundering and heat-drying all clothing and bedding at high temperatures eradicates the infestation, because body lice reside in clothing seams rather than on the body. For pubic lice, permethrin 1 percent cream rinse is first-line, and all sexual partners within the preceding month should be treated. All patients diagnosed with pubic lice should be screened for other sexually transmitted infections.

Arthropod Bites and Stings: Identification, Reactions, and Management

Bite Reaction Patterns and Identification

Arthropod bites produce cutaneous reactions through a combination of mechanical trauma, injection of salivary antigens, and host immune response. The clinical morphology of bite reactions varies by the causative arthropod and the host's prior sensitization. Mosquito bites produce pruritic, erythematous papules and wheals (immediate IgE-mediated reaction) followed by delayed papules (cell-mediated response); in unsensitized individuals (first exposure), no reaction occurs. Bedbug bites (Cimex lectularius) produce grouped, erythematous papules in a linear or clustered arrangement (the breakfast, lunch, and dinner pattern — three bites in a line), often on exposed skin during sleep. Flea bites (from cat or dog fleas) produce pruritic, erythematous papules predominantly on the ankles and lower legs, often in clusters. Spider bites are far less common than clinically suspected — most lesions diagnosed as spider bites are actually staphylococcal skin infections (MRSA abscesses), and a true spider bite etiology should only be accepted when the spider is captured and identified or when the clinical features are pathognomonic (e.g., the necrotic eschar of a brown recluse bite).

Hypersensitivity Reactions and Papular Urticaria

Papular urticaria is a chronic, recurrent, pruritic papular eruption that is the most common pediatric arthropod bite hypersensitivity — it occurs in children aged 2 to 7 who develop exaggerated, persistent papular and urticarial reactions to bites from fleas, mosquitoes, or bedbugs. Lesions are grouped, symmetrically distributed, and persist for days to weeks beyond the expected duration of a normal bite reaction. The condition reflects the child's immune maturation: as immunologic tolerance to arthropod salivary antigens develops with repeated exposure, papular urticaria gradually resolves. Severe allergic reactions to Hymenoptera stings (bees, wasps, hornets, fire ants) range from large local reactions (erythema and edema exceeding 10 cm at the sting site, peaking at 48 hours) to systemic anaphylaxis (urticaria, angioedema, bronchospasm, hypotension). Patients with a history of systemic Hymenoptera anaphylaxis should carry injectable epinephrine and be referred for venom immunotherapy, which is over 95 percent effective in preventing subsequent systemic reactions.

CAUTION: Most lesions diagnosed as spider bites are not spider bites. The most common cause of a lesion misdiagnosed as a spider bite is a staphylococcal skin abscess (particularly community-associated MRSA). Before attributing any skin lesion to a spider bite, the clinician should confirm that (1) the spider was seen and identified, (2) the clinical course is consistent with a known spider envenomation syndrome (brown recluse necrotic arachnidism or black widow neurotoxic syndrome), and (3) alternative diagnoses (MRSA abscess, necrotizing fasciitis, other infection) have been excluded by appropriate cultures and imaging.

KEY POINT: Papular urticaria is a diagnosis of exclusion in children: before attributing recurrent pruritic papules to arthropod bite hypersensitivity, exclude scabies (check the web spaces), dermatitis herpetiformis (check for IgA deposits on biopsy), and prurigo nodularis. The hallmark of papular urticaria is that lesions are grouped and recur in crops on exposed areas, with each crop representing new bites triggering an exaggerated immune response. The condition self-resolves over months to years as immunologic tolerance to arthropod salivary antigens develops with repeated exposure.

Arthropod	Typical Distribution	Morphology	Key Diagnostic Feature
Mosquito	Exposed skin (arms, legs, face)	Pruritic erythematous wheal → papule	Immediate wheal followed by delayed papule; seasonal variation
Bedbug (Cimex lectularius)	Exposed skin during sleep (arms, shoulders, face)	Grouped erythematous papules in linear clusters	Breakfast-lunch-dinner pattern (3 bites in a row); bites appear on waking

Flea	Ankles, lower legs	Clustered pruritic papules, often with central punctum	Predilection for ankles; association with pet ownership
Tick	Any site; scalp, hairline, groin common	Central attached tick or erythematous papule at bite site	Attached tick may be found; erythema migrans ring suggests Lyme disease
Brown recluse spider	Any site; single lesion	Necrotic ulcer with violaceous border (red-white-blue sign)	Spider must be identified; necrotic eschar develops over 3 to 7 days

Cutaneous Larva Migrans and Myiasis

Cutaneous Larva Migrans

Cutaneous larva migrans (creeping eruption) is caused by the percutaneous penetration and subsequent migration of hookworm larvae (Ancylostoma braziliense, Ancylostoma caninum) through human skin. The larvae are deposited in sandy or moist soil by the feces of infected dogs or cats, and they penetrate human skin on contact with contaminated ground — the feet, buttocks, and hands are the most common sites. The clinical hallmark is an intensely pruritic, erythematous, serpiginous (snakelike), elevated track that advances 1 to 2 cm per day as the larva migrates through the epidermis. The human is a dead-end host for these animal hookworms — the larva cannot complete its lifecycle and eventually dies within weeks, but the track can persist for weeks to months and secondary bacterial infection of excoriated tracks is common. Treatment is oral ivermectin (single dose) or albendazole, which rapidly kills the larva and resolves the eruption.

Myiasis

Myiasis is the infestation of living tissue by fly larvae (maggots). Cutaneous myiasis takes several forms: furuncular myiasis (the most common in travelers returning from Central and South America or sub-Saharan Africa) is caused by the bot fly (Dermatobia hominis) or tumbu fly (Cordylobia anthropophaga). The larva develops within a furuncle-like subcutaneous nodule with a central punctum through which the larva breathes — the patient may feel intermittent, sharp, lancinating pain and notice movement within the nodule. The diagnosis is made by visualizing the larva's posterior spiracles at the punctum or by extracting the larva after occluding the punctum with petroleum jelly or bacon fat (which forces the larva to the surface to breathe). Wound myiasis occurs when fly larvae infest open wounds or ulcers. Migratory myiasis (caused by Hypoderma species in cattle-raising regions) produces a migrating subcutaneous swelling similar to cutaneous larva migrans but deeper and larger.

Leishmaniasis: Cutaneous, Mucocutaneous, and Post-Kala-Azar Dermal Forms

Etiology, Epidemiology, and Pathogenesis

Leishmaniasis is a vector-borne parasitic infection caused by protozoa of the genus Leishmania, transmitted through the bite of infected female phlebotomine sandflies. The clinical form depends on the Leishmania species and the host immune response: cutaneous leishmaniasis (CL, caused by L. major, L. tropica, L. mexicana, and other species), mucocutaneous leishmaniasis (MCL, caused by L. braziliensis and other New World species), and visceral leishmaniasis (kala-azar, caused by L. donovani and L. infantum). Cutaneous leishmaniasis is endemic in parts of the Middle East, Central Asia, North Africa, and Central and South America, and is increasingly seen in travelers, military personnel, and refugees from these regions. The sandfly inoculates Leishmania promastigotes into the skin during a blood meal; the promastigotes are phagocytosed by macrophages and convert to amastigotes, which multiply within the phagolysosome — the host's cell-mediated immune response determines whether the infection self-resolves (Th1 response) or progresses (inadequate Th1 response).

Clinical Presentations

Cutaneous leishmaniasis presents as a papule at the sandfly bite site that enlarges over weeks to form a painless, indurated, well-demarcated nodule or plaque with a central crust or ulcer — the classic volcano-like ulcer with raised, rolled borders and a necrotic base. Old World CL (L. major) tends to produce wet ulcers that self-resolve within 6 to 12 months leaving a depressed scar. New World CL (L. mexicana complex) produces similar ulcers but carries a risk of progression to diffuse cutaneous leishmaniasis (DCL) in anergic patients. Mucocutaneous leishmaniasis (espundia, caused by L. braziliensis) develops months to years after the primary cutaneous lesion, with destructive, granulomatous involvement of the nasal mucosa, septum, palate, and pharynx — progressive nasal destruction produces the tapir nose deformity. Post-kala-azar dermal leishmaniasis (PKDL) occurs after treatment of visceral leishmaniasis, presenting as hypopigmented macules, papules, and nodules on the face and trunk that may serve as a reservoir for ongoing transmission.

Differential Diagnosis and Diagnostic Workup

The differential diagnosis of cutaneous leishmaniasis is broad and includes squamous cell carcinoma (the most important mimicker — both produce an indurated, ulcerated nodule with rolled borders on sun-exposed or trauma-prone skin), lupus vulgaris (cutaneous tuberculosis, which produces apple-jelly nodules on diascopy), sporotrichosis (lymphocutaneous nodular spread), deep fungal infections, foreign body granuloma, and sarcoidosis. Diagnosis is confirmed by demonstrating Leishmania amastigotes on Giemsa-stained smear or touch preparation from the ulcer margin (sensitivity 50 to 70 percent), tissue biopsy showing granulomatous inflammation with intracellular amastigotes (Donovan bodies), culture on NNN medium, or PCR (the most sensitive method for species identification, which is important because species determines the risk of mucocutaneous progression and guides therapy).

Treatment Approach and Species-Guided Decision-Making

Treatment of cutaneous leishmaniasis depends on the infecting species, number and size of lesions, anatomic location, and risk of mucocutaneous progression. Observation alone is appropriate for small, uncomplicated Old World CL lesions (L. major) in cosmetically acceptable locations, because most self-resolve within 6 to 12 months — the trade-off is a potentially larger scar if resolution is slow. Active treatment is indicated for lesions that are large (greater than 4 cm), multiple, cosmetically sensitive (face, hands), or caused by species with mucocutaneous risk (L. braziliensis, L. panamensis). Local therapies include intralesional pentavalent antimonials (injected into the base and margins of the ulcer, 1 to 5 sessions), cryotherapy (liquid nitrogen applied in two freeze-thaw cycles every 2 to 3 weeks), and thermotherapy (localized heat application at 50 degrees Celsius for 30 seconds, single session). Systemic therapy options include parenteral pentavalent antimonials (sodium stibogluconate or meglumine antimoniate, administered for 20 days with cardiac monitoring for QTc prolongation), oral miltefosine (28-day course, teratogenic and therefore contraindicated in pregnancy), and liposomal amphotericin B (for refractory or visceral cases). The critical treatment decision point is species identification: all patients with New World CL caused by Leishmania (Viannia) species require systemic therapy regardless of lesion size, because the risk of delayed mucocutaneous progression (espundia) persists for years after the cutaneous lesion heals.

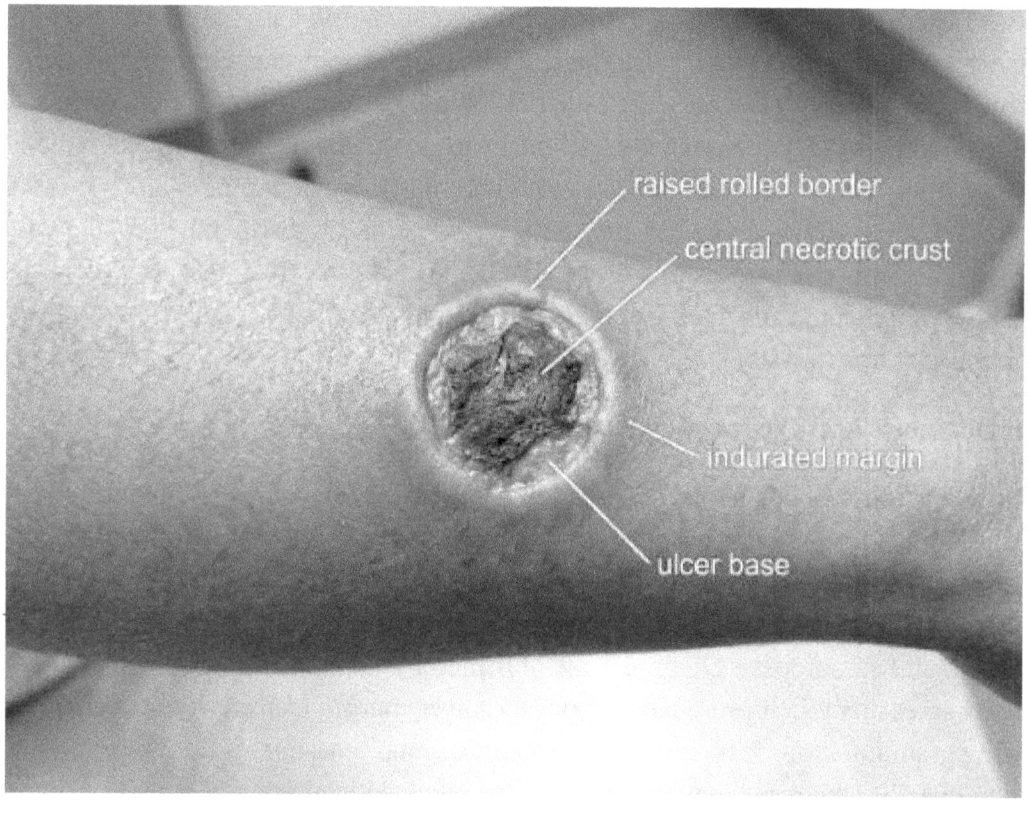

The Clinical Pattern: Scabies presents as intensely pruritic papules, vesicles, and excoriations in a characteristic distribution: interdigital web spaces, wrists (flexor), axillae, periareolar skin, periumbilical area, genitalia, and buttocks. Pruritus is worse at night. The pathognomonic finding is the burrow — a thin, serpentine, grey line in the web spaces or wrists. Household contacts or sexual partners are often symptomatic concurrently.

The Mimicker: Eczematous dermatitis (atopic dermatitis, nummular eczema, contact dermatitis) produces pruritic papules, vesicles, and excoriations that overlap with scabies morphology, particularly in patients with pre-existing eczema where the two conditions may coexist. Eczema tends to involve the antecubital and popliteal fossae, the face, and the neck — different from the scabies-characteristic interdigital, genital, and periumbilical distribution. Eczema pruritus is not specifically nocturnal, and household contacts are not simultaneously affected (unless they share the same allergen exposure).

Trap Logic: Treating generalized pruritus as eczema with topical corticosteroids without examining the interdigital web spaces for burrows or asking about contacts is the cognitive trap. Topical corticosteroids partially suppress the immune response to scabies mites, temporarily reducing the pruritus and masking the clinical picture (scabies incognito), while the infestation persists and household contacts continue to be infected. The reverse trap — over-diagnosing scabies in a patient with eczema who has coincidentally itchy family members — is less harmful but leads to unnecessary treatment.

The Decision Anchor: The discriminating features are **distribution (scabies affects the interdigital web spaces, wrists, genitalia, and periumbilical area — sites rarely involved in eczema), the burrow (pathognomonic for scabies, visible with dermoscopy showing the delta-wing jet sign), nocturnal predominance of itch (characteristic of scabies), and symptomatic close contacts (scabies is contagious; eczema is not)**. Dermoscopic examination of the web spaces for the delta-wing jet sign takes 30 seconds and is the single most efficient bedside test for scabies.

Onchocerciasis, Filariasis, and Other Helminthic Dermatoses

Onchocerciasis (River Blindness)

Onchocerciasis is caused by the filarial nematode Onchocerca volvulus, transmitted by the bite of Simulium blackflies that breed near fast-flowing rivers in sub-Saharan Africa and focal areas of Central and South America. Adult worms reside in subcutaneous nodules (onchocercomata) and release microfilariae that migrate through the skin and eyes. Cutaneous disease includes intensely pruritic papular dermatitis (onchodermatitis), lichenified plaques, premature skin aging and atrophy (presbyderma), and depigmentation (leopard skin — hypopigmented macules predominantly on the anterior shins). The most feared complication is visual impairment and blindness caused by microfilariae invading the cornea and posterior segment of the eye. Diagnosis is by skin snip microscopy (demonstrating microfilariae in bloodless skin snips from the iliac crest or scapula) or by PCR. Treatment is ivermectin (which kills microfilariae but not adult worms), administered as mass drug administration programs in endemic areas

— the Mectizan Donation Program has been one of the most successful public health partnerships in history.

Lymphatic Filariasis and Other Helminthic Skin Diseases

Lymphatic filariasis (caused by Wuchereria bancrofti, Brugia malayi, and Brugia timori, transmitted by mosquitoes) produces lymphatic obstruction leading to chronic lymphedema, elephantiasis (massive lymphedema of the extremities, genitalia, or breasts), and hydrocele. Acute filarial dermatolymphangioadenitis presents as recurrent episodes of fever, lymphangitis, and limb swelling. Loiasis (caused by Loa loa, transmitted by Chrysops deer flies in West and Central Africa) produces transient subcutaneous swellings (Calabar swellings) and the dramatic sign of an adult worm migrating across the subconjunctival space. Gnathostomiasis (caused by Gnathostoma species, acquired through consumption of undercooked freshwater fish in Southeast Asia) produces migratory subcutaneous swellings and serpiginous eruptions. Strongyloides stercoralis produces a pathognomonic cutaneous sign: larva currens (racing larva) — a rapidly migrating, serpiginous, urticarial track on the buttocks, groin, or trunk that advances up to 10 cm per hour (much faster than cutaneous larva migrans, which moves 1 to 2 cm per day), caused by autoinfective filariform larvae penetrating the perianal skin. In immunosuppressed patients (particularly those receiving systemic corticosteroids), Strongyloides can cause hyperinfection syndrome with disseminated larval migration and sepsis.

Evidence-Based Anti-Parasitic Management

Scabicides and Pediculicides

Permethrin 5 percent cream is the first-line topical treatment for scabies: applied from the neck down (including interdigital spaces, genitalia, and under the nails) for 8 to 14 hours, then washed off, with a repeat application at 1 week. All household contacts and sexual partners must be treated simultaneously, regardless of symptoms, because asymptomatic carriers perpetuate transmission. Oral ivermectin (single dose, repeated at 2 weeks) is an effective alternative with the advantage of systemic distribution, making it particularly useful for crusted scabies (where topical penetration through thick crusts is limited), institutional outbreaks, and patients who cannot apply topical treatment reliably. For crusted scabies, combined topical permethrin plus oral ivermectin (multiple doses), with keratolytic agents to reduce the crusted burden, is the standard approach, complemented by environmental decontamination (laundering bedding and clothing in hot water, vacuuming furniture). For head lice, permethrin 1 percent lotion is first-line, with malathion 0.5 percent or spinosad as alternatives for permethrin-resistant lice. Wet combing (bug busting) with a fine-toothed nit comb every 3 to 4 days for 2 weeks is a non-chemical alternative favored in some guidelines.

Patient Education and Counseling

Effective management of parasitic skin diseases requires patient education that addresses both treatment adherence and transmission prevention. For scabies, patients and their household contacts must understand that all close contacts require simultaneous treatment regardless of whether they are symptomatic, because the 4 to 6 week delay between infestation and symptom onset means asymptomatic carriers are actively transmitting mites. Patients should be counseled that pruritus may persist for 2 to 4 weeks after successful treatment (because the hypersensitivity reaction to dead mite antigens continues until antigen clearance), and that this persistent itch does not indicate treatment failure — re-treatment should be considered only if new burrows appear or pruritus fails to improve after 4 weeks. For travelers to tropical regions, preventive counseling includes wearing protective clothing (long sleeves, insect repellent containing DEET or picaridin) to reduce sandfly and mosquito exposure, avoiding walking barefoot on contaminated soil (cutaneous larva migrans prevention), and using insecticide-treated bed nets in areas endemic for leishmaniasis and filariasis. Patients treated for leishmaniasis should be informed about the importance of follow-up monitoring, as mucocutaneous progression from L. braziliensis can occur months to years after the primary lesion heals and may first manifest as nasal congestion or epistaxis.

Anti-Parasitic Agents for Tropical Infections

Ivermectin is the cornerstone of treatment for multiple cutaneous parasitic infections: scabies, onchocerciasis (microfilaricidal), strongyloidiasis, cutaneous larva migrans (single dose), and demodicosis. Antimonial compounds (sodium stibogluconate, meglumine antimoniate) remain first-line for cutaneous and mucocutaneous leishmaniasis in many endemic regions, despite their toxicity profile (cardiotoxicity, pancreatitis); alternatives include miltefosine (oral, effective for several Leishmania species), liposomal amphotericin B (for visceral and refractory cutaneous disease), and paromomycin (topical, for uncomplicated Old World CL). Treatment decisions for cutaneous leishmaniasis are species-dependent: L. major infections may be observed for spontaneous resolution (6 to 12 months), while L. braziliensis infections require systemic therapy to prevent mucocutaneous progression. Albendazole is used for cutaneous larva migrans (alternative to ivermectin), gnathostomiasis, and echinococcal cysts. Diethylcarbamazine (DEC) is the drug of choice for loiasis and lymphatic filariasis but is contraindicated in onchocerciasis co-endemic areas because of the risk of severe Mazzotti reaction (massive microfilarial death causing hypotension, encephalopathy, and death).

THE CUTANEOUS MIMICKER RECOGNITION ATLAS — Cutaneous Leishmaniasis versus Squamous Cell Carcinoma

The Clinical Pattern: Cutaneous leishmaniasis presents as a painless, indurated, well-demarcated nodule or plaque with raised, rolled borders and a central crust or ulcer — the classic volcano-like ulcer. It develops at the site of a sandfly bite over weeks, usually on exposed skin (face, arms, legs). The patient has a history of travel to or residence in an endemic region (Middle East, Central Asia, North Africa, Central/South America). The lesion is typically painless despite its ulcerated appearance.

The Mimicker: Squamous cell carcinoma (SCC) of the skin presents as an indurated, keratotic nodule or plaque that may ulcerate centrally, producing a lesion with raised, rolled borders and a necrotic or crusted center — morphologically overlapping with cutaneous leishmaniasis. SCC occurs on sun-exposed skin (face, ears, dorsal hands, forearms), particularly in fair-skinned individuals with chronic UV damage. SCC develops slowly over months and is typically in an older patient with actinic damage.

Trap Logic: Biopsying a suspicious ulcerated nodule and receiving a histopathology report showing granulomatous inflammation without recognizing that the pathologist must be alerted to look specifically for Leishmania amastigotes is the cognitive trap. In non-endemic settings, pathologists may not routinely search for intracellular organisms in granulomatous tissue, and the amastigotes (2 to 4 micrometer intracellular bodies) can be missed without directed examination or Giemsa staining. The reverse trap — assuming a painless, indurated, ulcerated nodule on the face of an elderly patient is CL when it is actually SCC — delays oncologic management.

The Decision Anchor: The discriminating features are **travel/endemic exposure history (essential for CL), age and UV damage profile (SCC favors elderly, sun-damaged skin), tissue biopsy with directed examination for Leishmania amastigotes (Giemsa stain, PCR), and the timeframe of lesion development (CL develops over weeks following a sandfly bite; SCC develops over months in a background of chronic actinic damage)**. When biopsying a suspicious ulcerated nodule in a patient with endemic area exposure, alert the pathologist to examine for Leishmania amastigotes with Giemsa staining and request tissue PCR for Leishmania species identification.

EVIDENCE: A Cochrane systematic review of interventions for cutaneous leishmaniasis found that oral miltefosine and intralesional antimonials showed similar efficacy to parenteral antimonials for uncomplicated Old World CL, with improved safety profiles. For New World CL caused by L. braziliensis, systemic therapy (pentavalent antimonials or miltefosine) is recommended over local treatment to prevent mucocutaneous progression. Thermotherapy and cryotherapy are effective physical treatments for small, uncomplicated lesions and avoid systemic drug toxicity.

Clinical Case: Generalized Pruritus in a Nursing Home Resident

An 82-year-old nursing home resident with dementia presents with generalized pruritus of 3 weeks duration. She has been treated with emollients and low-potency topical corticosteroids for presumed xerotic eczema without improvement. On examination, there are diffuse excoriations on the trunk, arms, and interdigital web spaces, with small papules in the web spaces, periumbilical area, and axillary folds. Two other residents and a nursing aide on the same unit have developed generalized pruritus in the past 2 weeks.

The clinical triad — pruritus worse at night, distribution involving the web spaces and typical scabies-predilection sites, and multiple symptomatic contacts in an institutional setting — is classic for scabies. Dermoscopic examination of the web spaces reveals the delta-wing jet sign at the leading edge of a serpentine burrow, confirming the diagnosis. Mineral oil preparation of a burrow scraping shows the mite, eggs, and fecal pellets under light microscopy. Given the institutional setting, the patient's skin is examined thoroughly for hyperkeratotic plaques suggesting crusted scabies — thick, scaly plaques are noted on both hands, confirming crusted scabies as the index case driving the facility outbreak. Treatment includes topical permethrin 5 percent cream plus oral ivermectin (multiple doses), keratolytic cream to reduce the crusted burden, and simultaneous treatment of all residents and staff on the affected unit. Environmental measures (hot-water laundering of bedding, vacuuming mattresses, bagging non-washable items for 72 hours) are implemented. This case demonstrates the institutional cascade: a single undiagnosed crusted scabies patient harboring millions of mites can sustain an outbreak affecting dozens of contacts.

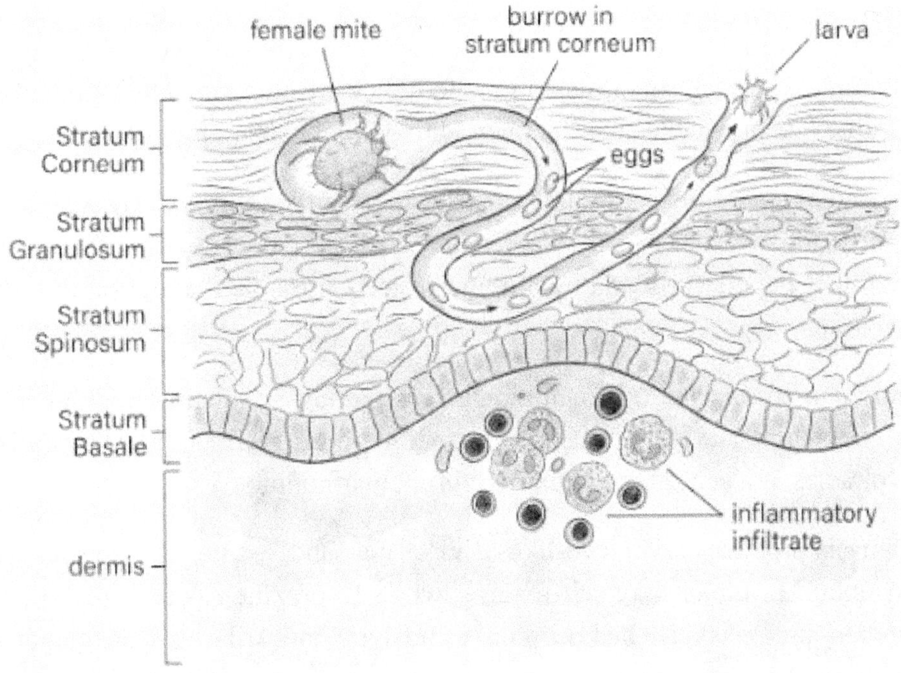

Scabies vs. Eczema: The discriminating features are distribution (scabies affects the interdigital web spaces, wrists, genitalia, and periumbilical area — sites rarely involved in eczema), the burrow (pathognomonic, visible with the delta-wing jet sign on dermoscopy), nocturnal predominance of pruritus, and symptomatic close contacts. Cognitive trap: treating generalized pruritus with topical corticosteroids without examining the web spaces, which partially suppresses the clinical picture (scabies incognito) while the infestation persists.

Cutaneous Leishmaniasis vs. Squamous Cell Carcinoma: The discriminating features are travel or endemic area exposure history (essential for CL), age and chronic actinic damage profile (SCC favors elderly, UV-damaged skin), and tissue biopsy with directed examination for Leishmania amastigotes (Giemsa stain, PCR). When biopsying an ulcerated nodule in a patient with endemic exposure, alert the pathologist to look for intracellular amastigotes — they are easily missed without directed examination.

Summary and Key Concepts

Scabies is diagnosed by the pathognomonic burrow and the delta-wing jet sign on dermoscopy. Classic scabies harbors 10 to 15 mites; crusted scabies harbors millions and requires combination therapy plus environmental decontamination. All household contacts must be treated simultaneously regardless of symptoms.

Body lice are medically significant as vectors for epidemic typhus, trench fever, and relapsing fever. Head lice are treated with topical permethrin or malathion; body lice are eradicated by laundering and replacing infested clothing. Pubic lice prevalence has declined with genital hair removal practices.

Most lesions diagnosed as spider bites are staphylococcal skin infections (MRSA abscesses). True spider envenomation requires identification of the spider and a clinical course consistent with a recognized envenomation syndrome. Papular urticaria in children reflects immune maturation to arthropod salivary antigens.

Cutaneous larva migrans produces a pathognomonic serpiginous, advancing track (1 to 2 cm per day) caused by animal hookworm larvae and responds to single-dose ivermectin. Myiasis is diagnosed by visualizing larval spiracles at a central punctum in a furuncular nodule.

Cutaneous leishmaniasis produces a volcano-like ulcer at the sandfly bite site. Species identification by PCR guides management: L. major may self-resolve, while L. braziliensis requires systemic therapy to prevent mucocutaneous progression. Onchocerciasis and lymphatic filariasis are major causes of skin disease in endemic tropical regions.

CHAPTER 13: BENIGN SKIN TUMORS AND CYSTS

Learning Objectives

1. Classify melanocytic nevi by histologic architecture (junctional, compound, intradermal) and recognize the clinical and dermoscopic features of special variants — Spitz nevi, dysplastic nevi, blue nevi, halo nevi, and congenital melanocytic nevi — that require careful clinical and histologic distinction from melanoma.
2. Distinguish seborrheic keratoses from melanocytic lesions and premalignant keratoses using clinical examination and dermoscopy, and recognize the sign of Leser-Trélat as a paraneoplastic phenomenon.
3. Identify the clinical features and histopathologic findings of common cystic lesions, benign fibrohistiocytic tumors, lipomas, vascular tumors, and adnexal neoplasms, and apply evidence-based management strategies for each.
4. Apply clinical criteria — the ABCDE framework, dermoscopic red flags, and growth pattern analysis — to distinguish benign from potentially malignant skin lesions and determine when biopsy is indicated.

Melanocytic Nevi: Junctional, Compound, Intradermal, and Special Variants (Spitz, Dysplastic, Blue, Halo, Congenital)

Classification by Histologic Architecture

Melanocytic nevi are benign proliferations of melanocytes that are classified by the location of melanocyte nests within the skin. Junctional nevi contain melanocyte nests at the dermoepidermal junction and present as flat, uniformly pigmented, well-circumscribed macules — they are most common in childhood and adolescence. Compound nevi contain melanocyte nests at both the junction and the dermis, presenting as slightly raised, dome-shaped papules that may retain peripheral pigmentation with a lighter center. Intradermal nevi contain melanocyte nests entirely within the dermis and present as flesh-colored or lightly pigmented, dome-shaped or pedunculated papules — they represent the most mature stage of nevus evolution and are the most common nevus type in adults. This junctional-to-intradermal progression reflects the Unna-Abtropfung concept of gradual nevus maturation: melanocyte nests migrate from the junction into the dermis over years, with progressive loss of pigment and increasing elevation.

Epidemiology and Natural History

The number of melanocytic nevi peaks in the third decade of life and gradually decreases thereafter, with a typical adult carrying 20 to 40 nevi. Nevus count is the strongest independent risk factor for melanoma — individuals with more than 100 nevi carry a 7-fold increased melanoma risk compared to those with fewer than 15. Nevus development is driven by ultraviolet radiation exposure (particularly intermittent, intense sun exposure in childhood), genetic factors (the MC1R gene variants associated with red hair and fair skin correlate with higher nevus counts), and immunosuppression (organ transplant recipients develop eruptive nevi). Most nevi are clinically stable and require no treatment; however, any nevus that demonstrates change in size, shape, color, or symptoms (the ABCDE criteria) warrants clinical evaluation and potential biopsy to exclude melanoma arising within a pre-existing nevus.

Special Variants

Spitz nevi (formerly spindle and epithelioid cell nevi) present as well-circumscribed, dome-shaped, pink to red-brown papules, most commonly on the face or lower extremities of children and young adults. Histologically, they show spindled and epithelioid melanocytes arranged in fascicles with Kamino bodies (eosinophilic globules at the dermoepidermal junction) and maturation with depth. Despite benign behavior in most cases, Spitz nevi are histologically challenging because they share features with melanoma — the atypical Spitz tumor (spitzoid tumor of uncertain malignant potential) occupies a diagnostic grey zone requiring expert dermatopathologic assessment and sometimes sentinel lymph node biopsy. Dysplastic (Clark) nevi are flat to slightly elevated, irregularly bordered, variably pigmented lesions larger than 5 mm that occur sporadically or as part of the dysplastic nevus syndrome (familial atypical mole and melanoma syndrome, FAMMM). Histologically, they show architectural disorder with shouldering of the junctional component beyond the dermal component, bridging of rete ridges, concentric and lamellar fibroplasia, and random cytologic atypia. Dysplastic nevi are melanoma risk markers: patients with the dysplastic nevus syndrome and a family history of melanoma carry a lifetime melanoma risk approaching 100 percent. Blue nevi are dermal melanocytic proliferations that appear clinically as blue-grey papules or nodules because the deep dermal melanin absorbs longer wavelengths and scatters shorter wavelengths (the Tyndall effect). Common blue nevi are small (less than 1 cm) and benign; cellular blue nevi are larger and may rarely undergo malignant transformation. Halo nevi (Sutton nevi) show a symmetric zone of depigmentation surrounding a central melanocytic nevus, caused by an immune-mediated lymphocytic attack against nevus melanocytes — they are benign and most common in adolescents, though their association with vitiligo warrants a skin examination for other depigmented patches.

Dermoscopic Assessment of Melanocytic Nevi

Dermoscopy provides structured criteria for evaluating melanocytic nevi beyond what is visible to the naked eye. Benign melanocytic nevi typically show a symmetric, regular pigment network (brown lines on a lighter background corresponding to melanin along the rete ridges), homogeneous globules (round, uniformly sized and spaced pigmented structures at the lesion periphery representing nests of melanocytes at the dermoepidermal junction), and central hypopigmentation in compound and intradermal nevi (reflecting dermal maturation). The global dermoscopic patterns of benign nevi include reticular (regular pigment network), globular (regular globules), cobblestone (closely packed, angulated globules in intradermal nevi), and homogeneous (diffuse, structureless pigmentation in blue nevi). A nevus that displays two different global patterns (combined pattern) or that shows any of the melanoma-specific structures (atypical network, blue-white veil, regression structures, irregular streaks) requires clinical correlation and potential biopsy. In children and adolescents, melanocytic nevi frequently show peripheral globules reflecting benign nevus growth — this is a normal finding in growing nevi and should not be confused with the irregular peripheral streaks of melanoma.

Congenital Melanocytic Nevi

Congenital melanocytic nevi (CMN) are present at birth or appear within the first few months of life and are classified by projected adult size: small (less than 1.5 cm), medium (1.5 to 20 cm), and giant (greater than 20 cm). Giant congenital nevi carry a 5 to 10 percent lifetime risk of melanoma, with the highest risk occurring in the first decade of life — melanoma arising in giant CMN often develops within the deeper dermal or subcutaneous component, making clinical surveillance of surface changes insufficient. Giant CMN of the posterior axial location (bathing trunk distribution) carry additional risk of neurocutaneous melanocytosis, a condition in which melanocyte proliferation occurs within the leptomeninges and may produce symptomatic CNS disease. Management of giant CMN remains controversial: serial excision or tissue expansion may be offered for cosmetic and oncologic reasons, but complete excision is often not feasible due to the lesion's extent, and melanoma can arise in the residual nevus cells deep to the excision plane.

Seborrheic Keratoses and Dermatosis Papulosa Nigra

Clinical Features and Dermoscopic Findings

Seborrheic keratoses are the most common benign epithelial tumors, affecting virtually all adults over age 50. They present as well-demarcated, waxy, verrucous, stuck-on papules and plaques ranging from skin-colored to dark brown or black, distributed on the trunk, face, and extremities (sparing the palms and soles). The surface shows horn cysts (keratin-filled invaginations) and fissures visible with dermoscopy. Dermoscopic features are distinctive: milia-like cysts (round, white-yellow globules representing intraepidermal horn cysts), comedo-like openings (irregular, dark crypts corresponding to keratin-filled follicular ostia), fat finger-like structures (thick, linear, light-brown ridges), and cerebriform pattern (gyrus-and-sulcus architecture). These dermoscopic features collectively produce the brain-like pattern that reliably distinguishes seborrheic keratoses from melanocytic lesions — this is critical because darkly pigmented seborrheic keratoses are one of the most common clinical mimickers of melanoma.

Variants and Clinical Significance

The irritated (inflamed) seborrheic keratosis develops when mechanical trauma or friction triggers an inflammatory response, producing erythema, crusting, and pruritus that may further mimic melanoma or squamous cell carcinoma clinically. Stucco keratoses are small, dry, white-grey, flat keratoses clustered on the distal lower extremities. Dermatosis papulosa nigra is a common variant seen in individuals with Fitzpatrick skin types IV through VI, presenting as multiple small (1 to 5 mm), smooth, pedunculated, dark-brown to black papules on the malar cheeks, forehead, and neck — Morgan Freeman's characteristic facial papules are the most publicly recognizable example of this benign condition. Treatment of seborrheic keratoses is indicated for cosmetic reasons or symptomatic relief and includes cryotherapy, curettage, electrodesiccation, and shave removal. The sign of Leser-Trélat — the sudden eruptive onset of multiple seborrheic keratoses, often pruritic — is a rare but important paraneoplastic phenomenon associated with internal malignancies (most commonly gastric adenocarcinoma), requiring an age-appropriate malignancy workup when recognized.

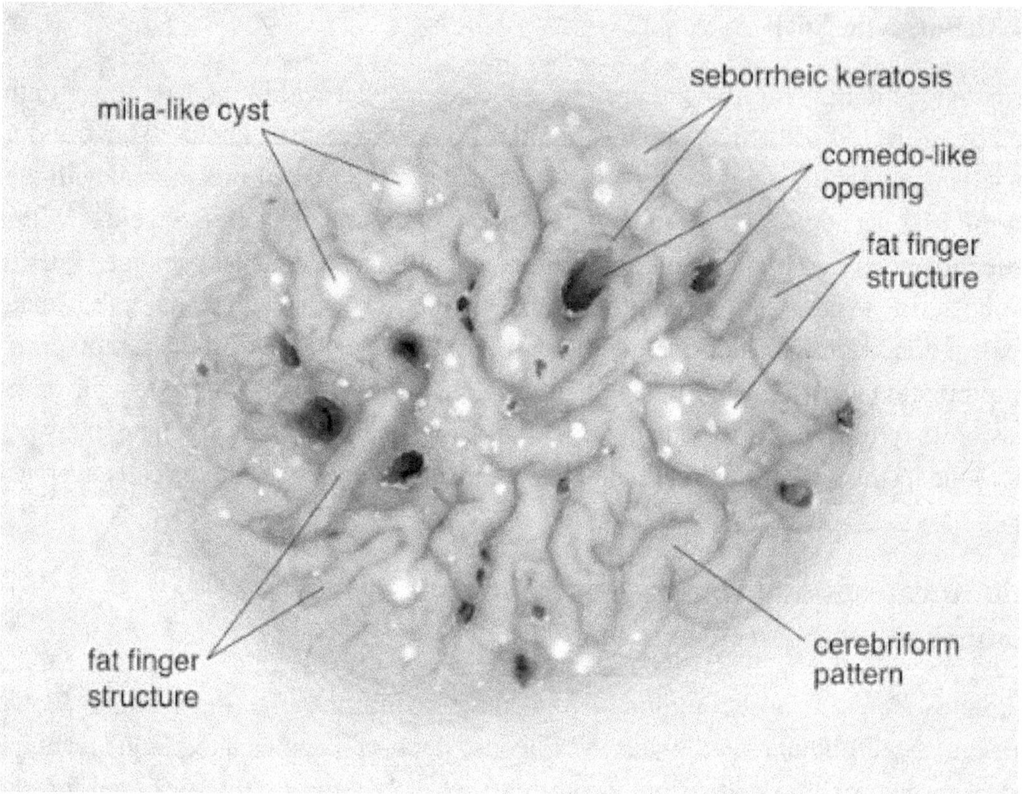

THE CUTANEOUS MIMICKER RECOGNITION ATLAS — Seborrheic Keratosis versus Melanoma

The Clinical Pattern: Seborrheic keratoses present as well-demarcated, waxy, stuck-on papules and plaques with a verrucous surface, ranging from skin-colored to dark brown or black. They are multiple, symmetrically distributed on the trunk and face, and show horn cysts and fissures on close inspection. The lesion surface has a dull, waxy quality — not the shiny surface of a melanocytic lesion. On dermoscopy, milia-like cysts, comedo-like openings, and the cerebriform pattern are diagnostic.

The Mimicker: Melanoma (particularly nodular melanoma) can present as a dark brown to black papule or nodule that superficially resembles a darkly pigmented seborrheic keratosis. Melanoma lacks the stuck-on quality and instead shows an asymmetric shape, irregular borders, color variegation (blue-white veil, regression structures, irregular pigment network on dermoscopy), and a history of change. A melanoma may present as a single new or changing lesion, unlike the typically stable and multiple seborrheic keratoses.

Trap Logic: Dismissing a darkly pigmented nodule as just another seborrheic keratosis without dermoscopic examination is the cognitive trap. The naked eye cannot reliably distinguish a dark seborrheic keratosis from a nodular melanoma, and clinicians who treat many seborrheic keratoses daily may develop complacency toward dark lesions. The reverse trap — biopsying every seborrheic keratosis — is resource-wasteful but less dangerous; a targeted approach using dermoscopy reduces unnecessary biopsies while catching the rare melanoma mimic.

The Decision Anchor: The discriminating features are **dermoscopic pattern (milia-like cysts, comedo-like openings, and cerebriform pattern are diagnostic of seborrheic keratosis; blue-white veil, atypical pigment network, irregular dots and globules, and regression structures indicate melanoma), surface quality (dull, waxy, stuck-on surface favors seborrheic keratosis; shiny, smooth surface favors melanocytic lesion), and history (stable or slowly growing over months to years favors benign; rapid change in size, shape, or color raises concern for melanoma)**. When in doubt, biopsy — the cost of missing a melanoma far exceeds the cost of excising a seborrheic keratosis.

Epidermal Cysts, Pilar Cysts, Dermoid Cysts, and Steatocystomas

Epidermal Inclusion Cysts

Epidermal inclusion cysts (infundibular cysts) are the most common cutaneous cysts, presenting as firm, round, mobile, subcutaneous nodules with a central punctum representing the occluded follicular ostium. They are filled with laminated keratin (not sebum — the historical term sebaceous cyst is a misnomer) and are lined by stratified squamous epithelium with a granular layer. They occur most commonly on the face, trunk, and neck. Rupture of the cyst wall into the surrounding dermis triggers an intense foreign body granulomatous reaction — the resulting inflamed, tender, erythematous nodule is often misdiagnosed as an infected cyst, but the inflammation is usually sterile (caused by keratin spillage, not bacterial infection), and antibiotics alone are inadequate without drainage of the keratin contents. Definitive treatment is complete surgical excision including the cyst wall; incision and drainage alone leaves the cyst wall in place and results in recurrence.

Pilar Cysts, Dermoid Cysts, and Steatocystomas

Pilar cysts (trichilemmal cysts) are the second most common cutaneous cyst and occur predominantly on the scalp, often as multiple lesions with autosomal dominant inheritance. They are lined by epithelium without a granular layer (trichilemmal keratinization, mimicking the outer root sheath of the hair follicle) and contain compact, homogeneous keratin. Dermoid cysts are congenital developmental cysts that present at birth or in early childhood as firm, subcutaneous nodules along embryonic fusion lines — the periorbital area (lateral brow) is the most common site. They are lined by keratinizing epithelium with adnexal structures (hair follicles, sebaceous glands, eccrine glands) within the cyst wall, and periorbital dermoid cysts require imaging before excision to exclude intracranial extension through a cranial suture. Steatocystoma multiplex is an autosomal dominant condition (mutation in keratin 17) presenting as multiple, small, yellowish, dermal cysts on the trunk, axillae, and proximal extremities, filled with oily, sebaceous material; individual lesions are termed steatocystoma simplex.

Dermatofibromas and Benign Fibrohistiocytic Tumors

Clinical Features and Pathogenesis

Dermatofibromas (benign fibrous histiocytomas) are among the most common benign skin tumors, presenting as firm, dome-shaped or slightly depressed, pink-brown to dark-brown papules, most commonly on the lower extremities of young to middle-aged women. The pathognomonic clinical finding is the dimple sign (Fitzpatrick sign): lateral compression of the lesion causes central dimpling because the tumor is tethered to the overlying epidermis. Most dermatofibromas are thought to arise as a reactive fibrohistiocytic proliferation following minor trauma (insect bites, folliculitis) — the lesion represents an exaggerated wound healing response rather than a true neoplasm. On dermoscopy, dermatofibromas show a central white scar-like patch with a peripheral delicate pigment network — this pattern is diagnostic and distinguishes dermatofibromas from melanocytic lesions. Histologically, they show a proliferation of fibroblasts and histiocytes arranged in a storiform pattern, trapping collagen bundles at the periphery (collagen trapping), with overlying epidermal hyperplasia (acanthosis) and basal layer hyperpigmentation (dirty feet sign on histology).

Differential Diagnosis and Management

The differential diagnosis of dermatofibroma includes dermatofibrosarcoma protuberans (DFSP — a locally aggressive fibroblastic tumor that is CD34-positive on immunohistochemistry, unlike dermatofibromas which are Factor XIIIa-positive and CD34-negative), melanoma (particularly amelanotic nodular melanoma), blue nevus, and Kaposi sarcoma. Multiple dermatofibromas (more than 15) can be associated with systemic lupus erythematosus and immunosuppression (HIV, immunosuppressive therapy). Dermatofibromas are benign and do not require treatment unless symptomatic; shave excision may be performed for cosmetically bothersome or pruritic lesions, though recurrence can occur if excision is incomplete. Surgical excision with clear margins is reserved for lesions where the clinical or dermoscopic features raise concern for DFSP.

Lipomas and Subcutaneous Benign Neoplasms

Lipomas

Lipomas are the most common soft tissue tumor, composed of mature adipocytes encapsulated by a thin fibrous capsule. They present as soft, mobile, non-tender, subcutaneous nodules most commonly on the trunk, proximal extremities, and neck. Lipomas are slow-growing and typically range from 1 to 5 cm in diameter. Multiple lipomas occur in familial multiple lipomatosis (autosomal dominant) and in Dercum disease (adiposis dolorosa — multiple painful lipomas associated with obesity, fatigue, and depression, predominantly in postmenopausal women). Angiolipomas are lipoma variants that contain a prominent vascular component and are characteristically painful or tender, distinguishing them from the typically painless ordinary lipoma. The primary clinical concern is distinguishing lipoma from liposarcoma: features suggesting liposarcoma include large size (greater than 5 cm), deep subfascial location, rapid growth, firmness on palpation, and fixation to underlying structures. Ultrasound or MRI is indicated for large or atypical lipomas, and excisional biopsy is performed if imaging features are concerning. Most lipomas are managed conservatively or excised for cosmetic reasons; recurrence after complete excision is uncommon.

EVIDENCE: A systematic review of lipoma management found that simple excision remains the standard of care for symptomatic lipomas, with recurrence rates below 5 percent after complete removal. Liposuction-assisted removal is an alternative for large or cosmetically sensitive lipomas, producing smaller scars but with higher incomplete removal rates. For large (greater than 5 cm) or deep-seated soft tissue masses, MRI is the imaging modality of choice for distinguishing lipoma from well-differentiated liposarcoma — the presence of thick septations (greater than 2 mm), non-adipose components, or contrast enhancement suggests liposarcoma and mandates excisional biopsy.

Other Subcutaneous Benign Neoplasms

Hibernomas are benign tumors of brown fat presenting as slow-growing, soft, deep subcutaneous masses, most commonly on the thigh, shoulder, and back. They are histologically distinct from lipomas, composed of multivacuolated brown fat cells, and are benign with no malignant potential. Neurofibromas are benign nerve sheath tumors presenting as soft, skin-colored, pedunculated papules or subcutaneous nodules that demonstrate the buttonhole sign (the lesion can be invaginated into the skin with finger pressure). Solitary neurofibromas are common and benign; multiple neurofibromas raise concern for neurofibromatosis type 1 (NF1), requiring assessment for diagnostic criteria (cafe-au-lait macules, axillary freckling, Lisch nodules, optic glioma, osseous dysplasia, first-degree relative with NF1). Schwannomas (neurilemmomas) are encapsulated nerve sheath tumors that present as firm, mobile, subcutaneous nodules along the course of a peripheral nerve, with a positive Tinel sign (paresthesias elicited by percussion).

Vascular Tumors: Cherry Angiomas, Pyogenic Granulomas, and Hemangiomas

Cherry Angiomas and Venous Lakes

Cherry angiomas (Campbell de Morgan spots) are the most common vascular tumors in adults, presenting as bright red, dome-shaped papules 1 to 5 mm in diameter on the trunk and proximal extremities. They increase in number and size with advancing age and are composed of dilated capillaries in the papillary dermis. Cherry angiomas are entirely benign and require no treatment; cosmetic removal is performed with electrodesiccation, laser ablation, or shave excision. Venous lakes are soft, dark-blue, compressible papules on sun-damaged skin of the lower lip, ears, and face in elderly patients — they represent dilated venules in the superficial dermis and are distinguished from melanoma by their complete compressibility with diascopy (a melanocytic lesion retains its color on compression).

Pyogenic Granulomas

Pyogenic granulomas (lobular capillary hemangiomas) are rapidly growing, friable, erythematous, dome-shaped or pedunculated nodules that bleed profusely with minor trauma. Despite their name, they are neither pyogenic (infectious) nor granulomatous — they represent a lobular proliferation of capillaries in a loose stroma. They occur at sites of prior trauma or within areas of chronic irritation, and are common in children, pregnant women (granuloma gravidarum of the gingiva), and patients taking retinoids or targeted cancer therapies (BRAF inhibitors, EGFR inhibitors). The key clinical concern is distinguishing pyogenic granuloma from amelanotic melanoma — both present as rapidly growing, pink to red, friable nodules that bleed easily. Shave excision with electrodesiccation of the base is curative; recurrence after incomplete removal may require full-thickness excision. All excised pyogenic granulomas should be submitted for histopathologic examination to exclude amelanotic melanoma.

Vascular Malformations Versus Vascular Tumors

The distinction between vascular tumors (true neoplasms with endothelial cell proliferation) and vascular malformations (structural anomalies of blood vessels without proliferation) is fundamental to correct diagnosis and management. Vascular tumors — including infantile hemangiomas, pyogenic granulomas, and kaposiform hemangioendotheliomas — demonstrate endothelial cell proliferation, express GLUT-1 (glucose transporter-1) on immunohistochemistry, and may involute spontaneously. Vascular malformations — including capillary malformations (port-wine stains), venous malformations, lymphatic malformations, and arteriovenous malformations — are present at birth, grow proportionately with the child, never involute spontaneously, and are GLUT-1 negative. This biological classification (Mulliken and Glowacki, refined by the International Society for the Study of Vascular Anomalies) replaced the confusing older terminology that used hemangioma as a catch-all for both tumors and malformations. Capillary malformations (port-wine stains) present as well-demarcated, pink-red, blanchable patches that darken and thicken with age; facial port-wine stains in the V1 trigeminal distribution carry a risk of Sturge-Weber syndrome (ipsilateral leptomeningeal and ocular vascular malformations), requiring ophthalmologic evaluation and brain MRI.

Infantile Hemangiomas

Infantile hemangiomas are the most common tumors of infancy, affecting 4 to 5 percent of infants (higher incidence in premature infants, females, and those of European descent). They follow a characteristic lifecycle: absence at birth or presence as a precursor mark (pale macule or telangiectatic patch), rapid proliferative phase during the first 3 to 6 months of life, plateau at 6 to 12 months, and slow spontaneous involution over 3 to 7 years. Most infantile hemangiomas are uncomplicated and require only observation and parental reassurance. Treatment with oral propranolol (the standard of care since its serendipitous discovery in 2008) is indicated for hemangiomas that are ulcerated, obstructing a vital structure (airway, visual axis), causing disfigurement (facial hemangiomas, particularly on the nose or lip), or extensive (associated with PHACE syndrome — posterior fossa anomalies, hemangioma, arterial anomalies, coarctation of the aorta, eye abnormalities).

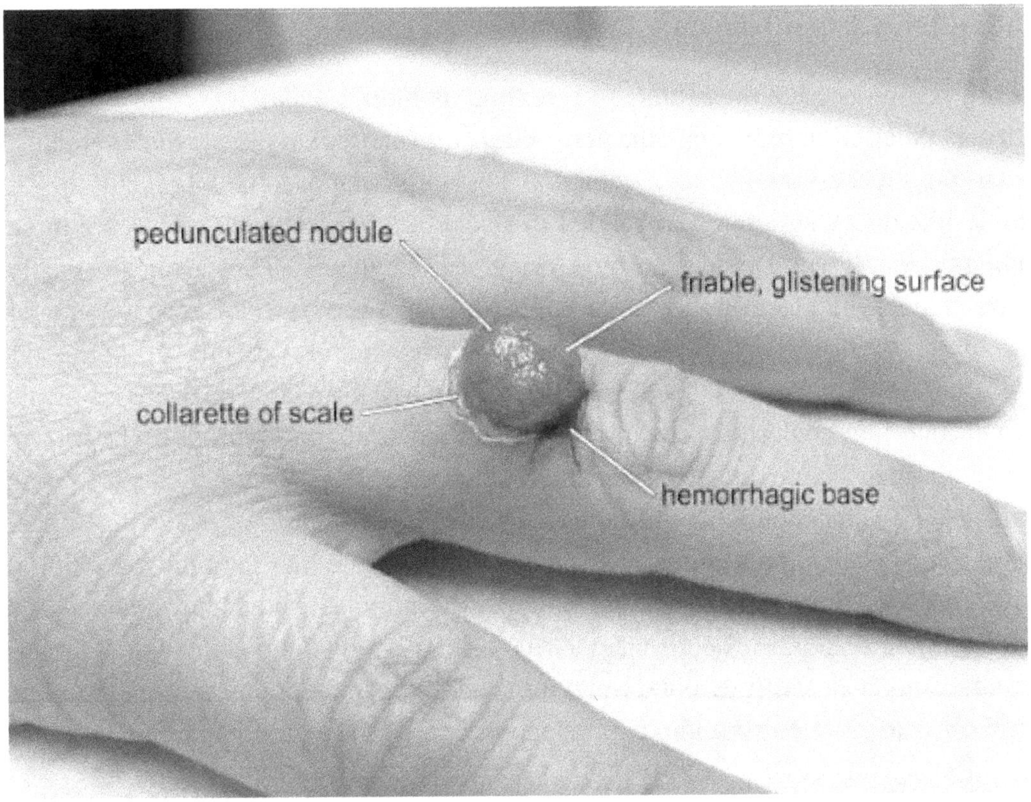

Adnexal Tumors: Trichoepithelioma, Syringoma, Cylindroma, and Pilomatricoma

Follicular Differentiation Tumors

Trichoepitheliomas are benign hair follicle tumors presenting as skin-colored to pink, dome-shaped papules on the central face (nasolabial folds, nose, upper lip). Solitary trichoepitheliomas are sporadic; multiple trichoepitheliomas (Brooke-Spiegler syndrome, when co-occurring with cylindromas and spiradenomas) are autosomal dominant (CYLD gene mutation on chromosome 16q). The critical clinical challenge is distinguishing trichoepithelioma from basal cell carcinoma (BCC): both present as translucent, skin-colored papules on the face, and histologic distinction requires careful assessment (trichoepitheliomas show basaloid epithelial islands with peripheral palisading similar to BCC but with papillary mesenchymal bodies, horn cysts, and absence of retraction artifact from the stroma). Trichoblastomas are related follicular tumors that are deeper and larger than trichoepitheliomas and may be even more histologically challenging to distinguish from BCC. Pilomatricomas (calcifying epitheliomas of Malherbe) are firm, rock-hard, subcutaneous nodules on the face, neck, or upper extremities of children, arising from hair matrix cells. They show a characteristic tent sign (the overlying skin tents over the hard tumor when compressed) and histologically contain basophilic cells transitioning to shadow (ghost) cells with calcification.

Sweat Gland Differentiation Tumors

Syringomas are benign eccrine duct tumors presenting as multiple, small (1 to 3 mm), skin-colored to yellowish, firm papules clustered around the periorbital area (particularly the lower eyelids), although they may also occur on the chest, axillae, and genitalia. They are composed histologically of small, comma-shaped, tadpole-like ductal structures embedded in a sclerotic stroma. Syringomas are more common in women and in individuals with Down syndrome (eruptive syringomas). They are cosmetically bothersome but benign; treatment with electrodesiccation, CO_2 laser ablation, or trichloroacetic acid chemical peel produces variable cosmetic improvement. Cylindromas (turban tumors) are benign eccrine-derived tumors presenting as smooth, pink, dome-shaped, rubbery nodules on the scalp. In Brooke-Spiegler syndrome, multiple cylindromas may coalesce to cover the scalp (turban tumor configuration). Eccrine poromas arise from the intraepidermal eccrine duct and present as solitary, red-pink, pedunculated or sessile nodules on the palms and soles. Hidradenoma papilliferum is a benign apocrine tumor occurring almost exclusively in the vulva of adult women, presenting as a subcutaneous nodule that may ulcerate. Spiradenomas are eccrine-derived tumors presenting as deep, tender, blue-grey subcutaneous nodules — the pain is characteristically intense and disproportionate to the lesion size, distinguishing spiradenomas from other painless subcutaneous nodules. In Brooke-Spiegler syndrome, spiradenomas co-occur with cylindromas and trichoepitheliomas, and long-standing spiradenomas carry a rare risk of malignant transformation to spiradenocarcinoma.

THE CUTANEOUS MIMICKER RECOGNITION ATLAS — Pyogenic Granuloma versus Amelanotic Melanoma

---

The Clinical Pattern: Pyogenic granuloma presents as a rapidly growing (days to weeks), friable, bright red, dome-shaped or pedunculated nodule that bleeds profusely with minor trauma. A collarette of scale is often visible at the base. It typically occurs at a site of prior trauma or chronic irritation. It is common in children, pregnant women, and patients on retinoids or targeted cancer therapies. On dermoscopy, it shows a homogeneous red pattern with white collarette and no melanocytic features.

The Mimicker: Amelanotic melanoma can present as a rapidly growing, pink to red, friable, dome-shaped or pedunculated nodule that bleeds easily — morphologically identical to a pyogenic granuloma on clinical inspection. Amelanotic melanoma lacks the typical brown-black pigmentation of conventional melanoma, making it one of the most diagnostically treacherous melanoma subtypes. It occurs on sun-exposed skin in older adults and shows irregular vascular patterns (polymorphous vessels, milky-red globules) on dermoscopy.

Trap Logic: Treating a friable, bleeding red nodule with shave excision and electrodesiccation without submitting tissue for histopathologic examination is the cognitive trap. The clinician who destroys a presumed pyogenic granuloma without biopsy may unknowingly destroy an amelanotic melanoma, eliminating the only opportunity for accurate staging and rendering the margins indeterminate. The reverse trap — referring every pyogenic granuloma for wide excision — creates unnecessary surgical morbidity, but the error is far less consequential.

The Decision Anchor: The discriminating features are **dermoscopic vascular pattern (pyogenic granuloma shows a homogeneous red structureless area with a white collarette; amelanotic melanoma shows polymorphous vessels — linear irregular, dotted, and hairpin vessels — with milky-red globules and possible remnant pigment structures), age and context (pyogenic granuloma is common in children and pregnancy; amelanotic melanoma is overwhelmingly an adult malignancy), and the critical rule: ALWAYS submit excised tissue for histopathologic examination**. A shaved pyogenic granuloma that recurs should raise immediate concern for amelanotic melanoma and requires re-excision with pathologic assessment.

When to Biopsy: Clinical Features Suggesting Malignant Transformation

The ABCDE Framework and Ugly Duckling Sign

The ABCDE criteria provide a systematic framework for identifying melanocytic lesions that warrant biopsy: Asymmetry (one half of the lesion does not mirror the other), Border irregularity (notched, scalloped, or poorly defined margins), Color variation (multiple shades of brown, black, red, white, or blue within a single lesion), Diameter greater than 6 mm, and Evolution (any change in size, shape, color, elevation, or symptoms — the single most sensitive criterion). The ugly duckling sign complements the ABCDE framework: a lesion that looks different from the patient's other nevi (the outlier) deserves heightened scrutiny regardless of whether it meets individual ABCDE criteria. In patients with few nevi, any new changing lesion is by definition an ugly duckling. In patients with many nevi, the ugly duckling is the one that stands out from the prevailing pattern — darker when most are light, larger when most are small, raised when most are flat.

Dermoscopic Red Flags

Dermoscopy improves diagnostic accuracy for pigmented lesions by 15 to 30 percent over naked-eye examination. Red flag dermoscopic features warranting biopsy include: atypical pigment network (irregularly thickened and distributed network lines with abrupt termination), blue-white veil (a confluent blue-white area overlying irregular structures, indicating melanin in the dermis with overlying acanthosis), irregular dots and globules (asymmetrically distributed pigmented structures of varying size), regression structures (grey-blue peppering and white scar-like areas indicating spontaneous regression of a melanocytic component), and polymorphous vessels (multiple different vascular morphologies within a single lesion). The 3-point checklist (asymmetry of pattern, atypical network, blue-white structures) and the 7-point checklist provide validated scoring systems for biopsy decisions. For non-melanocytic lesions, features warranting biopsy include rapid growth, ulceration, bleeding without trauma, and failure to respond to appropriate treatment.

Clinical Features Suggesting Malignant Transformation of Benign Lesions

Several benign tumors carry a small but clinically significant risk of malignant transformation, and recognizing the features that herald this change is essential for timely intervention. In melanocytic nevi, the development of asymmetry, border irregularity, new color (particularly blue-grey, white, or red), rapid enlargement, ulceration, or bleeding suggests possible melanoma arising within the nevus. Seborrheic keratoses do not undergo malignant transformation, but a dark, irregularly pigmented seborrheic keratosis may harbor a melanoma in situ on histopathologic examination — the collision tumor phenomenon. Giant congenital melanocytic nevi carry a lifetime melanoma risk of 5 to 10 percent, with nodularity, rapid growth, ulceration, or satellite lesions signaling malignant change. Dermatofibromas very rarely undergo malignant transformation, but lesions that are large (greater than 5 cm), rapidly growing, or show atypical histologic features should be re-evaluated as possible DFSP. Cylindromas and spiradenomas in Brooke-Spiegler syndrome can rarely transform into spiradenocarcinoma, heralded by rapid growth, pain, and ulceration in a previously stable tumor.

Biopsy Technique Selection

The biopsy technique should match the clinical concern. For lesions suspicious for melanoma, an excisional biopsy (narrow-margin elliptical excision or deep punch excision encompassing the entire lesion to the subcutaneous fat) is preferred to allow complete assessment of Breslow thickness, which determines staging and guides definitive surgical margins. Shave biopsy should be avoided for lesions where melanoma is in the differential, because a superficial shave may transect the deep margin and underestimate the true Breslow thickness, leading to understaging. Punch biopsy (3 to 4 mm) is appropriate for inflammatory lesions, rashes, and flat pigmented lesions when excisional biopsy is impractical (e.g., large lesions on the face); if punch biopsy is used for a pigmented lesion, it should target the most clinically atypical area. Shave biopsy is appropriate for lesions where melanoma is not in the differential (suspected seborrheic keratosis, basal cell carcinoma, squamous cell carcinoma, pyogenic granuloma) and provides adequate tissue for diagnosis while preserving cosmesis.

CLINICAL PEARL: The single most important clinical criterion for melanoma detection is evolution — any change in a melanocytic lesion. A patient who says a mole has changed should be believed even if the lesion appears bland on examination. The converse is equally important: a lesion that has been stable and unchanged for years is overwhelmingly likely to be benign, regardless of its clinical appearance. When examining a patient with many nevi, start by asking which lesions have changed — patient-reported change is a more sensitive indicator than any individual ABCDE criterion.

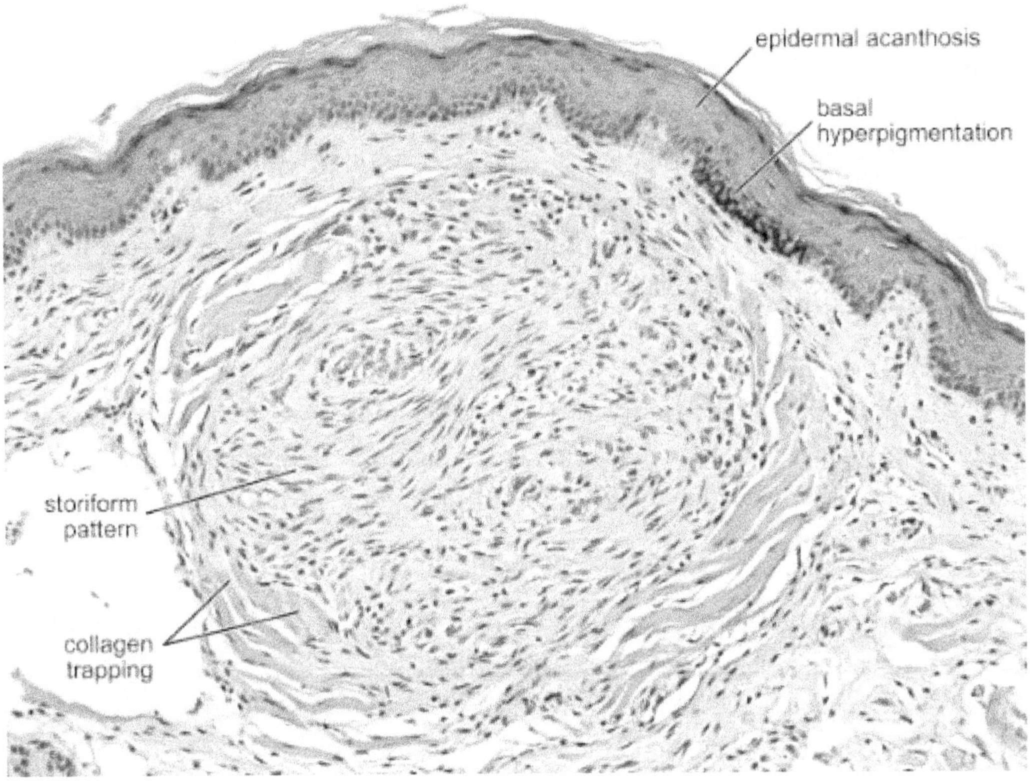

KEY POINT: The dimple sign (Fitzpatrick sign) is pathognomonic for dermatofibroma: lateral compression causes the overlying skin to dimple inward because the tumor is tethered to the epidermis. This 2-second clinical test reliably distinguishes a dermatofibroma from other firm dermal nodules (lipoma, cyst, DFSP). On dermoscopy, the central white scar-like patch surrounded by a peripheral delicate pigment network is the diagnostic pattern for dermatofibroma — if a pigmented network extends to the center of the lesion, the diagnosis is melanocytic and biopsy is warranted.

CAUTION: Never dismiss a rapidly growing, pink or red, friable nodule as a benign pyogenic granuloma without histopathologic confirmation. Amelanotic melanoma and amelanotic Merkel cell carcinoma can present identically. The rule is absolute: all tissue removed from a suspicious or ambiguous skin lesion must be submitted for pathologic examination — destruction of tissue without biopsy (electrodesiccation, laser ablation, cryotherapy) eliminates the only opportunity for histologic diagnosis and can delay cancer detection with life-threatening consequences.

Clinical Case: The Changing Mole in a Young Woman

A 28-year-old woman presents with a mole on her left calf that she reports has changed over the past 6 months, becoming darker and larger. She has fair skin (Fitzpatrick type II) and more than 50 melanocytic nevi on her trunk and extremities. On examination, the lesion is a 7 mm, asymmetric, irregularly bordered macule with color variegation — brown, dark brown, and a focal area of blue-grey at the periphery. It stands out from her other nevi, which are uniformly tan and well-circumscribed (ugly duckling sign positive). Dermoscopy reveals an atypical pigment network with irregular thickening and abrupt termination at the superior margin, irregular dots and globules at the inferior margin, and a blue-white veil in the area of blue-grey pigmentation.

Three dermoscopic red flags are present: atypical pigment network, irregular dots and globules, and blue-white veil. Combined with the clinical history of change (evolution), the ugly duckling appearance, and the ABCDE criteria (asymmetry, border irregularity, color variation, diameter greater than 6 mm), this lesion requires excisional biopsy. A narrow-margin (1 to 2 mm) elliptical excision to the subcutaneous fat is performed to allow full assessment of Breslow thickness. Histopathology reveals a superficial spreading melanoma, Breslow thickness 0.6 mm, no ulceration, mitotic rate less than 1 per square millimeter — stage T1a. The patient undergoes wide local excision with 1 cm margins (per current guidelines for melanomas with Breslow thickness 1.0 mm or less) with clear histologic margins. This case demonstrates the critical role of patient-reported change, the ugly duckling sign, and dermoscopy in identifying melanoma at a thin, curable stage among a background of multiple benign nevi.

THE CUTANEOUS MIMICKER RECOGNITION ATLAS — Benign Tumor Diagnostic Arcs

Seborrheic Keratosis vs. Melanoma: The discriminating features are dermoscopic pattern (milia-like cysts, comedo-like openings, and cerebriform pattern are diagnostic of seborrheic keratosis; atypical pigment network, blue-white veil, and regression structures indicate melanoma), surface quality (dull, waxy, stuck-on surface favors seborrheic keratosis), and history of change. Cognitive trap: dismissing a dark nodule as another seborrheic keratosis without dermoscopic examination, because the naked eye cannot reliably distinguish dark seborrheic keratoses from nodular melanoma.

Pyogenic Granuloma vs. Amelanotic Melanoma: The discriminating features are dermoscopic vascular pattern (homogeneous red with white collarette favors pyogenic granuloma; polymorphous vessels with milky-red globules and possible remnant pigment structures favor amelanotic melanoma), clinical context (pyogenic granuloma is common in children and pregnancy; amelanotic melanoma is an adult malignancy), and the absolute rule: always submit excised tissue for histopathologic examination, never destroy a skin lesion without biopsy when the diagnosis is uncertain.

Summary and Key Concepts

Melanocytic nevi are classified by nest location: junctional (flat, junction), compound (slightly raised, junction and dermis), and intradermal (dome-shaped, dermis only). Nevus count is the strongest independent risk factor for melanoma, and any nevus demonstrating change warrants clinical evaluation.

Seborrheic keratoses are the most common benign epithelial tumors and are distinguished from melanocytic lesions by dermoscopic findings — milia-like cysts, comedo-like openings, and cerebriform pattern. The sign of Leser-Trélat (eruptive seborrheic keratoses) is a paraneoplastic marker, most commonly associated with gastric adenocarcinoma.

Dermatofibromas are identified by the pathognomonic dimple sign (Fitzpatrick sign) and dermoscopic central white scar-like patch with peripheral pigment network. The key differential is dermatofibrosarcoma protuberans (DFSP), distinguished by CD34 positivity on immunohistochemistry.

Pyogenic granulomas must always be submitted for histopathologic examination because amelanotic melanoma is an important mimicker. All excised skin lesions should undergo pathologic assessment — destruction without biopsy eliminates the opportunity for diagnosis.

The ABCDE criteria, ugly duckling sign, and dermoscopic red flags (atypical network, blue-white veil, irregular dots and globules, regression structures, polymorphous vessels) guide biopsy decisions. Evolution is the single most sensitive criterion for melanoma detection.

CHAPTER 14: PREMALIGNANT LESIONS AND NON-MELANOMA SKIN CANCER

Learning Objectives

1. Describe the concept of field cancerization and apply risk stratification criteria to actinic keratoses, selecting appropriate management from observation, topical field therapy, and procedural destruction based on lesion burden and patient risk profile.
2. Recognize the clinical variants and histologic subtypes of squamous cell carcinoma and basal cell carcinoma, apply staging systems for cutaneous SCC, and determine which lesions meet criteria for high-risk management including Mohs micrographic surgery.
3. Identify Merkel cell carcinoma, dermatofibrosarcoma protuberans, and other rare cutaneous malignancies by their clinical presentations, and initiate appropriate diagnostic workup and referral pathways.
4. Compare the indications, techniques, cure rates, and limitations of surgical and non-surgical treatments for non-melanoma skin cancer, including Mohs micrographic surgery, standard excision, radiation therapy, topical immunotherapy, and hedgehog pathway inhibitors.

Actinic Keratosis: Field Cancerization, Risk Stratification, and Management

Epidemiology and Pathogenesis

Actinic keratoses (AKs) are the most common premalignant skin lesions, affecting over 58 million individuals in the United States alone, with prevalence exceeding 60 percent in fair-skinned adults over age 60 in high-UV environments. AKs arise from keratinocyte dysplasia induced by cumulative ultraviolet radiation (primarily UVB) damage to epidermal DNA — the same UV-induced p53 tumor suppressor gene mutations found in AKs are also present in cutaneous squamous cell carcinoma, establishing the AK-to-SCC continuum. The concept of field cancerization (Slaughter, 1953) recognizes that clinically visible AKs are focal manifestations of a broader field of UV-damaged, genetically altered epidermis — subclinical dysplastic keratinocytes extend well beyond the visible lesion margins, which is why isolated lesion-directed therapy (cryotherapy of individual AKs) does not address the surrounding field of premalignant change, and new AKs continue to develop in previously treated areas.

Clinical Features and Risk Stratification

AKs present as rough, scaly, erythematous macules and papules on chronically sun-exposed skin — the face (particularly the forehead, temples, nose, and ears), dorsal hands, forearms, and scalp (in bald or thinning-haired individuals). The gritty, sandpaper-like texture is often more palpable than visible, and patients frequently describe a rough area they can feel better than see. AKs are graded clinically by thickness: Grade I (slightly palpable, better felt than seen), Grade II (moderately thick, easily seen and felt), and Grade III (very thick, hyperkeratotic). The risk of an individual AK progressing to invasive SCC is estimated at 0.025 to 16 percent per year per lesion, but the cumulative risk across a patient's entire field of AKs is clinically significant — a patient with 10 AKs has a 10 to 15 percent risk of developing at least one SCC within 10 years. Risk factors for AK-to-SCC progression include lesion tenderness, induration, rapid growth, diameter greater than 1 cm, ulceration, and immunosuppression (organ transplant recipients have a 65-fold increased SCC risk and a more aggressive clinical course).

Management: Lesion-Directed and Field Therapy

Lesion-directed therapies target individual, clinically visible AKs: cryotherapy with liquid nitrogen (the most widely used; 10 to 30 second freeze, one or two freeze-thaw cycles, cure rate approximately 75 to 99 percent depending on freeze duration), curettage (scraping with a curette, often combined with electrodesiccation), and shave excision (provides tissue for histopathologic examination, recommended for thick or clinically atypical AKs where SCC must be excluded). Field-directed therapies treat both visible AKs and the surrounding subclinical field: topical 5-fluorouracil (5-FU, 5 percent cream applied twice daily for 2 to 4 weeks, causing a brisk inflammatory reaction that targets dysplastic cells), topical imiquimod (5 percent cream, an immune response modifier that stimulates innate and adaptive immunity against dysplastic keratinocytes, applied 2 to 3 times weekly for 12 to 16 weeks), topical diclofenac (3 percent gel, a COX-2 inhibitor with less inflammation but lower efficacy), ingenol mebutate gel (mechanism of direct cell death plus neutrophil-mediated antibody-dependent cellular cytotoxicity, though withdrawn from some markets due to increased skin cancer risk in one trial), and photodynamic therapy (PDT — application of a photosensitizing agent such as aminolevulinic acid followed by blue or red light activation, which produces reactive oxygen species that selectively destroy dysplastic cells). The choice between lesion-directed and field-directed therapy depends on AK count, distribution, and patient factors: isolated AKs on non-cosmetically sensitive areas respond well to cryotherapy; diffuse AKs across a large field (forehead, scalp, forearms) benefit from field therapy to treat subclinical disease.

CLINICAL PEARL: When evaluating a patient with actinic keratoses, do not simply count and treat the visible lesions — assess the entire field. Run your fingertips across the sun-exposed skin: the rough, sandpaper-like areas you feel but cannot see represent subclinical AKs that will become clinically apparent over time. A patient with multiple palpable AKs across a broad field is a candidate for field-directed therapy (5-FU, imiquimod, or PDT), not just serial cryotherapy of individual spots. This is the clinical application of the field cancerization concept: the problem is the field, not the individual lesion.

Bowen Disease (Squamous Cell Carcinoma In Situ)

Clinical Features and Histopathology

Bowen disease is squamous cell carcinoma in situ — full-thickness epidermal dysplasia confined to the epidermis without invasion through the basement membrane. It presents as a slowly enlarging, well-demarcated, erythematous, scaly plaque with an irregular but sharply defined border, most commonly on sun-exposed skin of the lower legs (women) and trunk (men). The surface may show crusting, fissuring, or slight elevation. Because Bowen disease grows slowly and lacks the rough, gritty texture of AKs, it is frequently misdiagnosed as eczema, psoriasis, or superficial fungal infection — the clinical clue is a persistent, well-demarcated, erythematous plaque that does not respond to topical corticosteroids or antifungals. Histologically, Bowen disease shows full-thickness epidermal dysplasia with atypical keratinocytes, mitotic figures at all levels of the epidermis, and an intact basement membrane. The risk of progression to invasive SCC is estimated at 3 to 5 percent. Erythroplasia of Queyrat is the genital variant of Bowen disease, presenting as a well-demarcated, velvety, erythematous plaque on the glans penis or vulva — it carries a higher risk of invasive progression than cutaneous Bowen disease.

Management

Treatment options for Bowen disease include topical 5-fluorouracil (effective for large or multiple lesions on the lower legs where surgical excision would require skin grafting), topical imiquimod, photodynamic therapy (particularly effective on the lower legs where healing is slow), cryotherapy (adequate for small lesions), curettage and electrodesiccation, and surgical excision (gold standard, with 5 mm clinical margins). For genital Bowen disease (erythroplasia of Queyrat), topical 5-FU or imiquimod is preferred to minimize surgical morbidity; circumcision is curative for glans lesions in uncircumcised men. Treatment selection for Bowen disease on the lower legs requires special consideration: wound healing on the lower legs is slow (particularly in elderly patients with venous insufficiency), and surgical excision of large plaques may require skin grafting. Non-surgical modalities — PDT, topical 5-FU, and imiquimod — offer complete clearance rates of 70 to 90 percent with the advantage of preserving tissue and avoiding the morbidity of leg wound healing. Follow-up after treatment of Bowen disease should continue for at least 12 months, as recurrence rates of 5 to 15 percent are reported across all modalities.

Squamous Cell Carcinoma: Risk Factors, Clinical Variants, Staging, and Management

Epidemiology and Risk Factors

Cutaneous squamous cell carcinoma (cSCC) is the second most common skin cancer after basal cell carcinoma, with an estimated 1.8 million new cases annually in the United States. The primary etiologic factor is cumulative ultraviolet radiation exposure, and the incidence increases sharply with latitude, skin phototype (highest in Fitzpatrick I–II), and age. Additional risk factors include immunosuppression (organ transplant recipients have a 65 to 250-fold increased risk, with SCC becoming the most common malignancy in this population — a reversal of the BCC-predominant pattern in immunocompetent individuals), human papillomavirus infection (particularly in periungual and genital SCC), chronic wounds and scars (Marjolin ulcer — SCC arising in a chronic burn scar, draining sinus tract, or chronic venous ulcer), arsenic exposure, and ionizing radiation. The molecular pathogenesis involves UV-induced p53 mutations (present in over 90 percent of cSCC), NOTCH1 mutations, and dysregulation of the Ras-MAPK and PI3K-AKT signaling pathways.

Clinical Variants and Histologic Subtypes

Classic cSCC presents as a firm, erythematous, keratotic papule, plaque, or nodule with a central keratin plug or ulcerated surface on sun-exposed skin. Clinical variants include verrucous carcinoma (a well-differentiated, slow-growing, exophytic variant with a warty surface that rarely metastasizes, occurring on the sole — epithelioma cuniculatum, oral mucosa — Ackerman tumor, or genitalia — Buschke-Lowenstein tumor), spindle cell SCC (a poorly differentiated variant with sarcomatoid morphology and aggressive behavior), and adenosquamous carcinoma (with glandular differentiation and high metastatic potential). Histologic grading uses the Broder classification (Grade 1, well-differentiated with abundant keratinization through Grade 4, anaplastic with minimal differentiation), though modern risk stratification relies more on specific high-risk histologic features than on the grading system alone.

Prevention, Screening, and Immunosuppression

Primary prevention of cutaneous SCC centers on UV exposure reduction: daily broad-spectrum sunscreen (SPF 30 or higher), protective clothing, and avoidance of peak UV hours. A landmark Australian randomized controlled trial demonstrated that regular sunscreen use reduced the incidence of cutaneous SCC by 40 percent over a 4.5-year period. In organ transplant recipients, chemoprevention with oral acitretin (a systemic retinoid) reduces the development of new SCCs by approximately 50 percent and is recommended for transplant patients who develop more than two SCCs per year or who have high-risk tumors. The mechanism involves retinoid-mediated normalization of keratinocyte differentiation and apoptosis in the UV-damaged field. Nicotinamide (vitamin B3, 500 mg twice daily) has also been shown to reduce the rate of new non-melanoma skin cancers by 23 percent in high-risk individuals through enhancement of cellular energy metabolism and DNA repair following UV damage. Immunosuppression modification — switching from calcineurin inhibitors (tacrolimus, cyclosporine) to mTOR inhibitors (sirolimus, everolimus) — reduces SCC incidence in transplant recipients because mTOR inhibitors have intrinsic antiproliferative properties and may enhance antitumor immune surveillance, but this decision must be balanced against the risk of allograft rejection in collaboration with the transplant team.

Staging and High-Risk Features

The AJCC 8th edition staging system for cSCC incorporates tumor diameter, depth of invasion, perineural invasion, and bone invasion. High-risk features that predict local recurrence, nodal metastasis, and disease-specific mortality include: tumor diameter greater than 2 cm, depth of invasion beyond subcutaneous fat, perineural invasion (particularly of named nerves with caliber 0.1 mm or greater), poorly differentiated histology, location on the ear or lip (metastatic rates 2 to 3 times higher than other sites), immunosuppression, recurrent tumor, and invasion of bone or cartilage. The Brigham and Women's Hospital staging system is an alternative that stratifies risk using four independent factors: tumor diameter 2 cm or greater, poorly differentiated histology, perineural invasion of nerves 0.1 mm or greater, and invasion beyond subcutaneous fat. Tumors with two or more of these factors have a 30 percent or higher risk of nodal metastasis and warrant aggressive management and close surveillance.

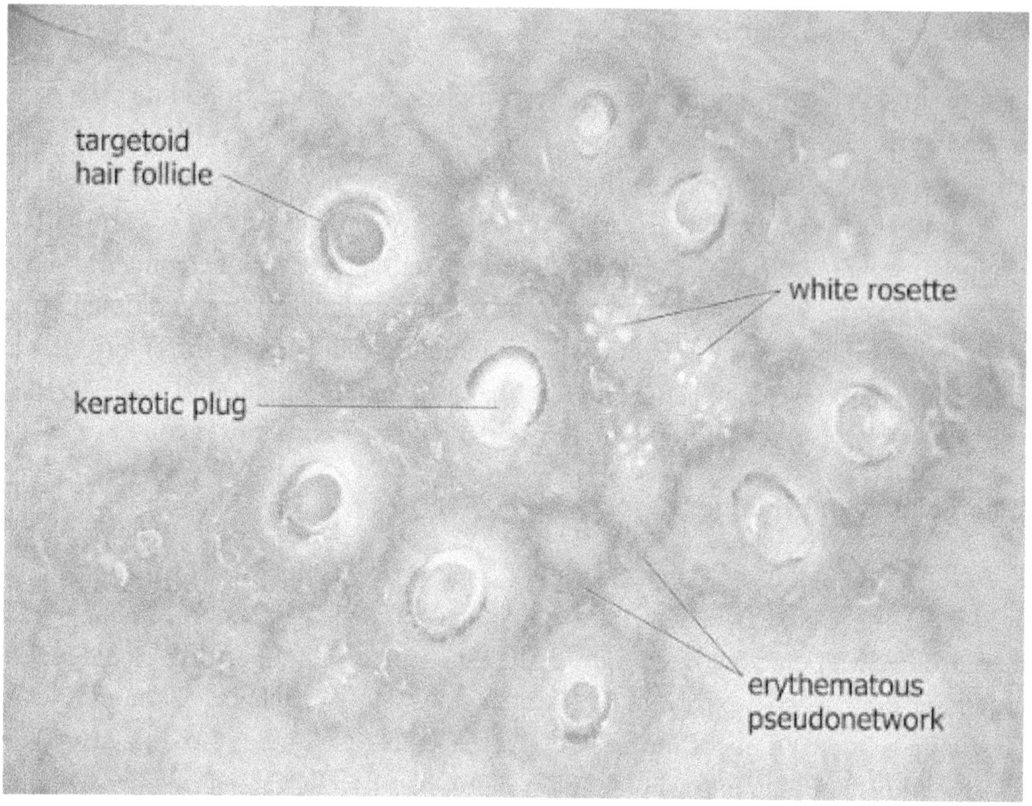

THE CUTANEOUS MIMICKER RECOGNITION ATLAS — Actinic Keratosis versus Bowen Disease

---

The Clinical Pattern: Actinic keratoses present as rough, scaly, erythematous macules and thin papules on chronically sun-exposed skin — often better felt than seen due to their gritty, sandpaper-like texture. They are typically small (2 to 6 mm), multiple, and poorly demarcated. On dermoscopy, AKs show the strawberry pattern (erythematous pseudonetwork with targetoid hair follicles and white rosettes).

The Mimicker: Bowen disease (SCC in situ) presents as a well-demarcated, erythematous, scaly plaque that is slowly enlarging. Unlike AKs, Bowen disease is sharply bordered, often larger (1 to 3 cm or more), and lacks the gritty texture. On dermoscopy, Bowen disease shows clustered glomerular vessels (coiled, dot-like vessels arranged in clusters) with a scaly surface, and the borders are more sharply defined than in AKs. Bowen disease is frequently misdiagnosed as eczema, psoriasis, or tinea.

Trap Logic: Treating a well-demarcated, persistent erythematous plaque with topical corticosteroids or antifungals for months without improvement, without considering biopsy to exclude Bowen disease is the cognitive trap. The sharp demarcation and treatment resistance are the clinical red flags that distinguish a premalignant plaque from inflammatory dermatosis. The reverse trap — biopsying every AK — is unnecessary but highlights the value of dermoscopy in distinguishing the strawberry pattern of AK from the glomerular vessel pattern of Bowen disease without biopsy.

The Decision Anchor: The discriminating features are **border quality (AKs are poorly demarcated; Bowen disease is sharply demarcated), texture (AKs are rough and gritty; Bowen disease is**

smoother and scaly), dermoscopic vascular pattern (AKs show the strawberry pattern; Bowen disease shows clustered glomerular vessels), and treatment response (AKs respond to cryotherapy and field therapy; a plaque that fails to respond to topical corticosteroids or antifungals warrants biopsy). A persistent, sharply demarcated, erythematous, scaly plaque on the lower leg of an older adult that does not respond to empiric therapy should be biopsied to exclude Bowen disease.

Basal Cell Carcinoma: Subtypes, Dermoscopic Features, and Treatment Algorithms

Epidemiology and Clinical Subtypes

Basal cell carcinoma (BCC) is the most common human malignancy, with an estimated 3.6 million new cases annually in the United States. It arises from aberrant activation of the Hedgehog signaling pathway — in over 90 percent of BCCs, loss-of-function mutations in the PTCH1 tumor suppressor gene or gain-of-function mutations in SMO result in constitutive activation of the Hedgehog pathway driving uncontrolled basal cell proliferation. BCC subtypes include: nodular BCC (the most common, presenting as a pearly, translucent, dome-shaped papule or nodule with surface telangiectasias and rolled borders, often with central ulceration — the classic rodent ulcer), superficial BCC (a thin, scaly, erythematous patch or plaque with a thread-like pearly border, most common on the trunk), morpheaform (sclerosing) BCC (a flat, indurated, scar-like plaque with ill-defined borders — the most aggressive subtype with the highest recurrence rate after conventional excision due to subclinical extension), and pigmented BCC (containing melanin pigment, which may mimic melanoma clinically, particularly in patients with darker skin phototypes).

Dermoscopic Features

Dermoscopy significantly improves diagnostic accuracy for BCC. Classic dermoscopic features include: arborizing (tree-like) vessels (thick-caliber branching vessels representing dilated arterioles in the tumor stroma — pathognomonic for nodular BCC), blue-grey ovoid nests (well-circumscribed ovoid structures corresponding to nests of basaloid cells in the dermis), leaf-like areas (bulbous extensions of pigment radiating from a common base), spoke-wheel structures (radial lines converging to a central pigmented hub), ulceration, and shiny white structures visible only under polarized dermoscopy (chrysalis structures — short, bright white, perpendicular or orthogonal lines corresponding to collagen remodeling). Superficial BCC shows short fine telangiectasias (rather than arborizing vessels), multiple small erosions, and a shiny white-red structureless background. The absence of a pigment network distinguishes BCC from melanocytic lesions, and the presence of arborizing vessels distinguishes BCC from SCC (which shows hairpin or glomerular vessels).

Treatment Algorithms and Margin Considerations

Management of BCC follows a risk-stratified approach. Low-risk BCC (small, nodular or superficial subtype, trunk or extremities, well-defined borders, no prior treatment) can be managed with standard surgical excision (3 to 5 mm margins), electrodesiccation and curettage (ED&C — effective for superficial and small nodular BCC on the trunk and extremities, with cure rates of 92 to 97 percent), or topical therapy (imiquimod or 5-FU for superficial BCC). High-risk BCC (morpheaform or infiltrative subtype, high-risk location such as central face, recurrent tumor, perineural invasion, large size, immunosuppression) requires Mohs micrographic surgery or wide excision with complete circumferential peripheral and deep margin assessment (CCPDMA). ED&C is contraindicated for morpheaform BCC because the indistinct clinical borders and aggressive histologic growth pattern produce unacceptably high recurrence rates. For patients with basal cell nevus syndrome (Gorlin syndrome — autosomal dominant PTCH1 mutation producing multiple BCCs beginning in adolescence, along with odontogenic keratocysts, skeletal anomalies, and calcified falx cerebri), management requires lifelong dermatologic surveillance and a combination of surgical and non-surgical approaches; hedgehog pathway inhibitors are particularly relevant in this population.

CAUTION: Morpheaform (sclerosing) basal cell carcinoma is the most diagnostically treacherous BCC subtype: it presents as a flat, indurated, scar-like, skin-colored plaque with ill-defined borders that can be clinically invisible to the untrained eye. Unlike nodular BCC, it lacks the pearly border, telangiectasia, and dome shape that trigger clinical suspicion. Its subclinical extension is typically far greater than the visible lesion suggests — what appears as a 1 cm scar-like plaque may have 2 to 3 cm of subclinical infiltration. Standard excision with predetermined margins has recurrence rates of 25 to 33 percent for morpheaform BCC. Mohs micrographic surgery is the treatment of choice because it traces the full extent of the tumor through serial margin examination.

Keratoacanthoma: Diagnosis, Natural History, and Management Controversies

Clinical Features and Natural History

Keratoacanthoma (KA) is a rapidly growing, dome-shaped, keratin-filled tumor that arises on sun-exposed skin and follows a characteristic three-phase lifecycle: rapid growth phase (the lesion expands to 1 to 2 cm or larger within 4 to 8 weeks), maturation phase (growth plateaus), and spontaneous involution phase (the tumor regresses over 2 to 6 months, leaving a depressed scar). It classically presents as a dome-shaped or crateriform nodule with a central keratin-filled crater (volcano-like morphology), sharply demarcated borders, and a flesh-colored to erythematous rim. The clinical and histologic relationship between KA and well-differentiated SCC remains controversial: some authorities classify KA as a distinct entity (a benign follicular neoplasm with self-limiting behavior), while others consider KA a subtype of well-differentiated SCC that happens to involute. Because histologic distinction between KA and well-differentiated SCC is unreliable (both show well-differentiated squamous proliferation with a ground-glass cytoplasmic quality and central keratinization), most dermatologists manage KA as if it were SCC — excision rather than observation — to avoid the risk of mistakenly observing a true SCC.

Management Approach

Surgical excision is the recommended treatment for KA, both for definitive histopathologic assessment and because the clinical distinction from invasive SCC is unreliable. For solitary KA, excision with 4 to 6 mm margins or Mohs micrographic surgery is curative. Intralesional methotrexate and intralesional 5-fluorouracil are alternatives for patients who are poor surgical candidates or who have multiple KAs (as seen in the Grzybowski and Ferguson-Smith variants). Observation alone (watching for spontaneous involution) is generally not recommended because of diagnostic uncertainty — a KA that does not involute as expected may be a well-differentiated SCC, and the delay in treatment allows continued growth and potential invasion.

Merkel Cell Carcinoma: Clinical Features, Staging, and Emerging Therapies

Epidemiology and Pathogenesis

Merkel cell carcinoma (MCC) is a rare but aggressive neuroendocrine carcinoma of the skin with a mortality rate exceeding that of melanoma. It arises from Merkel cells (mechanoreceptors in the basal epidermis) and has two distinct etiologic pathways: Merkel cell polyomavirus (MCPyV)-associated MCC (approximately 80 percent of cases, predominantly in immunosuppressed and elderly individuals) and UV-induced MCC (approximately 20 percent, characterized by a high tumor mutational burden from UV-induced DNA damage). Incidence has tripled over the past two decades, driven by population aging and increasing immunosuppression. Risk factors include advanced age (median age at diagnosis 75 to 80 years), fair skin, chronic UV exposure, immunosuppression (HIV, organ transplant — 13-fold increased risk, chronic lymphocytic leukemia), and MCPyV infection.

Clinical Features and Diagnosis

MCC presents as a rapidly growing, firm, non-tender, dome-shaped, red-violet or skin-colored nodule on sun-exposed skin (head, neck, and extremities). The clinical mnemonic AEIOU summarizes the features: Asymptomatic, Expanding rapidly, Immunosuppression, Older than 50, UV-exposed fair skin. MCC is often initially misdiagnosed as a cyst, lipoma, or BCC because of its non-specific clinical appearance. Histologically, MCC shows sheets of small, round, blue cells with scant cytoplasm and numerous mitotic figures — the neuroendocrine differentiation is confirmed by positive immunohistochemistry for CK20 (dot-like perinuclear pattern, highly characteristic), synaptophysin, and chromogranin A, and negative TTF-1 (which distinguishes MCC from metastatic small cell lung carcinoma). Sentinel lymph node biopsy is recommended for all MCC patients without clinically apparent nodal disease, as micrometastases are found in approximately 30 percent of clinically node-negative patients. Staging follows the AJCC 8th edition system, which incorporates primary tumor size, nodal status, and distant metastases.

Treatment and Emerging Therapies

Primary treatment of localized MCC is wide local excision with 1 to 2 cm margins (or Mohs micrographic surgery for head and neck lesions) combined with sentinel lymph node biopsy. Adjuvant radiation therapy to the primary site and regional nodal basin improves local control, particularly for high-risk features (positive margins, lymphovascular invasion, immunosuppression). For advanced and metastatic MCC, immune checkpoint inhibitors have transformed outcomes: avelumab (anti-PD-L1), pembrolizumab (anti-PD-1), and nivolumab (anti-PD-1) produce objective response rates of 33 to 62 percent in advanced MCC, with durable responses in many patients. The high immunogenicity of MCC (driven by either viral antigens in MCPyV-positive tumors or high mutational burden in MCPyV-negative tumors) explains the exceptional sensitivity to checkpoint inhibition — MCC is now a paradigm case for immunotherapy in rare cancers.

Dermatofibrosarcoma Protuberans and Other Rare Cutaneous Malignancies

Dermatofibrosarcoma Protuberans

Dermatofibrosarcoma protuberans (DFSP) is a low-to-intermediate grade fibroblastic sarcoma that presents as a slowly growing, indurated, pink to violaceous plaque or multinodular mass, most commonly on the trunk of young to middle-aged adults. It is characterized by a translocation t(17;22)(q22;q13) producing the COL1A1-PDGFB fusion gene, resulting in autocrine PDGFB-driven proliferation. DFSP infiltrates locally with extensive subclinical tentacle-like extensions through the dermis and subcutis (which is why standard excision has recurrence rates of 20 to 50 percent), but metastasis is rare (less than 5 percent). Histologically, DFSP shows a monotonous, densely cellular, storiform proliferation of spindle cells infiltrating the subcutaneous fat in a honeycomb pattern. Immunohistochemistry is CD34-positive (distinguishing it from dermatofibroma, which is CD34-negative and Factor XIIIa-positive). Mohs micrographic surgery is the treatment of choice for DFSP, with recurrence rates below 5 percent — far superior to conventional wide excision. Imatinib (a PDGFR tyrosine kinase inhibitor) is effective for unresectable or metastatic DFSP, directly targeting the COL1A1-PDGFB fusion-driven signaling.

Other Rare Cutaneous Malignancies

Atypical fibroxanthoma (AFX) is a low-grade superficial sarcoma presenting as a rapidly growing, dome-shaped, red nodule on sun-damaged skin of the head and neck in elderly patients. It is histologically indistinguishable from pleomorphic undifferentiated sarcoma (formerly malignant fibrous histiocytoma) but is defined by its superficial, dermis-confined location and excellent prognosis after excision. Microcystic adnexal carcinoma (MAC) is a rare, locally aggressive appendageal carcinoma that presents as a slow-growing, indurated, skin-colored plaque on the central face (nasolabial fold, upper lip) with perineural invasion as a hallmark feature — patients may present with numbness or paresthesias in the distribution of the involved nerve. MAC requires Mohs micrographic surgery for adequate clearance. Sebaceous carcinoma arises from sebaceous glands and is most common on the eyelid (from the meibomian glands), where it mimics chalazion or chronic blepharitis — the delayed diagnosis is typical, averaging 1 to 2 years. Periocular sebaceous carcinoma is associated with Muir-Torre syndrome (autosomal dominant, mismatch repair gene mutations) when accompanied by visceral malignancies.

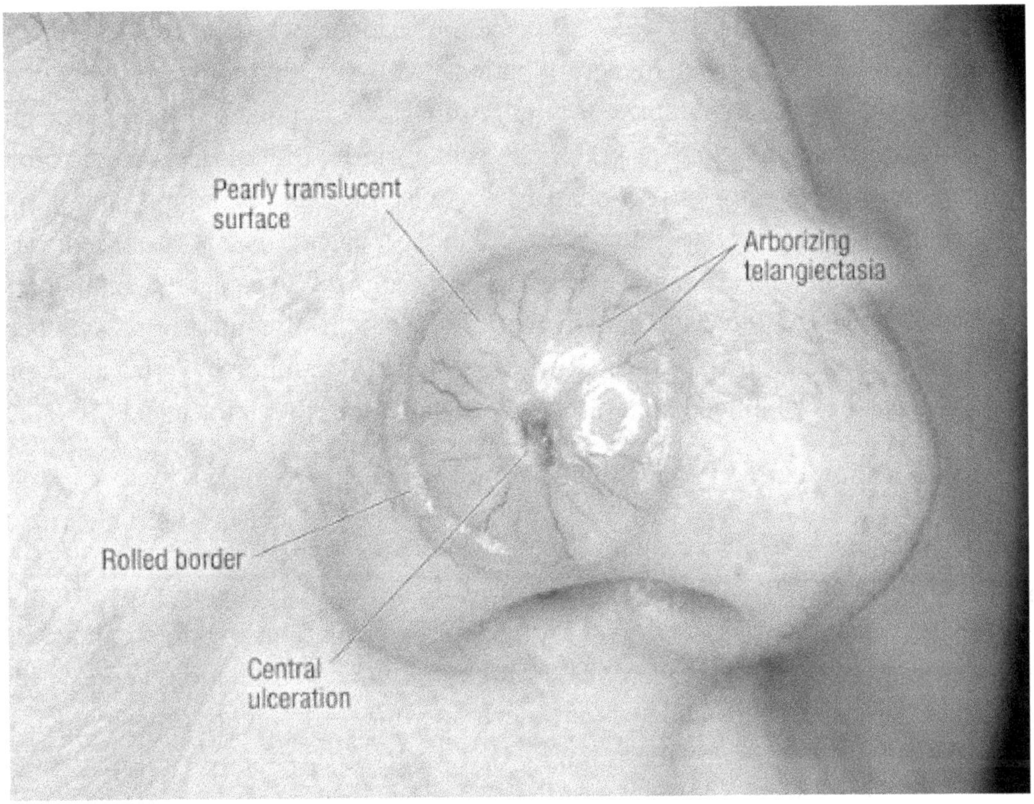

Surgical and Non-Surgical Management: Mohs Micrographic Surgery, Excision, Radiation, Topical Immunotherapy, and Hedgehog Pathway Inhibitors

Mohs Micrographic Surgery

Mohs micrographic surgery (MMS) is a tissue-sparing surgical technique that provides the highest cure rate for BCC and SCC by examining 100 percent of the surgical margin through horizontal frozen sections. The surgeon removes thin layers of tissue, maps the specimen, processes it with horizontal sectioning so that the entire peripheral and deep margin is examined microscopically, and identifies and re-excises any residual tumor in a targeted fashion — this process is repeated until all margins are clear. MMS achieves 5-year cure rates of 99 percent for primary BCC and 97 percent for primary SCC, compared with 90 to 95 percent for standard excision. Appropriate use criteria for MMS include: tumors in cosmetically or functionally sensitive locations (face, ears, eyelids, nose, lips, fingers, genitalia), tumors with high-risk histologic subtypes (morpheaform BCC, perineural invasion), recurrent tumors, large tumors (greater than 2 cm), tumors with poorly defined clinical borders, and tumors in immunosuppressed patients.

Patient Education and Surveillance

Patients diagnosed with any non-melanoma skin cancer carry a substantially elevated risk of developing subsequent skin cancers: approximately 40 to 50 percent of patients with one BCC will develop another BCC within 5 years, and the risk is even higher for patients with SCC or multiple primary cancers. Patient education should emphasize the importance of regular self-skin examination (monthly, using mirrors to inspect the entire skin surface including the scalp, ears, and posterior trunk), rigorous sun protection (daily broad-spectrum sunscreen, sun-protective clothing, avoidance of peak UV hours), and prompt reporting of any new, changing, or non-healing lesion. Surveillance frequency is risk-stratified: patients with a single, low-risk NMSC should be examined every 6 to 12 months for 2 years, then annually; patients with multiple or high-risk cancers require examination every 3 to 6 months. Immunosuppressed patients require the most intensive surveillance — every 3 to 6 months indefinitely — because their ongoing immunosuppression ensures continued high risk for new and aggressive skin cancers.

Standard Excision, Radiation, and Non-Surgical Options

Standard surgical excision with predetermined margins remains appropriate for low-risk BCC and SCC in non-cosmetically sensitive locations. Recommended margins for BCC are 3 to 5 mm for low-risk tumors and 5 to 10 mm for high-risk tumors (or Mohs). For SCC, margins of 4 to 6 mm are recommended for low-risk tumors and wider margins or Mohs for high-risk tumors. Radiation therapy is an alternative for patients who are not surgical candidates (advanced age, medical comorbidities, patient preference), with cure rates of 90 to 95 percent for primary BCC and SCC — however, radiation carries the disadvantage of a delayed recurrence pattern (failures may occur years to decades after treatment) and cosmetic deterioration of the irradiated field over time. Topical therapies (5-FU, imiquimod) are effective for superficial BCC and are approved alternatives when surgery or radiation is not appropriate. Hedgehog pathway inhibitors — vismodegib and sonidegib — are oral systemic therapies that target the constitutively activated Hedgehog signaling pathway driving BCC proliferation. They are indicated for locally advanced BCC that is not amenable to surgery or radiation, and for metastatic BCC. Response rates are approximately 30 to 60 percent, but side effects (muscle spasms, dysgeusia, alopecia, weight loss) limit tolerability and lead to treatment discontinuation in a substantial proportion of patients.

THE CUTANEOUS MIMICKER RECOGNITION ATLAS — Basal Cell Carcinoma versus Intradermal Nevus

---

The Clinical Pattern: Nodular basal cell carcinoma presents as a pearly, translucent, dome-shaped papule or nodule with surface telangiectasias and rolled borders. The pearlescent quality is visible when light is reflected at an oblique angle. There may be central ulceration or crusting. BCCs are typically solitary and occur on sun-exposed skin of the face, particularly the nose, periorbital area, and ears. On dermoscopy, arborizing vessels (thick, branching, tree-like vessels) and blue-grey ovoid nests are characteristic.

The Mimicker: Intradermal nevi present as flesh-colored to light-brown, dome-shaped or pedunculated papules on the face that can closely resemble nodular BCC clinically. Like BCC, they may have surface telangiectasias (thin, non-branching vessels). Intradermal nevi are typically stable, non-ulcerated, and present since young adulthood, whereas BCCs are new lesions in older adults that slowly enlarge. On dermoscopy, intradermal nevi show a cobblestone pattern or comma-shaped vessels — fundamentally different from the arborizing vessels of BCC.

Trap Logic: Reassuring a patient that a translucent papule on the nose is a benign mole without dermoscopic examination is the cognitive trap. The naked-eye distinction between a pearly BCC and a flesh-colored intradermal nevus is unreliable, particularly on the nose where both lesions are common. Dermoscopy provides the critical distinction in seconds: arborizing vessels indicate BCC; comma vessels and cobblestone pattern indicate intradermal nevus.

The Decision Anchor: The discriminating features are **dermoscopic vascular pattern (arborizing tree-like vessels are pathognomonic for BCC; comma-shaped vessels and cobblestone pattern indicate intradermal nevus), surface quality (pearly translucence with rolled borders suggests BCC; uniform dome shape without translucence suggests nevus), history (BCC is a new, slowly enlarging lesion; an intradermal nevus has been present for years and is stable), and ulceration (ulceration or crusting strongly favors BCC over nevus)**. A 2-second dermoscopic examination of the vascular pattern resolves the distinction in the majority of cases.

KEY POINT: Organ transplant recipients are the highest-risk population for cutaneous SCC: their risk is 65 to 250 times that of the general population, SCC becomes more common than BCC (reversing the normal ratio), and their SCCs are more aggressive with higher rates of local recurrence, metastasis, and mortality. All transplant recipients should undergo full-body skin examination every 6 to 12 months, with a low threshold for biopsy of suspicious lesions and aggressive management of confirmed cancers. Reduction or modification of immunosuppression (e.g., switching from calcineurin inhibitors to mTOR inhibitors such as sirolimus, which has antiproliferative properties) should be considered in collaboration with the transplant team for patients with multiple or high-risk skin cancers.

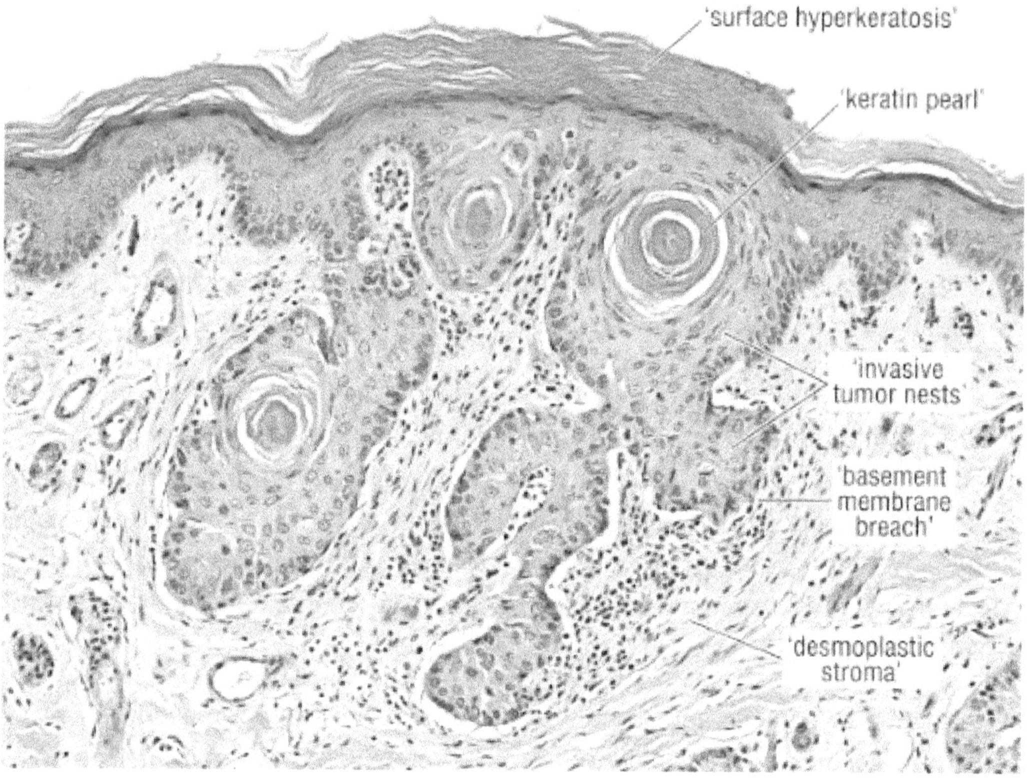

EVIDENCE: A multicenter randomized trial comparing Mohs micrographic surgery with standard surgical excision for primary facial BCC found that 10-year recurrence rates were 4.4 percent for standard excision versus 2.5 percent for Mohs (not statistically significant for primary tumors). However, for recurrent BCC, the difference was clinically significant: 12.1 percent recurrence with standard excision versus 3.9 percent with Mohs. These data support the use of Mohs particularly for recurrent tumors, where the distorted tissue planes and scar tissue make margin assessment more challenging for standard excision.

Clinical Case: The Non-Healing Lesion on the Ear

A 72-year-old man with a history of extensive sun exposure presents with a non-healing lesion on his left ear that has been present for 6 months. He reports that it occasionally bleeds and has been slowly enlarging. He has been applying antibiotic ointment without improvement. On examination, there is a 1.8 cm, indurated, erythematous nodule with a central ulceration and raised, rolled borders on the helix of the left ear. The surrounding skin shows solar elastosis and multiple AKs. Dermoscopy reveals polymorphous vessels (hairpin, linear irregular, and glomerular vessels), central ulceration, and white structureless areas — features consistent with SCC rather than BCC (which would show arborizing vessels).

The clinical presentation — an indurated, ulcerated, slowly enlarging nodule on the ear of an elderly sun-damaged patient — combined with dermoscopic features of polymorphous vessels is highly suspicious for squamous cell carcinoma. The ear is a high-risk location for SCC (metastatic rate 2 to 3 times higher than non-ear sites). Shave biopsy confirms moderately differentiated SCC. High-risk features are present: location on the ear, tumor diameter approaching 2 cm, and moderate differentiation. Mohs micrographic surgery is performed to achieve complete margin clearance with tissue preservation. Histology of the Mohs specimen shows no perineural invasion and the tumor is confined to the dermis. Postoperative surveillance includes full-body skin examination and regional lymph node assessment every 3 to 6 months for 2 years, then every 6 to 12 months for 3 additional years. This case demonstrates the importance of biopsying non-healing lesions on sun-exposed skin and applying high-risk criteria to guide treatment intensity.

THE CUTANEOUS MIMICKER RECOGNITION ATLAS — Premalignant and Non-Melanoma Skin Cancer Diagnostic Arcs

---

Actinic Keratosis vs. Bowen Disease: The discriminating features are border quality (AKs are poorly demarcated; Bowen disease is sharply demarcated), texture (AKs are rough and gritty; Bowen disease is smoother and scaly), dermoscopic vascular pattern (AKs show the strawberry pattern with targetoid follicles; Bowen disease shows clustered glomerular vessels), and treatment response. Cognitive trap: treating a persistent, well-demarcated plaque as eczema or tinea without considering biopsy to exclude Bowen disease.

Basal Cell Carcinoma vs. Intradermal Nevus: The discriminating features are dermoscopic vascular pattern (arborizing tree-like vessels are pathognomonic for BCC; comma-shaped vessels and cobblestone pattern indicate intradermal nevus), surface quality (pearly translucence with rolled borders suggests BCC), and history (BCC is a new enlarging lesion in older adults; intradermal nevi are stable and longstanding). Cognitive trap: reassuring a patient that a translucent papule is a mole without dermoscopic examination.

Summary and Key Concepts

Actinic keratoses are the most common premalignant lesions and exist within a field of UV-damaged epidermis (field cancerization). Management decisions between lesion-directed therapy (cryotherapy) and field-directed therapy (5-FU, imiquimod, PDT) depend on AK burden and distribution across the field.

Bowen disease (SCC in situ) is frequently misdiagnosed as eczema, psoriasis, or tinea. The clinical clues are sharp demarcation, treatment resistance, and dermoscopic glomerular vessels. Progression to invasive SCC occurs in 3 to 5 percent of untreated lesions.

Cutaneous SCC risk is dramatically elevated in organ transplant recipients (65 to 250-fold), with a reversal of the BCC-to-SCC ratio and more aggressive tumor behavior. High-risk SCC features (diameter greater than 2 cm, perineural invasion, poorly differentiated histology, ear or lip location) guide management intensity.

Basal cell carcinoma is driven by Hedgehog pathway mutations (PTCH1, SMO) and is diagnosed dermoscopically by arborizing vessels, blue-grey ovoid nests, and the absence of a pigment network. Hedgehog pathway inhibitors (vismodegib, sonidegib) provide systemic treatment for locally advanced or metastatic disease.

Mohs micrographic surgery achieves the highest cure rates (99 percent for primary BCC, 97 percent for primary SCC) by examining 100 percent of the surgical margin. Merkel cell carcinoma, though rare, has a higher mortality rate than melanoma and responds exceptionally well to immune checkpoint inhibitors due to its high immunogenicity.

CHAPTER 15: MELANOMA

Learning Objectives

1. Identify the major risk factors for melanoma — including nevus count, family history, UV exposure pattern, and genetic susceptibility — and apply evidence-based prevention strategies to reduce melanoma incidence in high-risk populations.
2. Distinguish the four principal clinical subtypes of melanoma (superficial spreading, nodular, lentigo maligna, and acral lentiginous) by their clinical presentations, anatomic predilections, growth patterns, and dermoscopic features, with particular attention to melanoma presentations in skin of color.
3. Apply the AJCC 8th edition TNM staging system to determine prognosis, interpret sentinel lymph node biopsy results, and select appropriate surgical margins based on Breslow thickness.
4. Compare the indications, mechanisms, response rates, and toxicity profiles of immune checkpoint inhibitors and BRAF/MEK-targeted therapy for advanced and adjuvant melanoma treatment, and outline evidence-based surveillance protocols for melanoma survivors.

Epidemiology, Risk Factors, and Prevention Strategies

Epidemiology and Global Burden

Melanoma is the fifth most common cancer in the United States, with an estimated 100,640 new invasive cases and 8,290 deaths annually. Incidence has risen steadily over the past four decades — a 3 to 7 percent annual increase in white populations — driven by increased UV exposure (both solar and artificial from tanning beds), improved detection through screening and dermoscopy, and population aging. Australia and New Zealand have the highest incidence worldwide (50 to 60 per 100,000), while rates are substantially lower in populations with darker skin phototypes. However, melanoma in individuals with skin of color (Fitzpatrick IV–VI) carries worse stage-specific survival, largely due to delayed diagnosis and a higher proportion of acral lentiginous melanoma, which occurs on non-sun-exposed sites and is not captured by UV-focused screening paradigms. The median age at diagnosis is 65 years, but melanoma is one of the most common cancers in young adults aged 25 to 29, with a striking female predominance in the younger age group (lower extremity melanoma in young women).

Risk Factors and Genetic Susceptibility

The strongest risk factor for melanoma is total nevus count: individuals with more than 100 common melanocytic nevi carry a 7-fold increased risk. Other major risk factors include: a personal or family history of melanoma (first-degree relative with melanoma confers a 2 to 3-fold risk increase), dysplastic nevus syndrome (FAMMM — lifetime risk approaching 100 percent in families with CDKN2A germline mutations), fair skin and sun sensitivity (Fitzpatrick I–II), red or blond hair (MC1R variants), a history of severe, blistering sunburns (particularly in childhood and adolescence), chronic immunosuppression, and giant congenital melanocytic nevi (5 to 10 percent lifetime risk). The genetic landscape includes high-penetrance susceptibility genes (CDKN2A, CDK4 — responsible for familial melanoma), intermediatepenetrance genes (MC1R, MITF), and a polygenic contribution from multiple low-penetrance susceptibility loci identified by genome-wide association studies. Intermittent, intense UV exposure (recreational sun exposure, tanning bed use) is more strongly associated with melanoma than cumulative UV exposure (which drives SCC), supporting the sunburn-melanoma hypothesis.

Prevention Strategies

Primary prevention targets UV exposure reduction: daily broad-spectrum sunscreen (SPF 30 or higher, applied 15 to 30 minutes before exposure and reapplied every 2 hours), sun-protective clothing (UPF 50+ fabric, wide-brimmed hats, UV-blocking sunglasses), shade-seeking behavior during peak UV hours (10 AM to 4 PM), and avoidance of indoor tanning (tanning bed use before age 35 increases melanoma risk by 59 percent; many countries have banned tanning bed use for minors). Secondary prevention relies on screening and early detection: regular self-skin examination (monthly, using the ABCDE criteria and the ugly duckling sign), annual full-body skin examination by a dermatologist for high-risk individuals, and total body photography with sequential digital dermoscopy for patients with multiple atypical nevi or a strong family history.

Clinical Types: Superficial Spreading, Nodular, Lentigo Maligna, and Acral Lentiginous Melanoma

Superficial Spreading Melanoma

Superficial spreading melanoma (SSM) is the most common subtype, accounting for approximately 70 percent of cutaneous melanomas. It occurs most frequently on the trunk in men and the lower extremities in women and presents as a flat or slightly elevated, irregularly bordered, variably pigmented macule or patch. SSM grows radially (horizontally within the epidermis) for months to years before entering a vertical growth phase (invasion into the dermis) — this prolonged radial growth phase is why SSM is often detected at a thin, curable stage. Color variation is the hallmark: shades of brown, black, blue-grey, red, and white may coexist within a single lesion. The white areas represent regression (spontaneous immune-mediated destruction of part of the tumor), while blue-grey areas indicate melanin in the dermis. Dermoscopy of SSM shows an atypical pigment network (irregularly thickened network lines with irregular holes), irregular dots and globules, blue-white veil (corresponding to melanin deep in the dermis with overlying acanthosis), regression structures (peppering and scar-like areas), and pseudopods or radial streaming at the periphery (indicating centrifugal growth).

Nodular Melanoma

Nodular melanoma (NM) accounts for 15 to 30 percent of melanomas but causes a disproportionate share of melanoma deaths because it lacks a prolonged radial growth phase — it enters the vertical growth phase immediately, presenting as a rapidly growing (weeks to months), elevated, dome-shaped, blue-black or uniformly dark nodule. Nodular melanoma often fails the ABCDE criteria: it may be symmetric, well-circumscribed, and uniformly colored (it can be amelanotic — flesh-colored or pink), which delays clinical suspicion. The EFG criteria (Elevated, Firm, Growing for more than 1 month) were developed specifically

to capture nodular melanomas that escape ABCDE screening. Dermoscopy may show a blue-white veil, atypical vascular patterns (polymorphous vessels — dotted, linear irregular, and hairpin vessels), milky-red globules, and homogeneous blue or blue-black pigmentation. Amelanotic nodular melanoma is the most diagnostically treacherous variant — a rapidly growing, pink-red, friable nodule that may mimic pyogenic granuloma, BCC, or SCC.

Lentigo Maligna and Acral Lentiginous Melanoma

Lentigo maligna (melanoma in situ of chronically sun-damaged skin) presents as a slowly expanding, irregularly pigmented macule or patch on the face, neck, or dorsal forearms of elderly patients with extensive solar damage. It may grow radially for years to decades before progressing to invasive lentigo maligna melanoma. Dermoscopy shows an asymmetric, annular-granular pattern with circle-within-a-circle structures, rhomboid structures, and obliteration of follicular openings by pigment (a key feature distinguishing lentigo maligna from solar lentigo). Acral lentiginous melanoma (ALM) is the least common subtype in white populations (5 percent of melanomas) but is the most common subtype in Black, Asian, and Hispanic populations (35 to 60 percent of melanomas in these groups). ALM arises on the palms, soles, and subungual regions — non-sun-exposed sites — and is not related to UV exposure. The parallel ridge pattern on dermoscopy (pigment following the sulci of dermatoglyphics — the ridges rather than the furrows of the fingerprint) is the pathognomonic dermoscopic feature of ALM, distinguishing it from benign acral melanocytic nevus (which shows the parallel furrow pattern — pigment following the furrows).

Histopathology and Molecular Pathology

Histopathological examination of melanoma reveals atypical melanocytes arranged in irregular nests at the dermoepidermal junction and, in invasive melanoma, extending into the dermis and subcutis. Pagetoid spread — individual atypical melanocytes scattered throughout the upper epidermis — is a hallmark feature of superficial spreading melanoma, distinguishing it from benign nevi (in which melanocytes are generally confined to the dermoepidermal junction and dermis). Cytologic features include enlarged, hyperchromatic nuclei with prominent nucleoli, irregular nuclear contours, dusty melanin pigment, and mitotic figures (mitotic rate was previously part of the AJCC staging system and remains a prognostic factor). Ulceration, defined histopathologically as full-thickness epidermal loss with fibrin deposition above the tumor, is an adverse prognostic feature that upstages within each T-category. Tumor-infiltrating lymphocytes (TILs) at the base of the tumor indicate a host immune response and are associated with more favorable prognosis. The molecular landscape of melanoma is dominated by four genomic subtypes: BRAF-mutant (approximately 50 percent — predominantly V600E, driven by intermittent UV exposure), NRAS-mutant (15 to 20 percent — associated with thicker tumors and nodular subtype), NF1-mutant (10 to 15 percent — associated with chronic sun damage and older patients), and triple-wild-type (no BRAF, NRAS, or NF1 mutation — includes KIT-mutant melanomas arising on acral, mucosal, and chronic sun-damaged skin, which may respond to KIT inhibitors such as imatinib). Molecular testing for BRAF mutation status is mandatory for all patients with Stage III or IV melanoma to determine eligibility for targeted therapy.

Subtype	Proportion	Typical Site	Dermoscopic Features	Growth Pattern
SSM	70%	Trunk (men), legs (women)	Atypical network, irregular dots/globules, blue-white veil, regression structures, pseudopods	Prolonged radial phase, then vertical invasion
Nodular	15–30%	Trunk, head/neck	Blue-white veil, polymorphous vessels, milky-red globules, homogeneous blue-black structureless	Vertical growth phase from onset — no radial phase
Lentigo maligna	10–15%	Face, chronically sun-damaged skin	Annular-granular pattern, rhomboid structures, obliterated follicular openings, circle-within-circle	Prolonged radial phase (years to decades)
ALM	5% (white); 35–60% (Black, Asian, Hispanic)	Palms, soles, nail unit	Parallel ridge pattern (acral), irregular band width and loss of parallelism (nail)	Radial then vertical; not UV-related

CLINICAL PEARL: Desmoplastic melanoma is a rare variant that deserves special attention because of its diagnostic difficulty. It presents as a flesh-colored or pink, firm, scar-like papule or plaque — often amelanotic — on chronically sun-damaged skin of the head and neck in elderly patients. Because it lacks pigment and mimics a scar, dermatofibroma, or morpheaform BCC, diagnosis is frequently delayed. Histopathology shows spindle-shaped melanocytes embedded in a collagenous stroma with perineural invasion (present in up to 40 percent of cases). Despite its thick Breslow depth at diagnosis, pure desmoplastic melanoma has a lower rate of lymph node metastasis than other melanoma subtypes of equivalent thickness, and SLNB is often omitted for pure desmoplastic melanoma. S-100 is the most reliable immunohistochemical marker — HMB-45 and Melan-A are frequently negative in desmoplastic variants.

Melanoma in Skin of Color: Unique Presentations and Diagnostic Challenges

Epidemiology and Anatomic Distribution

Although melanoma is less common in individuals with Fitzpatrick IV–VI skin phototypes, it carries worse prognosis in these populations — 5-year survival rates for Black patients are 70 percent compared to 94 percent for white patients. This disparity is driven primarily by delayed diagnosis: melanoma in skin of color is disproportionately acral lentiginous (palms, soles, nail unit), mucosal (oral cavity, vulvovaginal), or in sites not routinely screened during UV-focused skin examinations. The lower index of suspicion for melanoma in darker-skinned individuals — both among patients (who may believe melanoma does not affect people of color) and clinicians (whose training emphasizes melanoma on white skin) — compounds the diagnostic delay. By the time of diagnosis, melanoma in patients with skin of color is more likely to be at a later stage, with thicker Breslow depth and higher rates of nodal and distant metastasis.

Clinical Features and Diagnostic Approach

Subungual melanoma (a variant of ALM) presents as longitudinal melanonychia — a band of brown-black pigment extending from the nail matrix to the free edge. Hutchinson sign (periungual pigmentation extending from the nail fold onto the surrounding skin) is a clinical indicator of subungual melanoma, though it is not pathognomonic (it can be seen in benign causes of melanonychia). The nail matrix biopsy is the gold standard for diagnosis — a punch or incisional biopsy of the matrix at the proximal origin of the pigmented band. Dermoscopy of the nail plate (onychoscopy) shows irregular band width, irregular spacing of longitudinal lines, loss of parallelism, micro-Hutchinson sign (periungual pigment visible only dermoscopically), and brown-black background — features that distinguish melanoma from benign ethnic melanonychia (which shows regular, parallel lines on a grey background). Melanoma on the palms and soles may present as an irregularly pigmented macule or patch that evolves over months; the parallel ridge pattern on dermoscopy is the key diagnostic feature.

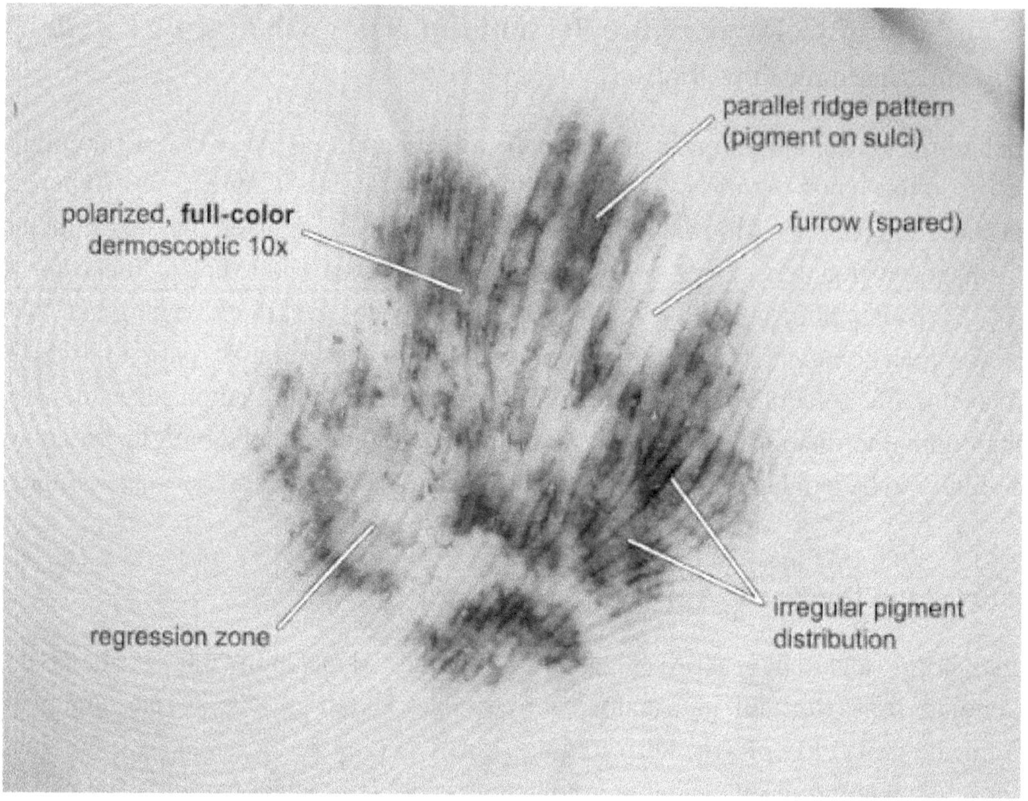

THE CUTANEOUS MIMICKER RECOGNITION ATLAS — Acral Melanoma versus Acral Nevus

---

The Clinical Pattern: Acral lentiginous melanoma presents as an irregularly pigmented, asymmetric, expanding macule or patch on the palm, sole, or nail unit. On the sole, it may present as a brown-black macule with irregular borders and color variation. Subungual melanoma presents as longitudinal melanonychia (a pigmented band in the nail) that is widening, irregular in color, and may show Hutchinson sign. ALM occurs most frequently in older adults and is not related to UV exposure.

The Mimicker: Acral melanocytic nevi present as well-circumscribed, uniformly pigmented macules on the palms and soles, and as regular longitudinal melanonychia on the nails. Acral nevi are common, particularly in individuals with darker skin phototypes — multiple longitudinal pigmented bands are a normal finding in Black and Asian individuals. Benign acral nevi are stable, symmetric, and uniformly colored, without the irregular borders and color variation of melanoma.

Trap Logic: Dismissing longitudinal melanonychia in a patient with darker skin as ethnic melanonychia without dermoscopic assessment is the cognitive trap. While melanonychia is common and usually benign in Fitzpatrick IV–VI skin, subungual melanoma does occur in these populations — and the assumption that melanoma does not affect darker-skinned individuals is the primary driver of diagnostic delay. The reverse trap — performing nail matrix biopsy on every pigmented band — is invasive and produces nail dystrophy, which is why dermoscopy is essential for risk stratification.

The Decision Anchor: The discriminating features are **dermoscopic pattern on the sole (parallel ridge pattern is pathognomonic for melanoma; parallel furrow pattern, lattice-like pattern, and fibrillar pattern indicate benign nevus), onychoscopic features (irregular band width, loss of parallelism, micro-Hutchinson sign indicate melanoma; regular, parallel lines on a grey background indicate benign melanonychia), clinical evolution (any change in a pigmented band — widening, darkening, or development of Hutchinson sign — warrants biopsy), and the ABCDEF rule for nail pigment (Age, Band width, Color, Digit most commonly affected, Extension to nail fold, Family history)**. Perform nail matrix biopsy for any single-digit, darkening, or widening pigmented band.

Dermoscopic Assessment and the ABCDE Criteria

Systematic Dermoscopic Evaluation

Dermoscopy improves diagnostic accuracy for melanoma by 15 to 30 percent over naked-eye examination. The two-step dermoscopic algorithm first determines whether a lesion is melanocytic (by identifying pigment network, aggregated globules, homogeneous blue pigment, or parallel pattern on acral skin), then evaluates melanocytic lesions for melanoma-specific features. The revised pattern analysis approach assesses: atypical pigment network (irregularly thickened lines with variable spacing and abrupt termination), irregular dots and globules (asymmetrically placed, varying in size and shape), blue-white veil (confluent blue-white structureless area indicating melanin in the dermis with overlying acanthosis — present in melanomas with Breslow thickness greater than 0.75 mm), regression structures (white scar-like areas and blue-grey peppering indicating spontaneous immune-mediated regression), pseudopods and radial streaming (irregular finger-like projections at the lesion periphery indicating centrifugal radial growth), and atypical vascular patterns (polymorphous vessels visible in amelanotic and hypomelanotic melanoma).

Scoring Systems and Clinical Decision-Making

Several validated dermoscopic scoring systems aid biopsy decisions. The 7-point checklist (Argenziano) assigns major criteria (atypical network, blue-white veil, atypical vascular pattern — 2 points each) and minor criteria (irregular streaks, irregular dots/globules, regression, irregular blotches — 1 point each); a total score of 3 or more triggers biopsy. The ABCD dermoscopy rule (Stolz) scores Asymmetry, Border, Color, and Differential structures to generate a total dermoscopy score (TDS): TDS below 4.75 favors benign; TDS above 5.45 suggests melanoma; intermediate scores warrant close monitoring or biopsy. The Menzies method uses a simplified two-rule approach: the presence of any positive feature (blue-white veil, pseudopods, radial streaming, scar-like depigmentation, irregular dots/globules, multiple colors, or atypical network) combined with the absence of both symmetry of pattern and single color (i.e., asymmetry and multiple colors must be present). In clinical practice, dermoscopy should be integrated into a comprehensive assessment that includes clinical context (patient age, risk factors, lesion history), the ABCDE criteria, and the ugly duckling sign.

Staging: AJCC TNM Classification and Sentinel Lymph Node Biopsy

AJCC 8th Edition TNM Classification

The AJCC 8th edition staging system for cutaneous melanoma is the standard for prognosis and treatment planning. T-stage is determined by Breslow thickness (the most important prognostic factor) and ulceration: T1 (1.0 mm or less; T1a if less than 0.8 mm without ulceration, T1b if 0.8 to 1.0 mm or less than 0.8 mm with ulceration), T2 (greater than 1.0 to 2.0 mm), T3 (greater than 2.0 to 4.0 mm), and T4 (greater than 4.0 mm). Ulceration upstages within each T-category (e.g., T2a is non-ulcerated, T2b is ulcerated). N-stage reflects regional lymph node involvement: N1 (1 node), N2 (2 to 3 nodes), N3 (4 or more nodes or in-transit/satellite/microsatellite metastases with nodal involvement). M-stage classifies distant metastases by site and LDH level: M1a (skin, soft tissue, non-regional nodes), M1b (lung), M1c (other visceral sites), M1d (CNS). Overall staging ranges from Stage I (localized, thin, non-ulcerated) through Stage IV (distant metastases).

Sentinel Lymph Node Biopsy

Sentinel lymph node biopsy (SLNB) identifies occult nodal micrometastases and is the most important staging procedure for melanoma. Current guidelines recommend SLNB for melanomas with Breslow thickness of 0.8 mm or greater (T1b or higher), or for thinner melanomas with adverse features (ulceration, mitotic rate of 1 or more per square millimeter, lymphovascular invasion, or younger patient age). The procedure involves peritumoral injection of radioactive tracer (technetium-99m sulfur colloid) and blue dye, followed by intraoperative gamma probe-guided identification and excision of the sentinel node(s). The sentinel node is sectioned and examined for micrometastatic melanoma using H&E staining and immunohistochemistry (S-100, HMB-45, Melan-A). A positive SLNB indicates Stage III disease and informs the need for adjuvant systemic therapy. The Multicenter Selective Lymphadenectomy Trial (MSLT-I) established that SLNB provides critical staging information and identifies patients who benefit from adjuvant therapy, though it did not demonstrate a melanoma-specific survival benefit from immediate completion lymph node dissection (CLND). The subsequent MSLT-II and DeCOG-SLT trials demonstrated that CLND does not improve survival over observation with nodal basin ultrasound surveillance in patients with positive SLNB — leading to a paradigm shift away from routine CLND.

Surgical Management: Excision Margins, Sentinel Node Assessment, and Lymphadenectomy

Wide Local Excision Margins

Definitive surgical management of primary melanoma is wide local excision (WLE) with margins determined by Breslow thickness. Current guideline-recommended margins (National Comprehensive Cancer Network, European Society for Medical Oncology) are: melanoma in situ — 5 mm (or modified Mohs for lentigo maligna on the face); Breslow thickness 1.0 mm or less — 1 cm; Breslow 1.01 to 2.0 mm — 1 to 2 cm; Breslow greater than 2.0 mm — 2 cm. These margins are based on prospective randomized trials (the WHO Melanoma Programme Trial, the Swedish Melanoma Study Group Trial, the Intergroup Melanoma Surgical Trial) that demonstrated no survival benefit from margins wider than those listed, while confirming that narrower margins carry higher local recurrence rates. For melanoma in situ (particularly lentigo maligna on the face), conventional 5 mm margins may be inadequate due to subclinical extension along adnexal structures — staged excision with complete margin assessment or Mohs micrographic surgery with immunohistochemical staining (MART-1/Melan-A) provides higher clearance rates while preserving tissue.

Lymph Node Management

For patients with a positive SLNB, the standard approach has shifted from immediate CLND to observation with regular nodal basin ultrasound surveillance (every 4 to 6 months for the first 2 years, then every 6 to 12 months). Therapeutic lymph node dissection (TLND) is reserved for patients who develop clinically detected nodal recurrence during surveillance. This shift was driven by the MSLT-II and DeCOG-SLT trials, which demonstrated equivalent melanoma-specific survival between CLND and observation while showing that CLND increases lymphedema and other surgical morbidity without survival benefit. For patients presenting with clinically palpable nodal disease (macrometastases detected by physical examination or imaging), TLND remains indicated, often followed by adjuvant systemic therapy.

Special Populations: Melanoma in Pregnancy, Pediatric, and Immunosuppressed Patients

Melanoma in pregnancy presents unique management challenges. Pregnancy does not increase the risk of developing melanoma, and hormonal influences on melanocytic nevi (darkening and enlargement during pregnancy) do not indicate malignant transformation. However, melanoma diagnosed during pregnancy tends to present at a later stage — partly because of delayed recognition (physiologic pigmentary changes are attributed to pregnancy) and partly because of reluctance to biopsy during pregnancy. The standard of care for melanoma in pregnancy is the same as for non-pregnant patients: excisional biopsy under local anesthesia is safe and should not be deferred. Wide local excision is performed with standard margins, and SLNB can be performed using technetium-99m tracer without blue dye (to avoid the anaphylaxis risk of isosulfan blue). Systemic therapy decisions are complex: immune checkpoint inhibitors and BRAF/MEK inhibitors carry teratogenic risk and are generally deferred until after delivery when possible. Transplacental metastasis is exceptionally rare but documented — the placenta should be examined histopathologically at delivery. Pediatric melanoma is uncommon (approximately 300 cases per year in the United States in patients under 20), but adolescents aged 15 to 19 have rising incidence rates. Spitzoid melanoma — a diagnostic challenge at the intersection of Spitz nevus and melanoma — predominates in younger patients. In organ transplant recipients, melanoma risk is 2 to 3-fold higher than the general population, and de novo melanomas in immunosuppressed patients tend to be thicker at diagnosis with worse outcomes. Reduction of immunosuppression should be discussed with the transplant team when melanoma is diagnosed.

Complications and Prognosis

The most critical prognostic factors for localized melanoma are Breslow thickness and ulceration status. Five-year melanoma-specific survival rates for localized disease range from 99 percent for T1a (less than 0.8 mm, non-ulcerated) to 82 percent for T4b (greater than 4.0 mm, ulcerated). For patients with regional nodal disease (Stage III), survival depends on the number of positive nodes, tumor burden within nodes (clinically occult micrometastasis detected by SLNB versus clinically detected macrometastasis), and the presence of in-transit or satellite metastases — 5-year survival ranges from 93 percent for Stage IIIA to 32 percent for Stage IIID. Common sites of distant metastasis include skin, soft tissue, and non-regional lymph nodes (most favorable), lung (intermediate prognosis), other visceral sites including liver and bone (poor prognosis), and the central nervous system (worst prognosis — brain metastases occur in 20 to 45 percent of patients with Stage IV disease and historically carried median survival of 4 to 6 months, though outcomes have improved with immunotherapy and stereotactic radiosurgery). Most melanoma recurrences occur within the first 3 years after diagnosis, but late recurrences (10 to 20 years after primary treatment) are well documented, particularly for thin melanomas — which is why lifelong surveillance is recommended.

CAUTION: Regression in a melanoma — clinically visible as a grey-white or blue-grey area within the lesion, and histopathologically as fibrosis, melanophages, and vascular proliferation replacing tumor cells — presents a diagnostic and prognostic paradox. A melanoma with extensive regression may have a thin measured Breslow thickness because the immune system has destroyed the thicker portion of the tumor, and the measured thickness underestimates the original tumor depth. This has implications for staging and SLNB decision-making: some experts recommend SLNB for thin melanomas (less than 0.8 mm) with extensive regression, because the original tumor may have been substantially thicker. Regression can also make diagnosis more difficult — a completely regressed melanoma may present as a blue-grey patch without identifiable melanoma cells on biopsy, yet may have already metastasized from the pre-regression primary tumor.

Systemic Therapy: Immune Checkpoint Inhibitors, Targeted Therapy (BRAF/MEK), and Adjuvant Protocols

Immune Checkpoint Inhibitors

Immune checkpoint inhibitors have revolutionized the treatment of advanced melanoma. Anti-PD-1 monotherapy (nivolumab or pembrolizumab) produces objective response rates of 40 to 45 percent in unresectable Stage III and Stage IV melanoma, with durable responses lasting years in many responders — a dramatic improvement over the 10 to 15 percent response rates of prior chemotherapy (dacarbazine). The combination of nivolumab plus ipilimumab (anti-PD-1 plus anti-CTLA-4) produces higher response rates (approximately 58 percent) and longer progression-free survival than either agent alone, but at the cost of significantly higher immune-related adverse events (60 to 65 percent Grade 3–4 toxicity, including colitis, hepatitis, pneumonitis, endocrinopathies, and nephritis). In the adjuvant setting (after complete surgical resection of Stage III melanoma), one year of pembrolizumab or nivolumab reduces the risk of recurrence by 35 to 40 percent compared to placebo. The landmark KEYNOTE-716 trial extended adjuvant pembrolizumab to Stage IIB and IIC melanoma (thick primary tumors without nodal involvement), demonstrating a recurrence-free survival benefit in this population.

BRAF/MEK-Targeted Therapy

Approximately 40 to 50 percent of cutaneous melanomas harbor activating BRAF V600E or V600K mutations, making them amenable to targeted therapy with BRAF inhibitors (vemurafenib, dabrafenib, encorafenib) combined with MEK inhibitors (cobimetinib, trametinib, binimetinib). Combination BRAF/MEK inhibition produces rapid responses (response rates of 65 to 70 percent, median time to response 2 to 3 months) and is preferred over BRAF monotherapy because the addition of MEK inhibition delays resistance and reduces paradoxical MAPK pathway activation (which causes cutaneous SCCs and keratoacanthomas — a side effect of BRAF inhibitor monotherapy). The choice between immunotherapy and targeted therapy for BRAF-mutant melanoma is guided by tumor burden and clinical urgency: patients with bulky, rapidly progressing disease may benefit from the rapid response of BRAF/MEK inhibition as initial therapy, while immunotherapy is often preferred for patients with lower tumor burden because of the durability of responses. Combined adjuvant dabrafenib plus trametinib for 12 months in resected Stage III BRAF-mutant melanoma improved relapse-free survival in the COMBI-AD trial.

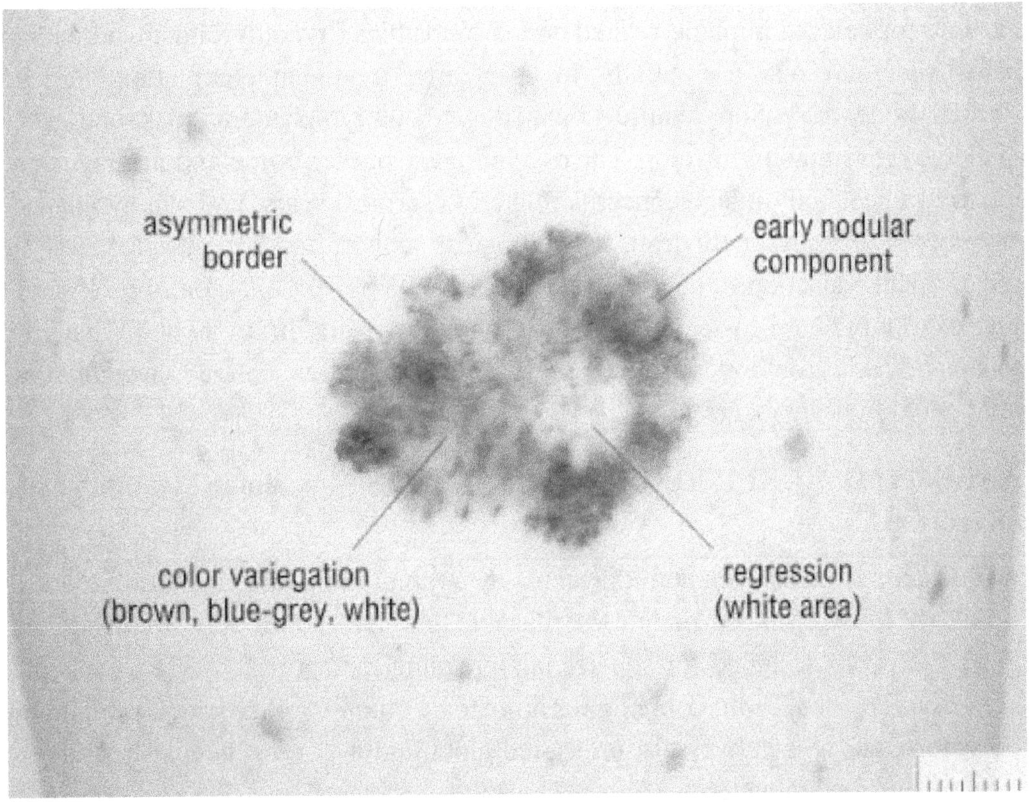

Surveillance, Recurrence Detection, and Survivorship

Evidence-Based Surveillance Protocols

Melanoma surveillance aims to detect recurrence early (when salvage treatment is most effective) and to identify new primary melanomas (patients with one melanoma have a 4 to 8 percent lifetime risk of developing a second primary). Surveillance intensity is stage-dependent: Stage I-IIA patients are followed with history, physical examination, and full-body skin examination every 6 to 12 months for 5 years, then annually. Stage IIB-III patients are followed every 3 to 6 months for the first 2 to 3 years (the highest-risk period for recurrence), then every 6 to 12 months for years 3 to 5, then annually. Routine imaging (CT, PET/CT, MRI) is recommended for Stage IIB and higher — specifically CT of the chest, abdomen, and pelvis, and brain MRI — at intervals guided by stage and risk factors. S-100B and LDH are serum biomarkers used in some surveillance protocols, though their sensitivity and specificity are limited for early recurrence detection.

Survivorship and Psychosocial Considerations

Melanoma survivorship extends beyond oncologic surveillance to include long-term management of treatment toxicities and psychosocial support. Patients who have received immune checkpoint inhibitors require monitoring for delayed immune-related endocrinopathies (hypothyroidism, adrenal insufficiency, type 1 diabetes) that may manifest months to years after treatment completion. Patients who have undergone lymph node dissection require counseling about lymphedema risk and early referral to lymphedema therapy if symptoms develop. The psychological burden of melanoma diagnosis — including anxiety about recurrence, body image concerns related to surgical scars, and sun avoidance behavior — is well documented and may benefit from psychological support and patient education about realistic recurrence risk. Patient education should reinforce lifelong sun protection, monthly self-skin examination (with a partner examining hard-to-see areas), and prompt reporting of any new or changing lesion, any new subcutaneous nodule, or any unexplained systemic symptom (fatigue, weight loss, neurologic symptoms) that could indicate recurrence.

THE CUTANEOUS MIMICKER RECOGNITION ATLAS — Nodular Melanoma versus Seborrheic Keratosis

---

The Clinical Pattern: Nodular melanoma presents as a rapidly growing, uniformly dark blue-black or amelanotic (pink-red) dome-shaped nodule. It may be symmetric and well-circumscribed, failing the ABCDE criteria that were designed for superficial spreading melanoma. It is a new, rapidly enlarging lesion (EFG criteria: Elevated, Firm, Growing for more than 1 month). On dermoscopy, it may show blue-white veil, polymorphous atypical vessels, milky-red globules, or homogeneous structureless blue-black pigmentation without a benign pattern.

The Mimicker: A darkly pigmented, dome-shaped seborrheic keratosis can closely resemble a pigmented nodular melanoma on clinical inspection. Both present as elevated, dark papules or nodules on the trunk and extremities. Seborrheic keratoses have a dull, waxy, stuck-on surface with visible horn cysts and fissures, while nodular melanoma has a smoother, shinier surface. On dermoscopy, seborrheic keratoses show milia-like cysts, comedo-like openings, and the cerebriform pattern — entirely different from the melanocytic features of melanoma.

Trap Logic: Assuming that any dark, dome-shaped papule on the trunk of an older adult is a seborrheic keratosis without dermoscopic examination is the cognitive trap. Nodular melanoma can be clinically indistinguishable from a dark seborrheic keratosis, and the error of dismissing a melanoma as a benign keratosis is catastrophic — nodular melanoma is the subtype most likely to be diagnosed at a thick, advanced stage precisely because of this complacency. The reverse trap — excising every seborrheic keratosis — is wasteful but avoids the lethal error.

The Decision Anchor: The discriminating features are **dermoscopic pattern (milia-like cysts and comedo-like openings are diagnostic of seborrheic keratosis; blue-white veil, polymorphous vessels, and structureless blue-black are melanocytic/malignant), surface quality (dull, waxy, stuck-on with visible horn cysts favors SK; shiny, smooth surface favors melanocytic lesion), and growth history (stable for months to years favors SK; rapid growth over weeks favors nodular melanoma)**. The clinical rule: any dark, elevated lesion that does not show unambiguous seborrheic keratosis features on dermoscopy must be biopsied to exclude melanoma.

KEY POINT: Nodular melanoma accounts for only 15 to 30 percent of melanomas but causes a disproportionate share of melanoma deaths because it lacks the prolonged radial growth phase that gives other subtypes time for early detection. The traditional ABCDE criteria often fail for nodular melanoma — it may be symmetric (not A), well-bordered (not B), uniformly colored (not C), and small (not D). The EFG criteria (Elevated, Firm, Growing for more than 1 month) were developed specifically to capture these lesions.

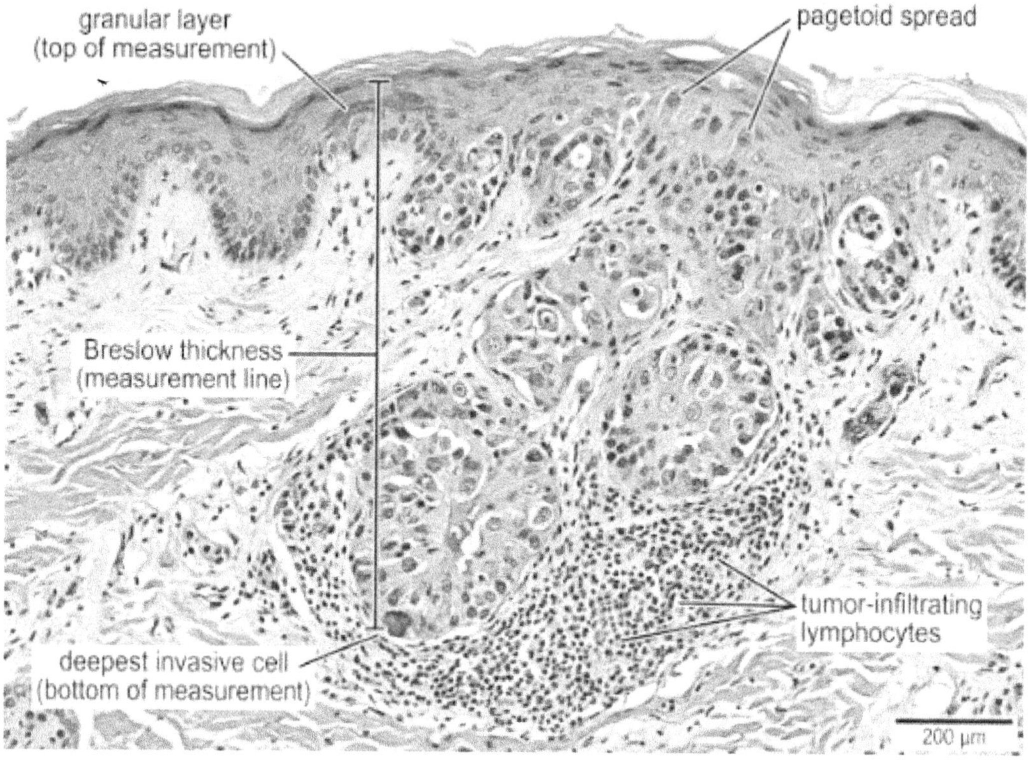

EVIDENCE: The CheckMate 067 trial established the long-term survival benefit of nivolumab plus ipilimumab for advanced melanoma: 10-year overall survival was 43 percent for the combination, compared to 36 percent for nivolumab alone and 18 percent for ipilimumab alone. These results demonstrate that durable, long-term disease control is achievable with immune checkpoint inhibition — a paradigm shift from the pre-immunotherapy era when median overall survival for metastatic melanoma was 6 to 9 months. Approximately 20 to 25 percent of patients achieve complete responses that are maintained without ongoing treatment.

Clinical Case: The Pigmented Band on the Thumbnail

A 58-year-old Black woman presents with a darkening, widening band of pigmentation on her right thumbnail that she first noticed 1 year ago. She has no history of nail trauma. On examination, the right thumbnail shows a 5 mm wide, irregular, dark-brown to black longitudinal band extending from the proximal nail fold to the free edge. The band shows variation in color intensity and irregular spacing of longitudinal lines. The proximal nail fold shows subtle brown pigmentation visible only with dermoscopy (micro-Hutchinson sign). The other nails are free of pigmentation.

The clinical features — a single-digit, widening, darkening, irregularly pigmented longitudinal band with micro-Hutchinson sign in a patient over 50 — are highly suspicious for subungual melanoma. Onychoscopy confirms irregular band width, loss of parallelism, multiple brown-black colors, and micro-Hutchinson sign. A nail matrix biopsy is performed: a 3 mm punch biopsy of the proximal nail matrix at the origin of the pigmented band. Histopathology reveals melanoma in situ with atypical melanocytic proliferation at the nail matrix epithelium. Wide local excision of the nail apparatus with 5 mm margins is curative for melanoma in situ. This case demonstrates the diagnostic algorithm for longitudinal melanonychia in a patient with darker skin: dermoscopy first (to stratify risk and avoid unnecessary biopsy of benign ethnic melanonychia), followed by nail matrix biopsy when dermoscopic features are suspicious, with definitive management guided by histologic diagnosis.

THE CUTANEOUS MIMICKER RECOGNITION ATLAS — Melanoma Diagnostic Arcs

Acral Melanoma vs. Acral Nevus: The discriminating features are dermoscopic pattern on acral skin (parallel ridge pattern is pathognomonic for melanoma; parallel furrow pattern indicates benign nevus), onychoscopic features for nail lesions (irregular band width, loss of parallelism, micro-Hutchinson sign indicate melanoma; regular, parallel lines on a grey background indicate benign melanonychia), and clinical evolution. Cognitive trap: dismissing melanonychia in darker-skinned patients as ethnic melanonychia without dermoscopic assessment — this assumption drives the diagnostic delay that produces worse stage-specific survival in skin of color.

Nodular Melanoma vs. Seborrheic Keratosis: The discriminating features are dermoscopic pattern (milia-like cysts and comedo-like openings are diagnostic of seborrheic keratosis; blue-white veil and polymorphous vessels indicate melanoma), surface quality (dull, waxy, stuck-on favors SK; shiny and smooth favors melanocytic), and growth history (rapid growth favors nodular melanoma). Cognitive trap: assuming any dark dome-shaped papule is a seborrheic keratosis without dermoscopy, because nodular melanoma is the subtype most commonly missed due to its failure to meet ABCDE criteria.

Summary and Key Concepts

Nevus count is the strongest independent risk factor for melanoma. Intermittent, intense UV exposure (sunburns) is more strongly associated with melanoma than cumulative UV, and indoor tanning before age 35 increases risk by 59 percent. Prevention relies on UV reduction and screening with dermoscopy and total body photography for high-risk individuals.

Nodular melanoma lacks a prolonged radial growth phase and often fails ABCDE criteria — the EFG criteria (Elevated, Firm, Growing) were developed specifically to detect this subtype, which causes a disproportionate share of melanoma deaths. Amelanotic nodular melanoma is the most diagnostically treacherous variant.

Acral lentiginous melanoma is the most common melanoma subtype in Black, Asian, and Hispanic populations. The parallel ridge pattern on dermoscopy is pathognomonic. Diagnostic delay in skin of color drives the survival disparity — clinicians must examine the palms, soles, and nail units regardless of skin phototype.

SLNB is recommended for melanomas with Breslow thickness of 0.8 mm or greater. Completion lymph node dissection no longer provides survival benefit over observation with ultrasound surveillance (MSLT-II, DeCOG-SLT trials). Wide excision margins are determined by Breslow thickness (1 cm for tumors 1 mm or less; 2 cm for tumors greater than 2 mm).

Immune checkpoint inhibitors (nivolumab, pembrolizumab, ipilimumab) have transformed advanced melanoma outcomes, with 10-year overall survival reaching 43 percent for combination nivolumab plus ipilimumab. BRAF/MEK-targeted therapy produces rapid responses in BRAF-mutant melanoma and is preferred when rapid tumor shrinkage is clinically urgent.

CHAPTER 16: CUTANEOUS LYMPHOMA AND LYMPHOPROLIFERATIVE DISORDERS

Learning Objectives

1. Classify cutaneous lymphomas using the WHO-EORTC system, distinguishing indolent from aggressive subtypes and primary cutaneous from secondary cutaneous involvement by systemic lymphoma.
2. Recognize the clinical stages and histopathologic features of mycosis fungoides, identify its clinical variants, and differentiate early-stage MF from its inflammatory mimickers using clinicopathologic correlation and immunophenotyping.
3. Apply the diagnostic criteria for Sézary syndrome, distinguish it from other causes of erythroderma, and outline the evidence-based treatment algorithm from skin-directed therapy through systemic immunotherapy, targeted agents, and allogeneic stem cell transplantation.
4. Differentiate primary cutaneous CD30+ lymphoproliferative disorders and primary cutaneous B-cell lymphomas from cutaneous pseudolymphoma and secondary cutaneous involvement by systemic lymphoma, using the integration of clinical, histopathologic, immunophenotypic, and molecular data.

Mycosis Fungoides: Stages, Variants, and Clinical Mimicry

Definition and Epidemiology

Mycosis fungoides (MF) is the most common primary cutaneous T-cell lymphoma (CTCL), accounting for approximately 50 percent of all primary cutaneous lymphomas. It is a neoplasm of mature, skin-homing CD4+ T-lymphocytes that demonstrates an epidermotropic growth pattern — malignant T-cells preferentially infiltrating the epidermis. MF has an annual incidence of approximately 5 to 6 per million population, with a median age at diagnosis of 55 to 60 years and a male-to-female ratio of approximately 2:1. African Americans have a higher incidence and present at a younger age compared to white patients. The etiology is unknown — chronic antigenic stimulation, retroviral infection (HTLV-1 has been investigated but not confirmed as causative), and occupational exposures have been proposed but not established as definitive risk factors.

Clinical Stages and Natural History

MF follows a characteristic clinical progression through three stages, though many patients remain in early stages for years or decades. The patch stage presents as flat, erythematous to violaceous, finely scaling patches with well-defined borders — classically affecting sun-protected areas (the bathing trunk distribution: buttocks, inner thighs, lower trunk, and axillae). Patches may be hypopigmented (particularly in patients with darker skin, where hypopigmented MF is the most common presentation) or poikilodermatous (with atrophy, telangiectasia, and mottled pigmentation — poikiloderma atrophicans vasculare). The plaque stage is characterized by thicker, more infiltrated, well-demarcated plaques with a dusky red-brown to violaceous color; plaques may develop central clearing, annular configuration, or follicular prominence. The tumor stage presents with dome-shaped to ulcerated nodules and tumors arising within existing plaques or de novo — tumor-stage disease carries a significantly worse prognosis. Large-cell transformation (the presence of large cells exceeding 25 percent of the dermal infiltrate, or forming microscopic nodules) indicates biological aggressiveness and is associated with rapid progression and shorter survival.

Clinical Variants

Several clinicopathologic variants of MF are recognized. Folliculotropic MF (pilotropic MF) preferentially involves hair follicles, presenting as grouped follicular papules, alopecia (often of the eyebrows — a diagnostically useful feature), acneiform lesions, and comedonal plugging, typically on the head and neck. The folliculotropic variant often lacks visible epidermotropism on biopsy (the malignant infiltrate surrounds and invades hair follicles rather than the interfollicular epidermis), may be associated with mucinous degeneration of the hair follicle (follicular mucinosis), and has a worse prognosis than classic patch/plaque MF. Pagetoid reticulosis (Woringer-Kolopp disease) is a localized variant presenting as a solitary, slowly expanding, psoriasiform or hyperkeratotic plaque, usually on an extremity — histopathology shows prominent pagetoid epidermotropism by atypical lymphocytes. Granulomatous slack skin is an exceptionally rare variant presenting as pendulous folds of lax, redundant skin in the axillae and groin, with a dense granulomatous infiltrate on biopsy. Syringotropic MF shows tropism for eccrine sweat glands and may present with anhidrosis.

Differential Diagnosis and Diagnostic Challenges in Early MF

Early-stage (patch-stage) MF is among the most diagnostically challenging entities in dermatopathology because the clinical and histopathologic features overlap extensively with benign inflammatory dermatoses. The median time from symptom onset to diagnosis of MF is 3 to 6 years, reflecting this diagnostic difficulty. Clinical mimickers include chronic eczematous dermatitis (atopic or nummular eczema), psoriasis (particularly small-plaque parapsoriasis/digitate dermatosis versus large-plaque parapsoriasis, which is considered a precursor of MF), drug eruptions, contact dermatitis, and tinea corporis. Histopathologic features that favor MF over benign inflammatory disease include epidermotropism of atypical lymphocytes without spongiosis (lymphocytes infiltrating the epidermis in the absence of the intercellular edema seen in eczema), Pautrier microabscesses (collections of atypical lymphocytes within the epidermis — a specific but insensitive finding), disproportionate epidermotropism relative to the dermal infiltrate, haloed lymphocytes (atypical lymphocytes surrounded by a clear halo in the epidermis), a band-like upper dermal infiltrate with fibrosis of the papillary dermis, and cerebriform lymphocyte nuclei. Immunophenotyping by immunohistochemistry demonstrates a CD3+/CD4+/CD8- T-cell population; loss of CD7 expression by the neoplastic T-cells (CD7-negative CD4+ T-cells) is a supportive finding but is not specific for MF. T-cell receptor (TCR) gene rearrangement studies demonstrating a clonal T-cell population support the diagnosis, though clonality can be found in some benign inflammatory conditions and is not diagnostic in isolation.

Histopathology and Immunophenotyping

Histopathologic confirmation of MF requires clinicopathologic correlation — the histologic features alone are often insufficient for diagnosis, particularly in early-stage disease. Multiple biopsies from different lesions (ideally 2 to 3 punch biopsies from the most clinically suspicious patches or plaques) increase diagnostic yield. The characteristic histopathologic features of established MF include a band-like (lichenoid) infiltrate of atypical lymphocytes in the papillary dermis with epidermotropism — atypical lymphocytes migrating into the epidermis, often preferentially aligning along the basal layer. Pautrier microabscesses (intraepidermal collections of 4 or more atypical lymphocytes) are the most specific finding but are present in only 15 to 40 percent of biopsies. The atypical lymphocytes have cerebriform nuclei — hyperconvoluted nuclear membranes that create a brain-like appearance on high-power examination. Papillary dermal fibrosis (wiry collagen bundles replacing the normal papillary dermis) develops in established lesions and is a supportive feature. Immunohistochemistry demonstrates a CD3+/CD4+/CD8- T-cell phenotype in most cases, with loss of CD7 expression (CD4+/CD7- population) supporting the diagnosis. TCR gene rearrangement analysis by PCR demonstrating identical clonal peaks in multiple anatomic sites strengthens the diagnostic confidence, though monoclonality alone does not confirm lymphoma, and polyclonality does not exclude it.

CLINICAL PEARL: Hypopigmented MF is the most common presentation of mycosis fungoides in children and adolescents, and in patients with Fitzpatrick IV–VI skin. It presents as well-demarcated, hypopigmented patches — often misdiagnosed as vitiligo, pityriasis alba, or post-inflammatory hypopigmentation. Unlike vitiligo, hypopigmented MF patches are not depigmented (they retain some melanin) and often show fine scaling. Biopsy shows the classic epidermotropic pattern of MF, with the hypopigmentation caused by cytotoxic damage to melanocytes by the CD8+ (rather than CD4+) atypical lymphocytes that characterize this variant. Hypopigmented MF has an excellent prognosis — it responds well to phototherapy (narrowband UVB or PUVA) and rarely progresses beyond early stage.

Sézary Syndrome: Diagnosis and Differentiation From Erythrodermic Dermatoses

Definition and Diagnostic Criteria

Sézary syndrome (SS) is the leukemic variant of CTCL — an aggressive, erythrodermic T-cell lymphoma characterized by the triad of erythroderma (confluent erythema affecting 80 percent or more of the body surface area), lymphadenopathy, and the presence of circulating neoplastic T-cells (Sézary cells) in the peripheral blood. The International Society for Cutaneous Lymphomas (ISCL) and EORTC diagnostic criteria require erythroderma plus one or more of: an absolute Sézary cell count of 1,000 per microliter or more in the peripheral blood, an expanded CD4+ T-cell population with a CD4:CD8 ratio of 10 or more (by flow cytometry), loss of one or more T-cell antigens (CD2, CD3, CD4, CD5, or CD7) on the circulating T-cells, or demonstration of a T-cell clone in the blood by molecular methods (identical to the clone in the skin). Sézary cells are characterized by their large, cerebriform nuclei — a highly convoluted nuclear membrane visible on peripheral blood smear and confirmed by electron microscopy.

Differentiating Sézary Syndrome From Other Causes of Erythroderma

Erythroderma (exfoliative dermatitis) is a clinical syndrome with multiple etiologies, and SS must be differentiated from drug-induced erythroderma, erythrodermic psoriasis, erythrodermic atopic dermatitis, pityriasis rubra pilaris, and other causes. The clinical features that favor SS over inflammatory erythroderma include generalized lymphadenopathy, severe pruritus (often intractable), palmoplantar keratoderma, leonine facies, alopecia, and ectropion. However, none of these features is pathognomonic — drug-induced erythroderma and erythrodermic psoriasis can produce identical clinical pictures. The diagnostic distinction rests on peripheral blood evaluation: flow cytometry demonstrating an expanded CD4+/CD7- or CD4+/CD26- population with a CD4:CD8 ratio exceeding 10, and TCR gene rearrangement demonstrating a blood clone matching the skin clone. A skin biopsy showing epidermotropic atypical lymphocytes with cerebriform nuclei supports the diagnosis but may be nonspecific in erythrodermic patients (spongiotic and psoriasiform patterns can obscure the lymphoma features). The distinction matters because SS has a significantly worse prognosis than inflammatory erythroderma — median survival for SS is 2 to 4 years, compared to the generally favorable prognosis of most inflammatory causes once the trigger is removed.

Pathophysiology and Immunologic Consequences

SS produces profound immunosuppression because the neoplastic T-cells are Th2-polarized, secreting IL-4, IL-5, IL-10, and IL-13 while suppressing Th1 immunity (IFN-gamma, IL-2). This Th2 skew results in impaired cell-mediated immunity, eosinophilia, elevated serum IgE, and increased susceptibility to infections — particularly Staphylococcus aureus skin infections, which are a major source of morbidity and mortality in SS. The pruritus of SS is severe and multifactorial, driven by IL-31 (a pruritogenic cytokine secreted by Th2 cells), neuropathic mechanisms, and skin barrier disruption from the erythroderma. Patients with SS often develop secondary bacterial sepsis originating from S. aureus colonization of the erythrodermic skin — infection management and skin barrier support are critical components of the care plan.

Complications and Infectious Morbidity

The immunosuppression inherent to SS — driven by the Th2-polarized neoplastic T-cell clone that suppresses cell-mediated Th1 immunity — renders patients profoundly susceptible to infections. Staphylococcus aureus colonizes the erythrodermic skin in up to 90 percent of SS patients, and bacterial sepsis originating from skin entry points is a leading cause of death. Management requires aggressive skin care (emollients to restore the barrier, dilute bleach baths to reduce S. aureus burden, prompt antibiotic treatment of clinical infection, and mupirocin for nares decolonization) alongside lymphoma-directed therapy. Herpes simplex and varicella-zoster reactivation, dermatophyte infections, and opportunistic infections (including Pneumocystis jirovecii pneumonia in heavily treated patients) contribute to morbidity. Erythrodermic skin failure — analogous to burn-related fluid and protein loss — causes thermoregulatory dysfunction, insensible fluid and electrolyte losses (particularly in hospitalized patients), hypoalbuminemia from protein loss through the skin, and high-output cardiac failure from the massively increased cutaneous blood flow. Peripheral edema is common and multifactorial: hypoalbuminemia, lymphatic obstruction from nodal disease, and cardiac strain. Thromboembolic events occur at increased rates in advanced CTCL, particularly in erythrodermic patients.

THE CUTANEOUS MIMICKER RECOGNITION ATLAS — Patch-Stage MF versus Chronic Eczema

The Clinical Pattern: Patch-stage mycosis fungoides presents as persistent, well-demarcated, erythematous to dusky patches with fine scaling, characteristically in a bathing trunk distribution (buttocks, inner thighs, lower trunk — sun-protected sites). Patches persist for months to years despite topical corticosteroid treatment, which may partially suppress the infiltrate but does not produce lasting clearance. In patients with darker skin, hypopigmented patches predominate. The clinical history of fixed, persistent patches in sun-protected areas that fail conventional eczema therapy is the earliest clinical warning sign.

The Mimicker: Chronic nummular or atopic eczema produces erythematous, scaling patches that can closely mimic early MF. Eczematous patches tend to be pruritic, symmetrically distributed, associated with a personal or family atopic history, and responsive to topical corticosteroids with sustained improvement. Eczema favors flexural sites (antecubital and popliteal fossae) and sun-exposed areas, unlike the sun-protected distribution of MF. Contact dermatitis can also produce chronic, persistent patches, but the distribution correlates with the contactant exposure.

Trap Logic: Treating persistent, fixed patches in a bathing trunk distribution as eczema for years without biopsy is the cognitive trap — the mean diagnostic delay for MF is 3 to 6 years precisely because clinicians default to an eczema diagnosis. The reverse trap — biopsying every eczema patient — would overwhelm pathology services. The clinical threshold for biopsy should lower when patches are fixed (same location for months), in a sun-protected distribution, unresponsive to topical therapy, or present in a patient without an atopic history.

The Decision Anchor: The discriminating features are **distribution (sun-protected bathing trunk distribution favors MF; flexural and sun-exposed favors eczema), clinical course (fixed, persistent patches unresponsive to topical corticosteroids favor MF; waxing-waning patches responsive to treatment favor eczema), histopathology (epidermotropism without spongiosis, haloed lymphocytes, and papillary dermal fibrosis favor MF; spongiosis with eosinophils favors eczema), and immunophenotype (CD4+/CD7- clone on immunohistochemistry and TCR gene rearrangement support MF)**. Biopsy any persistent scaling patch in a sun-protected distribution that fails to clear with appropriate topical therapy.

Primary Cutaneous CD30+ Lymphoproliferative Disorders

Classification and Clinical Spectrum

Primary cutaneous CD30+ lymphoproliferative disorders (LPD) comprise the second most common group of CTCLs and include a clinical spectrum ranging from lymphomatoid papulosis (LyP) to primary cutaneous anaplastic large cell lymphoma (pcALCL). These disorders share expression of the CD30 antigen (a member of the tumor necrosis factor receptor superfamily) by the neoplastic cells, but differ dramatically in clinical behavior. The distinction between LyP and pcALCL is primarily clinical, not histopathologic — both may show identical microscopic features, and the diagnosis depends on clinicopathologic correlation.

Lymphomatoid Papulosis

LyP is a chronic, recurrent, self-healing papulonodular skin disease characterized by crops of red-brown papules and small nodules that develop central necrosis and crust, then spontaneously regress over 3 to 12 weeks — leaving varioliform scars. Lesions occur in successive crops, so lesions at different stages of evolution coexist. LyP is histopathologically classified into types A through E: Type A (most common) shows a wedge-shaped dermal infiltrate with scattered CD30+ large cells amid inflammatory cells (eosinophils, neutrophils, histiocytes); Type B mimics MF with an epidermotropic infiltrate of small cerebriform T-cells; Type C shows sheets of CD30+ large cells resembling pcALCL; Type D mimics aggressive epidermotropic CD8+ CTCL; and Type E is an angioinvasive variant with extensive necrosis. Despite its alarming histopathology, LyP has an excellent prognosis — 5-year disease-specific survival exceeds 99 percent. However, 10 to 20 percent of patients with LyP develop a secondary lymphoid malignancy (MF, pcALCL, or Hodgkin lymphoma), requiring long-term clinical surveillance.

Primary Cutaneous Anaplastic Large Cell Lymphoma

PcALCL presents as a solitary or localized, rapidly growing, red-brown to violaceous nodule or tumor, often on the extremities or trunk, that may ulcerate. Unlike LyP, pcALCL does not spontaneously regress (though partial regression occurs in approximately 25 percent of cases). Histopathology shows cohesive sheets of large, anaplastic or pleomorphic CD30+ cells — more than 75 percent of tumor cells must express CD30 to meet the diagnostic threshold. PcALCL must be distinguished from systemic anaplastic large cell lymphoma (sALCL) with secondary skin involvement: sALCL is ALK-positive in most pediatric and young adult cases and ALK-negative in older adults, while pcALCL is almost always ALK-negative. Staging workup (CT, PET/CT, bone marrow biopsy) is mandatory to exclude systemic disease. Solitary pcALCL has an excellent prognosis (5-year survival exceeding 95 percent) and is treated with excision or local radiation therapy; multifocal disease may require low-dose methotrexate or brentuximab vedotin.

KEY POINT: The critical clinical distinction in cutaneous CD30+ LPD is between LyP (self-regressing papulonodular lesions) and pcALCL (persistent, growing nodules). Both are CD30+ and may be histopathologically identical — the diagnosis is CLINICAL, not histopathologic. LyP is a chronic disease managed with observation or low-dose methotrexate, while pcALCL is managed with excision or radiation for solitary lesions. The most important pitfall is mistaking either for systemic ALCL — which has a dramatically different prognosis and requires systemic chemotherapy. Staging workup is mandatory for any CD30+ cutaneous lymphoma to exclude systemic disease.

Primary Cutaneous B-Cell Lymphomas

Classification and Clinical Features

Primary cutaneous B-cell lymphomas (PCBCLs) account for approximately 20 to 25 percent of primary cutaneous lymphomas. The WHO-EORTC classification recognizes three main types: primary cutaneous marginal zone lymphoma (PCMZL), primary cutaneous follicle center lymphoma (PCFCL), and primary cutaneous diffuse large B-cell lymphoma, leg type (PCDLBCL-LT). PCMZL and PCFCL are indolent lymphomas with excellent prognosis (5-year survival exceeding 95 percent), while PCDLBCL-LT is an aggressive lymphoma with 5-year survival of approximately 50 to 60 percent.

Indolent Primary Cutaneous B-Cell Lymphomas

PCMZL (cutaneous MALT lymphoma) presents as solitary or multifocal, red-brown to violaceous papules, plaques, or nodules — often on the trunk or extremities. In Europe, an association with Borrelia burgdorferi infection has been reported, and antibiotic therapy may induce remission in Borrelia-associated cases. Histopathology shows a nodular to diffuse dermal infiltrate of small B-cells (marginal zone cells, lymphoplasmacytoid cells, and mature plasma cells) surrounding reactive germinal centers. PCFCL presents as grouped, flesh-colored to red-brown papules, plaques, or nodules, characteristically on the scalp, forehead, or trunk. Histopathology shows follicular, follicular and diffuse, or diffuse growth patterns composed of centrocytes (cleaved follicle center cells) and centroblasts. Treatment of indolent PCBCLs is local: radiation therapy (24 to 30 Gy) for solitary or localized disease, or observation for asymptomatic multifocal disease. Systemic therapy is rarely required. PCDLBCL-LT predominantly affects elderly women and presents as rapidly growing, red-blue nodules or tumors on the lower legs (though it can occur at other sites). Its aggressive biology is driven by MYC and BCL2 co-expression and inactivation of the CDKN2A locus. Treatment is R-CHOP (rituximab, cyclophosphamide, doxorubicin, vincristine, prednisone) with or without involved-field radiation — identical to the approach for systemic DLBCL.

Cutaneous Pseudolymphomas

Definition and Etiology

Cutaneous pseudolymphoma (lymphocytoma cutis) refers to benign reactive lymphoid proliferations in the skin that clinically and histopathologically mimic cutaneous lymphoma. Pseudolymphomas may be triggered by arthropod bites (particularly tick bites — borrelial lymphocytoma), tattoo pigments, medications (anticonvulsants, antidepressants, angiotensin-converting enzyme inhibitors), vaccination, foreign body reactions, or may be idiopathic. The clinical presentation is typically a solitary or grouped, dome-shaped, red-brown to violaceous papule or nodule — most commonly on the face (ear lobe, nose, cheek), breast, or arm. Borrelial lymphocytoma has a predilection for the ear lobe in children and the areola in adults.

Histopathologic Distinction From Lymphoma

The histopathologic distinction between pseudolymphoma and true cutaneous lymphoma is one of the most challenging areas in dermatopathology. Features favoring pseudolymphoma include a well-circumscribed, bottom-heavy (Grenz zone-sparing) dermal nodule with mixed cellular composition (a polyclonal population of B-cells, T-cells, histiocytes, eosinophils, and plasma cells), reactive germinal centers with tingible body macrophages, and the absence of cytologic atypia. Features favoring lymphoma include monomorphous cellular composition, effacement of normal dermal architecture, cytologic atypia, and an aberrant immunophenotype (loss of pan-T-cell or pan-B-cell markers). The definitive discriminator is clonality: polyclonal immunoglobulin or TCR gene rearrangement supports pseudolymphoma, while monoclonal rearrangement supports lymphoma — though interpretation requires caution, as small clones may be detected in benign reactive conditions (pseudoclonality) and a negative clonality study does not exclude lymphoma.

Diagnostic Workup: Distinguishing Primary From Secondary Cutaneous Lymphoma

The distinction between primary cutaneous lymphoma (arising in and confined to the skin) and secondary cutaneous involvement by systemic lymphoma is clinically critical because prognosis and treatment differ substantially. A cutaneous lymphoma is classified as primary only if it is confined to the skin at the time of diagnosis, with no evidence of extracutaneous disease on complete staging workup. The staging workup for any newly diagnosed cutaneous lymphoma includes: complete blood count with differential (looking for circulating atypical lymphocytes), comprehensive metabolic panel including LDH, peripheral blood flow cytometry (essential for SS; useful for MF with suspected blood involvement), CT of the chest, abdomen, and pelvis (PET/CT is more sensitive for nodal and extranodal disease), and bone marrow biopsy (for aggressive subtypes and when systemic involvement is suspected). For B-cell lymphomas, serum protein electrophoresis and immunofixation may identify a monoclonal gammopathy. Secondary cutaneous involvement by systemic lymphoma — particularly systemic ALCL, mantle cell lymphoma, and chronic lymphocytic leukemia — must be excluded because these entities require systemic chemotherapy rather than the skin-directed approaches appropriate for most primary cutaneous lymphomas.

Clinical Case: The Persistent Patches

A 52-year-old man is referred for evaluation of persistent, mildly pruritic, erythematous patches on his trunk and proximal thighs that have been present for 4 years. He has been treated with topical corticosteroids and emollients by his primary care physician with a diagnosis of eczema, with only partial and temporary improvement. He has no personal or family history of atopic disease. On examination, there are well-demarcated, finely scaling, erythematous to dusky red-brown patches on the buttocks, lower trunk, and inner thighs — a bathing trunk distribution. Several patches show poikilodermatous changes with mottled pigmentation, telangiectasia, and epidermal atrophy. There are no tumors, nodules, or palpable lymphadenopathy.

The fixed, persistent patches in a sun-protected distribution, the lack of atopic history, and the failure to respond to topical therapy raise clinical suspicion for early MF. Three punch biopsies are taken from the most clinically suspicious patches. Histopathology shows a band-like infiltrate of small to medium lymphocytes in the papillary dermis with epidermotropism — lymphocytes extending into the lower epidermis with pericellular halos. One biopsy shows a Pautrier microabscess. Immunohistochemistry demonstrates a CD3+/CD4+/CD8-/CD7- T-cell population. TCR gene rearrangement shows a monoclonal T-cell population, identical across all three biopsy sites. The diagnosis is mycosis fungoides, patch/early plaque stage. Staging evaluation (blood counts, flow cytometry, CT) shows no extracutaneous involvement — Stage IB (T2N0M0B0, generalized patches covering more than 10 percent of BSA). Treatment with narrowband UVB phototherapy three times weekly produces clearance of patches over 3 months. This case illustrates the typical diagnostic delay in MF, the importance of the clinical pattern (sun-protected distribution, treatment failure, absent atopic history), and the value of multiple biopsies with immunophenotyping and clonality studies.

CAUTION: Cutaneous pseudolymphoma caused by tattoo pigment — particularly red dye — can present years after the tattoo is placed and may show dense, atypical lymphoid infiltrates with monotypic features that closely mimic PCMZL or PCFCL. The clinical context (lesion confined to the tattoo, temporal association with tattooing) is the key diagnostic clue. However, true cutaneous lymphoma arising within a tattoo has been reported, and any persistent, growing nodule within a tattoo should be biopsied and evaluated with immunohistochemistry and clonality studies, not dismissed as a tattoo reaction.

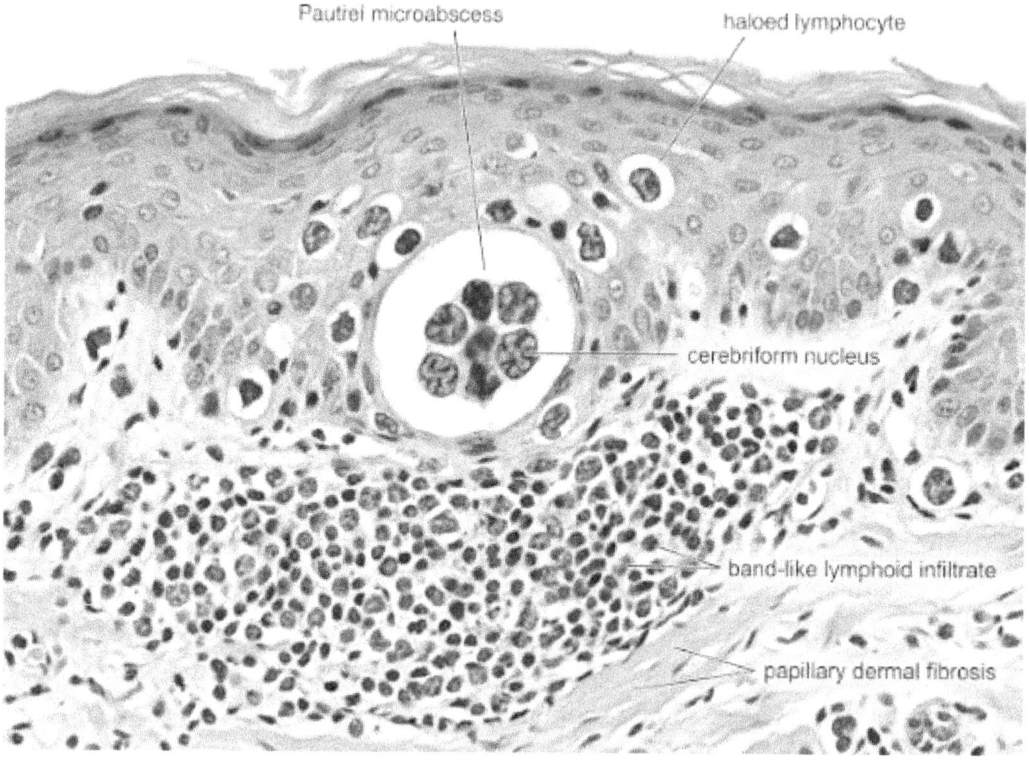

Staging, Prognosis, and Evidence-Based Treatment Algorithms: Skin-Directed and Systemic Therapies

TNMB Staging for MF and SS

Staging of MF and SS uses the TNMB system (Tumor/skin, Node, Metastasis, Blood). T-stage is based on the type and extent of skin involvement: T1 (limited patches, papules, or plaques covering less than 10 percent of skin surface), T2 (generalized patches, papules, or plaques covering 10 percent or more of skin surface), T3 (tumors — one or more cutaneous tumors 1 cm or more in diameter), and T4 (erythroderma — confluent erythema covering 80 percent or more of body surface). N-stage reflects lymph node involvement (clinically abnormal nodes confirmed by biopsy with partial or complete effacement by lymphoma cells). M-stage reflects visceral organ involvement. B-stage reflects blood involvement (Sézary cell count and flow cytometry-defined abnormal T-cell populations). Overall staging: Stage IA (T1N0M0B0 — limited patches/plaques without nodal, visceral, or blood involvement) carries 5-year survival exceeding 98 percent, while Stage IVB (any T, visceral involvement) carries 5-year survival of approximately 15 percent.

Molecular Diagnostics and Prognostic Biomarkers

Molecular diagnostics play an increasingly important role in CTCL diagnosis and prognostication. TCR gene rearrangement analysis by PCR — identifying identical clonal T-cell populations across multiple skin biopsy sites and, in SS, matching clones between skin and blood — is the most widely used molecular test. Next-generation sequencing has revealed recurrent genomic alterations in MF/SS, including mutations in epigenetic regulators (TET2, DNMT3A, IDH2), chromatin remodeling genes (ARID1A), signaling pathway genes (PLCG1, CARD11, STAT3, STAT5B), and the tumor suppressor TP53. JAK/STAT pathway activation is a particularly common finding in advanced MF/SS and has emerged as a therapeutic target. High-throughput TCR sequencing (TCR-seq) can quantify the tumor clone in skin and blood with greater sensitivity than flow cytometry, allowing more precise monitoring of disease burden and treatment response. Serum biomarkers under investigation include soluble IL-2 receptor (sIL-2R), which correlates with tumor burden and disease activity, thymidine kinase, and beta-2 microglobulin — elevated levels are associated with advanced stage and worse prognosis. The development of circulating tumor DNA (ctDNA) assays for CTCL is an active area of research that may enable non-invasive disease monitoring in the future.

Treatment Algorithms: Skin-Directed Therapies

Treatment of MF/SS is stage-directed, beginning with skin-directed therapies for early-stage disease and escalating to systemic therapy for advanced or refractory disease. Skin-directed therapies include topical corticosteroids (high-potency — the first-line treatment for limited patch/plaque MF, with complete response rates of 60 to 65 percent for T1 disease), topical nitrogen mustard (mechlorethamine — available as a commercial gel formulation for use in MF), topical retinoids (bexarotene gel), phototherapy (narrowband UVB for patch-stage disease, PUVA for plaque-stage disease — PUVA penetrates deeper into the dermis and is more effective for thicker plaques), localized radiation therapy (12 to 24 Gy for individual tumors or localized disease — MF is exquisitely radiosensitive), and total skin electron beam therapy (TSEBT — 12 to 36 Gy delivered to the entire skin surface for refractory or generalized disease). TSEBT produces high complete response rates but is associated with significant acute toxicity (erythema, desquamation, alopecia, nail loss) and is generally reserved for patients with generalized thick plaques or tumors who have failed less aggressive therapies.

Treatment Algorithms: Systemic Therapies

Systemic therapies are indicated for advanced-stage MF (Stage IIB and higher), SS, and refractory early-stage disease. Options include oral retinoids (bexarotene — an RXR-selective retinoid with response rates of 45 to 55 percent, associated with hypertriglyceridemia and central hypothyroidism requiring monitoring), histone deacetylase inhibitors (vorinostat, romidepsin — epigenetic modifiers with response rates of 30 to 35 percent), interferons (IFN-alpha, which may be combined with phototherapy or retinoids for synergistic effect), extracorporeal photopheresis (ECP — the standard first-line systemic therapy for SS, involving leukapheresis, ex vivo PUVA treatment of the buffy coat, and reinfusion — response rates of 30 to 80 percent with particularly good responses in early SS), antibody-based therapies (mogamulizumab — anti-CCR4 monoclonal antibody; brentuximab vedotin — anti-CD30 antibody-drug conjugate for CD30+ CTCL), and low-dose chemotherapy (gemcitabine, liposomal doxorubicin). Allogeneic hematopoietic stem cell transplantation is the only potentially curative therapy for advanced MF/SS and is considered for younger patients with refractory, aggressive disease, although transplant-related mortality and graft-versus-host disease limit its applicability.

Patient Education and Prognosis

Patient education in CTCL is essential because the diagnosis of lymphoma provokes significant anxiety, yet most patients with early-stage MF have an indolent, chronic disease with near-normal life expectancy. Patients with Stage IA MF have disease-specific survival equivalent to age-matched controls. It is critical to communicate that MF is not the same disease as nodal non-Hodgkin lymphoma — aggressive systemic chemotherapy is not appropriate for early-stage MF and does not improve outcomes compared to skin-directed therapy. Patients require counseling about the chronic, relapsing nature of MF, the need for regular skin surveillance (every 3 to 6 months), the importance of skin care to minimize barrier disruption and infection risk (particularly in erythrodermic patients), and the signs of disease progression that should prompt return (development of tumors, rapidly expanding disease, new systemic symptoms). The psychological impact of living with a cancer diagnosis that requires lifelong monitoring should not be underestimated — referral to psycho-oncology support services may benefit patients struggling with the chronic disease burden.

Subtype	Presentation	5-Year Survival	First-Line Treatment
MF, Stage IA	Limited patches/plaques (<10% BSA)	98%	Topical corticosteroids, phototherapy
MF, Stage IB-IIA	Generalized patches/plaques (≥10% BSA)	73–80%	Phototherapy (PUVA), topical mechlorethamine
MF, Stage IIB	Cutaneous tumors	40–65%	Local radiation, systemic retinoids, HDAC inhibitors
Sézary syndrome	Erythroderma + blood involvement	24–40%	ECP, mogamulizumab, combination regimens
pcALCL	Solitary/localized nodules (CD30+)	>95%	Excision or local radiation
PCDLBCL-LT	Rapidly growing leg nodules	50–60%	R-CHOP ± radiation

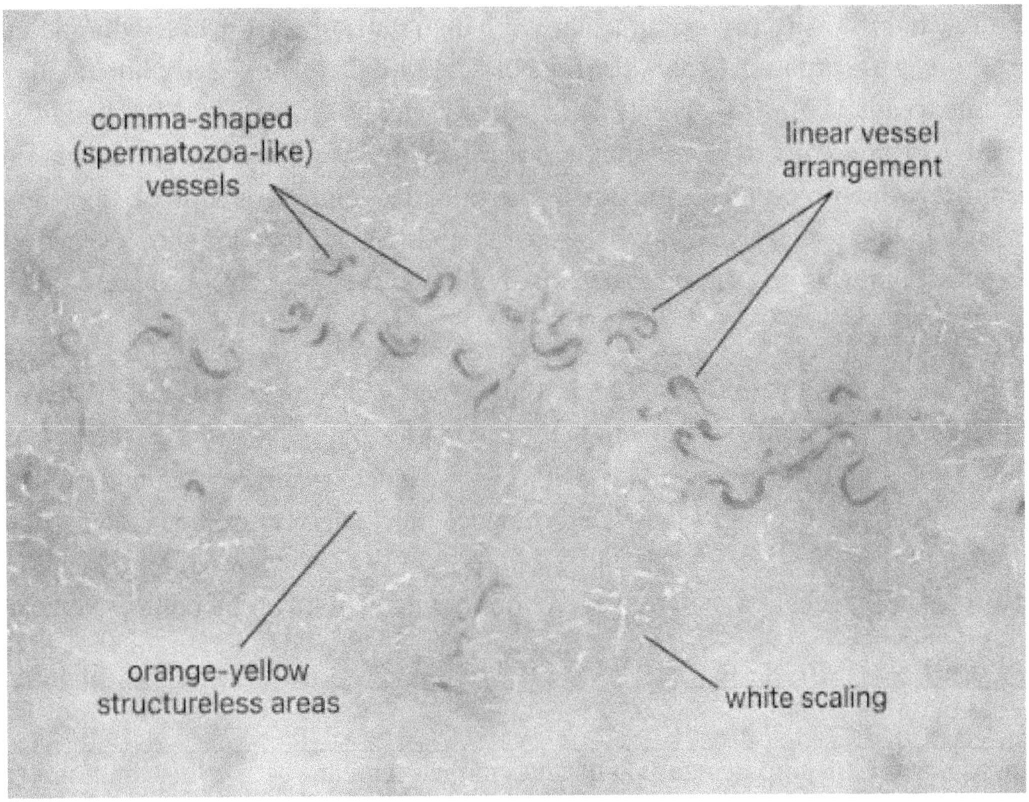

THE CUTANEOUS MIMICKER RECOGNITION ATLAS — Mycosis Fungoides Plaque versus Psoriasis Plaque

---

The Clinical Pattern: MF plaques are well-demarcated, dusky red-brown to violaceous, slightly infiltrated patches or plaques with fine scaling, typically in a bathing trunk distribution (sun-protected areas: buttocks, inner thighs, lower trunk). They are fixed — present in the same location for months to years — and only partially responsive to topical corticosteroids. The color tends toward dusky violaceous or red-brown rather than the bright salmon-pink of psoriasis. Dermoscopy shows spermatozoa-like (comma-shaped) vessels and orange-yellow structureless areas.

The Mimicker: Psoriasis plaques are erythematous, well-demarcated patches with thick, silvery-white micaceous scale, typically in an extensor distribution (elbows, knees, scalp, sacral area). Psoriasis plaques are symmetric and bilateral, respond well to topical corticosteroids and vitamin D analogs, show the Auspitz sign (punctate bleeding on scale removal), and demonstrate dotted or glomerular vessels on dermoscopy — a pattern distinct from the comma-shaped vessels of MF.

Trap Logic: Treating persistent, fixed, violaceous plaques with topical corticosteroids as psoriasis without biopsy is the cognitive trap. The partial response to corticosteroids (which suppress the T-cell infiltrate temporarily) reinforces the misdiagnosis. The clinical red flag is the distribution mismatch: psoriasis favors extensors and sun-exposed sites, while MF favors flexors and sun-protected sites. Additionally, psoriasis typically responds robustly to treatment, while MF produces only partial, unsustained improvement.

The Decision Anchor: The discriminating features are **distribution (sun-protected and flexural favors MF; extensor and sun-exposed favors psoriasis), scale quality (fine and thin favors MF; thick, silvery, and micaceous favors psoriasis), color (dusky violaceous favors MF; bright salmon-pink favors psoriasis), dermoscopy (comma-shaped vessels favor MF; dotted or glomerular vessels favor psoriasis), and treatment response (partial, unsustained response to topical steroids favors MF; robust clearance favors psoriasis)**. Biopsy any psoriasiform plaque that does not respond as expected to standard psoriasis therapy, is in a sun-protected distribution, or has a violaceous hue.

EVIDENCE: The ALCANZA trial demonstrated that brentuximab vedotin, an anti-CD30 antibody-drug conjugate, achieves an objective response rate lasting at least 4 months (ORR4) of 56 percent in CD30+ CTCL (pcALCL and CD30+ MF), compared to 13 percent for physician's choice therapy (methotrexate or bexarotene). This established brentuximab vedotin as a standard treatment option for CD30-expressing CTCL. Similarly, mogamulizumab (anti-CCR4 monoclonal antibody) demonstrated superiority over vorinostat in overall response rate for MF and SS in the MAVORIC trial, with particular benefit in the blood compartment — making it a preferred agent for SS with significant blood involvement.

THE CUTANEOUS MIMICKER RECOGNITION ATLAS — Cutaneous Lymphoma Diagnostic Arcs

---

Patch-Stage MF vs. Chronic Eczema: The discriminating features are distribution (sun-protected bathing trunk distribution favors MF; flexural and atopic distribution favors eczema), clinical course (fixed, persistent patches unresponsive to topical corticosteroids favor MF; waxing-waning and treatment-responsive favor eczema), histopathology (epidermotropism without spongiosis and Pautrier microabscesses favor MF; spongiosis with eosinophils favors eczema), and TCR clonality (monoclonal supports MF). Cognitive trap: treating persistent, fixed patches as eczema for years without biopsy — the mean diagnostic delay for MF is 3 to 6 years.

MF Plaque vs. Psoriasis Plaque: The discriminating features are distribution (sun-protected and flexural favors MF; extensor favors psoriasis), scale quality (fine and thin favors MF; thick, silvery, micaceous favors psoriasis), dermoscopy (comma-shaped vessels favor MF; dotted vessels favor psoriasis), and treatment response (partial, unsustained corticosteroid response favors MF; robust clearance favors psoriasis). Cognitive trap: the partial response to corticosteroids reinforces the psoriasis misdiagnosis by temporarily suppressing the lymphoid infiltrate.

Summary and Key Concepts

Mycosis fungoides is the most common CTCL, presenting as patches, plaques, and eventually tumors in a sun-protected (bathing trunk) distribution. The mean diagnostic delay is 3 to 6 years because patch-stage MF mimics chronic eczema and psoriasis. Biopsy should be performed for any persistent, fixed, scaling patch in a sun-protected distribution that fails to respond to topical therapy.

Sézary syndrome is the leukemic variant of CTCL characterized by erythroderma, lymphadenopathy, and circulating Sézary cells. Diagnosis requires peripheral blood flow cytometry demonstrating an expanded

CD4+/CD7- or CD4+/CD26- population with CD4:CD8 ratio exceeding 10. Median survival is 2 to 4 years despite therapy.

Primary cutaneous CD30+ LPD includes LyP (self-regressing papulonodules with excellent prognosis) and pcALCL (persistent nodules treated with excision or radiation). Both are CD30+ and may be histopathologically identical — the diagnosis is clinical. Staging workup is mandatory to exclude systemic ALCL.

Treatment of MF/SS is stage-directed: skin-directed therapies (topical corticosteroids, phototherapy, nitrogen mustard, local radiation) for early stages; systemic therapies (ECP, retinoids, HDAC inhibitors, mogamulizumab, brentuximab vedotin) for advanced or refractory disease. Early-stage MF has near-normal life expectancy.

Cutaneous pseudolymphoma mimics cutaneous lymphoma clinically and histopathologically. The distinction rests on polyclonal (pseudolymphoma) versus monoclonal (lymphoma) gene rearrangement, mixed cellular composition, and the presence of an identifiable trigger (arthropod bite, tattoo pigment, medication). Borrelia burgdorferi is an associated trigger for PCMZL in European populations.

CHAPTER 17: HAIR DISORDERS

Learning Objectives

1. Describe the hair cycle phases (anagen, catagen, telogen, exogen), the molecular regulators governing follicular cycling, and how disruption of each phase produces distinct patterns of hair loss.
2. Differentiate the major non-scarring alopecias — androgenetic alopecia, alopecia areata, telogen effluvium, and traction alopecia — by their clinical presentations, trichoscopic features, histopathologic findings, and evidence-based treatments.
3. Classify scarring (cicatricial) alopecias into lymphocytic and neutrophilic categories, recognize the clinical and trichoscopic features of lichen planopilaris, frontal fibrosing alopecia, central centrifugal cicatricial alopecia, and discoid lupus, and apply appropriate diagnostic workup and stage-directed management.
4. Evaluate hirsutism systematically using the modified Ferriman-Gallwey score, distinguish androgen-dependent hirsutism from hypertrichosis, and outline the hormonal workup and multimodal management approach incorporating pharmacotherapy, procedural hair removal, and emerging therapies.

Hair Biology: The Hair Cycle, Growth Regulation, and Hair Shaft Structure

Hair Follicle Anatomy and the Hair Cycle

The human scalp contains approximately 100,000 to 150,000 terminal hair follicles, each cycling independently through three principal phases. Anagen (the active growth phase) lasts 2 to 6 years on the scalp and determines final hair length — approximately 85 to 90 percent of scalp follicles are in anagen at any given time, growing at a rate of 0.3 to 0.4 mm per day. Catagen (the regression phase) is a brief transitional period lasting 2 to 3 weeks during which the lower follicle undergoes apoptosis-driven involution: the hair matrix ceases proliferating, the inner root sheath disintegrates, and the dermal papilla condenses and migrates upward. Telogen (the resting phase) lasts 2 to 3 months on the scalp; the follicle is quiescent, and the hair shaft (now a club hair with a white, bulb-shaped root) is retained loosely in the follicular canal. Exogen is the active shedding phase during which the club hair is released — normal shedding of 50 to 100 hairs per day reflects the orderly asynchronous cycling of individual follicles. The dermal papilla — a cluster of specialized mesenchymal cells at the base of the follicle — is the master regulator of the hair cycle, providing instructive signals (Wnt, BMP, FGF, Shh) to the hair matrix stem cells in the bulge region that drive regeneration at each new anagen.

Molecular Regulation and Hair Shaft Structure

The transition between hair cycle phases is governed by opposing signaling gradients. Anagen initiation requires activation of the Wnt/beta-catenin pathway and suppression of BMP signaling in the bulge stem cell niche — Wnt ligands from the dermal papilla activate follicular stem cells to proliferate and differentiate into the new hair shaft. Catagen is triggered by apoptotic signals (FGF5, TGF-beta, neurotrophins) that overcome the pro-growth environment. Telogen maintenance involves elevated BMP4 and BMP2 from the dermal papilla that keep bulge stem cells quiescent until the next anagen signal. Androgens modulate hair growth in a site-specific manner: dihydrotestosterone (DHT, converted from testosterone by 5-alpha-reductase type II in the dermal papilla) promotes terminal hair growth on the face (beard) and body but paradoxically induces follicular miniaturization on the scalp — the molecular basis of androgenetic alopecia. The hair shaft itself is composed of a medulla (central core, variably present), cortex (the bulk of the shaft, containing melanin and keratin intermediate filaments organized into macrofibrils), and cuticle (a protective layer of overlapping, scale-like cells). Hair shaft abnormalities — fractures, nodes, twists, or irregularities in the shaft diameter — produce the structural hair shaft disorders (trichorrhexis nodosa, monilethrix, pili torti, trichothiodystrophy) that present with brittle, easily fractured hair.

Non-Scarring Alopecias: Androgenetic Alopecia, Alopecia Areata, Telogen Effluvium, and Traction Alopecia

Androgenetic Alopecia

Androgenetic alopecia (AGA) is the most common cause of hair loss, affecting approximately 50 percent of men and 40 percent of women by age 50. In men, AGA follows the Hamilton-Norwood pattern: progressive bitemporal recession of the frontal hairline, thinning of the vertex, and eventual confluence of frontotemporal and vertex thinning, sparing the occipital and temporal fringes (where follicles lack androgen sensitivity). In women, AGA follows the Ludwig pattern: diffuse thinning over the crown with preservation of the frontal hairline — the part width widens progressively. The pathophysiology centers on follicular miniaturization: DHT binds to androgen receptors in the dermal papilla of genetically susceptible follicles, triggering a progressive shortening of anagen duration and reduction of the follicle size, converting terminal hairs (thick, pigmented) to vellus-like hairs (thin, unpigmented, short). The genetic susceptibility is polygenic, with the androgen receptor gene (AR, on the X chromosome) and other loci contributing to risk. Trichoscopy of AGA shows hair diameter diversity (the hallmark — a mix of thick and thin hairs in the same field, reflecting follicular miniaturization), peripilar sign (perifollicular brown halo, more prominent in early AGA), yellow dots (representing empty or sebum-filled follicular ostia), and a honeycomb pigment pattern of the scalp.

Alopecia Areata

Alopecia areata (AA) is an autoimmune, non-scarring alopecia characterized by sudden onset of well-circumscribed, smooth, round to oval patches of complete hair loss — without scarring, scaling, or follicular destruction. AA affects approximately 2 percent of the population over a lifetime, with peak onset in childhood and young adulthood. The pathogenesis involves collapse of the hair follicle's immune privilege: autoreactive CD8+ NKG2D+ T-lymphocytes attack the anagen hair bulb, causing premature catagen entry and hair shedding. The immune attack targets the hair matrix but does not destroy the follicular stem cells in the bulge, which is why regrowth potential is preserved — unlike scarring alopecias. Clinical variants include patchy AA (the most common — one or more discrete patches), alopecia totalis (complete loss of scalp hair), alopecia universalis (complete loss of all body hair), ophiasis pattern (band-like loss along the temporal and occipital scalp margins — a poor prognostic pattern), and diffuse AA (acute, diffuse thinning mimicking telogen effluvium). Exclamation point hairs (short, broken hairs that taper toward the proximal end, resembling !) are a pathognomonic clinical finding at the margins of active patches. Trichoscopy shows yellow dots, black dots (cadaverized hairs — broken hair shafts retained at the scalp surface), short vellus hairs, and exclamation point hairs. Nail involvement (fine pitting — the 'hammered brass' appearance — ridging, and trachyonychia) occurs in 10 to 20 percent of patients and can precede or accompany the alopecia.

Telogen Effluvium and Traction Alopecia

Telogen effluvium (TE) is a diffuse, non-scarring hair shedding caused by premature synchronized entry of anagen follicles into telogen, resulting in excessive daily hair loss (typically 150 to 400 hairs per day, compared to the normal 50 to 100). TE is triggered 2 to 3 months after a physiologic stressor — the latency reflects the duration of the telogen phase. Common triggers include childbirth (postpartum TE — the most common cause in young women), high fever, major surgery, severe illness, crash dieting or nutritional deficiency (iron, zinc, biotin, vitamin D), emotional stress, and medication initiation or discontinuation (anticoagulants, retinoids, beta-blockers, antidepressants). TE is self-limiting once the trigger resolves — regrowth begins within 3 to 6 months. Chronic TE (persisting beyond 6 months) exists and may represent ongoing low-grade triggering or a distinct entity with fluctuating shedding over years. Traction alopecia results from chronic, sustained tension on the hair follicle from tight hairstyles — braids, cornrows, weaves, ponytails, hair extensions, and chemical relaxers. The frontal and temporal hairlines and the areas of maximum tension are most affected. Early traction alopecia is reversible (hair regrows when the traction is eliminated), but prolonged traction produces irreversible follicular destruction and scarring — the fringe sign (retention of short, fine hairs along the frontal hairline where traction is least) is a characteristic clinical finding. Traction alopecia disproportionately affects Black women due to cultural hair care practices.

CLINICAL PEARL: The hair pull test is a simple bedside test for active hair shedding: grasp approximately 40 to 60 hairs between the thumb and forefinger near the scalp, then apply gentle traction from root to tip. A positive test (6 or more club hairs extracted) indicates active shedding and is typically positive in acute telogen effluvium and active alopecia areata. The test should be performed in multiple scalp regions. A negative pull test does not exclude hair loss — it simply means that shedding is not currently active. In androgenetic alopecia, the pull test is typically negative because the process is one of miniaturization rather than shedding.

Hair Shaft Disorders and Special Populations

Structural hair shaft disorders present with brittle, fragile hair that fractures easily, often without significant hair loss from the follicle itself. Trichorrhexis nodosa — the most common hair shaft abnormality — presents as white nodules along the hair shaft representing focal points of cortical cell fracture; it is usually acquired (caused by chemical treatments, heat styling, and mechanical trauma) but can be congenital (in citrullinemia and argininosuccinic aciduria). Trichorrhexis invaginata (bamboo hair) is pathognomonic for Netherton syndrome (an autosomal recessive ichthyosis caused by SPINK5 mutations), presenting as ball-and-socket invaginations of the hair shaft visible on light microscopy. Monilethrix (beaded hair) is caused by keratin gene mutations (KRT81, KRT83, KRT86) and presents with regular, periodic narrowing of the hair shaft producing a beaded appearance and hair breakage at the narrow points. Pregnancy-related hair changes are common and physiologic: during pregnancy, the proportion of anagen hairs increases (resulting in thicker, fuller hair), while postpartum, the synchronized re-entry of these follicles into telogen produces the dramatic shedding of postpartum telogen effluvium — typically 2 to 4 months after delivery, resolving spontaneously over 6 to 12 months. In children, the differential diagnosis of alopecia is weighted differently from adults: tinea capitis is the most common cause of patchy alopecia in prepubescent children (and must be excluded before diagnosing alopecia areata), while trichotillomania (compulsive hair pulling) produces irregular patches with broken hairs of varying lengths and should be considered in school-age children with focal alopecia and behavioral concerns.

CAUTION: Finasteride and dutasteride are absolutely contraindicated in women who are or may become pregnant — these 5-alpha-reductase inhibitors are FDA category X teratogens that can cause feminization of the external genitalia in male fetuses. Finasteride is absorbed through the skin, so pregnant women should not handle crushed or broken tablets. Reliable contraception must be established before prescribing finasteride or dutasteride to women of childbearing potential. Spironolactone, while not FDA-approved for alopecia, is also teratogenic (anti-androgenic effects on the developing fetus) and requires reliable contraception. When prescribing any anti-androgen for hair loss in premenopausal women, pregnancy prevention counseling and documentation are mandatory.

Clinical Case: The Receding Hairline

A 62-year-old postmenopausal woman presents with progressive recession of her frontal hairline over the past 3 years. She reports that her eyebrows have also thinned significantly, and she has noticed small bumps on her forehead. She has no history of tight hairstyles, chemical relaxers, or hair extensions. She has no personal or family history of autoimmune disease. On examination, the frontal hairline has receded symmetrically by approximately 3 cm. The band of alopecia behind the receding hairline is smooth, pale, and devoid of follicular ostia. Several isolated terminal hairs remain within the alopecic band (lonely hair sign). The lateral eyebrows are absent bilaterally. Small, flesh-colored, non-tender papules are present on the forehead and temples.

Trichoscopy of the hairline margin reveals perifollicular scaling (tubular casts around the proximal hair shafts), perifollicular erythema, and absence of follicular ostia behind the active margin. There is no poikiloderma, adherent scale, or carpet-tack sign to suggest DLE. The clinical and trichoscopic features — symmetric band-like hairline recession, eyebrow loss, facial papules, perifollicular scaling, and loss of ostia — are diagnostic of frontal fibrosing alopecia. Punch biopsy confirms a lichenoid lymphocytic infiltrate targeting the follicular isthmus and infundibulum with perifollicular lamellar fibrosis, consistent with LPP-pattern scarring alopecia. Treatment is initiated with topical clobetasol to the active hairline margin and oral hydroxychloroquine as systemic anti-inflammatory therapy to halt progression. The patient is counseled that the scarred, hair-free area will not regrow, but treatment aims to stabilize the hairline and prevent further recession. This case illustrates the importance of recognizing FFA as a distinct entity from age-related hairline thinning, and the role of eyebrow loss and facial papules as early diagnostic clues.

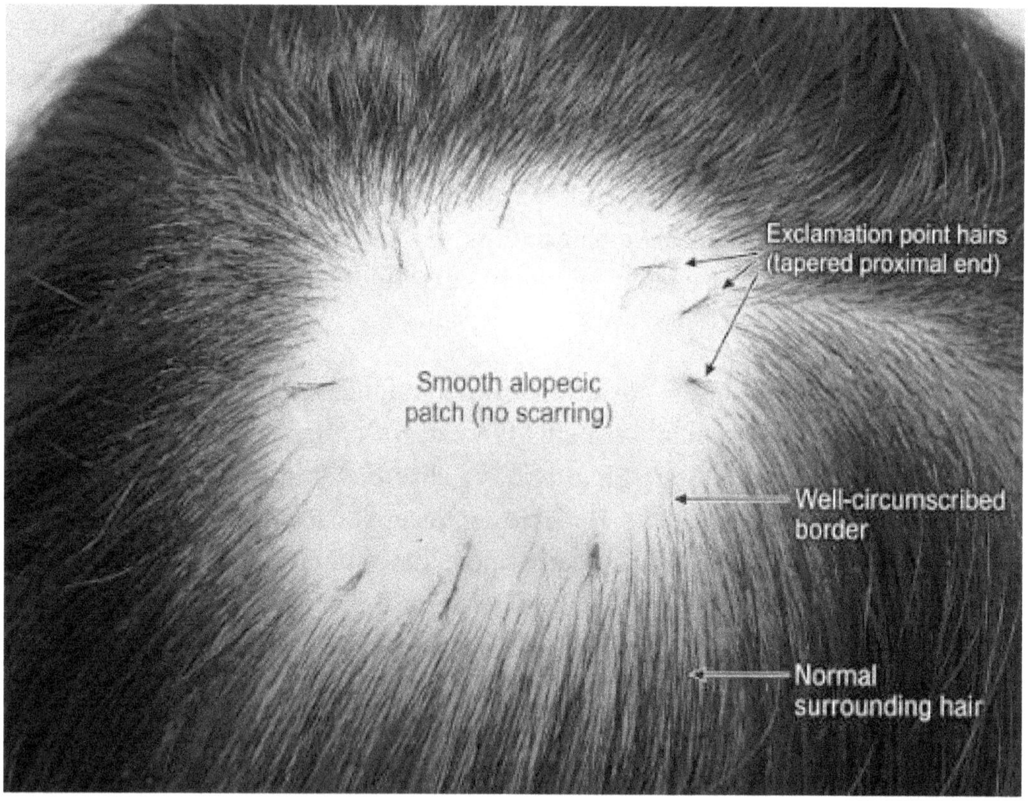

THE CUTANEOUS MIMICKER RECOGNITION ATLAS — Alopecia Areata versus Tinea Capitis

The Clinical Pattern: Alopecia areata presents as one or more well-circumscribed, smooth, round to oval patches of complete hair loss on the scalp, without scarring, scaling, or erythema. The patches appear suddenly and may expand over weeks. Exclamation point hairs at the margins and a positive hair pull test at the border indicate active disease. The scalp surface within the patch is entirely normal — smooth, supple, and free of inflammation.

The Mimicker: Tinea capitis produces patches of hair loss on the scalp that can closely mimic alopecia areata, particularly the non-inflammatory (grey patch) variant. However, tinea capitis produces scaling within the alopecic patch — fine, grey-white scale or more obvious annular scaling — and the hair within the patch is broken at the scalp surface (black dot pattern) rather than absent. Tinea capitis is a fungal infection that primarily affects children (rare in adults) and may be accompanied by occipital or posterior cervical lymphadenopathy.

Trap Logic: Diagnosing alopecia areata in a child without examining for scale or performing a fungal culture is the cognitive trap — tinea capitis is far more common than alopecia areata in prepubescent children, and misdiagnosis leads to months of unnecessary immunosuppressive treatment (topical or intralesional corticosteroids) while the fungal infection spreads. The reverse trap — treating every patchy alopecia as tinea — delays appropriate immunomodulatory therapy in true AA.

The Decision Anchor: The discriminating features are **scalp surface within the patch (smooth and scale-free in AA; scaling in tinea capitis), hair shaft appearance (exclamation point hairs in AA; broken hair shafts at the scalp surface producing black dots in tinea), patient age (tinea capitis primarily affects children aged 3 to 12; AA can occur at any age but does not have the same pediatric predominance as tinea), lymphadenopathy (occipital and cervical nodes favor tinea), and trichoscopy (comma hairs and corkscrew hairs are pathognomonic for tinea; exclamation point hairs and yellow dots favor AA)**. KOH preparation and fungal culture should be performed on any patchy alopecia with scaling, particularly in children.

Scarring (Cicatricial) Alopecias: Lichen Planopilaris, Frontal Fibrosing Alopecia, Central Centrifugal Cicatricial Alopecia, and Discoid Lupus

Classification and General Principles

Scarring (cicatricial) alopecias are a group of disorders characterized by permanent destruction of the hair follicle and its replacement by fibrous tissue — resulting in irreversible hair loss. The North American Hair Research Society classifies scarring alopecias by the predominant inflammatory infiltrate on histopathology: lymphocytic (lichen planopilaris, frontal fibrosing alopecia, CCCA, discoid lupus erythematosus, pseudopelade of Brocq), neutrophilic (dissecting cellulitis of the scalp, folliculitis decalvans), or mixed (folliculitis keloidalis nuchae, erosive pustular dermatosis). The clinical hallmark of scarring alopecia — and what distinguishes it from non-scarring forms — is the loss of follicular ostia: on close examination (or trichoscopy), the normal follicular openings are absent within the scarred area, replaced by smooth, atrophic, fibrotic skin. Because the follicular stem cells in the bulge region are destroyed, scarring alopecias are irreversible — treatment aims to halt disease progression and prevent further follicular destruction, not to regrow hair in already-scarred areas.

Lichen Planopilaris and Frontal Fibrosing Alopecia

Lichen planopilaris (LPP) is the most common primary lymphocytic scarring alopecia. It represents follicular lichen planus — a T-cell-mediated attack on the follicular epithelium, particularly targeting the bulge stem cells. LPP presents as multifocal patches of scarring alopecia on the vertex and parietal scalp, with perifollicular erythema and scale (follicular hyperkeratosis) at the active margins — the zone where inflammation is actively destroying follicles. Patients report scalp tenderness, burning, and pruritus. Trichoscopy at the active border shows perifollicular scaling (tubular casts around the hair shaft), perifollicular erythema, and loss of follicular ostia in the scarred center. Histopathology shows a lichenoid lymphocytic infiltrate targeting the isthmus and infundibulum of the hair follicle, with destruction of the outer root sheath and perifollicular lamellar fibrosis. Frontal fibrosing alopecia (FFA) is a clinical variant of LPP presenting as progressive recession of the frontal and temporal hairline in a band-like pattern, predominantly in postmenopausal women (though increasingly recognized in premenopausal women and men). FFA often affects the eyebrows (loss of the lateral eyebrows or complete eyebrow alopecia) before or concurrent with hairline recession — eyebrow loss is an important early diagnostic clue. The lonely hair sign (isolated hairs remaining in the frontal band of alopecia) and facial papules (small, flesh-colored papules on the temples and forehead representing affected vellus follicles) are characteristic features.

Central Centrifugal Cicatricial Alopecia and Discoid Lupus

Central centrifugal cicatricial alopecia (CCCA) is the most common scarring alopecia in Black women. It begins at the crown or vertex and expands centrifugally, producing a symmetric, oval area of scarring alopecia on the central scalp. The pathogenesis involves premature desquamation of the inner root sheath (PDIR — a characteristic histopathologic finding) with subsequent follicular destruction and fibrosis. Genetic susceptibility has been linked to mutations in PADI3 (peptidylarginine deiminase 3), an enzyme involved in inner root sheath formation. Hair care practices (chemical relaxers, high-heat styling, tight braiding) may exacerbate the condition but are not considered the primary cause — CCCA occurs in women who have never used chemical relaxers. Trichoscopy shows a reduction in follicular density on the central scalp, broken hairs, grey-white perifollicular halos, and the absence of follicular ostia in scarred areas. Discoid lupus erythematosus (DLE) of the scalp produces well-demarcated, erythematous, atrophic plaques with adherent follicular plugging (carpet-tack sign — keratotic plugs that produce a tack-like pattern when a removed scale is examined), dyspigmentation (central hypopigmentation with peripheral hyperpigmentation, particularly prominent in skin of color), and scarring alopecia with loss of follicular ostia. DLE of the scalp may occur in isolation (cutaneous lupus limited to the scalp) or as part of systemic lupus erythematosus — ANA and lupus band test (direct immunofluorescence) should be performed to assess for systemic disease.

Hirsutism and Hypertrichosis: Evaluation, Hormonal Workup, and Management

Definition and Differential Diagnosis

Hirsutism is the presence of terminal (coarse, pigmented) hair growth in women in a male-pattern distribution — face (upper lip, chin, sideburns), chest, abdomen (midline), back, and inner thighs — resulting from excess androgen activity at the hair follicle. It is distinct from hypertrichosis, which is a generalized or localized increase in hair growth that is not androgen-dependent and does not follow a male-pattern distribution. Hirsutism is assessed using the modified Ferriman-Gallwey score, which grades hair density at 9 body sites (upper lip, chin, chest, upper abdomen, lower abdomen, upper arms, thighs, upper back, lower back) on a 0 to 4 scale — a total score of 8 or more defines hirsutism in most populations (though ethnically adjusted thresholds exist, as baseline hair density varies among populations). Polycystic ovary syndrome (PCOS) is the cause in 70 to 80 percent of hirsute women, followed by idiopathic hirsutism (normal androgens with increased peripheral 5-alpha-reductase activity or androgen receptor sensitivity), non-classic congenital adrenal hyperplasia (21-hydroxylase deficiency), Cushing syndrome, and androgen-secreting tumors of the ovary or adrenal gland.

Hormonal Workup and Evaluation

The hormonal workup for hirsutism aims to identify the androgen source and exclude serious underlying pathology. Initial laboratory evaluation includes total and free testosterone (elevated in PCOS, ovarian tumors, and adrenal tumors), dehydroepiandrosterone sulfate (DHEA-S — elevated in adrenal sources), 17-hydroxyprogesterone (elevated in non-classic congenital adrenal hyperplasia — an early-morning follicular-phase level above a threshold value warrants ACTH stimulation testing), prolactin, thyroid function, and fasting glucose or HbA1c (insulin resistance is common in PCOS). Clinical red flags for an androgen-secreting tumor include rapid onset of virilization (deepening voice, clitoromegaly, male-pattern balding, increased muscle mass), markedly elevated testosterone (typically greater than 200 ng/dL), and onset in a patient with no prior history of hirsutism. Pelvic ultrasound evaluates ovarian morphology (polycystic ovaries: 12 or more follicles 2 to 9 mm in diameter and/or ovarian volume greater than 10 mL). CT or MRI of the adrenal glands is indicated when DHEA-S is markedly elevated or when an adrenal tumor is suspected clinically.

Management of Hirsutism

Management of hirsutism combines cosmetic hair removal with pharmacotherapy directed at the androgen pathway. Topical eflornithine (an ornithine decarboxylase inhibitor) reduces facial hair growth by inhibiting a key enzyme in hair follicle cell proliferation — it slows growth but does not remove existing hair, so it is used in combination with mechanical removal methods. Combined oral contraceptives (containing an anti-androgenic progestin — drospirenone, cyproterone acetate, chlormadinone) are first-line systemic therapy for hirsutism in premenopausal women; they suppress ovarian androgen production and increase sex hormone-binding globulin (SHBG), thereby reducing free testosterone. Spironolactone (an aldosterone antagonist with anti-androgenic properties — it blocks the androgen receptor and inhibits 5-alpha-reductase) is the most commonly prescribed anti-androgen in the United States for hirsutism and is used at doses that require reliable contraception due to teratogenicity risk. Finasteride (a 5-alpha-reductase type II inhibitor) reduces DHT levels and is effective for hirsutism, though it also requires contraception. Hypertrichosis — non-androgen-dependent excessive hair growth — is most commonly drug-induced (cyclosporine, minoxidil, diazoxide, phenytoin) and resolves with discontinuation of the causative medication. Congenital hypertrichosis syndromes are rare and may be associated with genetic conditions.

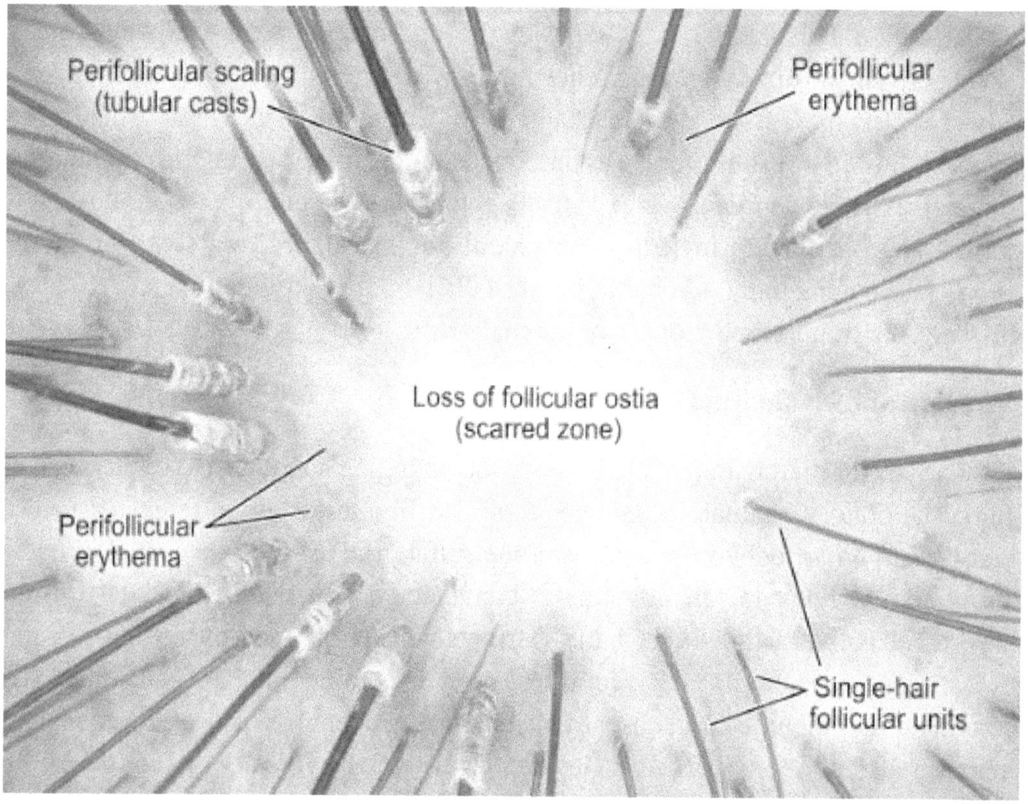

Trichoscopy: Diagnostic Patterns and Clinical Application

Trichoscopic Features of Common Alopecias

Trichoscopy (dermoscopy of the scalp and hair) has become an indispensable diagnostic tool for hair disorders, allowing non-invasive evaluation of the follicular ostia, hair shaft morphology, perifollicular signs, and scalp surface features. Each major alopecia has a characteristic trichoscopic signature. AGA shows hair diameter diversity (the hallmark — thick and thin hairs in the same field reflecting miniaturization), yellow dots, and the peripilar sign (a brown perifollicular halo representing perifollicular inflammation). AA shows yellow dots (empty follicles filled with sebum and keratinous material), black dots (cadaverized hairs — fractured hair shafts retained at the follicular opening), exclamation point hairs (short, distally thick hairs tapering toward the proximal end), and short regrowing vellus hairs (a sign of recovery). LPP/FFA shows perifollicular scaling (tubular casts), perifollicular erythema, loss of follicular ostia in scarred areas, and single-hair follicular units replacing the normal compound units. CCCA shows grey-white perifollicular halos, broken hairs, and progressive loss of follicular density on the central scalp. DLE shows large, yellow-brown dots (follicular keratotic plugs), thick arborizing vessels, and areas of blue-grey pigmentation (melanin in the dermis). Tinea capitis shows comma hairs (short, comma-shaped broken hairs), corkscrew hairs, and zigzag hairs — pathognomonic findings that distinguish fungal alopecia from other causes.

Clinical Decision-Making With Trichoscopy

Trichoscopy guides the clinical decision between observation, medical therapy, and biopsy. In non-scarring alopecias, trichoscopy can often confirm the diagnosis without biopsy: the combination of hair diameter diversity, yellow dots, and peripilar sign in a female patient with diffuse crown thinning is diagnostic of AGA without histopathologic confirmation. In scarring alopecias, trichoscopy identifies the active border (where inflammation is present and treatment should be directed) and monitors treatment response — reduction of perifollicular scaling and erythema indicates effective inflammation control. Trichoscopy also determines when biopsy is most informative: in scarring alopecia, biopsy should target the active, inflamed margin (where diagnostic histopathologic features are present), not the scarred center (which shows only end-stage fibrosis regardless of etiology). Serial trichoscopic photography enables objective monitoring of disease progression and treatment response over time — particularly valuable in slowly progressive conditions like FFA where clinical change may be difficult to appreciate.

Evidence-Based Management: Pharmacotherapy, Procedural Interventions, and Emerging Therapies

Medical Management of Androgenetic Alopecia

The two FDA-approved treatments for AGA are topical minoxidil and oral finasteride. Topical minoxidil (2 percent for women, 5 percent for men — applied twice daily) is a potassium channel opener that prolongs anagen, increases follicular size, and enhances perifollicular vascularity. Response is gradual (3 to 6 months for initial improvement, 12 months for maximum effect), and the effect is maintenance-dependent — hair loss resumes within 3 to 6 months of discontinuation. Oral minoxidil at low doses is increasingly used off-label for AGA, with doses typically ranging from 0.625 to 5 mg daily, and shows efficacy comparable or superior to topical formulations with improved adherence. Finasteride (1 mg daily for men) is a 5-alpha-reductase type II inhibitor that reduces scalp DHT levels by approximately 60 to 70 percent and produces meaningful hair regrowth or stabilization in 80 to 90 percent of men. Sexual side effects (decreased libido, erectile dysfunction) occur in 1 to 2 percent and are reversible in the vast majority upon discontinuation. Dutasteride (a dual 5-alpha-reductase type I and II inhibitor) is used off-label and may be more effective than finasteride but carries a similar side-effect profile. Spironolactone is the most commonly used anti-androgen for female AGA.

Treatment of Alopecia Areata

Treatment of AA is tailored to disease extent and patient age. For limited patchy AA, intralesional triamcinolone acetonide injections (concentration typically at a level confirmed per institutional protocol, injected into the dermis at 1 cm intervals) are first-line — response rates of 60 to 80 percent for limited patches. Topical immunotherapy with diphenylcyclopropenone (DPCP) or squaric acid dibutylester (SADBE) induces allergic contact dermatitis on the scalp, which is thought to redirect the immune attack away from the hair follicle — this is a second-line option for extensive AA, alopecia totalis, or alopecia universalis, with response rates of 30 to 50 percent. The JAK inhibitor revolution has transformed the treatment of moderate-to-severe AA: baricitinib (JAK1/JAK2 inhibitor) became the first FDA-approved systemic therapy for severe AA in adults, based on the BRAVE-AA1 and BRAVE-AA2 trials demonstrating clinically meaningful hair regrowth in 35 to 40 percent of patients at 36 weeks. Ritlecitinib (JAK3/TEC inhibitor) was subsequently approved. The mechanism of action is direct: JAK inhibitors block the IFN-gamma signaling that drives the CD8+ T-cell attack on the hair follicle. Response is dose-dependent and maintenance-dependent — hair loss typically recurs within months of discontinuation.

Management of Scarring Alopecias and Procedural Interventions

Treatment of scarring alopecias aims to halt progression — scarred follicles cannot be regenerated. LPP/FFA is treated with anti-inflammatory therapy: topical or intralesional corticosteroids for localized disease, hydroxychloroquine or doxycycline as first-line systemic therapy for progressive disease, and oral cyclosporine, mycophenolate mofetil, or methotrexate for refractory cases. CCCA management emphasizes gentle hair care practices (avoidance of chemical relaxers, high heat, and tight styling), topical and intralesional corticosteroids, and oral doxycycline or hydroxychloroquine for active disease. DLE of the scalp responds to potent topical corticosteroids, topical calcineurin inhibitors, and hydroxychloroquine — systemic immunosuppression is reserved for refractory cases. Hair transplantation is an option for stable scarring alopecias that have been quiescent for at least 1 to 2 years without evidence of active inflammation — transplanted follicles may be attacked by the same inflammatory process if disease is not adequately controlled. Platelet-rich plasma (PRP) injections are used as an adjunctive treatment for AGA and AA, with some evidence of benefit in increasing hair density, though standardization of preparation protocols and injection techniques remains an area of active research.

Alopecia Type	Pattern	Trichoscopy	Scarring	First-Line Treatment
AGA	Bitemporal/vertex (men); diffuse crown (women)	Hair diameter diversity, yellow dots, peripilar sign	No	Minoxidil, finasteride (men), spironolactone (women)
Alopecia areata	Well-circumscribed smooth patches	Yellow dots, black dots,	No	Intralesional corticosteroids;

		exclamation point hairs		JAK inhibitors for severe
Telogen effluvium	Diffuse shedding 2–3 months after trigger	Reduced density, no miniaturization, positive pull test	No	Remove trigger; self-limiting
LPP/FFA	Multifocal (LPP); band-like hairline recession (FFA)	Perifollicular scaling, perifollicular erythema, loss of ostia	Yes	Topical/intralesional steroids, hydroxychloroquine
CCCA	Central scalp, centrifugal expansion	Grey-white perifollicular halos, broken hairs	Yes	Gentle hair care, topical steroids, doxycycline

THE CUTANEOUS MIMICKER RECOGNITION ATLAS — Frontal Fibrosing Alopecia versus Traction Alopecia

The Clinical Pattern: Frontal fibrosing alopecia presents as progressive, symmetric, band-like recession of the frontal and temporal hairline in postmenopausal women (increasingly recognized in younger women and men). The hairline margin shows perifollicular erythema and scaling on trichoscopy, and the skin behind the receding hairline is smooth, pale, and devoid of follicular ostia — indicating scarring. Eyebrow loss (lateral or complete) often accompanies or precedes the scalp alopecia and is an important diagnostic clue. The lonely hair sign — scattered isolated terminal hairs remaining in the band of alopecia — is characteristic.

The Mimicker: Traction alopecia also produces frontal and temporal hairline recession and is common in women who wear tight braids, cornrows, weaves, or ponytails. The pattern of hair loss follows the areas of maximum tension — typically the frontotemporal hairline and the margins around braids or part lines. The fringe sign (retention of short, fine, vellus-like hairs along the frontal hairline) is characteristic of traction alopecia. In early traction alopecia, follicular ostia are preserved and the process is potentially reversible. Late traction alopecia produces follicular destruction and scarring.

Trap Logic: Attributing frontal hairline recession in a Black woman exclusively to traction alopecia without examining for perifollicular inflammation or eyebrow loss is the cognitive trap. FFA and traction alopecia coexist in the same patient populations (postmenopausal women, women of color), and FFA can be superimposed on traction alopecia. Trichoscopy is the discriminator: perifollicular scaling and erythema with loss of follicular ostia indicate FFA (a scarring, inflammatory process that needs immunosuppressive treatment), while retention of follicular ostia with perifollicular miniaturization indicates traction alopecia (managed by eliminating the traction).

The Decision Anchor: The discriminating features are **trichoscopy at the hairline margin (perifollicular scaling and erythema with loss of ostia indicate FFA; preserved ostia with miniaturization indicate traction), eyebrow involvement (eyebrow loss strongly favors FFA — traction alopecia does not affect the eyebrows), relationship to hairstyle (clear correlation with tight styling favors traction; progression despite style changes favors FFA), and facial papules (small flesh-colored papules on the forehead and temples favor FFA)**. Biopsy the active hairline margin when clinical and trichoscopic findings are ambiguous.

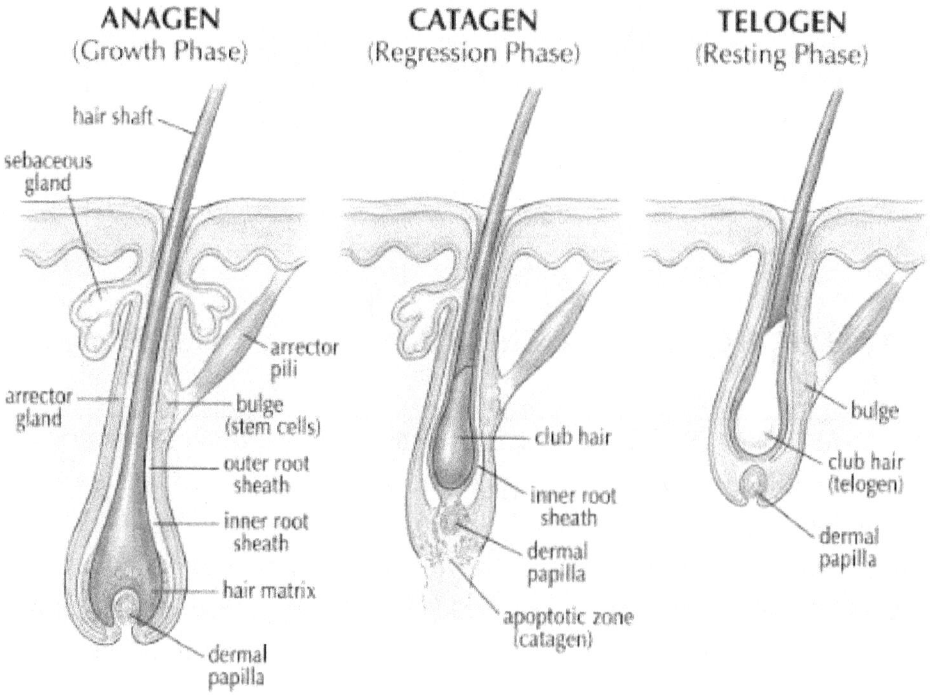

EVIDENCE: The BRAVE-AA1 and BRAVE-AA2 trials established baricitinib as the first FDA-approved systemic therapy for severe alopecia areata. In BRAVE-AA1, 35 percent of patients receiving baricitinib 4 mg achieved a Severity of Alopecia Tool (SALT) score of 20 or less (80 percent or more scalp coverage) at 36 weeks, compared to 5 percent with placebo. Ritlecitinib (JAK3/TEC inhibitor) was subsequently approved based on the ALLEGRO-2b/3 trial, demonstrating significant hair regrowth in patients with 50 percent or more scalp hair loss. These approvals represent a paradigm shift from off-label immunosuppression to targeted JAK inhibition for moderate-to-severe AA, though the maintenance-dependent nature of the response (hair loss recurs after discontinuation) and the need for long-term safety monitoring remain important considerations.

KEY POINT: The distinction between scarring and non-scarring alopecia is the single most important initial classification step, because it determines urgency and reversibility. Scarring alopecias destroy follicular stem cells permanently — early, aggressive anti-inflammatory treatment is essential to halt progression and preserve remaining follicles. Non-scarring alopecias preserve the follicular apparatus and are potentially reversible. The clinical clue is the presence or absence of follicular ostia on close inspection or trichoscopy: visible ostia indicate non-scarring; absent ostia within the alopecic area indicate scarring.

THE CUTANEOUS MIMICKER RECOGNITION ATLAS — Hair Disorder Diagnostic Arcs

Alopecia Areata vs. Tinea Capitis: The discriminating features are scalp surface (smooth and scale-free in AA; scaling in tinea), hair shaft appearance (exclamation point hairs in AA; comma and corkscrew hairs in tinea), patient age (tinea primarily affects children 3 to 12), lymphadenopathy (occipital nodes favor tinea), and trichoscopy (yellow and black dots in AA; comma and corkscrew hairs pathognomonic for tinea). Cognitive trap: diagnosing AA in a child without performing KOH and fungal culture to exclude tinea capitis, which is far more common in this age group.

FFA vs. Traction Alopecia: The discriminating features are trichoscopy at the hairline margin (perifollicular scaling and erythema with loss of ostia in FFA; preserved ostia with miniaturization in traction), eyebrow involvement (eyebrow loss strongly favors FFA), relationship to hairstyle (correlation with tight styling favors traction; progression despite style changes favors FFA), and facial papules (favor FFA). Cognitive trap: attributing hairline recession in a Black woman to traction without examining for perifollicular inflammation, especially since FFA and traction alopecia can coexist.

Summary and Key Concepts

The hair cycle (anagen, catagen, telogen, exogen) is independently regulated by each follicle through Wnt/beta-catenin (anagen initiation), BMP (telogen maintenance), and androgen (site-specific follicular miniaturization) signaling. Disruption at each phase produces distinct clinical patterns: shortened anagen causes AGA, premature telogen entry causes telogen effluvium, and immune-mediated catagen entry causes alopecia areata.

Androgenetic alopecia is caused by DHT-driven follicular miniaturization in genetically susceptible follicles, producing hair diameter diversity on trichoscopy. FDA-approved treatments include topical minoxidil and oral finasteride (men). Low-dose oral minoxidil is increasingly used off-label with efficacy comparable to topical formulations.

Alopecia areata is an autoimmune, CD8+ T-cell-mediated attack on the anagen hair bulb. JAK inhibitors (baricitinib, ritlecitinib) are now FDA-approved for severe AA, producing clinically meaningful regrowth in 35 to 40 percent of patients — a paradigm shift from off-label immunosuppression to targeted therapy.

Scarring alopecias (LPP, FFA, CCCA, DLE) permanently destroy follicular stem cells, making early anti-inflammatory treatment urgent. The key diagnostic step is the presence or absence of follicular ostia on trichoscopy. FFA (band-like hairline recession with eyebrow loss in postmenopausal women) must be distinguished from traction alopecia (hairstyle-related, preserved ostia).

Hirsutism in women is assessed by the modified Ferriman-Gallwey score and is caused by PCOS in 70 to 80 percent of cases. Hormonal workup (total/free testosterone, DHEA-S, 17-hydroxyprogesterone) identifies the androgen source. Management combines oral contraceptives, spironolactone, and procedural hair removal.

CHAPTER 18: NAIL DISORDERS

Learning Objectives

1. Describe the anatomy of the nail unit — matrix, nail bed, nail plate, nail folds, and hyponychium — and explain how the site of pathology within the nail unit determines the clinical pattern of nail disease.
2. Classify onychomycosis by clinical subtype (DLSO, WSO, PSO, TDO), select the appropriate diagnostic test (KOH, PAS, culture, PCR), and apply evidence-based treatment algorithms integrating topical, oral, and device-based therapies.
3. Evaluate longitudinal melanonychia systematically using the ABCDEF rule and dermoscopy, identify features that warrant nail matrix biopsy, and distinguish subungual melanoma from benign causes of nail pigmentation.
4. Recognize nail signs of systemic disease — clubbing, Beau lines, Muehrcke lines, Terry nails, splinter hemorrhages, and half-and-half nails — and correlate them with the underlying systemic conditions they indicate.

Nail Anatomy, Physiology, and Growth

Structural Anatomy of the Nail Unit

The nail unit is a specialized skin appendage composed of five anatomic components, each producing distinct clinical signs when diseased. The nail matrix — the germinative epithelium located beneath the proximal nail fold — is the source of the nail plate. The proximal matrix produces the dorsal (superficial) nail plate, while the distal matrix (visible as the lunula — the white, half-moon-shaped area at the nail base) produces the ventral (deep) nail plate. Disease of the proximal matrix produces surface abnormalities (pitting, ridging, roughness — as in nail psoriasis and nail alopecia areata), while disease of the distal matrix produces ventral nail plate abnormalities (thinning, onycholysis). The nail bed is the epithelium underlying and adherent to the ventral nail plate; it does not contribute to nail plate formation but provides the pink color visible through the translucent plate. Nail bed disease causes onycholysis (separation of the nail plate from the bed), subungual hyperkeratosis, and splinter hemorrhages. The proximal nail fold is a curtain of skin that overlies the proximal matrix and creates the cuticle (eponychium) — its seal prevents entry of moisture, microorganisms, and irritants. Loss of the cuticle (from chronic trauma, manicuring, or inflammation) predisposes to chronic paronychia. The hyponychium is the seal at the distal free edge where the nail bed epithelium transitions to fingertip skin.

Nail Growth and Physiology

Fingernails grow at approximately 3 mm per month (0.1 mm per day), requiring 4 to 6 months for complete replacement from lunula to free edge. Toenails grow more slowly — approximately 1 to 1.5 mm per month — and require 12 to 18 months for complete replacement. This slow growth has direct therapeutic implications: any treatment for nail disease (oral antifungals, systemic immunosuppressives for nail psoriasis) requires months before clinical improvement is visible, and complete nail replacement may take over a year. Nail growth rate decreases with age, increases during pregnancy, and is affected by systemic disease (slowed in peripheral vascular disease, hypothyroidism, and severe illness). Beau lines — transverse depressions in the nail plate corresponding to a temporary arrest of matrix activity — provide a clinical timestamp: their distance from the proximal nail fold, divided by the nail growth rate, estimates the timing of the systemic insult that caused the growth arrest (fever, chemotherapy, severe illness).

Onychomycosis: Diagnosis, Classification, and Treatment

Epidemiology and Classification

Onychomycosis is the most common nail disorder, affecting approximately 10 to 12 percent of the general population and up to 50 percent of individuals over age 70. Toenails are affected 4 to 10 times more frequently than fingernails. Risk factors include aging, diabetes mellitus, peripheral vascular disease, immunosuppression, tinea pedis (which serves as the fungal reservoir), and communal bathing facilities. The causative organisms include dermatophytes (Trichophyton rubrum accounts for 70 to 80 percent of cases; T. mentagrophytes for 10 to 20 percent), non-dermatophyte molds (Scopulariopsis brevicaulis, Aspergillus, Fusarium — more common in tropical climates and in toenails), and yeasts (Candida — more common in fingernails, particularly in chronic paronychia). Clinical subtypes are classified by the route of invasion: distal and lateral subungual onychomycosis (DLSO — the most common, entering through the hyponychium and spreading proximally), white superficial onychomycosis (WSO — invasion of the dorsal nail plate surface, producing chalky white patches), proximal subungual onychomycosis (PSO — invasion through the proximal nail fold, spreading distally — rare in immunocompetent patients and a potential marker of HIV infection), and total dystrophic onychomycosis (TDO — complete destruction of the nail plate, representing advanced disease of any subtype).

Diagnostic Approach

Clinical diagnosis of onychomycosis is unreliable — up to 50 percent of dystrophic nails are not fungal, and empiric treatment without mycologic confirmation is inappropriate given the duration, cost, and potential hepatotoxicity of systemic antifungals. Mycologic confirmation is mandatory before initiating oral antifungal therapy. Diagnostic methods include KOH preparation (direct microscopy of nail clippings or subungual debris dissolved in 10 to 20 percent KOH — sensitivity of 60 to 80 percent; fast but operator-dependent), PAS staining of nail clippings (more sensitive than KOH, 82 to 95 percent — a histopathologic technique using periodic acid-Schiff stain to identify fungal hyphae within the nail plate), fungal culture on Sabouraud dextrose agar (the gold standard for identifying the causative organism and species — but slow, requiring 3 to 4 weeks, and less sensitive than PAS due to non-viable organisms in clippings), and PCR-based assays (rapid, highly sensitive and specific — increasingly available commercially, though cost remains higher than conventional methods).

Treatment Algorithms

Treatment selection depends on the extent and severity of involvement, the number of nails affected, the causative organism, and patient comorbidities. Oral terbinafine is the first-line systemic treatment for dermatophyte onychomycosis: a fungicidal allylamine dosed continuously for 6 weeks (fingernails) or 12 weeks (toenails), producing mycologic cure rates of 70 to 80 percent. Oral itraconazole (a triazole antifungal) is used as pulse therapy (one week per month for 2 to 3 months) and is preferred for Candida and non-dermatophyte mold infections for which terbinafine has less activity. Both agents require baseline hepatic function testing. Topical antifungals (efinaconazole 10 percent solution, tavaborole 5 percent solution, ciclopirox 8 percent lacquer) are appropriate for mild-to-moderate disease (DLSO involving less than 50 percent of the nail plate, without matrix involvement) or as adjunctive therapy to oral agents. Topical monotherapy cure rates are modest (15 to 35 percent complete cure). Mechanical debridement of the thickened, dystrophic nail plate improves antifungal penetration and accelerates clinical improvement. Laser therapy (Nd:YAG) is marketed for onychomycosis but evidence for mycologic cure is limited, and it is not recommended as monotherapy.

KEY POINT: Never treat dystrophic nails with oral antifungals without mycologic confirmation (KOH, PAS, culture, or PCR). Up to 50 percent of dystrophic nails are not fungal — nail psoriasis, lichen planus, traumatic dystrophy, and onychogryphosis are common non-fungal mimickers. Empiric oral antifungal treatment without diagnosis exposes the patient to months of unnecessary medication, potential drug interactions, and hepatotoxicity risk for a condition that requires a completely different treatment approach.

Nail Psoriasis: Clinical Features, Severity Scoring, and Therapeutic Approach

Clinical Features

Nail involvement occurs in approximately 50 percent of psoriasis patients and up to 80 percent of patients with psoriatic arthritis. Nail psoriasis may precede skin psoriasis by years and is strongly associated with distal interphalangeal (DIP) joint disease in psoriatic arthritis — a clinically important correlation (the nail matrix and DIP joint share an entheseal connection). Clinical signs of nail psoriasis are classified by the site of pathology within the nail unit. Matrix disease produces pitting (the hallmark — small, regular, ice-pick depressions in the nail plate surface caused by foci of parakeratosis in the proximal matrix that crumble and fall off as the nail grows), ridging, crumbling, and trachyonychia (rough, sandpaper-like nail surface — twenty-nail dystrophy). Nail bed disease produces oil drop sign (salmon patches — translucent, yellow-red discoloration visible through the nail plate, representing psoriatic foci in the nail bed), onycholysis (separation of the nail plate from the bed, often with an erythematous border), subungual hyperkeratosis (accumulation of scale beneath the nail plate, lifting it), and splinter hemorrhages (dilated capillaries in the nail bed that thrombose and appear as thin, longitudinal, red-brown lines).

Severity Scoring and Therapeutic Approach

The Nail Psoriasis Severity Index (NAPSI) provides standardized severity assessment: each nail is divided into quadrants, and each quadrant is scored for matrix features (0 to 3) and nail bed features (0 to 3) — total NAPSI for all 20 nails ranges from 0 to 120. NAPSI is used in clinical trials to measure treatment response but has limited use in routine clinical practice due to its time-intensive nature. Treatment of nail psoriasis is challenging due to the slow growth of the nail plate — even effective therapies require 6 to 12 months for visible improvement. Topical therapy (potent corticosteroids under occlusion, calcipotriol, tazarotene) is first-line for mild disease. Intralesional triamcinolone injections into the proximal nail fold (targeting the matrix) and nail bed are effective for individual nails but are painful and require local anesthesia. Systemic therapy (methotrexate, cyclosporine, acitretin) improves nail psoriasis as part of their effect on overall psoriasis disease burden. Biologic agents — particularly the IL-17 inhibitors (ixekizumab, secukinumab) and IL-23 inhibitors (guselkumab) — have demonstrated the strongest efficacy for nail psoriasis in clinical trials, with ixekizumab showing near-complete nail clearance (NAPSI score reduction of 80 to 90 percent) at 52 weeks.

Nail Lichen Planus, Nail Alopecia Areata, and Other Inflammatory Nail Diseases

Nail Lichen Planus

Nail lichen planus (NLP) is a potentially destructive inflammatory nail disease that targets the nail matrix and may cause permanent scarring with loss of the nail plate (anonychia). NLP presents with longitudinal ridging, thinning of the nail plate, fissuring, and — in severe cases — dorsal pterygium (a V-shaped scar of the proximal nail fold fusing to the nail bed, splitting the nail plate). Dorsal pterygium is highly suggestive of NLP but is not pathognomonic. Twenty-nail dystrophy (trachyonychia — all 20 nails are rough and sandpaper-like) may represent a forme fruste of NLP or an idiopathic condition in children. NLP requires early treatment to prevent irreversible matrix destruction: systemic corticosteroids or intralesional triamcinolone for active disease, transitioning to systemic immunosuppression (methotrexate, mycophenolate) for maintenance. Unlike nail psoriasis, NLP causes permanent nail loss if the matrix is destroyed — early, aggressive treatment is essential.

Nail Alopecia Areata and Other Inflammatory Conditions

Nail involvement in alopecia areata occurs in 10 to 20 percent of patients and can precede, accompany, or follow the scalp alopecia. The hallmark finding is geometric pitting — regular, grid-like, shallow pitting of the nail surface (described as a hammered brass appearance) caused by focal areas of parakeratosis in the proximal matrix. Unlike the random, irregular pitting of psoriasis, AA pitting is regular and fine. Other AA nail findings include trachyonychia, Beau lines, onychorrhexis (longitudinal splitting), and punctate or transverse leukonychia (white spots or bands from transient matrix dysfunction). Chronic paronychia — a chronic, non-infectious inflammation of the proximal and lateral nail folds — is commonly misdiagnosed as a chronic fungal infection. It occurs in individuals with chronic wet-work exposure (dishwashers, bartenders, food handlers, healthcare workers) and is caused by loss of the cuticle seal, which allows moisture and irritants to penetrate beneath the proximal nail fold and produce chronic, low-grade inflammation. The proximal nail fold is swollen, erythematous, and tender, and the cuticle is absent. Superimposed Candida colonization is common but is a secondary event, not the primary pathology — treatment targets the underlying irritant dermatitis (cuticle protection, avoidance of wet work, topical steroids) rather than the Candida.

Melanonychia: Evaluation Algorithm, Nail Matrix Biopsy, and Subungual Melanoma

Differential Diagnosis of Melanonychia

Longitudinal melanonychia — a longitudinal brown-to-black pigmented band extending from the proximal nail fold to the free edge — is a common clinical finding with a differential diagnosis that ranges from benign (melanocyte activation, benign melanocytic nevus, ethnic melanonychia, drug-induced melanonychia, subungual hemorrhage) to malignant (subungual melanoma). Ethnic melanonychia (melanocyte activation by friction and melanin deposition in the nail plate) is extremely common in individuals with darker skin phototypes — multiple pigmented bands on multiple nails are normal in Black, Asian, and Hispanic individuals and should not trigger biopsy. Drug-induced melanonychia (caused by hydroxyurea, doxorubicin, cyclophosphamide, zidovudine, and other agents) is typically multifocal and resolves after discontinuation. Subungual hemorrhage (splinter hemorrhage or traumatic hemorrhage) can mimic melanonychia but moves distally with nail growth — a key distinguishing feature (melanonychia originating from the matrix remains fixed relative to the proximal nail fold as the nail grows).

The ABCDEF Rule and Biopsy Decision-Making

The ABCDEF mnemonic guides evaluation of longitudinal melanonychia for features suspicious for subungual melanoma: Age (peak incidence 50 to 70 years) and African American, Asian, or Native American ethnicity (higher risk of acral melanoma); Band (width greater than 3 mm, irregular borders, brown-black color); Change (evolution in width, color, or morphology); Digit (thumb, index finger, and great toe are most commonly affected by melanoma); Extension (Hutchinson sign — periungual pigmentation extending beyond the nail fold); and Family history of melanoma. Dermoscopy (onychoscopy) of the pigmented band provides critical diagnostic information: regular, parallel, equally spaced lines of uniform color and width on a grey background favor benign melanonychia, while irregular line spacing, irregular line width, loss of parallelism, polychromia (multiple shades of brown and black within the band), micro-Hutchinson sign (periungual pigment visible only dermoscopically), and a dark brown-black background favor melanoma. Nail matrix biopsy is indicated for any single-digit melanonychia that is new, widening, darkening, or shows suspicious dermoscopic features — particularly in adults over 40.

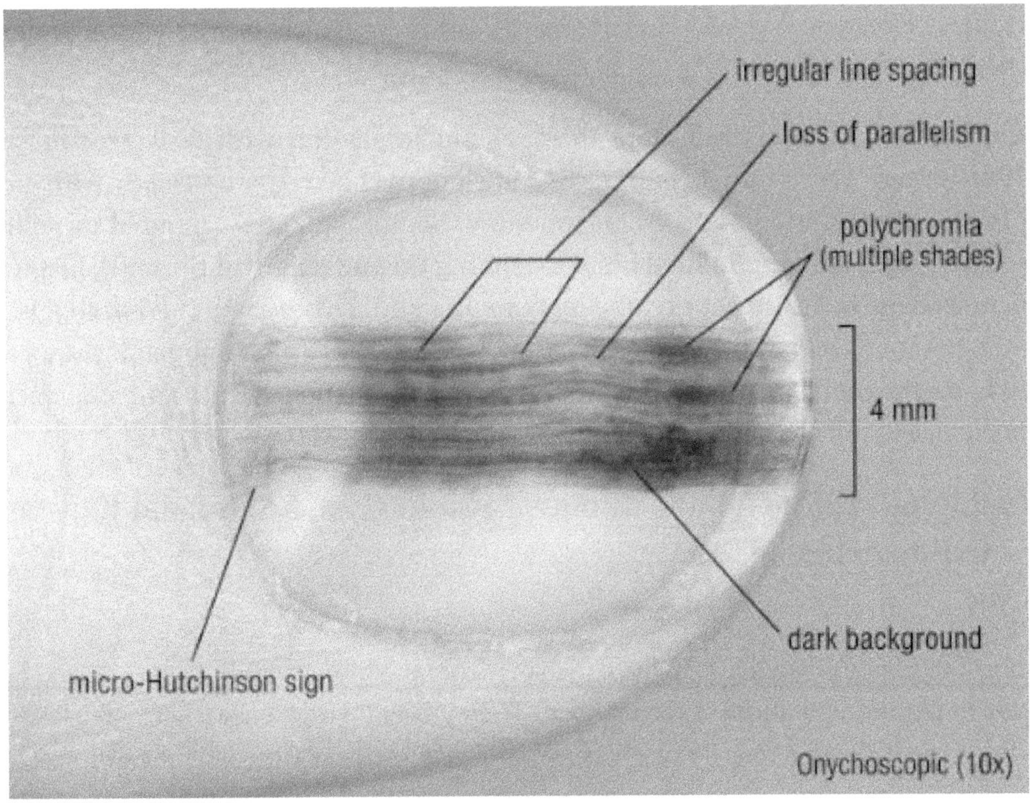

THE CUTANEOUS MIMICKER RECOGNITION ATLAS — Subungual Melanoma versus Subungual Hemorrhage

The Clinical Pattern: Subungual melanoma presents as longitudinal melanonychia — a persistent, widening, darkening band of brown-to-black pigment on the nail plate — originating from the nail matrix. The band is fixed relative to the proximal nail fold (it grows out with the nail but new pigment continues to emerge from the matrix). Hutchinson sign (periungual pigmentation) is an ominous finding. Subungual melanoma most commonly affects a single digit (thumb, index finger, or great toe), typically in adults over 50. It is the most common melanoma subtype in Black and Asian populations.

The Mimicker: Subungual hemorrhage (traumatic hemorrhage trapped beneath the nail plate) can produce dark brown-to-black discoloration that mimics melanonychia. Subungual hemorrhage typically follows trauma (which the patient may not recall) and is most common in active individuals and on toenails subject to repetitive microtrauma (runner's toe). The discoloration has a rounded or splinter-shaped border (not a longitudinal band arising from the matrix), and the key distinguishing behavior is that it migrates distally with nail growth — over weeks to months, the dark area moves toward the free edge and eventually grows out.

Trap Logic: Assuming that dark pigmentation under a nail is trauma-related hemorrhage without verifying that it migrates distally with nail growth is the cognitive trap. If the dark area does not migrate (remains fixed at or near the proximal nail fold), it is not hemorrhage — it is melanonychia arising from the matrix, and melanoma must be excluded. The reverse trap — biopsying every subungual hemorrhage

— produces unnecessary nail matrix damage and dystrophy, which is why the migration test is so clinically valuable.

The Decision Anchor: The discriminating features are **migration with nail growth (hemorrhage migrates distally and grows out over months; melanonychia remains fixed, with new pigment continuing to emerge from the matrix), morphology (hemorrhage has rounded or splinter-shaped borders; melanonychia is a longitudinal band extending the full length of the nail), history of trauma (supports hemorrhage but does not exclude melanoma), and dermoscopy (hemorrhage shows blood globules and a homogeneous red-brown color that fades distally; melanonychia shows longitudinal lines arising from the matrix)**. Any non-migrating dark pigmentation under a nail requires dermoscopic evaluation and consideration of nail matrix biopsy.

Tumors of the Nail Unit: Glomus Tumor, Myxoid Cyst, Subungual Exostosis, and Squamous Cell Carcinoma

Glomus Tumor

Glomus tumors are benign vascular neoplasms arising from the glomus body (a specialized arteriovenous shunt involved in thermoregulation) in the nail bed. They present with the classic triad: paroxysmal severe pain (often triggered by cold exposure or pressure), point tenderness (the patient can localize the pain to a precise point with a pin tip — the Love test), and temperature sensitivity (cold provocation reproduces the pain). The tumor appears as a small (2 to 5 mm), blue-red discoloration visible through the nail plate. MRI (with gadolinium enhancement) is the imaging modality of choice for confirming and localizing the tumor. Treatment is surgical excision through a transungual approach (removal of the nail plate overlying the tumor, excision of the tumor from the nail bed, and nail plate replacement) — recurrence after complete excision is uncommon.

Myxoid Cyst, Subungual Exostosis, and Squamous Cell Carcinoma

Myxoid (mucous) cysts are ganglion-like cysts arising from the distal interphalangeal joint capsule or the proximal nail fold, presenting as a translucent, dome-shaped, fluctuant papule on the proximal nail fold. Pressure on the underlying matrix produces a longitudinal groove in the nail plate. Treatment options include repeated drainage, intralesional corticosteroid injection, cryotherapy, and surgical excision (with osteophyte removal from the DIP joint if present — osteophytes contribute to cyst formation and recurrence). Subungual exostosis is a bony projection arising from the dorsal surface of the distal phalanx, presenting as a firm, painful nodule beneath the distal nail plate — it elevates and may destroy the overlying nail. Radiography confirms the diagnosis (visible as a bony outgrowth from the phalanx). Treatment is surgical excision. Subungual squamous cell carcinoma (Bowen disease of the nail unit) is the most common malignant tumor of the nail apparatus. It presents as a persistent, slowly growing, verrucous or hyperkeratotic lesion — often misdiagnosed as a viral wart, chronic paronychia, or onychomycosis for years before the correct diagnosis is established. HPV (particularly types 16 and 18) is implicated in a significant proportion of cases. Diagnosis requires biopsy. Treatment is surgical excision

(Mohs micrographic surgery provides the highest cure rate with nail apparatus preservation) or amputation of the distal phalanx for advanced disease.

CAUTION: Subungual SCC is frequently misdiagnosed as a wart for years — the mean time from onset to diagnosis exceeds 4 years in many series. Any verrucous, hyperkeratotic, or non-healing lesion of the nail unit that fails standard wart treatment (cryotherapy, topical salicylic acid) should be biopsied to exclude SCC. The presence of HPV in the etiology of subungual SCC means that wart-like morphology does not exclude malignancy — indeed, HPV-driven SCC may arise within a pre-existing wart.

Nail Signs of Systemic Disease

Diagnostic Nail Signs

The nail is a visible window to systemic health, and specific nail findings serve as clinical markers of underlying disease. Clubbing (bulbous enlargement of the distal digit with increased nail plate curvature, loss of the Lovibond angle, and a spongy feel of the nail bed on palpation — Schamroth sign positive: loss of the normal diamond-shaped window when the dorsal surfaces of opposite terminal phalanges are opposed) is associated with pulmonary disease (lung cancer, interstitial pulmonary fibrosis, bronchiectasis, cystic fibrosis, empyema), cardiovascular disease (endocarditis, cyanotic congenital heart disease), gastrointestinal disease (inflammatory bowel disease, celiac disease, hepatic cirrhosis), and may be hereditary (pachydermoperiostosis). Koilonychia (spoon-shaped nails — the nail plate is concave rather than convex) is the classic nail sign of iron deficiency anemia, though it also occurs in hemochromatosis, hypothyroidism, and Raynaud phenomenon. Beau lines — transverse depressions representing temporary matrix arrest — follow any systemic insult severe enough to interrupt nail growth: high fever, chemotherapy, severe illness, emotional shock. Mees lines (true leukonychia — transverse white bands within the nail plate that do not blanch with pressure and grow out with the nail) are associated with arsenic poisoning, thallium poisoning, chemotherapy, and severe systemic illness.

Vascular and Metabolic Nail Signs

Terry nails (proximal two-thirds of the nail plate is white with a distal band of normal pink — caused by reduced vascularity and increased connective tissue in the nail bed) are associated with hepatic cirrhosis, congestive heart failure, and diabetes. Muehrcke lines (paired, narrow, transverse white bands that disappear with pressure on the nail plate — indicating they are in the nail bed, not the plate) are associated with hypoalbuminemia (nephrotic syndrome, liver disease, malnutrition). Half-and-half nails (Lindsay nails — proximal half white, distal half brown — caused by melanin deposition in the distal nail bed) are associated with chronic kidney disease and uremia. Splinter hemorrhages — thin, longitudinal, red-brown lines in the nail bed caused by thrombosed capillaries — are nonspecific when in the distal nail (trauma is the most common cause), but when proximal (near the lunula), they are a clinical marker of vasculitis, endocarditis, antiphospholipid syndrome, and cholesterol emboli. Yellow nail syndrome (thick, slow-growing, excessively curved, yellow nails with absent lunulae) is a rare triad of yellow nails, lymphedema, and pulmonary disease (pleural effusion, bronchiectasis).

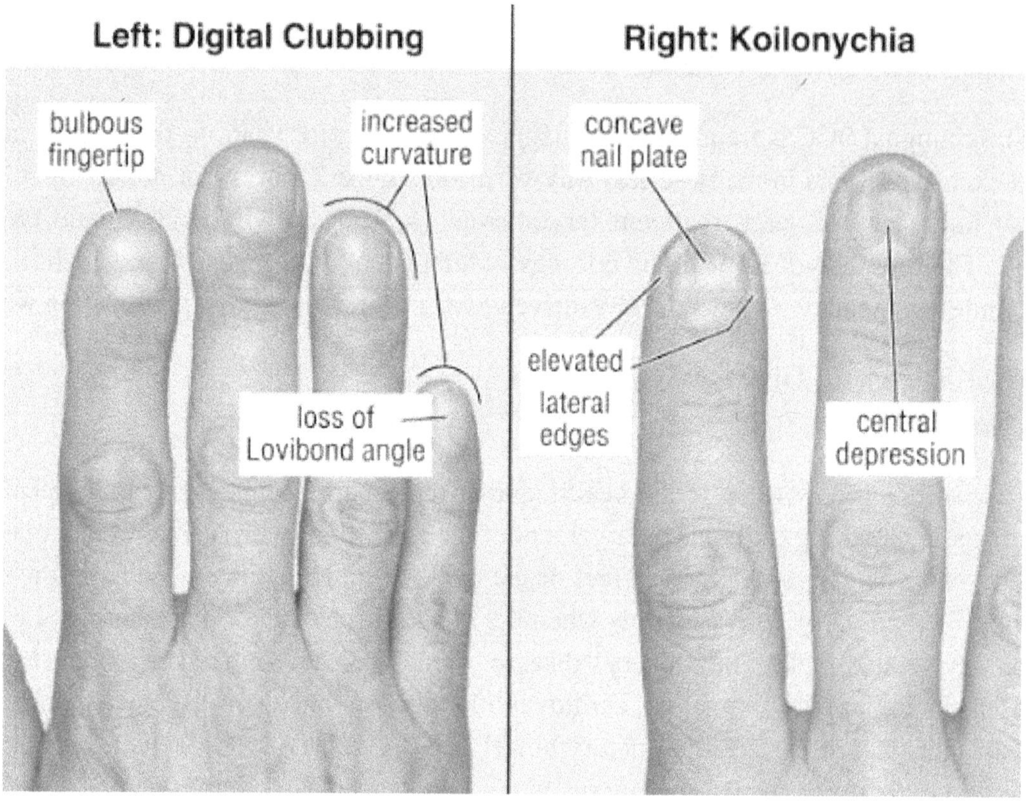

Nail Surgery: Biopsy Techniques, Matricectomy, and Nail Avulsion

Nail Biopsy Techniques

Nail biopsy is indicated when the clinical diagnosis is uncertain, when melanonychia requires histopathologic evaluation, or when nail unit tumors need tissue confirmation. The biopsy technique depends on the site of pathology. Nail plate biopsy (nail clipping) is the simplest technique — clipping the free edge of the nail plate for PAS staining (onychomycosis confirmation) or histopathologic examination of nail plate abnormalities. Nail bed biopsy (punch biopsy through the nail plate into the nail bed, typically 3 to 4 mm) is used for nail bed pathology (onycholysis, subungual hyperkeratosis, nail bed tumors). Nail matrix biopsy is the most technically demanding and carries the highest risk of permanent nail dystrophy — it requires reflection of the proximal nail fold, avulsion of the proximal nail plate to expose the matrix, and punch or fusiform excision of the matrix tissue. Matrix biopsies should be oriented longitudinally (parallel to the nail growth axis) to minimize the risk of a permanent nail plate split. For melanonychia evaluation, the biopsy must sample the matrix at the proximal origin of the pigmented band — the exact site where melanocytes are producing the pigment.

Matricectomy and Nail Avulsion

Nail avulsion (complete or partial removal of the nail plate) is performed for diagnostic purposes (exposing the nail bed or matrix for biopsy), therapeutic purposes (facilitating treatment of nail bed or matrix pathology), or as part of definitive surgical management. Partial nail avulsion removes only the portion of the nail plate overlying the area of interest. Matricectomy — permanent destruction of the nail matrix to prevent nail regrowth — is indicated for recurrent ingrown toenails (lateral matricectomy of the affected lateral horn using phenol cauterization or surgical excision) and for conditions requiring permanent nail elimination (severe, treatment-refractory onychomycosis in elderly patients, painful nail dystrophies). Chemical matricectomy with phenol (88 percent liquefied phenol applied to the exposed matrix after nail avulsion) is the most commonly performed technique for ingrown toenails: it produces permanent destruction of the lateral matrix horn, preventing regrowth of the offending lateral nail plate edge, with recurrence rates of approximately 2 to 5 percent. Postoperative wound care involves daily cleansing and application of topical antiseptic until the phenol burn heals — typically 4 to 6 weeks.

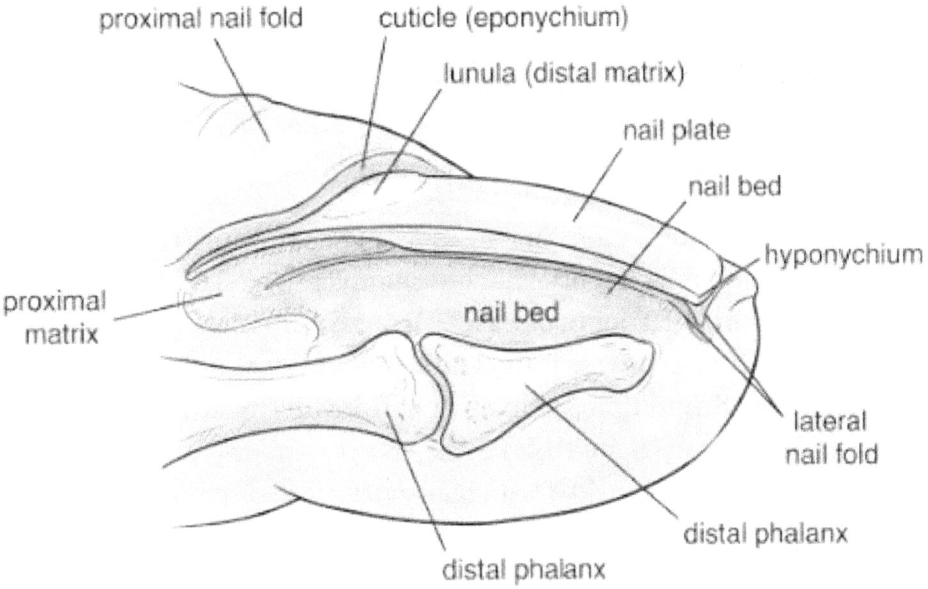

THE CUTANEOUS MIMICKER RECOGNITION ATLAS — Nail Psoriasis versus Onychomycosis

The Clinical Pattern: Nail psoriasis produces pitting (regular, ice-pick depressions in the nail surface from matrix disease), oil drop sign (salmon-colored translucent patches in the nail bed), onycholysis (often with an erythematous border), and subungual hyperkeratosis. Multiple nails are usually affected, and there is often concurrent skin psoriasis or psoriatic arthritis involving the DIP joints. The nails show a combination of matrix signs (surface changes) and bed signs (subungual changes), distinguishing it from pure onychomycosis which primarily affects the subungual region.

The Mimicker: Onychomycosis (particularly DLSO) produces subungual hyperkeratosis, onycholysis, yellow-brown discoloration, and nail plate thickening and dystrophy — features that overlap substantially with nail psoriasis. The two conditions coexist in up to 18 percent of patients (psoriatic nails are more susceptible to fungal colonization). Onychomycosis typically affects toenails more than fingernails, favors the great toenail, and involves fewer nails than psoriasis. It does not produce the characteristic matrix signs of psoriasis (regular pitting, Beau lines).

Trap Logic: Treating dystrophic nails empirically with oral antifungals without mycologic confirmation is the most common cognitive trap. The clinical overlap between nail psoriasis and onychomycosis is so extensive that clinical diagnosis alone is unreliable — studies show that up to 50 percent of clinically dystrophic nails in psoriasis patients do not have fungal infection. Conversely, treating fungally infected psoriatic nails with immunosuppression alone (without antifungals) allows the fungal infection to worsen. The dual trap requires dual testing.

The Decision Anchor: The discriminating features are **pitting (regular, ice-pick pitting is characteristic of psoriasis and does not occur in onychomycosis), oil drop sign (specific to psoriasis), concurrent skin psoriasis or DIP joint disease (strongly supports psoriasis), mycologic testing (KOH, PAS, or culture positive confirms fungal infection but does not exclude coexistent psoriasis), and number of nails affected (multiple symmetric nail involvement favors psoriasis; asymmetric, toenail-predominant favors onychomycosis)**. Always perform mycologic testing before treating dystrophic nails — and test psoriatic nails for fungal superinfection before attributing all dystrophy to psoriasis.

Histopathology of Nail Disorders

Nail biopsy interpretation requires familiarity with the unique histologic architecture of the nail unit. In onychomycosis, PAS staining of nail plate clippings reveals fungal hyphae and spores within the nail plate or between the nail plate and the nail bed — PAS is the most sensitive histologic method (82 to 95 percent) because it detects both viable and non-viable organisms. In nail psoriasis, histopathology of the nail bed shows features analogous to skin psoriasis: parakeratosis, neutrophilic collections (analogous to Munro microabscesses), dilated tortuous capillaries, and psoriasiform hyperplasia of the nail bed epithelium. Matrix biopsy in nail lichen planus reveals a lichenoid band-like lymphocytic infiltrate at the dermoepidermal junction of the matrix epithelium, with basal cell degeneration, civatte bodies (apoptotic keratinocytes), and eventual fibrosis that replaces the germinative matrix — this fibrotic replacement is the histologic correlate of irreversible nail loss and dorsal pterygium. In melanonychia evaluation, nail matrix biopsy must demonstrate the melanocyte population: benign activation shows increased melanin production by a normal number of regularly spaced melanocytes along the basal layer, while melanocytic nevus shows a nested proliferation of bland melanocytes, and melanoma in situ shows an irregular, crowded proliferation of atypical melanocytes with pagetoid scatter. Immunohistochemistry (SOX10, Melan-A, HMB-45) aids in identifying melanocytes and assessing architectural disorder.

Special Populations: Pediatric and Geriatric Nail Disease

Pediatric nail disorders present a distinct spectrum. Nail pitting and twenty-nail dystrophy (trachyonychia) in children may be idiopathic and self-resolving rather than indicative of psoriasis or lichen planus — watchful waiting with reassurance is appropriate when the child has no other dermatologic or systemic findings. Congenital nail abnormalities (anonychia, micronychia, malalignment of the great toenail) are uncommon but important to recognize: congenital malalignment of the great toenail — where the nail plate grows in a laterally deviated direction relative to the longitudinal axis of the toe — may self-correct by age 2 but can cause chronic ingrown toenails if persistent. Nail biting (onychophagia) and thumb sucking produce characteristic nail plate irregularities, paronychia, and periungual warts. In elderly patients, nail changes are nearly universal: decreased growth rate (toenails may take 18 to 24 months for complete replacement), increased thickness and brittleness (onychogryphosis — ram-horn dystrophy — is common on great toenails in elderly patients with reduced mobility and peripheral vascular disease), yellow discoloration, and increased susceptibility to onychomycosis. The thickened, dystrophic nails of elderly patients are frequently overtreated with oral antifungals when the dystrophy is mechanical or vascular rather than fungal — mycologic confirmation is especially important in this population.

Nail Sign	Mechanism	Associated Systemic Conditions	Clinical Significance
Clubbing	Increased vascularity and connective tissue in the nail bed; VEGF and platelet-derived growth factor implicated	Lung cancer, IPF, bronchiectasis, endocarditis, cyanotic CHD, IBD, cirrhosis	Screen for underlying pulmonary or cardiac disease; new-onset clubbing warrants chest imaging
Koilonychia	Softening and thinning of the nail plate with concave deformation	Iron deficiency anemia, hemochromatosis, hypothyroidism, Raynaud phenomenon	Check serum ferritin and iron studies; physiologic in infants
Terry Nails	Reduced vascularity with increased connective tissue in proximal nail bed	Hepatic cirrhosis, CHF, diabetes mellitus, advanced age	Evaluate hepatic and cardiac function

Muehrcke Lines	Vascular bed edema from hypoalbuminemia; disappear with pressure	Nephrotic syndrome, liver disease, malnutrition	Check serum albumin; resolve when albumin normalizes
Half-and-Half Nails	Melanin deposition in distal nail bed from uremia	Chronic kidney disease, uremia	Evaluate renal function; present in 20 to 40 percent of dialysis patients
Beau Lines	Temporary arrest of nail matrix proliferation	Severe illness, high fever, chemotherapy, emotional shock, Raynaud phenomenon	Distance from proximal nail fold estimates timing of causative insult

Patient Education and Counseling

Patient education is essential for nail disorders because treatment timelines are measured in months rather than weeks, and unrealistic expectations are a leading cause of treatment abandonment. Patients starting oral antifungal therapy for toenail onychomycosis should understand that the medication course (12 weeks for terbinafine) ends long before the nail appears normal — complete cosmetic improvement may require 12 to 18 months as the healthy nail slowly replaces the dystrophic plate. Counseling should address fungal reservoirs: concurrent tinea pedis must be treated, footwear should be rotated and treated with antifungal powder, and communal shower facilities require protective footwear. For nail psoriasis patients, counseling emphasizes that nail disease responds more slowly than skin psoriasis, that even with effective biologic therapy the nail may take 6 to 12 months to show improvement, and that the DIP joint connection means persistent nail disease may warrant rheumatologic evaluation. Patients with melanonychia — particularly those with darker skin phototypes who may have benign ethnic melanonychia — benefit from education about the difference between reassuring (multiple bands, symmetric, stable) and concerning (single band, widening, darkening, new in adult) patterns, empowering self-monitoring without causing unnecessary alarm.

CLINICAL PEARL: The oil drop sign (salmon patch) — a translucent, yellow-red to salmon-colored area visible through the nail plate — is the most specific clinical sign of nail psoriasis. It represents a focus of psoriatic inflammation in the nail bed, with serum and glycoprotein accumulation beneath the nail plate. While not present in every psoriatic nail, when present it is virtually diagnostic of nail psoriasis and is not seen in onychomycosis, lichen planus, or other nail dystrophies. The oil drop sign should be specifically sought on examination of any dystrophic nail, as it often provides the clinical clue that distinguishes psoriasis from fungal infection.

EVIDENCE: The TRANSFIGURE trial and subsequent studies demonstrated that ixekizumab (an IL-17A inhibitor) produces near-complete nail clearance in psoriasis patients with nail involvement. At 52 weeks, ixekizumab reduced NAPSI scores by 80 to 90 percent from baseline — a level of efficacy not previously achieved by traditional systemic therapies. Secukinumab and guselkumab have shown similar high-efficacy nail outcomes. These results have positioned IL-17 and IL-23 pathway inhibitors as preferred biologics for patients in whom nail psoriasis is a treatment priority, particularly those with coexistent psoriatic arthritis (which shares the entheseal connection with nail disease).

Clinical Case: Recurrent Subungual Pain

A 42-year-old woman presents with a 2-year history of episodic, lancinating pain beneath the left ring fingernail. The pain is triggered by cold exposure (opening the refrigerator, holding cold drinks) and by direct pressure on the nail. She has seen multiple providers who attributed her symptoms to trauma, and she was treated empirically with oral antifungals for presumed onychomycosis despite a normal-appearing nail. On examination, the nail plate is intact and appears normal except for a small, 3 mm, blue-red discoloration visible through the nail plate in the proximal nail bed region. The Love test (application of a pin tip to the nail surface over the discolored area) reproduces severe, sharp pain. The Hildreth test (pain relief when a tourniquet is inflated above systolic pressure on the ipsilateral arm) is positive. MRI with gadolinium enhancement reveals a well-circumscribed, 4 mm, enhancing lesion in the nail bed — consistent with a glomus tumor. The tumor is excised through a transungual approach under digital block anesthesia: the nail plate overlying the tumor is reflected, the encapsulated blue-red tumor is dissected from the nail bed, and the nail plate is replaced as a biologic dressing. The patient's pain resolves immediately and completely. Histopathology confirms a glomus tumor (sheets of uniform, round, glomus cells surrounding vascular channels). At 6-month follow-up, the nail has regrown normally with no recurrence of pain. This case illustrates the diagnostic triad (paroxysmal pain, point tenderness, cold sensitivity), the importance of careful nail bed inspection for subtle discoloration, and the curative nature of surgical excision.

THE CUTANEOUS MIMICKER RECOGNITION ATLAS — Nail Disorder Diagnostic Arcs

Subungual Melanoma vs. Subungual Hemorrhage: The discriminating features are migration with nail growth (hemorrhage migrates distally and grows out; melanonychia remains fixed, with new pigment continuing to emerge from the matrix), morphology (hemorrhage has rounded or splinter-shaped borders; melanonychia is a longitudinal band), and dermoscopy (hemorrhage shows homogeneous red-brown color; melanonychia shows longitudinal lines from the matrix). Cognitive trap: assuming dark subungual pigmentation is traumatic without verifying distal migration — non-migrating pigmentation is melanonychia, not hemorrhage, and melanoma must be excluded.

Nail Psoriasis vs. Onychomycosis: The discriminating features are pitting (regular pitting is specific to psoriasis), oil drop sign (specific to psoriasis), concurrent skin psoriasis or DIP arthritis (supports psoriasis), mycologic testing (confirms fungal infection but does not exclude coexistent psoriasis), and distribution (multiple symmetric nails favor psoriasis; asymmetric toenail involvement favors onychomycosis). Cognitive trap: treating dystrophic nails empirically with antifungals without mycologic confirmation — up to 50 percent of dystrophic nails are not fungal.

Summary and Key Concepts

The nail unit has five anatomic components (matrix, nail bed, nail plate, nail folds, hyponychium), and the site of pathology determines the clinical pattern: proximal matrix disease produces surface abnormalities (pitting, ridging), nail bed disease produces onycholysis and subungual changes, and matrix destruction causes permanent nail loss.

Onychomycosis affects 10 to 12 percent of the population, with T. rubrum causing 70 to 80 percent of cases. Mycologic confirmation (KOH, PAS, culture, or PCR) is mandatory before initiating oral antifungals. Oral terbinafine is first-line for dermatophyte onychomycosis (70 to 80 percent mycologic cure).

Nail psoriasis affects 50 percent of psoriasis patients and is strongly associated with DIP joint psoriatic arthritis. The oil drop sign is the most specific clinical feature. IL-17 inhibitors (ixekizumab, secukinumab) produce near-complete nail clearance at 52 weeks, positioning them as preferred biologics for nail-predominant psoriasis.

Longitudinal melanonychia is evaluated using the ABCDEF rule and dermoscopy. Irregular line spacing, loss of parallelism, polychromia, and micro-Hutchinson sign on onychoscopy favor melanoma. Nail matrix biopsy is indicated for any single-digit, widening, or dermoscopically suspicious band, particularly in adults over 40.

Nail signs of systemic disease include clubbing (pulmonary, cardiac, GI disease), koilonychia (iron deficiency), Terry nails (cirrhosis, CHF), Muehrcke lines (hypoalbuminemia), and half-and-half nails (CKD). Proximal splinter hemorrhages suggest vasculitis or endocarditis, while distal splinter hemorrhages are usually traumatic.

CHAPTER 19: LUPUS ERYTHEMATOSUS AND SCLERODERMA

Learning Objectives

1. Classify cutaneous lupus erythematosus into acute, subacute, and chronic (discoid) forms based on morphology, distribution, histopathology, and risk of systemic disease progression.
2. Apply the 2019 EULAR/ACR classification criteria for systemic lupus erythematosus, identify the weighted cutaneous domains, and recognize when skin-limited disease warrants systemic serologic and organ-targeted screening.
3. Distinguish systemic sclerosis (limited and diffuse subtypes) from localized scleroderma (morphea) based on clinical features, autoantibody profiles, and capillaroscopic patterns, and initiate appropriate organ-specific surveillance.
4. Select evidence-based management for cutaneous lupus and scleroderma, integrating topical, systemic, and biologic therapies while applying the clinical-accuracy drug-dose guardrail for immunosuppressives.

Cutaneous Lupus Erythematosus: Acute, Subacute, and Chronic (Discoid) Forms

Epidemiology and Risk Factors

Cutaneous lupus erythematosus affects approximately 70 per 100,000 people, with a female predominance (3:1 for DLE, higher for SCLE). DLE is the most common subtype and accounts for 70 to 80 percent of CLE cases. The disease shows significant racial disparities: DLE is 2 to 3 times more common in Black women, who develop more severe scarring, more widespread disease, and greater cosmetic morbidity due to the prominent dyspigmentation in darker skin phototypes. SCLE affects predominantly White women and is strongly associated with HLA-DR3. Ultraviolet radiation is the principal environmental trigger — UVB induces keratinocyte apoptosis and translocation of intracellular autoantigens (Ro/SSA and La/SSB) to the cell surface, initiating the autoimmune cascade. Smoking is an independent risk factor for CLE (particularly DLE) and reduces the therapeutic efficacy of antimalarials. Drug-induced SCLE has an expanding list of culprits: hydrochlorothiazide, terbinafine, proton pump inhibitors, TNF-alpha inhibitors, and immune checkpoint inhibitors are among the most commonly implicated agents.

Definition and Classification

Cutaneous lupus erythematosus (CLE) encompasses a spectrum of autoimmune skin diseases that may occur independently or in association with systemic lupus erythematosus (SLE). The Gilliam classification divides CLE into three subtypes based on clinical morphology, histopathology, and prognostic implications. Acute cutaneous lupus erythematosus (ACLE) presents as the classic malar (butterfly) rash — bilateral, symmetric erythema over the cheeks and nasal bridge, sparing the nasolabial folds — and occurs almost exclusively in the setting of active SLE. The malar rash is photosensitive, often triggered or worsened by ultraviolet exposure, and resolves without scarring (unlike discoid lupus). Generalized ACLE can present as a widespread morbilliform or photodistributed eruption mimicking a drug reaction or viral exanthem. Subacute cutaneous lupus erythematosus (SCLE) presents in two morphologic patterns: annular-polycyclic (the more common — expanding rings with central clearing, often confluent) and papulosquamous (psoriasiform plaques resembling psoriasis or dermatophyte infection). SCLE is characteristically photodistributed (V of chest, upper back, lateral arms) and heals without scarring but frequently leaves persistent post-inflammatory hypopigmentation or hyperpigmentation. SCLE is strongly associated with anti-Ro/SSA antibodies (present in 70 to 90 percent of cases) and can be drug-induced (hydrochlorothiazide, terbinafine, proton pump inhibitors, TNF-alpha inhibitors).

Chronic Cutaneous Lupus: Discoid Lupus Erythematosus

Chronic cutaneous lupus erythematosus, the most common form of CLE, presents primarily as discoid lupus erythematosus (DLE). DLE lesions are well-demarcated, indurated, erythematous plaques with adherent scale and follicular plugging (keratotic spicules that, when removed, show follicular-shaped keratotic projections on the undersurface — the carpet-tack sign). As DLE lesions evolve, they develop central atrophic scarring, dyspigmentation (central hypopigmentation with a peripheral hyperpigmented rim — particularly conspicuous in darker skin phototypes), and follicular destruction causing permanent scarring alopecia when the scalp is involved. Scalp DLE is one of the most common causes of scarring alopecia in women of African descent. DLE most commonly affects the face (especially the conchal bowl of the ears, the nose, and the malar cheeks), scalp, and ears, though generalized DLE can involve the trunk and extremities. The distinction between localized DLE (lesions above the neck only) and generalized DLE (lesions above and below the neck) has prognostic significance: generalized DLE carries a higher risk (approximately 20 percent) of progression to SLE, compared with 5 to 10 percent for localized DLE. Other chronic CLE variants include lupus panniculitis (lupus profundus — deep, firm subcutaneous nodules and plaques that heal with lipoatrophy and depressed scars) and chilblain lupus (painful, violaceous papules on acral sites precipitated by cold exposure — overlapping clinically with chilblains but associated with lupus serologies).

Histopathology of Cutaneous Lupus

The histopathologic hallmark shared across all CLE subtypes is an interface dermatitis — vacuolar degeneration of the basal layer with a superficial and deep perivascular and periadnexal lymphocytic infiltrate. DLE additionally shows epidermal atrophy, follicular plugging, basement membrane thickening (visible on PAS staining), and increased dermal mucin. Direct immunofluorescence (DIF) of lesional skin in DLE reveals a lupus band — granular deposition of IgG, IgM, IgA, and complement (C3) at the dermoepidermal junction. A positive lupus band in non-lesional, sun-protected skin (typically the volar forearm) is specific for SLE and may help distinguish skin-limited CLE from systemic disease. SCLE shows a less dense, more superficial infiltrate with epidermal atrophy but minimal follicular changes and minimal scarring — consistent with its clinical behavior (resolves without permanent scarring).

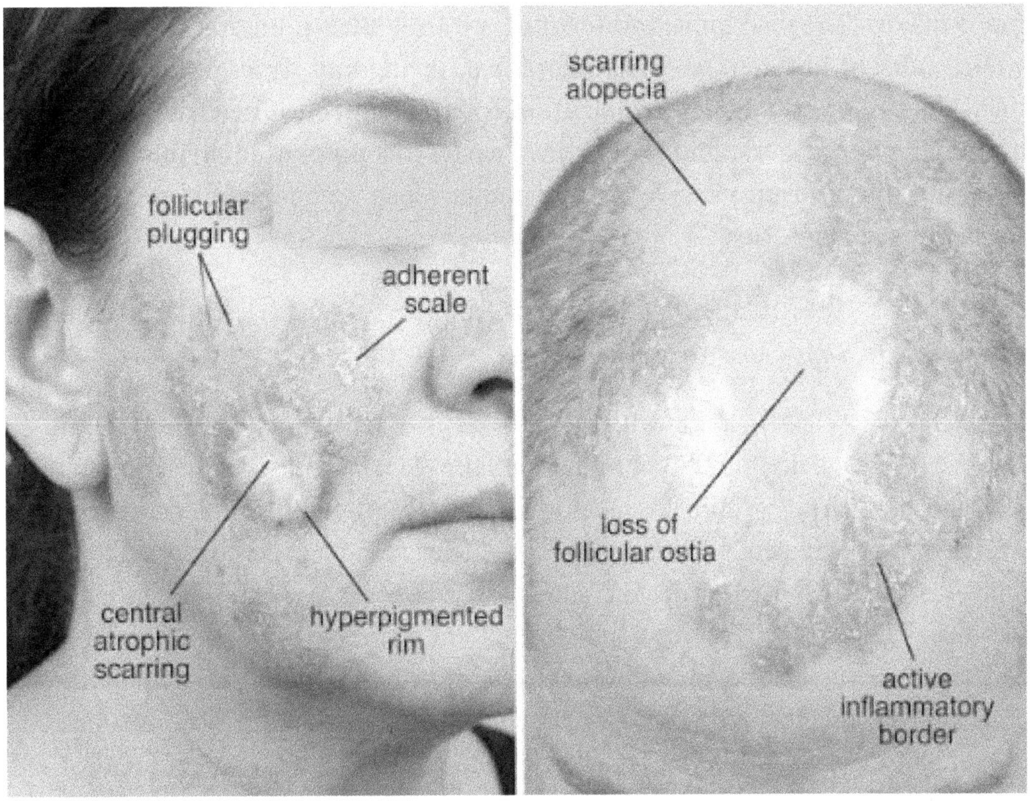

THE CUTANEOUS MIMICKER RECOGNITION ATLAS — Discoid Lupus versus Tinea Faciei

The Clinical Pattern: Discoid lupus erythematosus presents as well-demarcated, erythematous, indurated plaques with adherent scale and follicular plugging on the face. The lesions are characteristically photodistributed (malar cheeks, nose, ears) and develop central atrophic scarring with dyspigmentation as they evolve. The carpet-tack sign (keratotic follicular projections on the undersurface of removed scale) is a clinical hallmark. DLE is chronic, progressive, and — if untreated — causes permanent scarring with follicular destruction.

The Mimicker: Tinea faciei (dermatophyte infection of the face) presents as annular or polycyclic, erythematous, scaly plaques with raised, advancing borders and relative central clearing — morphology that closely mimics the annular variant of DLE or SCLE, particularly when the lesions are on the cheeks or nose. Tinea faciei is frequently misdiagnosed and inappropriately treated with topical corticosteroids (tinea incognito), which suppresses the scaling and inflammatory border while allowing the fungal infection to expand.

Trap Logic: Prescribing topical corticosteroids for an annular facial plaque without considering tinea faciei (and performing KOH) is the initial trap — corticosteroids suppress the clinical features of tinea and allow expansion (tinea incognito). The reverse trap is treating a lupus plaque empirically with topical antifungals, delaying the diagnosis of CLE and allowing scarring progression. The key is that DLE has follicular plugging and the carpet-tack sign (tinea does not), while tinea has a positive KOH scraping and an annular morphology with a truly clear center (DLE's center is atrophic and scarred, not simply clear).

The Decision Anchor: The discriminating features are **follicular plugging and the carpet-tack sign (present in DLE, absent in tinea), central atrophic scarring and dyspigmentation (DLE evolves to scarring; tinea does not scar), KOH preparation (positive in tinea, negative in DLE), distribution (DLE favors malar cheeks, ears, and scalp; tinea faciei has no photodistribution), and response to antifungals versus immunosuppressives**. Any annular facial plaque should receive a KOH scraping before corticosteroids are prescribed.

Systemic Lupus Erythematosus: Cutaneous Criteria and Systemic Assessment

Cutaneous Domains in SLE Classification

The 2019 EULAR/ACR classification criteria for SLE use a weighted scoring system with an entry criterion (positive ANA at a titer of 1:80 or higher on HEp-2 cells) followed by additive weighted criteria across clinical and immunologic domains. Among the clinical domains, mucocutaneous findings carry significant weight: acute cutaneous lupus (ACLE — malar rash or generalized ACLE) scores 6 points, subacute cutaneous lupus (SCLE) or discoid lupus (DLE) scores 4 points, oral or nasal ulcers score 2 points, and non-scarring alopecia scores 2 points. A total score of 10 or more classifies the patient as having SLE. The cutaneous criteria are important because skin manifestations may be the first presenting feature of SLE and can predate systemic involvement by years — ACLE accompanies active systemic disease in 90 percent of cases, while DLE progresses to SLE in 5 to 20 percent and SCLE in 10 to 15 percent.

Systemic Screening in Cutaneous Lupus

All patients with any CLE subtype require baseline serologic evaluation to assess for underlying or evolving systemic disease. The minimum panel includes ANA, anti-dsDNA antibodies (specific for SLE, associated with lupus nephritis), anti-Ro/SSA and anti-La/SSB antibodies (associated with SCLE, neonatal lupus, and Sjogren syndrome), anti-Smith antibodies (highly specific for SLE), complement levels (C3, C4 — consumed in active SLE), complete blood count (cytopenias — lymphopenia, thrombocytopenia, hemolytic anemia), serum creatinine, and urinalysis with microscopy (proteinuria, hematuria, and cellular casts suggest lupus nephritis). Patients with ACLE require comprehensive organ-targeted screening because ACLE virtually always accompanies systemic disease. Patients with isolated DLE and negative serologies can be monitored clinically, but generalized DLE, lupus panniculitis, or development of new serologic abnormalities warrants escalation of systemic surveillance.

KEY POINT: The nasolabial folds are characteristically spared in the malar rash of acute cutaneous lupus — erythema extends across the cheeks and nasal bridge but does not involve the nasolabial creases. This sparing distinguishes the lupus malar rash from the malar erythema of rosacea (which involves the nasolabial folds and has papules and pustules), seborrheic dermatitis (which concentrates in the nasolabial folds and has greasy scale), and contact dermatitis (which follows the pattern of exposure). Photosensitivity history and ANA testing further clarify the diagnosis.

Systemic Sclerosis and Localized Scleroderma (Morphea): Clinical Spectrum and Classification

Systemic Sclerosis: Limited and Diffuse Subtypes

Systemic sclerosis (SSc) is a multisystem autoimmune disease characterized by progressive fibrosis of the skin and internal organs, vasculopathy (Raynaud phenomenon and digital ischemia), and immune dysregulation. SSc is classified into two major subtypes based on the extent of skin involvement. Limited cutaneous SSc (lcSSc — formerly CREST syndrome) involves skin sclerosis distal to the elbows and knees and may affect the face, but spares the trunk and proximal extremities. The CREST acronym describes its five cardinal features: Calcinosis cutis (calcium deposits in the skin and subcutaneous tissue), Raynaud phenomenon (virtually universal in SSc — often the earliest manifestation, preceding skin sclerosis by years), Esophageal dysmotility (reflux, dysphagia from smooth muscle fibrosis), Sclerodactyly (skin tightening of the fingers producing tapered, sausage-like digits with limited mobility), and Telangiectasias (matte, non-pulsatile telangiectasias on the face, lips, tongue, and hands). The hallmark autoantibody of lcSSc is anti-centromere antibody (ACA — present in 50 to 80 percent), which is associated with a lower risk of interstitial lung disease but a significant risk of pulmonary arterial hypertension over time. Diffuse cutaneous SSc (dcSSc) involves skin sclerosis extending proximal to the elbows and knees and affecting the trunk. Diffuse disease has a more aggressive course with higher risk of early interstitial lung disease (anti-Scl-70/anti-topoisomerase I antibody — present in 20 to 40 percent) and scleroderma renal crisis (anti-RNA polymerase III antibody). Skin involvement is assessed using the modified Rodnan skin score (mRSS) — a semiquantitative measure of skin thickness at 17 body sites scored 0 to 3 each (maximum 51).

Localized Scleroderma: Morphea

Localized scleroderma (morphea) is a fibrotic disorder confined to the skin and subcutaneous tissue, without systemic organ involvement or Raynaud phenomenon. Morphea and systemic sclerosis are distinct diseases — morphea does not evolve into SSc. Morphea presents as circumscribed, indurated, sclerotic plaques with an ivory-white center surrounded by an inflammatory violaceous border (lilac ring) during the active phase. As the inflammation subsides, the plaques become firm, waxy, and atrophic. Subtypes include plaque morphea (the most common — one or a few discrete oval plaques), generalized morphea (four or more plaques or involvement of two or more body regions), linear morphea (band-like sclerosis along an extremity — the most common subtype in children — which can extend to fascia, muscle, and bone, causing growth restriction and limb-length discrepancy), en coup de sabre (linear morphea of the frontoparietal scalp and forehead, producing a depressed, atrophic, linear furrow with overlying alopecia — may be associated with Parry-Romberg syndrome, progressive hemifacial atrophy), and deep morphea (sclerosis extending to fascia and muscle). Morphea is typically diagnosed clinically, though biopsy can confirm the diagnosis (deep dermal and subcutaneous sclerosis with dense collagen bundles replacing fat, with loss of adnexal structures). Autoantibodies (ANA — positive in 20 to 40 percent, anti-ssDNA, anti-histone) may be present but do not correlate with disease extent or prognosis.

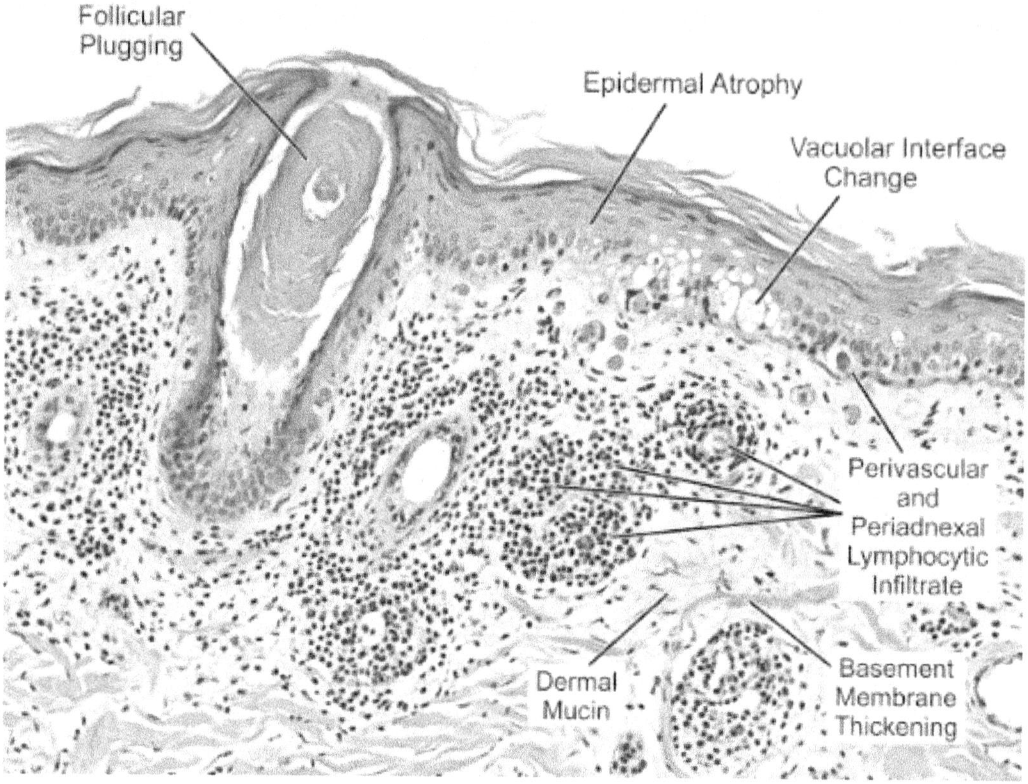

Mixed Connective Tissue Disease: Overlapping Cutaneous Features

Clinical Overlap Syndrome

Mixed connective tissue disease (MCTD) is an overlap syndrome with clinical features of SLE, systemic sclerosis, and polymyositis occurring together or sequentially, defined by the presence of high-titer anti-U1 RNP antibodies. Cutaneous findings in MCTD reflect the overlapping components: malar rash and photosensitivity (lupus component), sclerodactyly and Raynaud phenomenon (scleroderma component), and heliotrope rash or Gottron papules (dermatomyositis component). The hands are often the most informative anatomic site: patients may exhibit puffy, swollen fingers (sausage digits) in the early edematous phase, progressing to sclerodactyly, with periungual telangiectasias visible on nailfold capillaroscopy and Raynaud phenomenon present in 85 to 95 percent of patients. MCTD must be distinguished from undifferentiated connective tissue disease (UCTD — an early-stage or incomplete connective tissue disease that does not meet criteria for any specific diagnosis) and from overlap syndromes without the high-titer anti-U1 RNP that defines MCTD.

Prognosis and Disease Evolution

The prognosis of MCTD is generally more favorable than SLE or diffuse SSc, though a subset of patients develop serious complications: pulmonary arterial hypertension (the leading cause of mortality in MCTD, occurring in 10 to 25 percent), interstitial lung disease, esophageal dysmotility, and trigeminal neuropathy. Over time, some patients with MCTD evolve into a more defined connective tissue disease (most commonly SSc or SLE), while others maintain the overlap pattern. Pulmonary function testing (including

DLCO) and echocardiography should be performed at baseline and periodically to screen for pulmonary hypertension and ILD.

Diagnostic Workup: Autoantibody Panels, Nailfold Capillaroscopy, and Histopathology

Autoantibody Profiles and Disease Correlation

Autoantibody	Associated Disease	Clinical Significance	Prevalence
ANA	SLE, SSc, MCTD, DM	Entry criterion for SLE classification; non-specific — present in many autoimmune diseases and 5 to 15 percent of healthy individuals	Greater than 95% in SLE; 85 to 95% in SSc
Anti-dsDNA	SLE	Highly specific for SLE; titers correlate with lupus nephritis activity and predict renal flares	60 to 70% of SLE
Anti-Ro/SSA	SCLE, neonatal lupus, Sjogren syndrome	Associated with photosensitivity, annular SCLE, neonatal lupus with congenital heart block risk	70 to 90% of SCLE
Anti-Smith	SLE	Most specific antibody for SLE (virtually pathognomonic); associated with lupus nephritis	20 to 30% of SLE
Anti-centromere	Limited cutaneous SSc	Associated with CREST features, pulmonary arterial hypertension risk, milder skin disease	50 to 80% of lcSSc
Anti-Scl-70 (anti-topoisomerase I)	Diffuse cutaneous SSc	Associated with diffuse skin sclerosis and interstitial lung disease	20 to 40% of dcSSc

Anti-RNA polymerase III	Diffuse cutaneous SSc	Associated with rapidly progressive skin thickening and scleroderma renal crisis	10 to 25% of dcSSc
Anti-U1 RNP	MCTD	Defines MCTD at high titer; associated with Raynaud, puffy fingers, overlap features	100% of MCTD (by definition)

Autoantibody testing is central to the diagnosis and classification of lupus and scleroderma spectrum diseases. In SLE, ANA is the entry criterion (sensitivity greater than 95 percent but low specificity); anti-dsDNA antibodies are highly specific and correlate with lupus nephritis activity (rising titers predict renal flares); anti-Smith antibodies are the most specific for SLE (present in only 20 to 30 percent but virtually pathognomonic); and anti-Ro/SSA and anti-La/SSB antibodies are associated with SCLE, photosensitivity, neonatal lupus (congenital heart block in the fetus of an anti-Ro-positive mother), and Sjogren syndrome. In systemic sclerosis, anti-centromere antibody (ACA) associates with limited cutaneous SSc and pulmonary arterial hypertension risk; anti-Scl-70 (anti-topoisomerase I) associates with diffuse cutaneous SSc and interstitial lung disease; and anti-RNA polymerase III associates with diffuse SSc, rapidly progressive skin thickening, and scleroderma renal crisis. Anti-U1 RNP defines MCTD when present at high titer with the appropriate clinical overlap.

Nailfold Capillaroscopy

Nailfold capillaroscopy (NFC) is a non-invasive technique for visualizing the capillary loops at the nailfold — the only site where capillaries are visible en face through the translucent skin. In systemic sclerosis, NFC reveals a characteristic scleroderma pattern: early (few enlarged capillaries with no capillary loss), active (numerous enlarged and giant capillaries with capillary hemorrhages, moderate capillary loss, and mild disorganization of the capillary architecture), and late (few or no giant capillaries, severe capillary loss producing avascular areas, ramified/bushy neocapillaries representing neoangiogenesis). NFC findings in SSc are included in the 2013 ACR/EULAR classification criteria and help distinguish primary Raynaud phenomenon (normal capillaroscopy) from SSc-associated Raynaud (abnormal capillaroscopy). NFC is also abnormal in dermatomyositis (dilated, tortuous capillaries with dropout) and MCTD, but is typically normal in SLE.

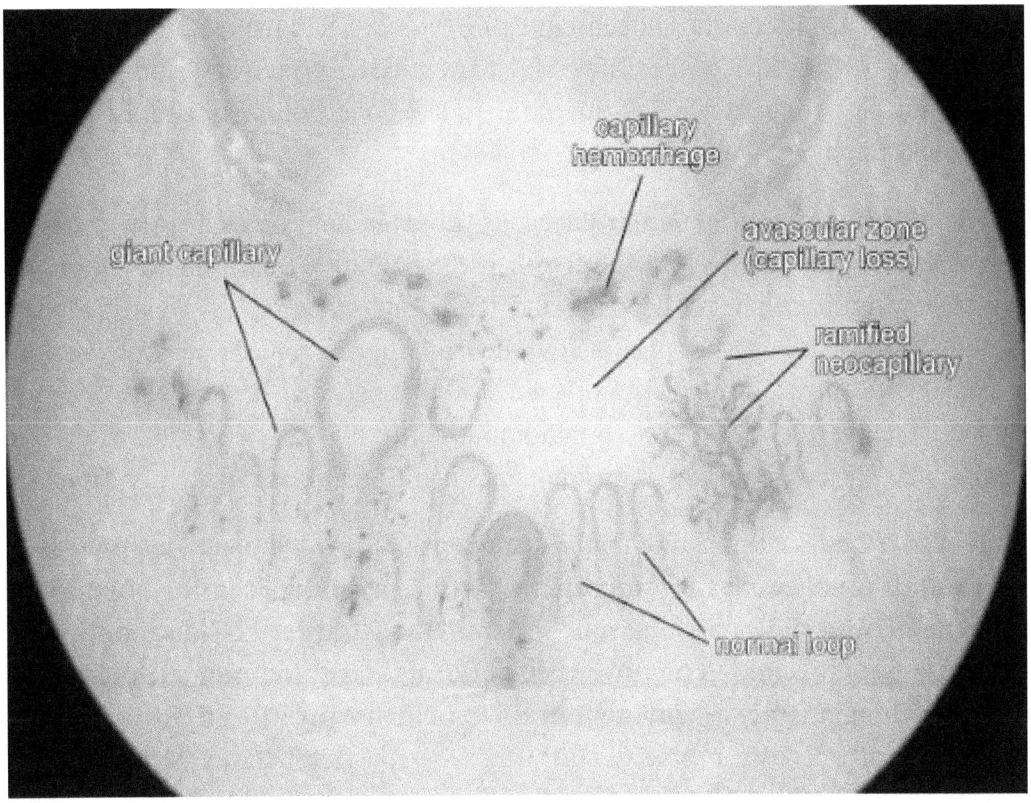

Histopathologic Features and Biopsy Indications

Biopsy is indicated in CLE when the clinical presentation is atypical or when distinguishing CLE from mimickers (rosacea, tinea, psoriasis, dermatomyositis). CLE histopathology was described above (interface dermatitis, periadnexal infiltrate, follicular plugging in DLE, basement membrane thickening, mucin deposition). In scleroderma, early morphea biopsy shows a perivascular lymphocytic and eosinophilic infiltrate in the lower dermis and subcutis, while established lesions show dense, homogenized collagen replacing the normal reticular dermis and extending into the subcutis, with loss of adnexal structures and entrapment of eccrine glands within the sclerotic collagen. Systemic sclerosis skin biopsy is similar but typically shows thinner epidermis, more extensive fibrosis, and vascular changes (intimal proliferation and luminal narrowing of dermal arterioles). Direct immunofluorescence is useful in CLE (lupus band test) but is not helpful in scleroderma.

THE CUTANEOUS MIMICKER RECOGNITION ATLAS — Morphea versus Lichen Sclerosus

The Clinical Pattern: Morphea (localized scleroderma) presents as circumscribed, indurated, sclerotic plaques with an ivory-white center and an inflammatory lilac ring at the active border. The plaques are firm and bound down — the skin cannot be pinched. Morphea favors the trunk and proximal extremities and can involve the dermis, subcutis, fascia, and even muscle in deep variants. Over time, active inflammation subsides and the plaques become atrophic and firm without the lilac border.

The Mimicker: Lichen sclerosus (LS) presents as porcelain-white, atrophic, sclerotic patches — often with a wrinkled, cigarette-paper texture and follicular plugging that can mimic the ivory-white center of morphea. LS predominantly affects the anogenital region (vulvar LS in women, foreskin in uncircumcised men) but extragenital LS can affect the trunk and extremities — precisely the same sites as plaque morphea. Both conditions produce white, firm, atrophic skin, and both may coexist in the same patient (morphea with concurrent LS is well described).

Trap Logic: Mistaking extragenital lichen sclerosus for morphea (or vice versa) when both present as white, sclerotic, atrophic plaques on the trunk is the cognitive trap. The conditions have different depth of involvement (morphea extends deep into the dermis and subcutis; LS is confined to the superficial dermis), different histopathology (morphea shows dense collagen replacement of the full dermis; LS shows a band of homogenized, hyalinized collagen in the superficial dermis with a zone of follicular plugging), and different associations (LS — autoimmune thyroid disease, morphea — no consistent systemic association). The consequence of misdiagnosis is different treatment and different surveillance.

The Decision Anchor: The discriminating features are **depth of involvement (morphea is deep — firm, bound-down, extends to subcutis; LS is superficial — thin, wrinkled, confined to upper dermis), the lilac ring (active morphea shows a violaceous inflammatory border; LS does not), surface texture (LS has a cigarette-paper, crinkled texture with epidermal atrophy; morphea has a smooth, waxy surface), follicular plugging (more prominent in LS than in morphea), and histopathology (morphea — dense deep dermal sclerosis replacing fat; LS — superficial band of hyalinization with an underlying lymphocytic infiltrate)**. Both conditions are managed differently, and biopsy resolves ambiguous cases.

Evidence-Based Management: Topical, Systemic, and Biologic Therapies

Management of Cutaneous Lupus Erythematosus

Photoprotection is the foundation of CLE management — strict broad-spectrum (UVA and UVB) sunscreen use, sun-protective clothing, and ultraviolet avoidance reduce disease activity and prevent flares in all CLE subtypes. First-line pharmacologic therapy is topical corticosteroids (medium to high potency for body; low to medium potency for the face) and topical calcineurin inhibitors (tacrolimus, pimecrolimus — particularly useful on the face to avoid corticosteroid-induced atrophy). Antimalarials are the systemic backbone of CLE treatment: hydroxychloroquine is first-line systemic therapy for all CLE subtypes, with dose-related retinal toxicity requiring baseline and annual ophthalmologic screening (dose should not exceed 5 mg per kg actual body weight per day — confirm against current guidelines). For hydroxychloroquine-refractory CLE, options include adding quinacrine (which does not carry the retinal toxicity risk of hydroxychloroquine or chloroquine), methotrexate, mycophenolate mofetil, dapsone (particularly effective for bullous lupus), and thalidomide or lenalidomide (highly effective but with teratogenicity and neuropathy risks requiring strict risk management). Belimumab (anti-BAFF monoclonal antibody) and anifrolumab (anti-type I interferon receptor antibody) are approved for SLE and have demonstrated efficacy in improving cutaneous disease activity scores — anifrolumab has shown particular efficacy for active skin disease in SLE.

Management of Scleroderma Spectrum Disorders

For morphea, treatment depends on the subtype and extent. Plaque morphea is managed with potent topical corticosteroids, topical calcineurin inhibitors, or topical calcipotriol. Active, inflammatory morphea (lilac ring present) benefits from phototherapy (UVA1 phototherapy — the treatment of choice for morphea when available — penetrates to the deep dermis and subcutis, targeting fibrosis at its origin; narrowband UVB for superficial disease). Linear morphea in children and deep or generalized morphea require systemic therapy: methotrexate (with or without an initial course of systemic corticosteroids to halt disease progression) is the first-line systemic agent, with mycophenolate mofetil as a second-line alternative. For systemic sclerosis, management is organ-specific and multidisciplinary. Skin fibrosis is addressed with methotrexate (for early, progressive skin disease) and mycophenolate mofetil (which also treats SSc-ILD). Raynaud phenomenon requires calcium channel blockers (nifedipine, amlodipine) as first-line, with phosphodiesterase-5 inhibitors (sildenafil) and intravenous iloprost for severe disease. Pulmonary arterial hypertension requires pulmonary vasodilators (endothelin receptor antagonists, phosphodiesterase-5 inhibitors, prostacyclin analogues). Scleroderma renal crisis — a life-threatening emergency presenting with abrupt-onset severe hypertension, renal failure, and microangiopathic hemolytic anemia — is treated with ACE inhibitors (the only class shown to improve outcomes in renal crisis). Nintedanib and tocilizumab have emerged as treatment options for SSc-ILD based on clinical trial evidence (SENSCIS and focuSSced trials, respectively).

CAUTION: Anti-RNA polymerase III antibody-positive patients with diffuse systemic sclerosis carry a significant risk of scleroderma renal crisis — a hypertensive emergency that can cause rapid renal failure and microangiopathic hemolytic anemia. Corticosteroids in moderate-to-high doses (prednisone equivalent greater than 15 mg per day) are an independent risk factor for precipitating renal crisis in SSc and should be avoided in patients with diffuse disease whenever possible. If renal crisis occurs, ACE inhibitors (captopril) must be initiated immediately and continued even if renal function initially worsens — they are the only agents with proven mortality benefit in this setting.

EVIDENCE: The TULIP-1 and TULIP-2 trials demonstrated that anifrolumab (a monoclonal antibody targeting the type I interferon receptor subunit IFNAR1) significantly improved cutaneous lupus disease activity in patients with moderate-to-severe SLE. In TULIP-2, anifrolumab achieved a significantly higher BICLA response rate versus placebo at 52 weeks, with notable improvement in skin-specific endpoints (CLASI activity score). These results led to FDA approval of anifrolumab for SLE and positioned type I interferon pathway inhibition as a mechanism-based therapy particularly relevant to patients with prominent cutaneous disease, given that interferon-driven gene expression signatures are strongly associated with CLE activity.

Complications of Systemic Sclerosis

Calcinosis cutis — subcutaneous calcium deposits that form painful, hard nodules under the skin, most commonly on the fingers, forearms, elbows, and knees — is one of the most distressing and treatment-resistant complications of limited cutaneous SSc. The calcium deposits may ulcerate through the skin, producing chronic wounds susceptible to secondary infection and significant functional impairment of the hands. No consistently effective medical therapy exists for calcinosis; options with anecdotal or limited evidence include diltiazem, colchicine, minocycline, and sodium thiosulfate (topical or intralesional). Surgical excision is considered for symptomatic, localized deposits but recurrence is common. Digital ulcers — ischemic ulcers on the fingertips resulting from obliterative vasculopathy of the digital arteries — occur in approximately 50 percent of SSc patients and cause severe pain, tissue loss, and functional disability. Bosentan (an endothelin receptor antagonist) reduces the development of new digital ulcers in SSc. Iloprost (intravenous prostacyclin analogue) is used for active ischemic digital ulcers and critical digital ischemia refractory to calcium channel blockers.

CLINICAL PEARL: The lupus band test — direct immunofluorescence of non-lesional, sun-protected skin (typically the volar forearm) — is a useful diagnostic tool for distinguishing cutaneous-limited lupus from systemic disease. A positive lupus band (granular IgG, IgM, and C3 deposition at the dermoepidermal junction) in non-lesional skin is specific for SLE and indicates systemic immune complex deposition beyond the skin. In DLE without systemic disease, the lupus band is positive only in lesional skin. A positive band in non-lesional skin in a patient with otherwise skin-limited CLE should prompt comprehensive serologic and organ-targeted screening for evolving SLE.

Special Populations and Pregnancy Considerations

Lupus in pregnancy presents specific dermatologic concerns: anti-Ro/SSA antibody-positive women carry a risk of neonatal lupus in the offspring (characterized by transient annular skin lesions in the newborn and, in 2 percent of cases, permanent congenital complete heart block — fetal echocardiographic monitoring is recommended from 16 to 26 weeks of gestation). Hydroxychloroquine should be continued throughout pregnancy (it reduces the risk of lupus flares, and discontinuation during pregnancy increases flare risk). Pediatric morphea (linear morphea is the most common subtype in children) requires particular attention to growth disturbance — linear morphea crossing a joint or involving an extremity can cause limb-length discrepancy, contractures, and functional disability if fibrosis extends to fascia and muscle. Aggressive systemic therapy with methotrexate is indicated early in pediatric linear morphea to prevent irreversible skeletal complications. Drug-induced CLE — particularly drug-induced SCLE — is an important consideration: hydrochlorothiazide, terbinafine, proton pump inhibitors, TNF-alpha inhibitors, and checkpoint inhibitors (pembrolizumab, nivolumab) are common causes. Drug-induced SCLE typically resolves within weeks to months after the offending agent is discontinued, though some cases persist.

Patient Education and Counseling

Patient education is central to the management of lupus and scleroderma spectrum diseases because both are chronic conditions that require ongoing self-management. CLE patients must understand the critical role of photoprotection — strict, daily, broad-spectrum sunscreen use (SPF 30 or higher, reapplied every 2 hours during sun exposure), sun-protective clothing including wide-brimmed hats, and avoidance of peak ultraviolet hours. Patients should be counseled that window glass blocks UVB but transmits UVA, and that fluorescent lighting and some LED sources emit small amounts of UV that can trigger photosensitive CLE. The emotional impact of scarring CLE, particularly DLE causing facial dyspigmentation and scarring alopecia, requires acknowledgment and referral to dermatologic camouflage services and psychological support where indicated. Hydroxychloroquine counseling should address the importance of adherence (full therapeutic effect may take 2 to 3 months), the need for baseline and annual retinal screening (OCT and visual field testing), and the reassurance that at recommended doses retinal toxicity is rare in the first 5 years. SSc patients benefit from detailed counseling on Raynaud management (hand warming techniques, avoidance of cold exposure, smoking cessation as an absolute priority), skin care for sclerotic skin (emollients, gentle stretching exercises to maintain hand function and prevent contractures), and the rationale for ongoing organ surveillance — pulmonary function testing and echocardiography detect interstitial lung disease and pulmonary arterial hypertension at a stage where treatment can modify outcomes. Patients with morphea should be reassured that morphea does not evolve into systemic sclerosis, though they should understand that active disease (indicated by the lilac ring) warrants treatment to limit fibrosis before it becomes irreversible.

Clinical Case: Progressive Skin Tightening

A 48-year-old woman presents with a 6-month history of progressive skin tightening of the fingers, hands, and forearms, and a 3-year history of Raynaud phenomenon. On examination, the skin of the hands and fingers is taut, shiny, and indurated — the fingers are tapered (sclerodactyly) with limited flexion. Matte telangiectasias are present on the face and lips. Nailfold capillaroscopy reveals enlarged, giant capillaries with areas of capillary dropout — the active scleroderma pattern. The skin proximal to the elbows is normal. The modified Rodnan skin score is 12. Serologies reveal a positive ANA (1:640, centromere pattern) and positive anti-centromere antibody. Anti-Scl-70 and anti-RNA polymerase III are negative. Pulmonary function tests show a mildly reduced DLCO. Echocardiography is normal. The clinical and serologic picture is consistent with limited cutaneous systemic sclerosis (lcSSc). Management includes nifedipine for Raynaud phenomenon, proton pump inhibitor for esophageal reflux, and annual pulmonary function testing and echocardiography to screen for pulmonary arterial hypertension — the principal long-term risk in ACA-positive lcSSc. The patient is counseled that skin involvement in lcSSc is typically limited in extent and progresses slowly, but that ongoing organ surveillance is essential because pulmonary arterial hypertension may develop years after the initial presentation.

Discoid Lupus vs. Tinea Faciei: The discriminating features are follicular plugging and the carpet-tack sign (present in DLE, absent in tinea), central atrophic scarring (DLE scars, tinea does not), KOH preparation (positive in tinea, negative in DLE), and photodistribution (DLE follows sun-exposed sites, tinea does not). Cognitive trap: prescribing topical corticosteroids for an annular facial plaque without performing KOH — creating tinea incognito and delaying both diagnoses.

Morphea vs. Lichen Sclerosus: The discriminating features are depth of involvement (morphea is deep, firm, and bound-down; LS is superficial and thin), the lilac ring (active morphea only), surface texture (LS is wrinkled and cigarette-paper; morphea is waxy and smooth), follicular plugging (more prominent in LS), and histopathology (morphea — dense deep sclerosis; LS — superficial hyalinized band). The conditions can coexist, and biopsy resolves ambiguous cases.

Summary and Key Concepts

Cutaneous lupus erythematosus is classified into acute (malar rash — almost always accompanies SLE), subacute (annular-polycyclic or papulosquamous, strongly associated with anti-Ro/SSA, heals without scarring), and chronic (discoid — follicular plugging, scarring alopecia, dyspigmentation, 5 to 20 percent risk of SLE progression).

The 2019 EULAR/ACR SLE classification criteria weight mucocutaneous findings significantly: ACLE scores 6 points, SCLE/DLE scores 4 points, oral ulcers 2 points, and non-scarring alopecia 2 points. All CLE patients require baseline serologic screening (ANA, dsDNA, Ro/SSA, Smith, complement, CBC, urinalysis).

Systemic sclerosis is classified into limited (skin distal to elbows/knees, anti-centromere, PAH risk) and diffuse (proximal skin, anti-Scl-70, ILD and renal crisis risk). Nailfold capillaroscopy identifies the scleroderma pattern (giant capillaries, capillary loss, neoangiogenesis) and distinguishes SSc-Raynaud from primary Raynaud.

Morphea is a localized fibrotic disease distinct from systemic sclerosis. The lilac ring indicates active disease. UVA1 phototherapy is the treatment of choice; linear morphea in children requires systemic methotrexate to prevent growth disturbance.

CLE management is built on photoprotection, topical corticosteroids/calcineurin inhibitors, and hydroxychloroquine as systemic backbone. Anifrolumab (anti-IFNAR1) has demonstrated particular efficacy for cutaneous lupus activity. In SSc, organ-specific management includes methotrexate/mycophenolate for skin fibrosis and ILD, calcium channel blockers for Raynaud, and ACE inhibitors for scleroderma renal crisis.

CHAPTER 20: CUTANEOUS VASCULITIS AND VASCULAR DISORDERS

Learning Objectives

1. Classify cutaneous vasculitis by vessel size (small, medium, large) using the Chapel Hill Consensus nomenclature, correlate vessel caliber with clinical morphology, and distinguish primary cutaneous vasculitis from systemic vasculitis with skin involvement.
2. Recognize the clinical features, histopathologic findings, and systemic associations of leukocytoclastic vasculitis, IgA vasculitis, and cutaneous polyarteritis nodosa, and apply appropriate diagnostic workups for each.
3. Differentiate livedo reticularis from livedo racemosa, evaluate for antiphospholipid syndrome, and manage Raynaud phenomenon and digital ischemia using a stepwise pharmacologic approach.
4. Classify leg ulcers by etiology (venous, arterial, neuropathic, inflammatory), apply evidence-based wound care principles, and integrate compression therapy, debridement, and advanced wound care modalities.

Classification of Cutaneous Vasculitis: Small-Vessel, Medium-Vessel, and Large-Vessel

Definition and the Chapel Hill Consensus Nomenclature

Vasculitis is defined as inflammation and destruction of blood vessel walls. Cutaneous vasculitis may be a skin-limited process (primary cutaneous vasculitis) or the cutaneous manifestation of systemic vasculitis. The revised Chapel Hill Consensus Conference (CHCC 2012) nomenclature classifies vasculitis by the caliber of the predominantly affected vessels: small-vessel vasculitis (arterioles, venules, capillaries), medium-vessel vasculitis (medium-sized muscular arteries), and large-vessel vasculitis (aorta and major branches). This vessel-size classification has direct clinical relevance because the size of the affected vessel determines the clinical morphology of the skin lesion. Small-vessel vasculitis produces palpable purpura — the hallmark lesion — because extravasation of red blood cells from damaged postcapillary venules creates non-blanching, elevated, purpuric papules. Medium-vessel vasculitis produces livedo reticularis, nodules, ulcers, and digital gangrene because inflammation of deeper muscular arteries causes tissue ischemia. Large-vessel vasculitis rarely produces primary skin lesions but may cause limb ischemia, absent pulses, or secondary ischemic skin changes.

Epidemiology and Etiology

Cutaneous small-vessel vasculitis (CSVV) is the most common form of skin vasculitis, with an estimated annual incidence of 15 to 30 per million. Identifiable triggers are found in approximately 50 percent of cases and include infections (upper respiratory tract infections, hepatitis B and C, HIV, streptococcal pharyngitis), medications (beta-lactam antibiotics, NSAIDs, thiazides, allopurinol, sulfonamides), autoimmune diseases (SLE, rheumatoid arthritis, Sjogren syndrome, inflammatory bowel disease), and malignancy (particularly hematologic malignancies). In 50 percent of cases, no trigger is identified (idiopathic CSVV). The typical clinical course of idiopathic CSVV is self-limited — resolving within 2 to 4 weeks — though post-inflammatory hyperpigmentation may persist for months. Chronic or recurrent CSVV should prompt re-evaluation for an underlying cause, particularly occult connective tissue disease, chronic infection, or malignancy.

Pathophysiology

The pathogenesis of most small-vessel vasculitis involves immune complex deposition in postcapillary venule walls (type III hypersensitivity — Arthus reaction). Circulating antigen-antibody complexes lodge in vessel walls, activate complement (C3a, C5a), recruit neutrophils, and trigger neutrophil degranulation with release of lysosomal enzymes that destroy the vessel wall — a process called leukocytoclasis (fragmentation of neutrophil nuclei into nuclear dust). The damaged vessel walls become permeable, allowing extravasation of red blood cells into the surrounding dermis — producing the clinically visible purpura. IgA-dominant immune complex deposition defines IgA vasculitis (Henoch-Schönlein purpura). ANCA-associated vasculitis (granulomatosis with polyangiitis, microscopic polyangiitis, eosinophilic granulomatosis with polyangiitis) operates through a different mechanism: ANCA antibodies (anti-PR3, anti-MPO) directly activate neutrophils, which adhere to and damage vessel walls without immune complex deposition — this is pauci-immune vasculitis (few or no immune deposits on DIF).

Leukocytoclastic Vasculitis and IgA Vasculitis (Henoch-Schönlein Purpura)

Clinical Features of Leukocytoclastic Vasculitis

Leukocytoclastic vasculitis (LCV) — also called cutaneous small-vessel vasculitis — presents as palpable purpura: crops of non-blanching, erythematous-to-violaceous papules ranging from 1 to 3 mm. The lesions are symmetric, gravity-dependent, and concentrated on the lower extremities (ankles, shins, calves) because hydrostatic pressure promotes immune complex deposition in dependent vessels. In ambulatory patients, the lower legs are predominantly affected; in bedridden patients, the buttocks and dependent surfaces are involved. Individual lesions evolve over 24 to 48 hours from initially blanching erythematous papules to non-blanching palpable purpura, and may progress to vesicles, bullae, pustules, or necrotic ulcers in severe cases. Associated symptoms include low-grade fever, arthralgias, and myalgias. The key diagnostic principle is timing: biopsy should be performed on a lesion 24 to 48 hours old for optimal histopathologic yield — early lesions show neutrophilic infiltration and leukocytoclasis; late lesions show lymphocytic infiltration and may be misinterpreted as a lymphocytic vasculitis.

IgA Vasculitis: Clinical Spectrum and Systemic Involvement

IgA vasculitis (IgAV, formerly Henoch-Schönlein purpura) is the most common vasculitis of childhood, with a peak incidence between ages 3 and 10 years. The classic tetrad is palpable purpura (100 percent — typically on the buttocks and lower extremities in children), arthritis or arthralgias (60 to 80 percent — large joints, migratory, non-deforming), gastrointestinal involvement (50 to 75 percent — colicky abdominal pain, GI bleeding, intussusception), and renal involvement (20 to 50 percent — hematuria, proteinuria, IgA nephropathy). IgAV in children is usually self-limited and resolves within 4 to 6 weeks, though recurrences occur in 30 to 40 percent. The principal prognostic concern is renal involvement: most children recover completely, but 1 to 5 percent develop chronic kidney disease. IgAV in adults is less common but more severe — adults have a higher rate of renal involvement (50 to 80 percent), a higher incidence of renal impairment, and a more prolonged course. Urinalysis monitoring for proteinuria and hematuria should continue for 6 months after resolution of skin lesions.

KEY POINT: The diagnosis of IgA vasculitis requires demonstration of IgA-dominant immune deposits in vessel walls on direct immunofluorescence (DIF) of a skin biopsy. While the clinical tetrad (purpura, arthritis, GI involvement, nephritis) is often sufficient for clinical diagnosis in children, DIF-confirmed IgA deposition is the definitive diagnostic criterion and is essential in adults, where the differential diagnosis of palpable purpura is broader (LCV, cryoglobulinemic vasculitis, ANCA-associated vasculitis). DIF should be performed on a lesion less than 24 hours old for optimal sensitivity, as IgA deposits may be cleared by the time late lesions are biopsied.

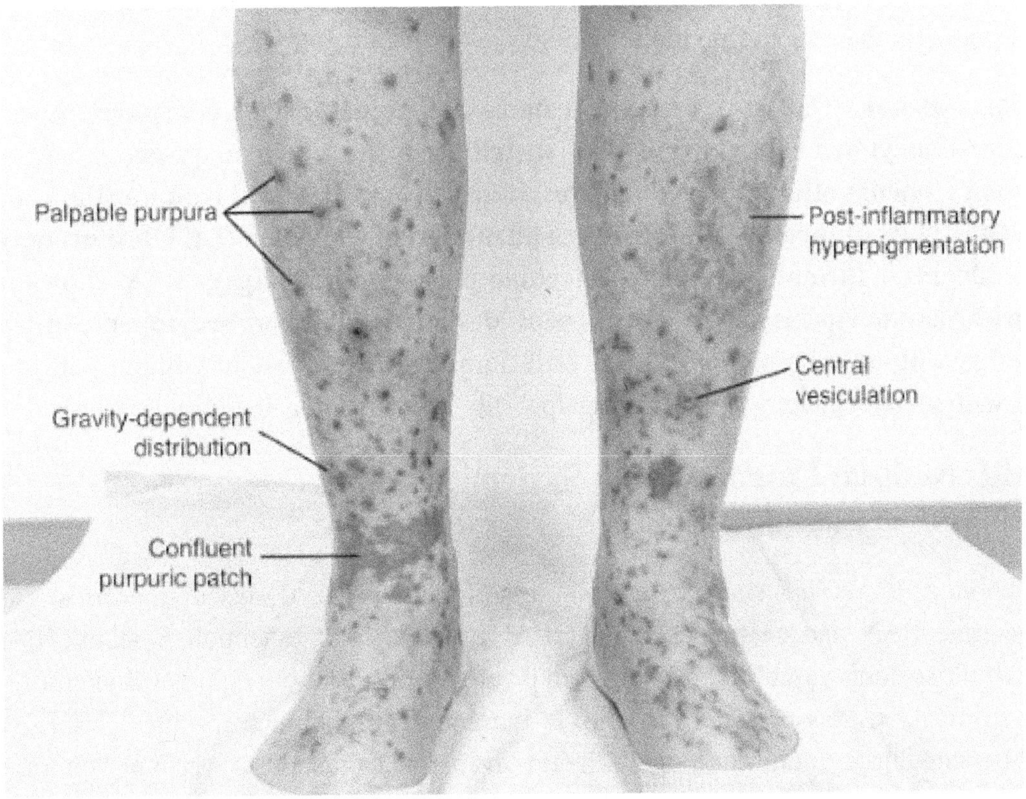

THE CUTANEOUS MIMICKER RECOGNITION ATLAS — Palpable Purpura (LCV) versus Thrombocytopenic Purpura

The Clinical Pattern: Palpable purpura of leukocytoclastic vasculitis presents as raised, non-blanching, erythematous-to-violaceous papules on the lower extremities. The lesions are palpable because the inflammatory infiltrate and extravasated blood cells create tissue swelling around the damaged vessel walls. The distribution is symmetric and gravity-dependent (ankles, shins, calves). Individual lesions may progress to vesicles, bullae, or necrotic ulcers, reflecting the severity of vessel wall damage.

The Mimicker: Thrombocytopenic purpura (from immune thrombocytopenia, bone marrow failure, DIC, or TTP/HUS) produces non-blanching purpura that is flat (non-palpable). Petechiae (pinpoint, less than 2 mm) and ecchymoses (larger areas of bruising) appear on dependent areas and sites of trauma but can also involve mucous membranes (oral, conjunctival). Thrombocytopenic purpura reflects a bleeding diathesis from low platelet count or function — NOT vessel wall inflammation. The lesions are flat because there is no perivascular inflammatory infiltrate.

Trap Logic: Attributing flat purpura to vasculitis without checking a platelet count delays recognition of potentially life-threatening thrombocytopenia (TTP, DIC, hematologic malignancy). Conversely, **assuming all purpura is thrombocytopenic and checking only a CBC without biopsy** misses vasculitis entirely — platelet counts are normal in LCV. The physical examination distinction between palpable (raised, indicating vasculitis) and non-palpable (flat, indicating coagulopathy or thrombocytopenia) is the critical first branch point.

The Decision Anchor: The discriminating features are **palpability (LCV purpura is raised and palpable; thrombocytopenic purpura is flat), distribution (LCV is gravity-dependent on the lower legs; thrombocytopenia affects dependent sites, mucosal surfaces, and trauma sites), platelet count (normal in LCV; low in thrombocytopenic purpura), lesion evolution (LCV lesions may vesiculate, necrose, or ulcerate; thrombocytopenic petechiae do not), and biopsy (LCV shows neutrophilic infiltrate with leukocytoclasis and vessel wall destruction; thrombocytopenic purpura shows extravasated red blood cells without vessel wall damage)**. Every patient with purpura should receive both a CBC with platelet count and a clinical palpability assessment as the initial triage.

Polyarteritis Nodosa: Cutaneous and Systemic Forms

Clinical Features and Pathophysiology

Polyarteritis nodosa (PAN) is a necrotizing vasculitis of medium-sized muscular arteries. The distinction between systemic PAN and cutaneous PAN (cPAN) is clinically essential. Systemic PAN is a life-threatening multisystem vasculitis causing renal infarction (without glomerulonephritis — a key distinction from ANCA-associated vasculitis), mesenteric ischemia, coronary arteritis, peripheral neuropathy (mononeuritis multiplex), and skin involvement. Cutaneous PAN is a benign, skin-limited form presenting with painful, subcutaneous nodules (1 to 2 cm) along the course of arteries — most commonly on the lower legs — accompanied by livedo reticularis and, in some cases, ulceration at the site of skin infarction. Cutaneous PAN does not progress to systemic PAN, though mild extracutaneous features (arthralgias, myalgias, peripheral neuropathy) may occur. The association between PAN and hepatitis B has declined with widespread vaccination, though hepatitis B serology should still be checked in all PAN patients.

Histopathology and Diagnostic Workup

Histopathology of PAN shows fibrinoid necrosis of the media of medium-sized muscular arteries with a mixed inflammatory infiltrate (neutrophils predominating in acute lesions, lymphocytes and macrophages in chronic lesions). The inflammation is segmental (affecting part of the vessel circumference) and transmural (extending through all vessel wall layers). Aneurysm formation at the site of vessel wall destruction is characteristic and may be visualized on CT angiography or conventional angiography (microaneurysms of renal, mesenteric, or hepatic arteries are virtually diagnostic of systemic PAN). Importantly, PAN is ANCA-negative — a positive ANCA (anti-PR3 or anti-MPO) should redirect the diagnosis toward granulomatosis with polyangiitis or microscopic polyangiitis. Biopsy of a subcutaneous nodule in cutaneous PAN should be deep (incisional or excisional) to sample the medium-sized arteries at the dermal-subcutaneous junction — superficial punch biopsies miss the affected vessels.

CLINICAL PEARL: Cryoglobulinemia should be considered in any patient presenting with palpable purpura, particularly when associated with arthralgias, peripheral neuropathy, and renal dysfunction. Type II mixed cryoglobulinemia (monoclonal IgM with rheumatoid factor activity against polyclonal IgG) is strongly associated with hepatitis C infection — HCV drives B-cell lymphoproliferation producing the monoclonal IgM. The cryoglobulins precipitate in cold-dependent dermal vessels, activating complement and causing immune complex vasculitis. Diagnosis requires proper specimen handling: blood must be drawn in a warm tube, transported at 37 degrees Celsius, and allowed to clot at 37 degrees before refrigeration to allow cryoprecipitate formation. Improper cold-chain handling produces false-negative results. Treatment targets the underlying HCV (direct-acting antivirals) and the B-cell clone (rituximab for severe disease).

Livedo Reticularis, Livedoid Vasculopathy, and Antiphospholipid Syndrome

Livedo Reticularis Versus Livedo Racemosa

Livedo reticularis is a net-like, violaceous, reticular (mesh-shaped) mottling of the skin caused by reduced blood flow in the dermal venous plexus. Physiologic livedo reticularis (cutis marmorata) is a benign, symmetric, regular, reversible pattern seen in cold environments or in infants — it resolves with warming and requires no workup. Pathologic livedo is persistent, asymmetric, and irregular in pattern and is called livedo racemosa — broken, branching, irregular, open-ended rings (unlike the closed, regular rings of physiologic livedo). Livedo racemosa suggests an underlying vasculopathy or vasculitis and warrants evaluation for antiphospholipid syndrome (APS), Sneddon syndrome (livedo racemosa with stroke), cholesterol crystal embolization, cryoglobulinemia, systemic vasculitis (PAN, SLE), and hypercoagulable states.

Antiphospholipid Syndrome and Livedoid Vasculopathy

Antiphospholipid syndrome (APS) is a prothrombotic autoimmune disorder defined by the combination of thrombotic events (arterial or venous thrombosis) or pregnancy morbidity (recurrent miscarriage, preeclampsia, intrauterine growth restriction) with persistently positive antiphospholipid antibodies (lupus anticoagulant, anticardiolipin antibodies, anti-beta2-glycoprotein I antibodies — positive on two occasions at least 12 weeks apart). Cutaneous manifestations of APS include livedo racemosa (the most common skin finding), skin necrosis and ulceration, digital gangrene, splinter hemorrhages, and superficial thrombophlebitis. Catastrophic APS (CAPS) is a rare, life-threatening variant with simultaneous multiorgan thrombosis occurring over days. Livedoid vasculopathy is a distinct thrombotic disorder (not a true vasculitis) presenting as painful, recurrent, punched-out ulcers on the lower legs and ankles that heal with characteristic porcelain-white stellate scars (atrophie blanche). Histopathology shows thrombosis of dermal vessels with hyalinization of the vessel walls — no vasculitis. Treatment is anticoagulation (rivaroxaban, warfarin) or antiplatelet therapy, not immunosuppression.

Raynaud Phenomenon and Digital Ischemia

Primary Versus Secondary Raynaud

Raynaud phenomenon is episodic, reversible digital vasospasm producing the classic triphasic color change: white (pallor — vasospasm and ischemia), blue (cyanosis — deoxygenation of stagnant blood), and red (rubor — reactive hyperemia on reperfusion). Primary Raynaud (Raynaud disease) occurs without an underlying cause, typically begins before age 30, is symmetric, and has normal nailfold capillaroscopy and negative autoantibodies. Secondary Raynaud occurs in the setting of connective tissue disease (SSc in particular — Raynaud is the most common initial symptom of SSc, preceding skin fibrosis by years), atherosclerosis, thoracic outlet syndrome, or medication/drug use (beta-blockers, ergotamines, stimulants, vinyl chloride exposure). The critical distinction between primary and secondary Raynaud is made by nailfold capillaroscopy (abnormal scleroderma pattern in SSc-associated Raynaud), autoantibody testing (ANA, anti-centromere, anti-Scl-70), and clinical assessment for digital pitting scars, skin sclerosis, or ulceration. Secondary Raynaud may progress to critical digital ischemia with ulceration and acral gangrene — a vascular emergency.

Management of Raynaud and Digital Ischemia

First-line management of Raynaud includes behavioral measures (hand warming, avoiding cold exposure, smoking cessation) and pharmacotherapy with dihydropyridine calcium channel blockers (nifedipine extended-release or amlodipine). For refractory Raynaud, phosphodiesterase-5 inhibitors (sildenafil, tadalafil) provide additional vasodilation and are used as second-line agents. Topical nitroglycerin applied to the digits may provide local vasodilation but is limited by headache. For severe Raynaud with digital ulceration, intravenous iloprost (a prostacyclin analogue) promotes vasodilation and platelet inhibition. Bosentan (an endothelin receptor antagonist) is approved for the prevention of new digital ulcers in SSc. Sympathectomy (chemical or surgical) of the digital arteries is reserved for severe, refractory cases with impending tissue loss.

Leg Ulcers: Venous, Arterial, Neuropathic, and Inflammatory Etiologies

Classification and Clinical Features

Leg ulcers affect approximately 1 to 2 percent of the adult population and carry significant morbidity. Venous ulcers (70 to 80 percent of all leg ulcers) result from chronic venous insufficiency with sustained venous hypertension. They are characteristically located on the medial malleolus (gaiter area), have irregular, shallow margins with a fibrinous or granulating base, and are associated with surrounding venous stasis changes: hemosiderin deposition (brawny brownish discoloration), lipodermatosclerosis (fibrosis of subcutaneous fat producing an inverted champagne-bottle leg contour), stasis dermatitis (pruritic, eczematous changes), and varicose veins. Arterial ulcers (10 to 15 percent) result from peripheral arterial disease. They are located on the toes, foot, and lateral malleolus (distal territory of the affected artery), have punched-out margins with a pale, necrotic base, and are painful — particularly with leg elevation (relieved by dependency). The foot is cool, hairless, and pale, with diminished or absent pulses. The ankle-brachial index (ABI — ratio of ankle systolic pressure to brachial systolic pressure) is the key diagnostic test: ABI less than 0.9 indicates PAD, and ABI less than 0.5 indicates critical limb ischemia. Neuropathic ulcers (diabetic foot ulcers) occur at pressure points on the plantar foot (metatarsal heads, heel), are painless (due to peripheral neuropathy), and develop because the loss of protective sensation allows repetitive trauma to go undetected. Inflammatory ulcers (pyoderma gangrenosum, vasculitic ulcers, livedoid vasculopathy) have distinct morphologies and are treated with immunosuppression rather than wound care alone.

Ulcer Type	Location	Morphology	Key Clinical Features	Diagnostic Test
Venous	Medial malleolus (gaiter area)	Shallow, irregular margins, granulating or fibrinous base	Hemosiderin, lipodermatosclerosis, stasis dermatitis, varicosities; pain relieved by elevation	Duplex ultrasound for venous reflux; ABI greater than 0.8 confirms safe for compression
Arterial	Toes, foot, lateral malleolus	Punched-out, pale necrotic base, well-defined margins	Cool foot, absent pulses, pallor on elevation, dependent rubor; pain worsened by elevation	ABI less than 0.9 indicates PAD; less than 0.5 critical ischemia; angiography for revascularization planning
Neuropathic	Plantar pressure points (metatarsal heads, heel)	Punched-out, surrounded by callus, may have sinus tract	Painless (peripheral neuropathy), loss of protective	Monofilament testing (5.07 Semmes-Weinstein); tuning fork

			sensation, associated with diabetes	vibration; HbA1c
Pyoderma gangrenosum	Lower legs, peristomal	Violaceous undermined borders, cribriform or necrotic base	Pathergy (worsens with debridement), severe pain; associated with IBD, RA, hematologic malignancy	Biopsy (neutrophilic dermatosis, no vasculitis); diagnosis of exclusion — rule out infection
Livedoid vasculopathy	Lower legs, ankles	Punched-out, painful; heals with porcelain-white stellate scars (atrophie blanche)	Livedo racemosa, recurrent; thrombotic — not inflammatory; mostly young women	Biopsy: thrombosis and hyalinization without vasculitis; coagulation workup

Differential Diagnosis of Leg Ulcers

The location, morphology, and associated signs reliably distinguish ulcer etiology in most cases. Pyoderma gangrenosum (PG) presents as a rapidly enlarging ulcer with violaceous, undermined borders and a cribriform or necrotic base — classically on the lower leg or peristomal skin. PG demonstrates pathergy (worsening of the ulcer after surgical debridement or trauma — a critical clinical trap, as debridement is the standard wound care approach for most ulcers but exacerbates PG). PG is associated with inflammatory bowel disease, rheumatoid arthritis, and hematologic malignancy. Martorell hypertensive ischemic ulcer (MHIU) occurs in patients with poorly controlled hypertension and diabetes, presenting as exquisitely painful ulcers on the posterolateral or anterolateral lower leg — a location that distinguishes it from venous ulcers (medial malleolus). Histopathology shows arteriolosclerosis and thrombosis of subcutaneous arterioles.

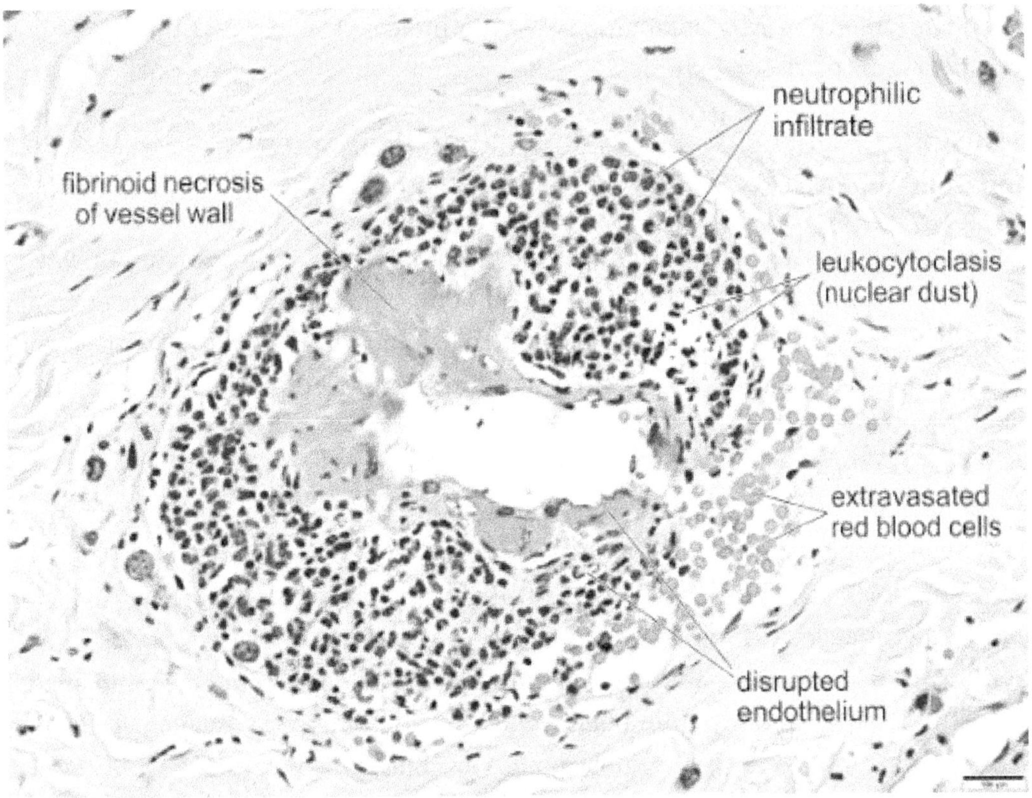

Diagnostic Approach: Biopsy, Serology, and Imaging

Biopsy Technique and Timing

Skin biopsy is essential for the definitive diagnosis of cutaneous vasculitis. The optimal biopsy technique and timing depend on the suspected diagnosis. For small-vessel vasculitis, a punch biopsy (4 mm) of a lesion 24 to 48 hours old is ideal — it captures the diagnostic neutrophilic infiltrate with leukocytoclasis and fibrinoid necrosis of postcapillary venules. Biopsies of lesions older than 48 hours show a lymphocytic infiltrate and may lack the diagnostic neutrophilic features. A second biopsy from an early lesion (less than 24 hours old) should be sent for direct immunofluorescence (DIF) — IgA-dominant vessel wall deposits confirm IgA vasculitis, while IgG/IgM/C3 deposition suggests immune complex vasculitis. For medium-vessel vasculitis (suspected PAN), deep incisional or excisional biopsy is required to sample the medium-sized arteries at the dermal-subcutaneous junction — superficial punch biopsies do not reach these vessels.

Serologic and Systemic Workup

The serologic workup for cutaneous vasculitis is guided by the clinical presentation and vessel size. A standard panel includes complete blood count, comprehensive metabolic panel (renal and hepatic function), urinalysis (to detect renal vasculitis), erythrocyte sedimentation rate and C-reactive protein, complement levels (C3, C4 — low in SLE, cryoglobulinemia, hypocomplementemic urticarial vasculitis), ANA, ANCA (anti-PR3, anti-MPO), cryoglobulins (draw in a warm tube and transport at 37 degrees Celsius), hepatitis B and C serologies, and antiphospholipid antibodies (for livedo racemosa). Imaging studies — CT angiography or MR angiography — are indicated when systemic PAN is suspected, to identify microaneurysms of visceral arteries.

Evidence-Based Management and Wound Care Principles

Special Populations and ANCA-Associated Vasculitis

ANCA-associated vasculitis (AAV) — comprising granulomatosis with polyangiitis (GPA, formerly Wegener), microscopic polyangiitis (MPA), and eosinophilic granulomatosis with polyangiitis (EGPA, formerly Churg-Strauss) — may present with cutaneous findings that overlap with isolated cutaneous small-vessel vasculitis. GPA produces palpable purpura, papulonecrotic lesions (papules with central necrosis), pyoderma gangrenosum-like ulcers, and strawberry gingival hyperplasia — coupled with anti-PR3 (c-ANCA) positivity and upper and lower respiratory tract involvement (saddle-nose deformity, pulmonary nodules, cavitary lesions). MPA produces palpable purpura and livedo with anti-MPO (p-ANCA) positivity and rapidly progressive glomerulonephritis. EGPA presents with palpable purpura and extravascular granulomas in a patient with adult-onset asthma, peripheral eosinophilia, and eosinophilic tissue infiltration. The cutaneous findings of AAV are not specific — they overlap with idiopathic CSVV — and ANCA testing is essential for any patient with palpable purpura accompanied by systemic symptoms (constitutional symptoms, pulmonary, renal, or neurologic involvement). Pediatric vasculitis presents its own spectrum: IgAV is the most common childhood vasculitis, while Kawasaki disease (medium-vessel vasculitis with coronary artery aneurysm risk) presents with fever, polymorphous rash, conjunctival injection, strawberry tongue, cervical lymphadenopathy, and palmar/plantar erythema with desquamation — requiring urgent echocardiography and intravenous immunoglobulin therapy.

Urticarial Vasculitis

Urticarial vasculitis is an important mimicker of chronic spontaneous urticaria. While both present with urticarial wheals, urticarial vasculitis is distinguished by lesions that persist in the same location for more than 24 hours (ordinary urticaria resolves within 24 hours and migrates), leave residual purpura or hemosiderin staining after resolution (ordinary urticaria resolves without a trace), are painful or burning rather than pruritic, and show leukocytoclastic vasculitis on biopsy (ordinary urticaria shows dermal edema without vessel wall damage). Urticarial vasculitis may be normocomplementemic (generally benign, skin-limited) or hypocomplementemic (hypocomplementemic urticarial vasculitis syndrome — HUVS — associated with SLE, anti-C1q antibodies, and systemic involvement including glomerulonephritis, obstructive pulmonary disease, and ocular inflammation). HUVS requires systemic immunosuppression and carries a more guarded prognosis.

Management of Cutaneous Vasculitis

For idiopathic cutaneous small-vessel vasculitis with no systemic involvement, management is supportive: leg elevation, compression stockings, NSAIDs for arthralgias, and observation (most episodes resolve within 2 to 4 weeks). Identification and removal of the offending trigger (medication, infection) is the most important intervention. For chronic or recurrent CSVV, colchicine and dapsone are first-line steroid-sparing agents. Systemic corticosteroids may be used for severe or rapidly progressive cutaneous vasculitis but should be tapered promptly to avoid rebound. For ANCA-associated vasculitis with systemic involvement, rituximab or cyclophosphamide with corticosteroids is the standard induction regimen, with azathioprine or rituximab for maintenance. Avacopan (a complement C5a receptor inhibitor) has been approved as an adjunctive therapy for ANCA-associated vasculitis based on the ADVOCATE trial, reducing corticosteroid exposure.

Wound Care for Leg Ulcers

Venous ulcer management is built on compression therapy — sustained graduated compression (30 to 40 mmHg at the ankle) is the single most important intervention and must be applied consistently to achieve healing. Compression is delivered via multilayer compression bandaging (for active ulceration) or compression stockings (for healed ulcers — lifelong to prevent recurrence). Wound bed preparation follows the TIME framework: Tissue management (debridement of non-viable tissue — sharp, enzymatic, or autolytic), Infection and inflammation control (topical antiseptics for biofilm, systemic antibiotics only for clinical infection with spreading cellulitis), Moisture balance (moist wound healing with appropriate dressings — foam, alginate, hydrofiber for exudative wounds; hydrogel for dry wounds), and Edge advancement (monitoring for epithelial migration from wound edges as a marker of healing). Arterial ulcers require vascular assessment (ABI, duplex ultrasonography, angiography) and revascularization (endovascular or surgical) before wound healing can be achieved — compression is contraindicated in arterial insufficiency (ABI less than 0.5). Neuropathic (diabetic) ulcers require offloading (total contact casting or removable cast walkers), glycemic optimization, and multidisciplinary foot care.

CAUTION: Pyoderma gangrenosum demonstrates pathergy — the ulcer worsens with surgical debridement, incision, or trauma. Because debridement is standard wound care for most ulcers, clinicians who do not recognize PG may inadvertently cause dramatic ulcer expansion. Any rapidly enlarging ulcer with violaceous, undermined borders — particularly in a patient with IBD, rheumatoid arthritis, or hematologic malignancy — should prompt consideration of PG before debridement is performed. PG is a diagnosis of exclusion confirmed by clinical pattern and biopsy (neutrophilic dermatosis without infection); treatment is immunosuppression (systemic corticosteroids, cyclosporine, biologics), not wound care alone.

EVIDENCE: The ADVOCATE trial demonstrated that avacopan (a selective complement C5a receptor inhibitor) was non-inferior to prednisone taper for induction of remission in ANCA-associated vasculitis and was superior for sustained remission at 52 weeks. Avacopan significantly reduced glucocorticoid exposure and its associated side effects (weight gain, glucose intolerance, osteoporosis, infection). These results positioned complement inhibition as a mechanism-based strategy for reducing corticosteroid dependence in ANCA-associated vasculitis — a disease historically treated with prolonged high-dose glucocorticoids carrying substantial cumulative toxicity.

THE CUTANEOUS MIMICKER RECOGNITION ATLAS — Venous Ulcer versus Pyoderma Gangrenosum

The Clinical Pattern: Venous ulcers are located on the medial malleolus (gaiter area), have irregular, shallow margins with a granulating or fibrinous base, and are surrounded by venous stasis changes: hemosiderin staining (brawny discoloration), lipodermatosclerosis (firm, fibrotic subcutaneous tissue producing an inverted champagne-bottle contour), and stasis dermatitis. Pain is typically mild and improves with leg elevation and compression.

The Mimicker: Pyoderma gangrenosum can present on the lower legs — the same location as venous ulcers — but has violaceous, undermined, overhanging borders with a cribriform (sieve-like) or necrotic base. The surrounding skin may show pustules at the advancing edge. PG is markedly painful (often out of proportion to ulcer size) and worsens with surgical debridement (pathergy). PG is associated with IBD, RA, and hematologic malignancy.

Trap Logic: Debriding a pyoderma gangrenosum ulcer because it looks like a venous ulcer that needs wound bed preparation is the catastrophic trap. Standard wound care debridement of PG triggers pathergy — explosive ulcer expansion that worsens the tissue loss. The reverse trap — refusing to debride an infected venous ulcer because of fear of PG — allows infection to propagate. The key is recognizing the violaceous, undermined border morphology of PG (venous ulcers have flat, irregular margins without undermining) and performing biopsy before debridement when PG is in the differential.

The Decision Anchor: The discriminating features are **border morphology (PG — violaceous, undermined, overhanging; venous ulcer — flat, irregular, not undermined), surrounding skin (venous ulcer — hemosiderin, lipodermatosclerosis, stasis dermatitis; PG — pustules, pathergy sites), pain character (PG — severe, out of proportion; venous — mild, improved by elevation), response to debridement (PG — pathergy/worsening; venous — healing), and systemic associations (PG — IBD, RA, hematologic malignancy; venous — venous insufficiency, varicosities, DVT history)**. Biopsy before debridement is mandatory when the clinical picture suggests PG.

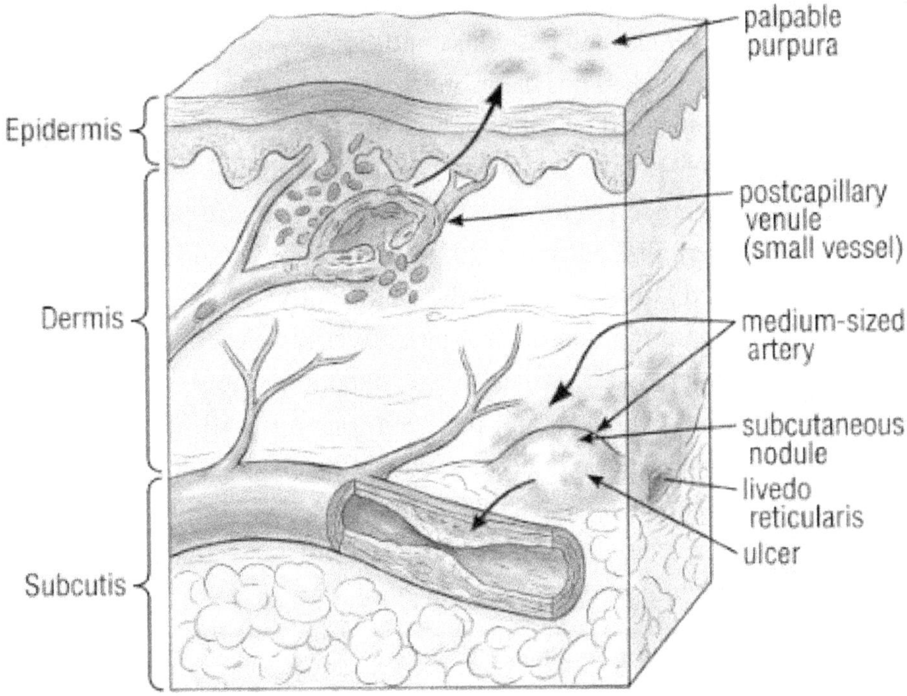

Complications and Prognosis

Chronic venous insufficiency producing recurrent venous ulcers carries significant long-term morbidity. Post-thrombotic syndrome (PTS) — the chronic sequelae of deep venous thrombosis — causes persistent venous hypertension with pain, edema, skin changes, and recurrent ulceration in 20 to 50 percent of DVT patients. Prevention of PTS focuses on adequate anticoagulation duration and early mobilization after DVT. Lipodermatosclerosis, once established, is irreversible — the fibrotic subcutaneous tissue creates a rigid cuff that impairs venous return and predisposes to recurrent ulceration. Secondary lymphedema may develop in the affected limb due to chronic inflammation and fibrosis of lymphatic channels. Arterial ulcers in the setting of critical limb ischemia (ABI less than 0.5) carry a risk of progressive tissue loss, gangrene, and amputation if revascularization is not achieved. Systemic vasculitis with cutaneous involvement (ANCA-associated vasculitis, systemic PAN) requires aggressive immunosuppression and carries long-term risks of treatment-related toxicity (corticosteroid side effects, cyclophosphamide-associated malignancy, infection from immunosuppression) balanced against the risk of uncontrolled vasculitis causing organ damage.

Patient Education and Self-Management

Patient education is essential for chronic vascular conditions. Venous ulcer patients must understand that compression therapy is not optional — it is the primary therapeutic intervention, and adherence determines healing. Patients should be counseled on proper application of compression stockings, the importance of replacing stockings every 3 to 6 months as elasticity decreases, and the need for lifelong compression after ulcer healing to prevent recurrence (recurrence rate without compression exceeds 70 percent within 12 months). Raynaud patients benefit from practical advice on cold avoidance strategies: layered clothing, chemical hand warmers, heated gloves, warming the whole body (not just the hands) before cold exposure, and absolute avoidance of smoking (nicotine is a potent vasoconstrictor that directly worsens Raynaud). Patients with antiphospholipid syndrome require education about thrombosis warning signs, the importance of anticoagulation adherence, and the need to inform all healthcare providers of their APS status before any surgical procedure. Wound care education for leg ulcer patients includes recognizing signs of wound infection (increasing pain, erythema, purulent discharge, fever), understanding the expected timeline for healing (venous ulcers typically require 12 to 24 weeks for complete healing with optimal compression), and the importance of leg elevation during rest.

Clinical Case: Recurrent Painful Leg Ulcers

A 38-year-old woman with a history of ulcerative colitis presents with a 3-week history of a rapidly enlarging, painful ulcer on the left anterior shin. The ulcer began as a small pustule after minor trauma (bumping her leg on a table) and has expanded rapidly to 6 cm despite oral antibiotics prescribed by her primary care physician. On examination, the ulcer has violaceous, undermined, overhanging borders with a necrotic base. Several satellite pustules are present at the advancing edge. The surrounding skin is erythematous and exquisitely tender. There are no signs of venous insufficiency (no hemosiderin, no lipodermatosclerosis, no varicosities). The clinical presentation — rapidly expanding ulcer with undermined violaceous borders, history of pathergy, underlying IBD — is highly suggestive of pyoderma gangrenosum. Punch biopsy from the ulcer edge shows a dense neutrophilic infiltrate without vasculitis, consistent with neutrophilic dermatosis. Tissue culture and special stains are negative for infection. The patient is started on systemic corticosteroids with rapid clinical improvement — the ulcer border flattens, pain decreases, and expansion arrests within 72 hours. Cyclosporine is initiated as a steroid-sparing agent for long-term maintenance. This case illustrates the importance of recognizing PG before debridement is attempted — the enlargement after initial trauma represents pathergy, and standard wound debridement would have caused further expansion.

Palpable Purpura (LCV) vs. Thrombocytopenic Purpura: The discriminating features are palpability (LCV is raised; thrombocytopenic is flat), distribution (LCV is gravity-dependent on the legs; thrombocytopenia involves mucosal surfaces and trauma sites), platelet count (normal in LCV; low in thrombocytopenia), lesion evolution (LCV may vesiculate or ulcerate; petechiae do not), and biopsy (LCV shows vessel wall destruction with leukocytoclasis; thrombocytopenic purpura shows extravasation without vessel damage). Cognitive trap: attributing flat purpura to vasculitis without checking a platelet count.

Venous Ulcer vs. Pyoderma Gangrenosum: The discriminating features are border morphology (PG is undermined and violaceous; venous is flat and irregular), surrounding skin (venous shows hemosiderin and stasis changes; PG shows satellite pustules), pain character (PG is severe and disproportionate; venous is mild), pathergy (PG worsens with debridement; venous improves), and associations (PG with IBD/RA/malignancy; venous with venous insufficiency). Cognitive trap: debriding a PG ulcer because it looks like a wound care case — pathergy causes explosive expansion.

Summary and Key Concepts

Cutaneous vasculitis is classified by vessel size: small-vessel vasculitis (postcapillary venules) produces palpable purpura, medium-vessel vasculitis (muscular arteries) produces nodules, livedo, and ulcers. Biopsy timing is critical — 24 to 48 hours old for H&E, less than 24 hours for DIF.

IgA vasculitis is the most common vasculitis of childhood, defined by IgA-dominant immune deposits on DIF. The classic tetrad is purpura, arthritis, GI involvement, and nephritis. Adult IgAV is more severe with higher rates of renal involvement. Urinalysis monitoring should continue for 6 months after skin resolution.

Livedo racemosa (pathologic, irregular, asymmetric) must be distinguished from physiologic livedo reticularis (symmetric, reversible with warming). Livedo racemosa warrants evaluation for antiphospholipid syndrome, Sneddon syndrome, cryoglobulinemia, and PAN.

Leg ulcers are classified by etiology: venous (medial malleolus, shallow, stasis changes — treat with compression), arterial (distal, punched-out, ischemic — ABI less than 0.9 indicates PAD, revascularize before wound care), neuropathic (plantar pressure points, painless — offload), and inflammatory (PG — DO NOT debride, treat with immunosuppression).

Pyoderma gangrenosum demonstrates pathergy — debridement causes explosive worsening. The violaceous, undermined border and association with IBD, RA, or hematologic malignancy distinguish it from venous ulcers. Always biopsy before debridement when PG is in the differential.

CHAPTER 21: PEDIATRIC DERMATOLOGY

Learning Objectives

1. Distinguish transient benign neonatal dermatoses (erythema toxicum neonatorum, transient neonatal pustular melanosis, miliaria) from pathologic neonatal eruptions (neonatal herpes, neonatal candidiasis, incontinentia pigmenti) that require urgent evaluation and treatment.
2. Classify infantile hemangiomas by morphology and depth, apply the PHACE and LUMBAR criteria for associated anomalies, and implement evidence-based treatment with oral propranolol based on the 2019 AAP clinical practice guideline.
3. Recognize the major genodermatoses (ichthyoses, epidermolysis bullosa, neurofibromatosis, tuberous sclerosis) by their cutaneous phenotypes and implement appropriate genetic counseling and multidisciplinary surveillance.
4. Identify the cutaneous signs of child abuse — including patterned bruising, burns in stocking-glove distribution, and injuries at unusual sites — and understand the mandatory reporting obligations.

Neonatal Dermatoses: Transient and Pathologic Eruptions

Benign Transient Neonatal Eruptions

Several benign, self-limited eruptions occur in the neonatal period and must be distinguished from infections and other pathologic conditions to avoid unnecessary workup and parental anxiety. Erythema toxicum neonatorum (ETN) is the most common neonatal eruption, affecting 30 to 70 percent of term neonates. It presents between 24 and 72 hours of life as blotchy erythematous macules, papules, and pustules on the trunk, proximal extremities, and face — sparing the palms and soles. Wright-stained smear of the pustule contents reveals abundant eosinophils (no organisms). ETN resolves spontaneously within 5 to 14 days and requires no treatment. Transient neonatal pustular melanosis (TNPM) presents at birth (unlike ETN, which appears after 24 hours) as superficial vesicles and pustules on a non-erythematous base, most commonly on the chin, forehead, nape, lower back, and shins. The pustules rupture easily, leaving a collarette of scale surrounding a hyperpigmented macule that persists for weeks to months. Smear shows neutrophils (no organisms). TNPM is more common in Black neonates. Miliaria (heat rash) results from eccrine duct obstruction: miliaria crystallina (superficial obstruction — tiny, fragile, clear vesicles on a non-erythematous base), miliaria rubra (mid-epidermal obstruction — erythematous papulovesicles, the classic prickly heat), and miliaria profunda (deep obstruction — flesh-colored papules). Treatment is environmental cooling and avoidance of excessive swaddling. Milia are tiny (1 to 2 mm), pearly-white, firm papules on the face (nose, cheeks, chin) caused by retention of keratin within the pilosebaceous unit — present in up to 50 percent of neonates and resolve spontaneously.

Pathologic Neonatal Eruptions Requiring Urgent Evaluation

Neonatal herpes simplex virus (HSV) infection is the most important pathologic eruption to exclude in any neonate with vesicles or pustules. Neonatal HSV presents in three forms: skin, eye, and mouth disease (SEM — clustered vesicles on an erythematous base, keratoconjunctivitis, oral ulcers); CNS disease (encephalitis with seizures, lethargy, CSF pleocytosis); and disseminated disease (hepatitis, pneumonitis, DIC — the most lethal form). Onset is typically between 5 and 14 days of life. Tzanck smear shows multinucleated giant cells, and viral PCR of vesicle fluid and blood confirms the diagnosis. Intravenous acyclovir must be initiated immediately at the first suspicion of neonatal HSV — delay increases morbidity and mortality. Neonatal candidiasis presents as oral thrush (white plaques on the buccal mucosa, palate, and tongue) and diaper dermatitis (beefy-red erythema with satellite pustules at the periphery of the diaper area — the satellite lesions distinguish candidal diaper dermatitis from irritant contact dermatitis). Congenital candidiasis (acquired in utero from ascending chorioamnionitis) presents at birth as a widespread papulopustular eruption. Incontinentia pigmenti (IP) is an X-linked dominant genodermatosis (lethal in males) presenting in neonatal girls as linear vesicles along Blaschko lines — stage 1 (vesicular) is followed by verrucous papules (stage 2), swirling hyperpigmentation (stage 3), and hypopigmented atrophic streaks (stage 4). IP requires ophthalmologic and neurologic screening.

KEY POINT: The critical distinction in neonatal vesiculopustular eruptions is between benign (ETN — eosinophils on smear, presents after 24 hours, resolves spontaneously) and dangerous (neonatal HSV — multinucleated giant cells on Tzanck, presents 5 to 14 days, requires immediate IV acyclovir). Any neonate with grouped vesicles on an erythematous base must be evaluated for HSV with Tzanck smear and viral PCR, and empiric IV acyclovir should be started while results are pending. The cost of missing neonatal HSV — encephalitis, disseminated disease, death — far outweighs the cost of a brief empiric course of acyclovir.

Eruption	Onset	Morphology	Smear Finding	Distribution	Course
Erythema toxicum neonatorum	24–72 hours of life	Blotchy erythematous macules, papules, and pustules on non-erythematous background	Eosinophils; no organisms	Trunk, proximal extremities, face; spares palms and soles	Self-limited; resolves 5–14 days
Transient neonatal pustular melanosis	At birth	Superficial vesicles and pustules on non-erythematous base; rupture leaves	Neutrophils; no organisms	Chin, forehead, nape, lower back, shins	Self-limited; pigmented macules may persist weeks to months

		collarette of scale and hyperpigmented macule			
Miliaria crystallina	Variable (heat-related)	Tiny, fragile, clear vesicles on non-erythematous base	Not indicated	Areas of occlusion — trunk, scalp, skin folds	Self-limited; resolves with cooling
Neonatal HSV	5–14 days of life	Grouped vesicles on erythematous base; may progress to erosions	Multinucleated giant cells (Tzanck); viral PCR positive	Any site; may be localized (SEM) or disseminated	Progressive without treatment; requires immediate IV acyclovir
Neonatal candidiasis	Variable; congenital form at birth	Oral thrush (white plaques on buccal mucosa); diaper — beefy-red erythema with satellite pustules	Budding yeast and pseudohyphae on KOH	Oral mucosa, diaper area; congenital form diffuse	Responds to topical nystatin (oral/diaper) or systemic fluconazole (congenital/disseminated)
Incontinentia pigmenti (stage 1)	At birth or first weeks	Linear vesicles and pustules along Blaschko lines	Eosinophils	Linear, following Blaschko lines on trunk and extremities	Progresses through 4 stages; requires ophthalmologic and neurologic screening

Infantile Hemangiomas and Vascular Malformations

Classification and Natural History

The distinction between infantile hemangiomas (IH) and vascular malformations is fundamental. Infantile hemangiomas are benign vascular tumors that follow a characteristic lifecycle: they are absent at birth or present as a precursor lesion (pale macule, telangiectatic patch, or bruise-like area), undergo rapid proliferation during the first 3 to 6 months of life (superficial IH — bright red, raised, compressible; deep IH — bluish, soft, subcutaneous; mixed — features of both), plateau between 6 and 12 months, and then slowly involute over years (50 percent involuted by age 5, 90 percent by age 9). Post-involution residua include telangiectasias, fibrofatty tissue, and redundant skin. IH are the most common tumor of infancy (4 to 5 percent of infants), with risk factors including female sex (3:1), prematurity, low birth weight, White race, and multiple gestation. Vascular malformations, in contrast, are structural anomalies of blood vessels present at birth that grow proportionately with the child and never involute. They are classified by the predominant vessel type: capillary malformations (port-wine stains — nevus flammeus), venous malformations, lymphatic malformations, arteriovenous malformations, and combined forms.

PHACE Syndrome, LUMBAR Syndrome, and Treatment

Large segmental facial IH (greater than 5 cm) warrant evaluation for PHACE syndrome: Posterior fossa malformations, Hemangioma (large facial), Arterial anomalies (cerebrovascular), Cardiac defects (coarctation of the aorta), and Eye anomalies. MRI/MRA of the brain and echocardiography are indicated. Similarly, large segmental IH of the lower body and perineum warrant evaluation for LUMBAR syndrome: Lower body hemangioma, Urogenital anomalies, Myelopathy, Bony deformities, Anorectal malformations, and Renal anomalies — requiring spinal MRI, renal ultrasound, and urologic evaluation. Treatment of IH follows the 2019 AAP clinical practice guideline: oral propranolol (a non-selective beta-blocker) is the first-line systemic therapy for problematic IH (those threatening vision, airway, or feeding, causing ulceration, or at risk for permanent disfigurement). Propranolol should be initiated between 1 and 3 months of age (during the proliferative phase) and continued until at least 12 months of age. Monitoring includes heart rate and blood pressure at initiation. Topical timolol (a beta-blocker) is used for small, superficial, non-ulcerated IH. Capillary malformations (port-wine stains) in the V1 trigeminal distribution warrant evaluation for Sturge-Weber syndrome (leptomeningeal angioma, glaucoma, seizures) — MRI of the brain and ophthalmologic evaluation are indicated.

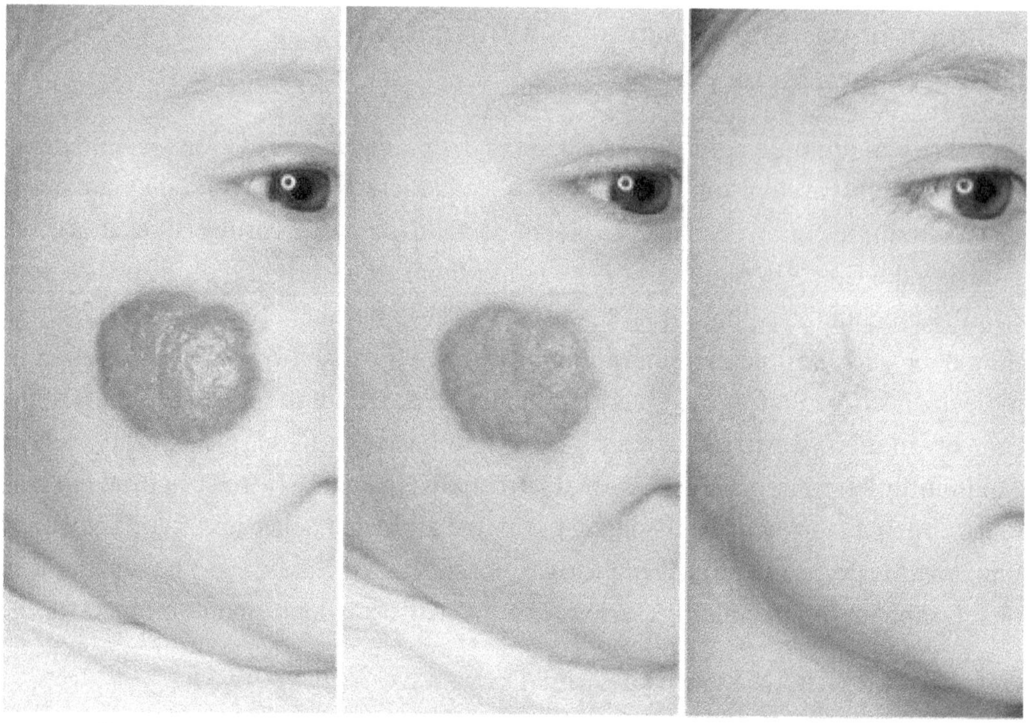

proliferative phase (3 months) | plateau phase (12 months) | involution (4 years), residual telangiectasia

EVIDENCE: The landmark randomized controlled trial by Léauté-Labrèze and colleagues (2015) established oral propranolol as the standard of care for problematic infantile hemangiomas. The trial demonstrated that propranolol at 3 mg/kg/day for 6 months achieved complete or near-complete resolution in 60 percent of treated infants compared to 4 percent in the placebo group. Subsequent studies confirmed the safety profile — the most common adverse effects are sleep disturbance, cold extremities, and bronchospasm in predisposed infants, while hypoglycemia remains the most serious risk (parents should be counseled to ensure regular feeding schedules). The 2019 AAP clinical practice guideline codified propranolol as first-line systemic therapy and provided detailed initiation and monitoring protocols, including heart rate and blood pressure assessment at each dose escalation.

Atopic Dermatitis in Children: Age-Specific Presentations and Management

Age-Specific Distribution Patterns

Atopic dermatitis (AD) is the most common chronic inflammatory skin disease of childhood, affecting 15 to 20 percent of children in developed countries. The distribution of AD lesions is strongly age-dependent. In infants (0 to 2 years), AD involves the face (cheeks, forehead — sparing the nose), scalp, and extensor surfaces of the extremities. In children (2 to 12 years), the classic flexural distribution emerges — antecubital and popliteal fossae, wrists, ankles, and neck. In adolescents, AD favors the face (periorbital, perioral), neck, and hands (hand eczema). Morphologically, infantile AD is more exudative (weeping, crusting), while childhood and adolescent AD is more lichenified (thickened, leathery skin from chronic scratching). The itch-scratch cycle is the central feature — pruritus is the sine qua non of AD, and the resulting scratching perpetuates barrier disruption, inflammation, and infection.

Pathogenesis and Filaggrin

The pathogenesis of AD involves the convergence of epidermal barrier dysfunction, immune dysregulation, and environmental triggers. Loss-of-function mutations in the filaggrin gene (FLG) are the strongest known genetic risk factor for AD — filaggrin is a structural protein essential for epidermal barrier integrity, and its deficiency leads to increased transepidermal water loss, allergen penetration, and microbial colonization. Approximately 20 to 30 percent of European AD patients carry FLG mutations (the R501X and 2282del4 variants are most common), and these patients develop earlier-onset, more severe AD with a higher risk of progression to asthma and allergic rhinitis (the atopic march). The immune response in AD is Th2-dominant in the acute phase (IL-4, IL-13, IL-31 — IL-31 is the principal pruritogen driving the itch), with Th1 and Th22 contributions in chronic disease. Staphylococcus aureus colonizes the skin of 70 to 90 percent of AD patients (compared to 5 to 10 percent of healthy individuals), exploiting the defective barrier and producing superantigens that exacerbate inflammation.

Management: Stepwise Approach

AD management follows a stepwise approach: (1) baseline for all patients — emollient therapy (frequent application of fragrance-free moisturizers to restore the epidermal barrier, applied immediately after bathing), trigger avoidance (irritants, known allergens, excessive heat), and daily bathing followed by immediate emollient application (soak and seal). (2) Mild AD — low-potency topical corticosteroids (hydrocortisone for the face and skin folds) or topical calcineurin inhibitors (pimecrolimus, tacrolimus — preferred for sensitive areas to avoid steroid atrophy). (3) Moderate AD — medium-potency topical corticosteroids, topical calcineurin inhibitors, topical PDE4 inhibitors (crisaborole), or topical JAK inhibitors (ruxolitinib). Proactive maintenance therapy (applying topical anti-inflammatory agents twice weekly to previously affected areas even after clearing) reduces flare frequency. (4) Severe AD — systemic therapy: dupilumab (anti-IL-4R-alpha monoclonal antibody, approved for children aged 6 months and older — the first biologic approved for pediatric AD), tralokinumab (anti-IL-13), JAK inhibitors (abrocitinib, upadacitinib — approved for adolescents and adults), and traditional immunosuppressives (cyclosporine, methotrexate, azathioprine — used off-label in children when biologics are unavailable or contraindicated).

CLINICAL PEARL: The headlight sign is a useful clinical clue in infantile atopic dermatitis: the tip of the nose is characteristically spared, appearing as a pale island within the surrounding facial erythema — as if the headlights are off while the rest of the face is lit up. This nose-sparing pattern reflects the relative paucity of the type of immune cells and the thicker, more sebaceous skin of the nasal tip. The headlight sign helps distinguish infantile AD from seborrheic dermatitis (which prominently involves the nasolabial folds) and from contact dermatitis (which follows the pattern of the contactant). When the nose IS prominently involved in an infant's facial eruption, reconsider the diagnosis — think seborrheic dermatitis, contact dermatitis to a pacifier or topical agent, or less commonly, zinc deficiency (acrodermatitis enteropathica).

Patient Education and Counseling

Effective management of pediatric AD requires sustained caregiver education and partnership. Parents should understand that AD is a chronic, relapsing condition with a genetic basis — it is not caused by poor hygiene, food allergy (though food allergy may coexist and exacerbate AD in a subset of patients, particularly those with severe early-onset disease), or parental neglect. The soak-and-seal technique should be demonstrated: bathe the child in lukewarm water for 5 to 10 minutes using a gentle, fragrance-free, soap-free cleanser, then immediately (within 3 minutes of patting dry) apply a thick layer of emollient to seal in moisture. Emollients should be applied at least twice daily and after every water exposure. Parents should be counseled on the safe use of topical corticosteroids — fears of skin thinning (steroid phobia) are the most common reason for non-adherence, and clinicians should acknowledge these concerns while explaining that appropriate use of the correct potency for the correct duration on the correct body site is safe. The fingertip unit (FTU) system helps standardize application: one FTU (from the distal interphalangeal crease to the fingertip) covers an area equivalent to two adult palms. Environmental modification includes cotton clothing (avoid wool and synthetic fibers), maintaining a cool room temperature, keeping nails short to minimize excoriation damage, and identifying and avoiding individual triggers (certain foods if confirmed by supervised oral food challenge, dust mites, pet dander, irritant soaps). Parents of children on systemic therapy (dupilumab, JAK inhibitors) require education on injection technique or medication administration, monitoring schedules, and signs of adverse effects.

THE CUTANEOUS MIMICKER RECOGNITION ATLAS — Infantile Atopic Dermatitis versus Seborrheic Dermatitis

The Clinical Pattern: Infantile atopic dermatitis presents as intensely pruritic, erythematous, exudative patches and plaques on the face (cheeks, forehead — characteristically sparing the nose), scalp, and extensor surfaces. The infant is irritable, scratching, and may have a family history of atopy (asthma, allergic rhinitis, AD). The lesions are poorly demarcated and associated with xerosis (dry skin). Onset is typically after 3 months of age.

The Mimicker: Infantile seborrheic dermatitis (cradle cap) presents as greasy, yellowish, adherent scale on the scalp (cradle cap), face (particularly the nasolabial folds and eyebrows — areas typically spared in AD), and intertriginous areas (axillae, groin, neck folds). Onset is typically before 3 months of age. The infant is NOT pruritic — seborrheic dermatitis is characteristically non-itchy, in contrast to the intense itch of AD. The lesions are well-demarcated with a greasy rather than dry quality.

Trap Logic: Treating an infant's facial rash as AD when it involves the nasolabial folds and is non-pruritic misclassifies seborrheic dermatitis and leads to unnecessary topical corticosteroid escalation. **Conversely, dismissing cheek eczema as cradle cap when the infant is actively scratching and the skin is dry rather than greasy** delays the diagnosis of AD and misses the window for early aggressive barrier repair and emollient therapy. Both conditions may coexist in the same infant, further complicating the distinction.

The Decision Anchor: The discriminating features are **pruritus (AD — intense itch, scratching, irritability; seborrheic — non-pruritic), distribution (AD — cheeks with nose sparing, extensors; seborrheic — scalp, nasolabial folds, intertriginous areas), age of onset (AD — typically after 3 months; seborrheic — typically before 3 months), morphology (AD — dry, exudative, poorly demarcated; seborrheic — greasy, well-demarcated, adherent yellow scale), and family atopic history (supports AD)**. Seborrheic dermatitis is self-limited and resolves by 6 to 12 months; AD is chronic and requires long-term management.

Genodermatoses: Ichthyoses, Epidermolysis Bullosa, Neurofibromatosis, and Tuberous Sclerosis

Ichthyoses

The ichthyoses are a group of hereditary disorders of cornification characterized by generalized scaling. Ichthyosis vulgaris — the most common (1 in 250 to 300 people) — is autosomal dominant (caused by FLG mutations, linking it pathogenetically to AD) and presents in early childhood with fine, white, fish-scale-like scaling on the extensor surfaces and trunk, with hyperlinear palms and keratosis pilaris. The flexures are characteristically spared. X-linked recessive ichthyosis (1 in 2,000 to 6,000 males, caused by steroid sulfatase deficiency) presents with larger, darker, brown-grey scales (dirty appearance) that involve the neck, trunk, and extremities — unlike ichthyosis vulgaris, it may involve the flexures. Lamellar ichthyosis and congenital ichthyosiform erythroderma (CIE) are autosomal recessive disorders presenting at birth: the collodion baby phenotype (the neonate is encased in a tight, shiny, cellophane-like membrane that cracks and sheds over the first weeks of life) can be the initial presentation of several underlying ichthyoses. Harlequin ichthyosis is the most severe form — thick, plate-like armor of hyperkeratosis with deep fissures, ectropion, eclabium, and flexion contractures — historically fatal but survival has improved with neonatal intensive care and systemic retinoids.

Epidermolysis Bullosa

Epidermolysis bullosa (EB) is a group of inherited mechanobullous disorders caused by mutations in structural proteins of the dermoepidermal junction, resulting in skin fragility and blistering from minimal mechanical trauma. EB is classified by the ultrastructural level of cleavage: EB simplex (intraepidermal — mutations in keratins 5 and 14; blisters heal without scarring), junctional EB (within the lamina lucida — mutations in laminin-332, type XVII collagen; severe, often lethal forms), and dystrophic EB (sublamina densa — mutations in type VII collagen; blisters heal with scarring, milia, and in severe forms, mitten deformities of the hands from recurrent blistering and fusion of the digits). Recessive dystrophic EB carries a lifetime risk of aggressive squamous cell carcinoma in chronically scarred skin. Management is multidisciplinary: wound care (non-adherent dressings, pain management), nutritional support (iron and protein supplementation), occupational therapy, and surveillance for complications (esophageal strictures, cardiomyopathy in junctional EB, SCC in dystrophic EB).

Neurofibromatosis and Tuberous Sclerosis

Neurofibromatosis type 1 (NF1 — autosomal dominant, 1 in 3,000) is diagnosed by the presence of two or more NIH criteria: 6 or more café-au-lait macules (greater than 5 mm prepubertal, greater than 15 mm postpubertal), axillary or inguinal freckling (Crowe sign), 2 or more neurofibromas or 1 plexiform neurofibroma, optic pathway glioma, 2 or more Lisch nodules (iris hamartomas), a distinctive osseous lesion (sphenoid dysplasia, tibial pseudoarthrosis), and a first-degree relative with NF1. Café-au-lait macules are often the first sign, present in early infancy. Plexiform neurofibromas carry a 10 to 15 percent lifetime risk of malignant transformation to malignant peripheral nerve sheath tumor (MPNST). Selumetinib (a MEK inhibitor) is approved for inoperable plexiform neurofibromas in NF1. Tuberous sclerosis complex (TSC — autosomal dominant, mutations in TSC1/hamartin or TSC2/tuberin) produces hamartomas in multiple organs. Cutaneous features include hypomelanotic macules (ash-leaf spots — the earliest sign, visible under Wood lamp in fair-skinned neonates), facial angiofibromas (adenoma sebaceum — red-pink papules on the nasolabial folds and cheeks, developing in childhood), shagreen patch (a connective tissue hamartoma — a flesh-colored, cobblestone-textured plaque on the lower back), and periungual fibromas (Koenen tumors — developing in adolescence). TSC requires surveillance for renal angiomyolipomas, cardiac rhabdomyomas, and cortical tubers causing seizures. mTOR inhibitors (sirolimus, everolimus) reduce angiomyolipoma size and are used topically for facial angiofibromas.

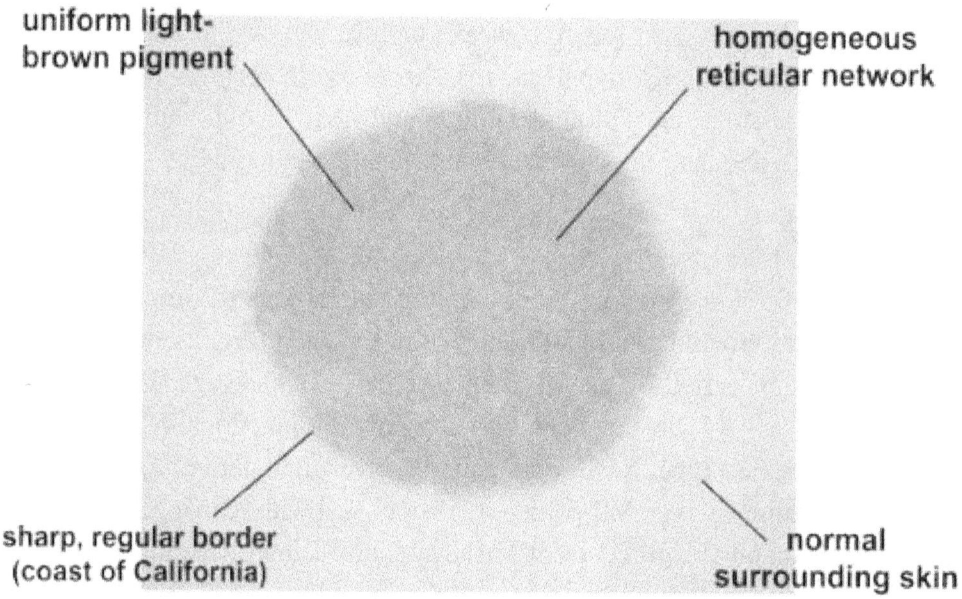

Childhood Exanthems and Viral Infections

Classic Childhood Exanthems

The classic childhood exanthems are numbered by historical convention. Measles (first disease — paramyxovirus) presents with prodromal fever, cough, coryza, and conjunctivitis (the three Cs), followed by Koplik spots (pathognomonic — blue-white papules on the buccal mucosa opposite the molars) and a morbilliform (measles-like) rash that begins on the face and spreads cephalocaudally to the trunk and extremities over 3 days. Scarlet fever (second disease — group A streptococcal pharyngitis with erythrogenic toxin) presents with a sandpaper-textured, diffuse erythematous rash beginning on the trunk, strawberry tongue, Pastia lines (linear petechiae in the antecubital and inguinal creases), and facial flushing with circumoral pallor. Rubella (third disease — togavirus) presents with a fine, pink, maculopapular rash beginning on the face and spreading downward, with posterior auricular and postoccipital lymphadenopathy. Erythema infectiosum (fifth disease — parvovirus B19) presents with the slapped-cheek sign (bilateral facial erythema sparing the nose) followed by a lacy, reticular, erythematous rash on the trunk and extremities. Parvovirus B19 causes transient aplastic crisis in patients with hemolytic anemias (sickle cell disease) and hydrops fetalis in the fetus if maternal infection occurs during pregnancy. Roseola infantum (sixth disease — HHV-6) presents with 3 to 5 days of high fever in a well-appearing infant, followed by the sudden defervescence and appearance of a diffuse, pink, maculopapular rash (fever breaks, rash comes). Hand, foot, and mouth disease (coxsackievirus A16, enterovirus 71) presents with oral vesicles and ulcers on the palate and pharynx, and oval, grey vesicles on the palms, soles, and buttocks.

Complications and Prognosis of Childhood Viral Exanthems

While most childhood exanthems are self-limited, serious complications can occur and must be anticipated. Measles carries the highest complication burden: pneumonia (the leading cause of measles-related mortality in children), acute encephalitis (1 in 1,000 cases — seizures, altered consciousness, focal neurologic deficits), and subacute sclerosing panencephalitis (SSPE — a uniformly fatal degenerative CNS disease that develops 7 to 10 years after initial measles infection, caused by persistent mutant measles virus in the brain). Measles also causes immune amnesia — it depletes the existing memory lymphocyte repertoire, leaving the child vulnerable to other infections for months to years after recovery. Varicella-zoster virus complications in children include secondary bacterial skin infection (the most common complication — group A streptococcal or staphylococcal superinfection of vesicles, which can progress to necrotizing fasciitis), cerebellar ataxia (the most common neurologic complication — self-limited in most cases), pneumonia (more common in adults and immunocompromised children), and Reye syndrome (associated with aspirin use during varicella — aspirin is absolutely contraindicated in children with varicella or influenza). Parvovirus B19 in children with sickle cell disease or other chronic hemolytic anemias can precipitate transient aplastic crisis (abrupt cessation of erythropoiesis with profound anemia requiring transfusion), because parvovirus B19 specifically infects erythroid progenitor cells via the P antigen (globoside) receptor. Maternal parvovirus B19 infection during the first or second trimester can cause hydrops fetalis due to severe fetal anemia.

Common Pediatric Infections: Impetigo, Tinea Capitis, Molluscum, and Scabies

Impetigo and Tinea Capitis

Impetigo is the most common bacterial skin infection of childhood, caused by Staphylococcus aureus (including MRSA) and group A Streptococcus. Non-bullous impetigo (the more common form) presents as honey-colored crusted erosions, typically on the face (perioral, perinasal). Bullous impetigo (caused by staphylococcal exfoliative toxins) presents as flaccid bullae that rupture to leave polycyclic erosions with a collarette of scale. Treatment is topical mupirocin or retapamulin for limited disease, oral antibiotics (cephalexin, or TMP-SMX/clindamycin if MRSA is suspected) for extensive disease. Tinea capitis is the most common dermatophyte infection in prepubescent children, caused predominantly by Trichophyton tonsurans in North America (endothrix infection — spores within the hair shaft, black dot pattern on scalp) and Microsporum canis in parts of Europe and Asia (ectothrix — fluorescent under Wood lamp). It presents as patchy alopecia with scaling, broken hairs (black dots), and cervical lymphadenopathy. KOH preparation of plucked hairs and fungal culture confirm the diagnosis. Systemic antifungal therapy is required (griseofulvin or terbinafine) because topical agents do not penetrate the hair follicle. Kerion — a boggy, inflammatory, tender mass with pustules and draining sinuses — is a severe inflammatory response to the dermatophyte and should be treated with oral antifungals (not incision and drainage, which is both unnecessary and harmful).

Molluscum Contagiosum and Scabies

Molluscum contagiosum (poxvirus) presents as firm, dome-shaped, flesh-colored papules with central umbilication, typically on the trunk, axillae, and extremities. The disease is self-limited (resolving over 6 to 18 months as the immune system clears the virus), and in immunocompetent children, observation is a valid approach. Treatment options for symptomatic or persistent lesions include curettage, cryotherapy, cantharidin (a topical vesicant), and topical retinoids. Extensive, confluent, or giant molluscum in an older child or adolescent should prompt evaluation for immunodeficiency (HIV). Scabies (Sarcoptes scabiei infestation) presents as intensely pruritic papules and burrows, with a distribution that is age-specific: in infants, scabies involves the palms, soles, face, and scalp (sites typically spared in older children and adults), while in older children and adults, the classic distribution includes the web spaces of the fingers, wrists, axillary folds, periumbilical area, waistband, and genitalia. The pathognomonic finding is the burrow — a thin, serpiginous, slightly elevated track representing the mite's tunnel in the stratum corneum. Microscopic identification of the mite, eggs, or fecal pellets (scybala) on skin scraping confirms the diagnosis. Treatment is topical permethrin 5 percent cream (applied from neck to toes, left on overnight, repeated at 1 week) — in infants, the scalp and face must also be treated. Oral ivermectin is used for crusted (Norwegian) scabies and in institutional outbreaks.

Clinical Case: Vesicular Eruption in a 10-Day-Old Neonate

A 10-day-old full-term neonate is brought to the emergency department by her parents with a 12-hour history of a vesicular eruption on her trunk and left thigh. She was born via vaginal delivery at 39 weeks to a 26-year-old mother with no reported history of genital herpes. The neonate was feeding well until the morning of presentation, when she became increasingly irritable and lethargic, with poor latch during breastfeeding. On examination, the neonate has a temperature of 38.4 degrees Celsius. There are approximately 15 to 20 grouped vesicles on an erythematous base distributed over the left lateral trunk and left anterior thigh, some of which have ruptured to form shallow erosions. The remainder of the skin examination shows a few scattered erythematous papules on the trunk without surrounding erythema or pustulation — consistent with residual erythema toxicum neonatorum. The oropharynx shows no ulcerations. The eyes are clear without conjunctival injection.

The clinical reasoning begins with recognizing that grouped vesicles on an erythematous base in a neonate between 5 and 14 days of life constitute a neonatal HSV emergency until proven otherwise. The fever, irritability, and lethargy raise concern for disseminated disease or early CNS involvement. A Tzanck smear is performed from the base of a fresh vesicle and reveals multinucleated giant cells — highly suggestive of herpesvirus infection. Intravenous acyclovir is initiated immediately at a dose appropriate for neonatal HSV (clinicians should confirm current dosing against the AAP Red Book or institutional protocol). Vesicle fluid is sent for HSV PCR (to distinguish HSV-1 from HSV-2), blood is sent for HSV PCR and hepatic transaminases, and a lumbar puncture is performed (CSF for HSV PCR and cell count). The scattered papules elsewhere are recognized as residual ETN — benign, eosinophil-rich, and unrelated to the herpetic eruption. The mother reports no history of genital herpes, but approximately 70 percent of neonatal HSV cases occur in mothers with no recognized history of genital herpes (most are caused by subclinical viral shedding from undiagnosed genital HSV). HSV PCR returns positive for HSV-2 from vesicle fluid and blood. CSF HSV PCR is negative. The diagnosis is neonatal HSV — SEM disease with possible early dissemination (positive blood viremia). The neonate completes a 14-day course of IV acyclovir for SEM disease (21 days would be indicated for CNS or disseminated disease) and is subsequently placed on oral acyclovir suppressive therapy for 6 months per the AAP recommendation to prevent recurrence and improve neurodevelopmental outcomes.

Child Abuse: Cutaneous Signs and Reporting Obligations

Cutaneous Indicators of Non-Accidental Injury

The skin is the most commonly injured organ in child abuse, and dermatologists play a critical role in recognizing abuse-related lesions. Bruising is the most common cutaneous manifestation of physical abuse. Features that raise suspicion include bruising in non-mobile infants (infants who cannot roll, crawl, or cruise should not have bruises — the TEN-4 rule: bruising on the Torso, Ears, or Neck in a child under 4 years, or any bruising in an infant under 4 months, is concerning), patterned bruising (loop marks from cords, linear marks from belts, hand prints, bite marks — a bite mark with an intercanine distance greater than 3 cm is likely from an adult), and bruising in unusual locations (ears, neck, buttocks, trunk — as opposed to typical accidental bruising over bony prominences such as shins and forehead). Burns account for approximately 10 percent of physical abuse injuries. Suspicious patterns include stocking-glove distribution burns (forced immersion — sharp lines of demarcation with sparing of flexural creases where the child reflexively flexed), circular burns (cigarette), and patterned contact burns (iron, curling iron, stove grate). Injuries at different stages of healing suggest repeated abuse over time.

Differential Diagnosis and Mandatory Reporting

Several dermatologic conditions can mimic the bruising of child abuse and must be considered in the differential diagnosis: Mongolian spots (dermal melanocytosis — blue-grey patches on the lumbosacral area, buttocks, and occasionally extremities, present at birth in 80 to 100 percent of Asian, Black, Hispanic, and Native American neonates — can be mistaken for bruises), phytophotodermatitis (linear and geometric areas of hyperpigmentation following contact with psoralen-containing plants and sun exposure — can mimic patterned burn marks), coining and cupping marks (cultural healing practices producing patterned bruising), bleeding disorders (idiopathic thrombocytopenic purpura, hemophilia, von Willebrand disease — should be excluded with coagulation studies when abuse is suspected), and Ehlers-Danlos syndrome (easy bruisability from connective tissue fragility). Despite these mimickers, clinicians must maintain a high index of suspicion. In all states and territories, healthcare providers are mandated reporters — they are legally required to report suspected child abuse to child protective services. The reporting threshold is reasonable suspicion, not certainty of diagnosis. Failure to report is both a legal violation and a clinical failure that leaves the child in danger.

THE CUTANEOUS MIMICKER RECOGNITION ATLAS — Mongolian Spots versus Non-Accidental Bruising

---

The Clinical Pattern: Non-accidental bruising (child abuse) produces ecchymoses in unusual locations — ears, neck, trunk, buttocks, and inner thighs — that are not consistent with the typical pattern of accidental injury over bony prominences. The bruises may show different stages of color evolution (indicating repeated injury over time), may be patterned (loop marks, hand prints, bite marks), and the history provided by the caregiver is inconsistent with the pattern or developmental stage of the child.

The Mimicker: Mongolian spots (dermal melanocytosis) are blue-grey patches on the lumbosacral area, buttocks, and occasionally the extremities, present at birth and caused by dermal melanocytes that failed to reach the epidermis during embryonic migration. They are present in 80 to 100 percent of Asian, Black, Hispanic, and Native American neonates and 1 to 10 percent of White neonates. Mongolian spots are flat, non-tender, and stable (they do not change color over days the way bruises do) — they may persist for years or fade gradually during childhood.

Trap Logic: Misidentifying Mongolian spots as bruises and reporting suspected child abuse causes devastating consequences for innocent families — invasive investigations, family separation, and lasting psychological harm. **Conversely, dismissing genuine bruises as Mongolian spots** leaves an abused child in danger. The trap is bidirectional, and the stakes in both directions are high. Documentation of Mongolian spots at birth or at the first well-child visit is the simplest preventive measure.

The Decision Anchor: The discriminating features are **color evolution (bruises change color over days — red to purple to green to yellow; Mongolian spots remain stable blue-grey), palpation (bruises may be tender and slightly raised; Mongolian spots are flat and non-tender), location consistency (Mongolian spots are present from birth in typical locations; new bruises in unusual locations are concerning), and documentation (if Mongolian spots were documented at birth, the diagnosis is clear)**. When in doubt, a coagulation workup excludes a bleeding diathesis, and serial photography documents whether the lesion changes (bruise) or remains stable (Mongolian spot).

CAUTION: A kerion — a boggy, inflammatory, pustular mass on the scalp of a child — is a severe immune response to dermatophyte infection (tinea capitis), NOT an abscess requiring incision and drainage. Incision and drainage of a kerion is painful, unnecessary, and may cause permanent scarring alopecia. The correct treatment is systemic antifungal therapy (griseofulvin or terbinafine) with or without a short course of systemic corticosteroids to reduce the inflammatory response. Fungal culture confirms the diagnosis. The clinical distinction from a bacterial abscess is the presence of associated alopecia, broken hairs, and cervical lymphadenopathy — features consistent with tinea capitis.

THE CUTANEOUS MIMICKER RECOGNITION ATLAS — Pediatric Dermatology Diagnostic Arcs

Infantile AD vs. Seborrheic Dermatitis: The discriminating features are pruritus (AD — intense itch; seborrheic — non-pruritic), distribution (AD — cheeks with nose sparing, extensors; seborrheic — scalp, nasolabial folds, intertriginous areas), age of onset (AD — after 3 months; seborrheic — before 3 months), and morphology (AD — dry, exudative; seborrheic — greasy yellow scale). Cognitive trap: treating non-pruritic greasy scalp and nasolabial fold involvement as AD — this is seborrheic dermatitis and is self-limited.

Mongolian Spots vs. Non-Accidental Bruising: The discriminating features are color evolution (bruises change color over days; Mongolian spots are stable), tenderness (bruises may be tender; spots are non-tender), birth documentation (spots are present from birth), and pattern (patterned marks — loops, hand prints, bite marks — are never Mongolian spots). Cognitive trap: both directions carry high stakes — misidentifying spots as bruises harms families; dismissing bruises as spots leaves children in danger.

Summary and Key Concepts

Benign transient neonatal eruptions (ETN — eosinophils, after 24 hours; TNPM — neutrophils, at birth; miliaria — eccrine duct obstruction) must be distinguished from neonatal HSV (grouped vesicles, 5 to 14 days, requires immediate IV acyclovir). The stakes of missing neonatal HSV are encephalitis and death.

Infantile hemangiomas follow a characteristic lifecycle: absent at birth, proliferate 3 to 6 months, plateau, then involute over years. Oral propranolol is first-line treatment for problematic IH. Large segmental facial IH warrant PHACE evaluation; perineal IH warrant LUMBAR evaluation.

Atopic dermatitis has age-specific distributions: infant (face, extensors), child (flexures), adolescent (face, hands). Filaggrin mutations are the strongest genetic risk factor. Dupilumab is approved for children aged 6 months and older with moderate-to-severe AD.

The major genodermatoses have pathognomonic cutaneous features: NF1 (café-au-lait macules, neurofibromas, Crowe sign), TSC (ash-leaf spots, facial angiofibromas, shagreen patch), ichthyosis vulgaris (fine white scaling, hyperlinear palms), and EB (fragility and blistering at sites of trauma).

Cutaneous signs of child abuse include bruising in non-mobile infants, patterned injuries, burns in stocking-glove distribution, and injuries at different healing stages. Mongolian spots are the most common mimicker. Mandatory reporting is triggered by reasonable suspicion, not diagnostic certainty.

CHAPTER 22: CUTANEOUS MANIFESTATIONS OF SYSTEMIC DISEASE

Learning Objectives

1. Recognize the major cutaneous signs of endocrine disease — including necrobiosis lipoidica, diabetic dermopathy, pretibial myxedema, and striae — and correlate them with the underlying systemic disorder to guide targeted evaluation.
2. Identify paraneoplastic dermatoses (sign of Leser-Trelat, acanthosis nigricans, dermatomyositis, necrolytic migratory erythema) as potential harbingers of internal malignancy and initiate appropriate malignancy workup.
3. Classify drug eruptions by morphologic pattern (morbilliform, fixed, lichenoid, photosensitive) and severity (SJS/TEN, DRESS, AGEP), apply the SCORTEN prognostic index, and implement evidence-based management including identification and withdrawal of the culprit medication.
4. Distinguish psychocutaneous disorders (delusional infestation, dermatitis artefacta, neurotic excoriations, trichotillomania) from primary dermatologic disease, and implement a therapeutic approach that integrates dermatologic care with psychiatric treatment.

Skin Signs of Endocrine Disease: Diabetes, Thyroid Disorders, and Adrenal Conditions

Cutaneous Manifestations of Diabetes Mellitus

Diabetes mellitus produces a wide spectrum of cutaneous manifestations through the interrelated mechanisms of microangiopathy, neuropathy, immune dysfunction, and metabolic derangement. Diabetic dermopathy (shin spots) is the most common cutaneous finding in diabetes, affecting 30 to 60 percent of diabetic patients. It presents as bilateral, asymmetric, round or oval, atrophic, hyperpigmented macules and patches on the pretibial surfaces — representing small-vessel microangiopathy with hemosiderin deposition. Diabetic dermopathy is clinically insignificant but serves as a marker of microvascular disease and correlates with the presence of retinopathy, nephropathy, and neuropathy. Necrobiosis lipoidica (NL) is a granulomatous dermatosis classically associated with diabetes (although only 0.3 to 1.2 percent of diabetic patients develop NL, and up to one-third of NL patients are not diabetic). It presents as well-demarcated, yellowish-brown, waxy plaques with prominent telangiectasias on the pretibial surfaces — the central atrophy produces a characteristic translucent, porcelain-like quality through which dermal vessels are visible. NL plaques are prone to ulceration (approximately 35 percent), which can be painful and difficult to manage. The pathology shows palisading and interstitial granulomatous inflammation with necrobiosis (degeneration of collagen) in the dermis, surrounded by lymphocytes, histiocytes, and multinucleated giant cells. Acanthosis nigricans (AN) presents as velvety, hyperpigmented, papillomatous plaques in the flexural areas — axillae, posterior neck, groin, and inframammary folds. In the context of diabetes and metabolic syndrome, AN is driven by hyperinsulinemia: insulin at supraphysiologic concentrations binds to insulin-like growth factor-1 (IGF-1) receptors on keratinocytes and dermal fibroblasts, stimulating proliferation. AN in obesity and type 2 diabetes is the benign, insulin-resistant form — the most common type. However, AN can also be paraneoplastic (see Cutaneous Paraneoplastic Syndromes section below).

Cutaneous Manifestations of Thyroid Disease

Thyroid disease produces distinctive cutaneous findings that often precede the biochemical diagnosis. Hyperthyroidism (Graves disease) causes warm, moist, smooth skin with hyperhidrosis, diffuse non-scarring alopecia (telogen effluvium from accelerated hair cycling), and onycholysis (Plummer nails — separation of the nail plate from the nail bed, beginning distally). Pretibial myxedema (thyroid dermopathy) is specific to Graves disease, occurring in 1 to 4 percent of patients, almost always in association with thyroid eye disease and elevated TSH receptor antibodies. It presents as firm, non-pitting, waxy, skin-colored to pink-brown plaques and nodules on the anterolateral shins with a characteristic peau d'orange (orange-peel) surface texture. Histologically, pretibial myxedema shows massive dermal mucin deposition (hyaluronic acid and chondroitin sulfate), caused by TSH receptor antibody-mediated stimulation of dermal fibroblasts. First-line treatment is high-potency topical corticosteroids under occlusion. Hypothyroidism produces cool, dry, pale skin with generalized non-pitting edema (myxedema — from dermal mucin deposition, distinct from the localized pretibial form in Graves disease), coarse and brittle hair, lateral eyebrow thinning (madarosis — loss of the outer third), and xanthomas in patients with secondary hyperlipidemia. Carotenoderma — a yellowish discoloration of the skin (particularly the palms, soles, and nasolabial folds) from impaired hepatic conversion of carotene to vitamin A — occurs in hypothyroidism and can mimic jaundice, but the sclerae remain white (jaundice causes scleral icterus; carotenoderma does not).

Adrenal Disease and Cushing Syndrome

Addison disease (primary adrenal insufficiency) produces diffuse hyperpigmentation, most prominent on sun-exposed areas, palmar creases, buccal mucosa, pressure points, and recent scars. The hyperpigmentation results from elevated ACTH and melanocyte-stimulating hormone (MSH) — both derived from the same precursor molecule (proopiomelanocortin, POMC) — which stimulate melanocortin-1 receptors on melanocytes in the compensatory response to low cortisol. Cushing syndrome (glucocorticoid excess) produces a constellation of cutaneous findings: wide (greater than 1 cm), violaceous (red-purple) striae on the abdomen, thighs, breasts, and axillae — distinct from the narrow, pale striae of pregnancy or simple weight gain; thin, fragile skin with easy bruising from cortisol-mediated suppression of collagen synthesis; facial plethora (moon facies); dorsocervical fat pad (buffalo hump); and proximal muscle wasting. Iatrogenic Cushing syndrome from chronic systemic corticosteroid therapy produces the same findings. Steroid-induced acne (monomorphic papulopustular eruption without comedones on the trunk) and steroid rosacea (perioral and periocular erythema and papulopustules from prolonged topical corticosteroid use on the face) are additional corticosteroid-related dermatoses.

KEY POINT: The color of striae is a critical diagnostic clue: wide, violaceous (purple-red) striae suggest Cushing syndrome (glucocorticoid excess), because cortisol thins the dermis and weakens connective tissue, allowing the underlying vasculature to show through. Narrow, pale or silvery striae are the common stretch marks of pregnancy, adolescent growth, or simple weight gain. When wide purple striae are found on the abdomen, thighs, or breasts — especially if accompanied by thin skin, easy bruising, proximal weakness, and facial plethora — a cortisol workup (24-hour urinary free cortisol, overnight dexamethasone suppression test, or late-night salivary cortisol) is indicated.

Skin Signs of Hepatic, Renal, and Gastrointestinal Disease

Cutaneous Manifestations of Liver Disease

Chronic liver disease produces a characteristic constellation of cutaneous findings that reflect the liver's role in estrogen metabolism, coagulation, and bile acid clearance. Spider angiomas (spider nevi) are arterial vascular lesions consisting of a central arteriole with radiating capillary branches — they blanch with pressure on the central point and refill centrifugally. When multiple spider angiomas are present in the distribution of the superior vena cava (face, neck, upper chest, arms), they suggest hyperestrogenism from impaired hepatic estrogen metabolism and correlate with the severity of cirrhosis. Palmar erythema — symmetric reddening of the thenar and hypothenar eminences — similarly reflects hyperestrogenism and occurs in 25 percent of patients with cirrhosis. Jaundice becomes clinically detectable when serum bilirubin exceeds approximately 2.5 to 3 mg/dL (43 to 51 micromol/L), appearing first in the sclerae (scleral icterus) and then progressing to the skin. Pruritus of cholestasis — generalized, often severe, and worst on the palms and soles — results from bile acid deposition in the skin and affects patients with obstructive and intrahepatic cholestatic diseases (primary biliary cholangitis, primary sclerosing cholangitis, drug-induced cholestasis). Terry nails (white nails with a narrow distal pink-brown band) and Muehrcke lines (paired white transverse bands on the nails reflecting hypoalbuminemia) are additional nail findings of chronic liver disease.

Cutaneous Manifestations of Renal Disease

Chronic kidney disease produces cutaneous changes that worsen with declining glomerular filtration rate. Uremic pruritus is the most common and debilitating cutaneous symptom, affecting 40 to 70 percent of dialysis patients. The pathogenesis is multifactorial — accumulation of uremic toxins, secondary hyperparathyroidism with calcium-phosphate deposition in the skin, peripheral neuropathy, and immune dysregulation. Half-and-half nails (Lindsay nails — proximal white and distal brown, with the distal band occupying 20 to 60 percent of the nail) are characteristic of uremia. Acquired perforating dermatosis (Kyrle disease, reactive perforating collagenosis) presents as umbilicated papules and nodules with central keratotic plugs, most commonly on the legs and trunk of dialysis patients — the pathology shows transepidermal elimination of collagen or elastic fibers. Calciphylaxis (calcific uremic arteriolopathy) is a life-threatening condition in patients with end-stage renal disease, characterized by painful, violaceous, reticular plaques (livedo racemosa pattern) that rapidly progress to ischemic necrosis and eschars, predominantly on adipose-rich areas (abdomen, thighs, buttocks). Calciphylaxis carries a mortality rate of 60 to 80 percent, primarily from sepsis of infected wounds. Risk factors include secondary hyperparathyroidism, hyperphosphatemia, warfarin use, obesity, and hypoalbuminemia. Management involves wound care, pain management, correction of calcium-phosphate product, and sodium thiosulfate (which chelates calcium deposits).

Cutaneous Manifestations of Gastrointestinal Disease

Inflammatory bowel disease (IBD) produces both specific and reactive cutaneous manifestations. Erythema nodosum — tender, erythematous, subcutaneous nodules on the anterior shins (the prototype of septal panniculitis) — is the most common cutaneous manifestation of IBD, correlating with disease activity in Crohn disease. Pyoderma gangrenosum (PG) — painful, rapidly expanding ulcers with undermined, violaceous borders — is associated with IBD (particularly ulcerative colitis), rheumatoid arthritis, and hematologic malignancies. PG exhibits pathergy (worsening at sites of trauma), and surgical debridement must be avoided because it triggers further ulceration. Dermatitis herpetiformis (DH) is the cutaneous manifestation of celiac disease, presenting as intensely pruritic, grouped papulovesicles on the elbows, knees, buttocks, and posterior scalp — mirroring the distribution of pressure points. The diagnosis is confirmed by direct immunofluorescence (DIF) showing granular IgA deposits at the dermal papillae. Treatment is dapsone (which provides rapid symptomatic relief within 24 to 48 hours) and a lifelong gluten-free diet (which treats the underlying celiac disease and reduces the long-term risk of intestinal lymphoma). Peutz-Jeghers syndrome — an autosomal dominant disorder caused by STK11 mutations — presents with mucocutaneous lentigines on the lips, buccal mucosa, and perioral skin in childhood, combined with hamartomatous gastrointestinal polyps and an increased risk of gastrointestinal and extraintestinal malignancies.

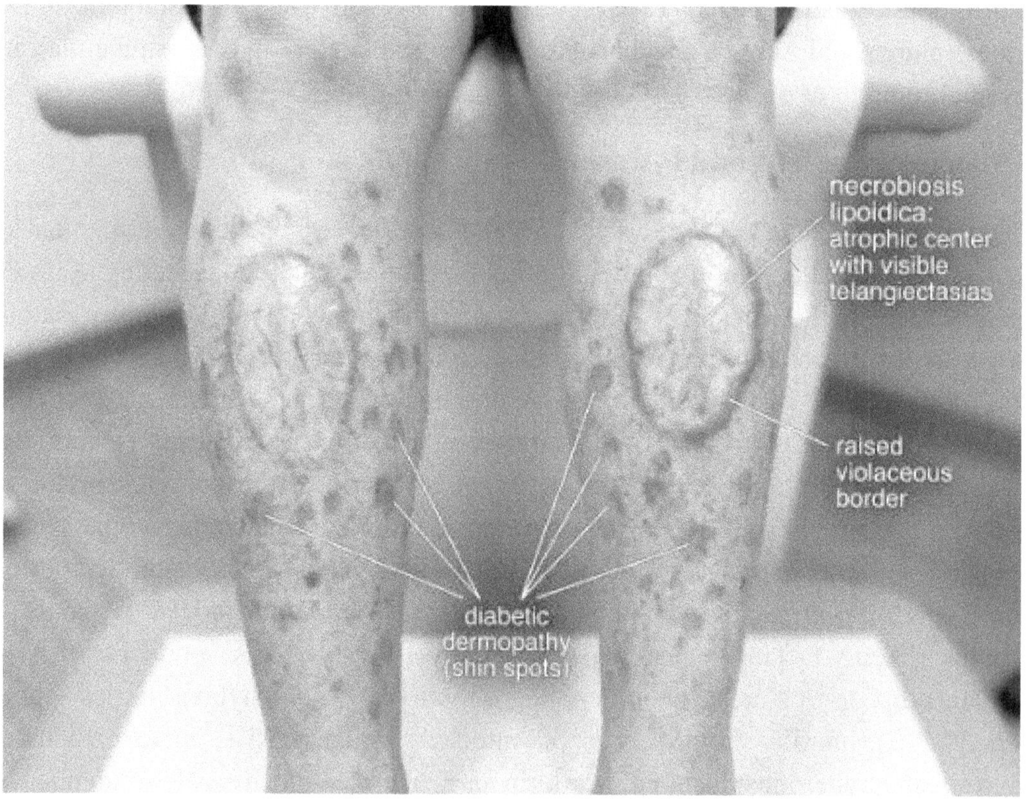

Skin Signs of Hematologic Disease: Purpura, Petechiae, and Coagulopathies

Pathophysiology of Cutaneous Hemorrhage

Cutaneous hemorrhage reflects failure of one or more components of hemostasis: the vessel wall, platelets, or coagulation factors. The morphology and distribution of the cutaneous hemorrhage provide diagnostic clues to the underlying mechanism. Petechiae (pinpoint, non-blanching, red-purple macules less than 2 mm) and purpura (non-blanching purple patches greater than 2 mm) that are non-palpable suggest thrombocytopenia or platelet dysfunction. Palpable purpura (raised, non-blanching lesions) indicates small-vessel vasculitis — the inflammatory infiltrate and vascular damage create the palpable component. Ecchymoses (bruises greater than 1 cm) in unusual locations or with minimal trauma suggest coagulation factor deficiency (hemophilia) or anticoagulant use. The distinction between blanching and non-blanching is fundamental: erythema blanches with pressure (blood is still within intact vessels and can be displaced), while purpura does not blanch (blood has extravasated into the tissue and cannot be displaced). The diascopy test (pressing a glass slide against the lesion) is the bedside method for making this distinction.

Thrombocytopenic and Non-Thrombocytopenic Purpura

Immune thrombocytopenic purpura (ITP) presents with generalized petechiae and purpura in a patient with isolated thrombocytopenia and no other identifiable cause. In children, ITP is typically acute and self-limited (often following a viral illness), while adult ITP tends to be chronic. Thrombotic thrombocytopenic purpura (TTP) produces the classic pentad of microangiopathic hemolytic anemia, thrombocytopenia, neurologic symptoms, renal dysfunction, and fever — though the full pentad is present in only a minority of cases. The peripheral blood smear shows schistocytes (fragmented red blood cells), confirming the microangiopathic process. TTP is caused by severe deficiency of ADAMTS13 (the von Willebrand factor-cleaving protease), leading to uncontrolled platelet aggregation, and is treated with urgent plasma exchange. Disseminated intravascular coagulation (DIC) produces widespread purpura, ecchymoses, oozing from venipuncture sites, and ischemic necrosis of the extremities and digits (purpura fulminans) in the context of an underlying trigger (sepsis, trauma, obstetric complications, malignancy). Warfarin-induced skin necrosis is a paradoxical thrombotic complication occurring in the first 3 to 10 days of warfarin initiation — it presents as painful, well-demarcated, purpuric plaques progressing to necrosis on adipose-rich areas (breasts, buttocks, thighs). The mechanism is the rapid depletion of protein C (which has a shorter half-life than the procoagulant factors) creating a transient hypercoagulable state. Risk factors include protein C deficiency, protein S deficiency, and initiation of warfarin without heparin bridging.

CAUTION: Purpura fulminans — symmetric, rapidly progressive, non-blanching purpura of the extremities and digits progressing to hemorrhagic necrosis — is a dermatologic emergency. The most common triggers are meningococcemia (Neisseria meningitidis sepsis, especially in children and young adults) and DIC from any cause. Purpura fulminans reflects widespread intravascular thrombosis of dermal and subcutaneous vessels. Immediate management includes aggressive fluid resuscitation, empiric broad-spectrum antibiotics (before blood culture results), correction of coagulopathy with fresh frozen plasma and cryoprecipitate, and ICU-level care. The characteristic morphology — geometric, reticular, well-demarcated purpuric patches that do not follow any vascular territory — combined with shock, mental status changes, and coagulopathy should trigger the clinician to act within minutes, not hours.

Cutaneous Paraneoplastic Syndromes: Sign of Leser-Trelat, Acanthosis Nigricans, Dermatomyositis, and Necrolytic Migratory Erythema

Paraneoplastic Acanthosis Nigricans and the Sign of Leser-Trelat

Paraneoplastic acanthosis nigricans (AN) differs from the benign insulin-resistant form in several critical respects: it is sudden in onset, rapidly progressive, extensive (involving mucosal surfaces — the lips, tongue, palms, and soles — in addition to the typical flexural sites), and occurs in an older patient without obesity or diabetes. Paraneoplastic AN is most commonly associated with gastric adenocarcinoma (the most frequent underlying malignancy) and other intra-abdominal carcinomas. The mechanism involves tumor-derived growth factors — transforming growth factor-alpha (TGF-alpha), which binds epidermal growth factor receptors on keratinocytes, and other mitogenic peptides — driving epidermal proliferation. The sign of Leser-Trelat is the sudden eruption of multiple seborrheic keratoses (or the rapid increase in size and number of pre-existing seborrheic keratoses), often accompanied by pruritus, signaling an underlying malignancy. It is most commonly associated with gastrointestinal adenocarcinomas and lymphomas. The sign of Leser-Trelat frequently coexists with paraneoplastic AN in the same patient. Both dermatoses may precede the diagnosis of the malignancy by months and can regress with successful treatment of the underlying cancer.

Dermatomyositis as a Paraneoplastic Marker

Dermatomyositis (DM) is an inflammatory myopathy with characteristic cutaneous findings. The pathognomonic skin findings include the heliotrope rash (violaceous erythema and edema of the upper eyelids — the lilac color is distinctive) and Gottron papules (violaceous, flat-topped papules over the metacarpophalangeal and interphalangeal joints, elbows, and knees — overlying bony prominences). Characteristic but non-pathognomonic findings include the shawl sign (erythema of the posterior shoulders and upper back), the V-sign (erythema of the anterior neck and upper chest), mechanic's hands (hyperkeratotic, fissured, rough skin of the radial and palmar surfaces of the fingers), and periungual telangiectasias with ragged cuticles. The malignancy risk in dermatomyositis is substantial: adult-onset DM carries a 15 to 30 percent risk of occult malignancy within 3 years of diagnosis (compared to roughly 5 percent in polymyositis). The most commonly associated malignancies are ovarian cancer (the highest risk of any DM-associated cancer), lung, breast, colorectal, and nasopharyngeal carcinoma. Anti-TIF1-gamma (anti-p155/140) autoantibodies are strongly associated with cancer-associated DM and can guide the intensity of malignancy screening. All adult patients with newly diagnosed DM require a comprehensive malignancy workup: CT of the chest, abdomen, and pelvis; age-appropriate cancer screening (mammography, colonoscopy); consideration of PET-CT; and for women, pelvic ultrasound and CA-125.

Necrolytic Migratory Erythema and Other Paraneoplastic Dermatoses

Necrolytic migratory erythema (NME) is the cutaneous marker of glucagonoma — a rare islet cell tumor of the pancreas that secretes excess glucagon. NME presents as erythematous, annular and polycyclic plaques with superficial erosions, crusting, and a characteristic trailing scale at the advancing border, predominantly on the perineum, groin, buttocks, lower abdomen, and lower extremities. The lesions follow a migratory pattern: they arise, expand centrifugally, and heal centrally over 7 to 14 days, only to recur elsewhere. The glucagonoma syndrome includes NME, diabetes mellitus (from glucagon-mediated gluconeogenesis), weight loss, anemia, diarrhea, venous thrombosis, and neuropsychiatric symptoms. Serum glucagon levels are markedly elevated (typically greater than 1,000 pg/mL; normal is less than 200 pg/mL), and imaging reveals a pancreatic mass. Other paraneoplastic dermatoses include Bazex syndrome (acrokeratosis paraneoplastica — psoriasiform, violaceous, keratotic plaques on the acral surfaces, helices of the ears, and nose, associated with upper aerodigestive tract squamous cell carcinomas), Sweet syndrome (acute febrile neutrophilic dermatosis — painful, edematous, red-purple plaques and nodules, associated with hematologic malignancies, particularly acute myeloid leukemia), and paraneoplastic pemphigus (a blistering disease with intractable, painful mucosal erosions, associated with lymphoproliferative disorders — distinguished by the characteristic finding of lichenoid interface dermatitis combined with suprabasal acantholysis on histology).

THE CUTANEOUS MIMICKER RECOGNITION ATLAS — Paraneoplastic Acanthosis Nigricans versus Benign Insulin-Resistant Acanthosis Nigricans

The Clinical Pattern: Benign acanthosis nigricans (the insulin-resistant form) presents as velvety, hyperpigmented plaques in the axillae, posterior neck, and groin of an obese patient with metabolic syndrome or type 2 diabetes. The onset is gradual, the distribution is limited to classic flexural sites, and the degree of acanthosis correlates with the degree of insulin resistance. It is common in adolescents with obesity and may improve with weight loss and insulin-sensitizing therapy. The mucosal surfaces and palms are NOT involved.

The Mimicker: Paraneoplastic acanthosis nigricans presents with sudden-onset, rapidly progressive, extensive velvety hyperpigmentation that extends BEYOND the typical flexural sites — involving the mucosal surfaces (lips, tongue, esophagus), palms (tripe palms — a rugose, ridged, velvety texture of the palmar surfaces), and soles. The patient is typically older, non-obese, and without diabetes. Paraneoplastic AN is most commonly associated with gastric adenocarcinoma. The rapid onset and unusual extent are the clinical red flags that distinguish the paraneoplastic form from the benign form.

Trap Logic: Dismissing new-onset acanthosis nigricans in an older, non-obese patient as a benign cosmetic finding delays the diagnosis of an underlying gastrointestinal malignancy — sometimes by months. The clinical red flags that mandate malignancy workup are sudden onset, rapid progression, mucosal involvement, tripe palms, and the absence of obesity or insulin resistance. **Conversely, initiating a malignancy workup in every obese adolescent with axillary AN** is unnecessary and anxiety-provoking — benign AN in the setting of obesity and metabolic syndrome is extremely common.

The Decision Anchor: The discriminating features are **onset (benign — gradual; paraneoplastic — sudden and rapidly progressive), extent (benign — flexural only; paraneoplastic — flexural plus mucosal, palmar, and solear involvement), patient profile (benign — young, obese, insulin-resistant; paraneoplastic — older, non-obese, no metabolic syndrome), and associated findings (benign — metabolic syndrome; paraneoplastic — weight loss, GI symptoms, sign of Leser-Trelat)**. Tripe palms are nearly pathognomonic for paraneoplastic AN and mandate a GI malignancy workup.

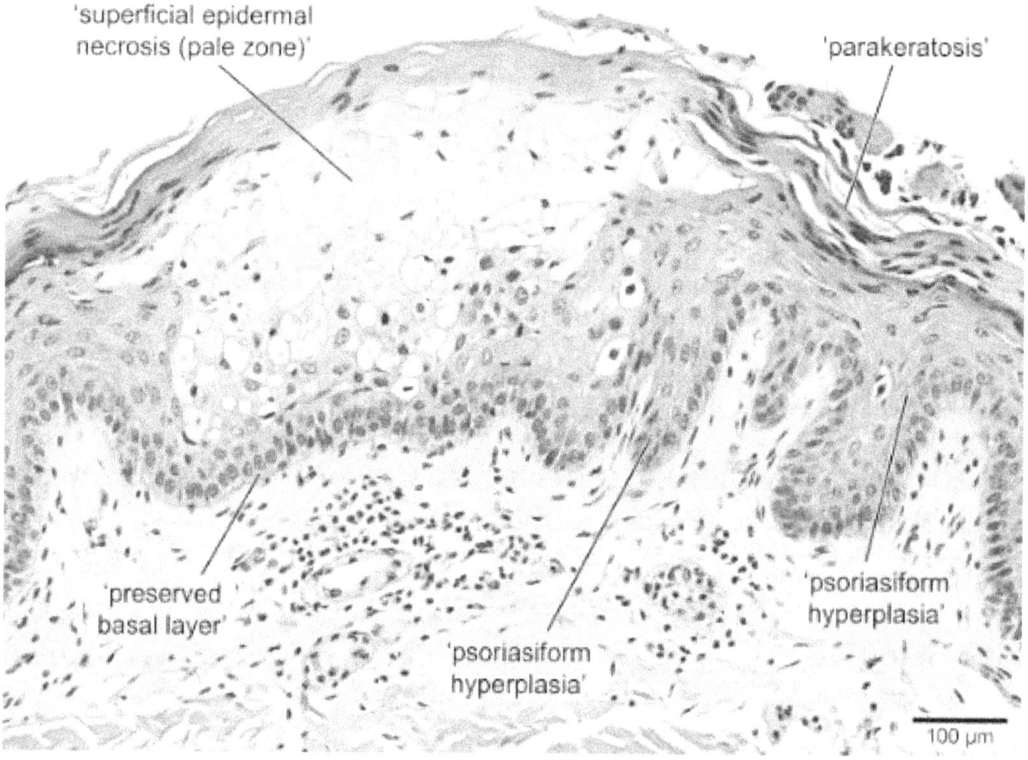

Drug Eruptions: Morbilliform, Fixed, Lichenoid, Photosensitive, and Severe Adverse Reactions (SJS/TEN, DRESS, AGEP)

Morbilliform Drug Eruptions and Fixed Drug Eruptions

Morbilliform (exanthematous) drug eruptions are the most common cutaneous adverse drug reaction, accounting for 40 to 75 percent of all drug eruptions. They present as symmetric, erythematous macules and papules that begin on the trunk and spread centrifugally to the extremities, typically 7 to 14 days after starting a new medication (or 1 to 3 days on re-exposure). The face, palms, soles, and mucous membranes are usually spared in uncomplicated morbilliform eruptions — mucous membrane involvement suggests a more severe reaction and should prompt reassessment. Common culprit medications include beta-lactam antibiotics (amoxicillin, ampicillin), sulfonamides, allopurinol, and anticonvulsants. The rash is typically self-limited, resolving within 1 to 2 weeks after drug discontinuation, and treatment is supportive (topical corticosteroids, antihistamines for pruritus). Fixed drug eruption (FDE) presents as one or more well-demarcated, round or oval, erythematous to violaceous patches or plaques that appear at the SAME anatomical location each time the offending drug is taken. The lips, genitalia, and acral surfaces are classic sites. After resolution, a characteristic post-inflammatory hyperpigmented macule remains, marking the site for future recurrences. Common culprits include TMP-SMX, NSAIDs, tetracyclines, and phenolphthalein. Generalized bullous FDE — an extensive form with widespread bullae — can mimic SJS/TEN and must be distinguished from it, as the management and prognosis differ.

Severe Cutaneous Adverse Reactions: SJS/TEN

Stevens-Johnson syndrome (SJS) and toxic epidermal necrolysis (TEN) represent a spectrum of the same life-threatening mucocutaneous reaction, classified by the percentage of body surface area (BSA) of epidermal detachment: SJS (less than 10 percent BSA), SJS-TEN overlap (10 to 30 percent BSA), and TEN (greater than 30 percent BSA). The hallmark is full-thickness epidermal necrosis and detachment — the Nikolsky sign (lateral pressure on uninvolved skin causes the epidermis to separate) is positive, and Asboe-Hansen sign (extension of a blister with lateral pressure on its edge) is present. Mucosal involvement (oral, ocular, and genital erosions) occurs in greater than 90 percent of cases and distinguishes SJS/TEN from other causes of widespread blistering. The most common culprit medications are allopurinol (the single most common cause worldwide), anticonvulsants (carbamazepine, phenytoin, lamotrigine, phenobarbital), sulfonamide antibiotics, and nevirapine. HLA-B*5801 is strongly associated with allopurinol-induced SJS/TEN, particularly in Southeast Asian, African American, and Korean populations — HLA-B*5801 screening before initiating allopurinol is recommended by the ACR in these groups. Mortality is estimated by the SCORTEN prognostic index (age greater than 40, malignancy, heart rate greater than 120, serum urea greater than 28 mg/dL, glucose greater than 252 mg/dL, bicarbonate less than 20 mEq/L, BSA detachment greater than 10 percent — each scores 1 point; SCORTEN 0-1 carries 3 percent mortality, SCORTEN 5+ carries greater than 90 percent mortality). Management requires immediate withdrawal of the culprit drug, transfer to a burn unit or ICU, meticulous wound care, fluid resuscitation, pain management, ophthalmology consultation (to prevent symblepharon and corneal damage), and nutritional support.

DRESS Syndrome and AGEP

Drug reaction with eosinophilia and systemic symptoms (DRESS), also known as drug-induced hypersensitivity syndrome (DiHS), is a severe, potentially fatal drug reaction with a delayed onset (2 to 8 weeks after starting the culprit medication — the longest latency of any drug eruption). DRESS is characterized by a widespread morbilliform or exfoliative eruption, facial edema (a distinctive early sign), fever, lymphadenopathy, eosinophilia (typically greater than 1,500 per microliter), atypical lymphocytosis, and visceral involvement — hepatitis is the most common organ involvement (70 percent of cases), followed by nephritis, pneumonitis, myocarditis, and thyroiditis. The most common culprit drugs are anticonvulsants (carbamazepine, phenytoin, lamotrigine, phenobarbital), allopurinol, sulfonamides, and dapsone. HHV-6 reactivation is detected in many DRESS cases and may contribute to the severity of organ involvement. Treatment is systemic corticosteroids (the mainstay, unlike SJS/TEN where corticosteroids are controversial), drug withdrawal, and organ-specific supportive care. Thyroid function should be monitored for months after DRESS resolution, as autoimmune thyroiditis is a recognized late complication. Acute generalized exanthematous pustulosis (AGEP) presents as a sudden eruption of hundreds of small, non-follicular, sterile pustules on a background of diffuse erythema, most prominently on the trunk and intertriginous areas. AGEP occurs 1 to 5 days after starting the culprit medication (the shortest latency of any drug eruption), is accompanied by fever and neutrophilic leukocytosis, and resolves rapidly after drug withdrawal with characteristic widespread desquamation. The most common culprits are beta-lactam antibiotics and macrolides.

CLINICAL PEARL: The timeline of drug eruption onset is a powerful diagnostic clue that helps identify the culprit medication. AGEP has the shortest latency (1 to 5 days), morbilliform eruptions appear at 7 to 14 days, SJS/TEN at 1 to 4 weeks, and DRESS has the longest latency (2 to 8 weeks). When a patient has been on multiple medications, identifying which drug was started within the expected latency window for the reaction pattern narrows the differential dramatically. The ALDEN algorithm for SJS/TEN and the RegiSCAR scoring systems for DRESS and AGEP are validated tools for determining drug causality.

Reaction	Latency	Key Morphology	Mucosal Involvement	Systemic Features	Mortality
Morbilliform	7–14 days	Symmetric maculopapular eruption, trunk to extremities	Usually absent	Rare; low-grade fever possible	Very low (less than 0.1%)
Fixed drug eruption	Hours to days on re-exposure	Well-demarcated round plaques at the same site each time; post-inflammatory hyperpigmentation	Possible in generalized bullous FDE	Absent in localized form	Very low; generalized bullous FDE has higher risk
SJS/TEN	1–4 weeks	Epidermal necrosis and detachment; targetoid macules; positive Nikolsky sign	Greater than 90% — oral, ocular, genital erosions	Fever, elevated transaminases	SJS 1–5%; TEN 25–35%; SCORTEN-dependent
DRESS	2–8 weeks	Widespread morbilliform or exfoliative eruption; facial edema	Variable	Eosinophilia, hepatitis, lymphadenopathy,	5–10%

				nephritis, myocarditis	
AGEP	1–5 days	Hundreds of small sterile pustules on erythematous background	Rare	Fever, neutrophilic leukocytosis	Less than 5%

THE CUTANEOUS MIMICKER RECOGNITION ATLAS — SJS/TEN versus Generalized Bullous Fixed Drug Eruption

The Clinical Pattern: Stevens-Johnson syndrome and toxic epidermal necrolysis present with widespread dusky erythematous or targetoid macules that progress to full-thickness epidermal necrosis and detachment. The Nikolsky sign is positive. Mucosal involvement (oral, ocular, genital erosions) occurs in greater than 90 percent of cases. The patient is febrile, in pain, and systemically ill. The clinical appearance resembles a large-area burn. The culprit medication was typically started 1 to 4 weeks before onset.

The Mimicker: Generalized bullous fixed drug eruption (GBFDE) presents with widespread, well-demarcated, round or oval, erythematous to dusky plaques with central bullae and erosions — it can mimic SJS/TEN in extent and severity. However, GBFDE characteristically spares the mucosal surfaces (or involves them minimally), the individual lesions are more well-demarcated and round than the confluent sheets of necrosis in TEN, and post-inflammatory hyperpigmentation is prominent. Onset is typically faster (hours to 1 to 2 days on re-exposure) than SJS/TEN.

Trap Logic: Treating GBFDE as TEN and transferring to a burn unit for aggressive wound management is not harmful per se — the supportive care is appropriate. But the distinction matters because GBFDE has a significantly better prognosis than true TEN (mortality approximately 5 percent vs. 25 to 35 percent for TEN), and the culprit drug identification differs. **Conversely, dismissing early SJS/TEN as a fixed drug eruption** delays transfer to an appropriate burn or ICU setting and delays the critical step of stopping the offending medication.

The Decision Anchor: The discriminating features are **mucosal involvement (SJS/TEN — prominent oral, ocular, and genital erosions in greater than 90%; GBFDE — absent or minimal mucosal disease), lesion morphology (SJS/TEN — confluent dusky macules progressing to sheets of necrosis; GBFDE — discrete, well-demarcated round plaques with central bullae), post-inflammatory hyperpigmentation (marked in GBFDE; absent in acute SJS/TEN), and timeline (GBFDE — rapid onset within hours on re-exposure; SJS/TEN — 1 to 4 weeks after starting the culprit)**. Biopsy can help: SJS/TEN shows full-thickness epidermal necrosis; GBFDE shows a mixed lichenoid and interface pattern with more eosinophils.

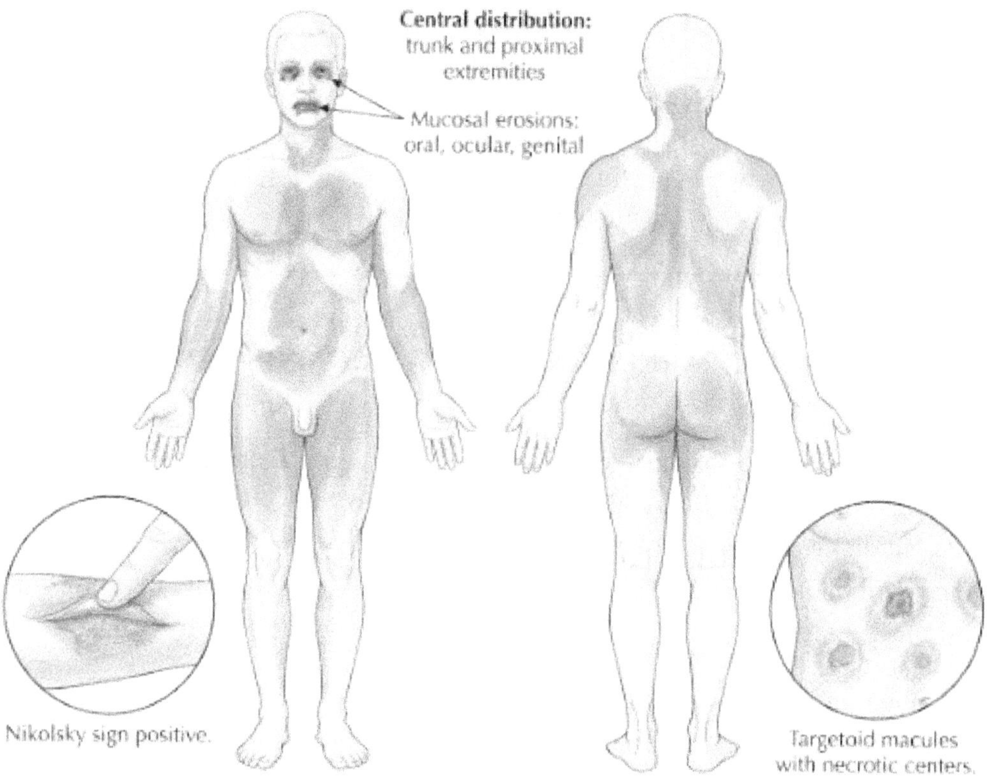

Psychodermatology: Delusional Infestation, Dermatitis Artefacta, Neurotic Excoriations, and Trichotillomania

Delusional Infestation

Delusional infestation (also known as delusional parasitosis or Morgellons disease in some formulations) is a fixed, monosymptomatic delusional disorder in which the patient is unshakably convinced that their skin is infested with parasites, insects, fibers, or other organisms, despite no objective evidence. Patients present with excoriations, erosions, and ulcerations that are entirely self-inflicted from picking, digging, and scratching to remove the perceived organisms. They frequently bring specimens (the matchbox sign or specimen sign) — collections of skin debris, lint, scabs, or fibers presented as evidence of the infestation. The delusion is fixed and cannot be corrected by reassurance, negative workup results, or demonstration that the specimens contain no organisms. The differential diagnosis includes actual infestation (scabies, lice, bed bugs — always exclude with appropriate testing), pruritic dermatoses that might drive the false belief (atopic dermatitis, contact dermatitis, xerosis), substance use (methamphetamine-induced formication, cocaine bugs), and secondary causes (hypothyroidism, hepatic or renal disease, vitamin B12 deficiency, HIV, lymphoma). Treatment is antipsychotic medication — pimozide was traditionally first-line but has been largely replaced by second-generation antipsychotics (risperidone, olanzapine, aripiprazole) because of pimozide's risk of QT prolongation and extrapyramidal side effects. Establishing therapeutic rapport is essential: patients with delusional infestation are often hostile to psychiatric referral and may doctor-shop, so dermatologists must engage empathetically, treat the skin symptoms, and introduce antipsychotic medication carefully (framing it as helping with itch or distress rather than psychosis).

Dermatitis Artefacta and Neurotic Excoriations

Dermatitis artefacta (factitious dermatitis) is the deliberate self-infliction of skin lesions to assume the sick role, typically denied by the patient. The lesions have characteristic features: they are geometric or angular (not following any natural dermatologic pattern), sharply demarcated (as if stamped onto the skin), located only in areas accessible to the dominant hand, and surrounded by normal skin. Common methods include burning (cigarettes, chemicals), cutting, applying caustic substances, and injection of foreign material. The patient typically denies self-infliction and may present with an elaborate, inconsistent history. The lesions often appear overnight or during periods of emotional stress. The diagnosis is clinical (biopsy is non-specific, showing tissue damage without a characteristic inflammatory pattern). Treatment requires a non-confrontational approach — directly accusing the patient of self-harm is counterproductive and leads to disengagement. Psychiatric referral is essential but must be introduced carefully. Neurotic excoriations (skin picking disorder, excoriation disorder in DSM-5-TR) differ from dermatitis artefacta in that the patient acknowledges the behavior: they compulsively pick, scratch, or dig at their skin, producing excoriations, ulcers, and scars, and they cannot stop despite wanting to. The face, arms, and upper back are common sites. Excoriation disorder falls within the obsessive-compulsive and related disorders spectrum in DSM-5-TR. Treatment includes cognitive-behavioral therapy (habit reversal training), SSRIs, and N-acetylcysteine.

Trichotillomania and Body-Focused Repetitive Behaviors

Trichotillomania (hair-pulling disorder) is a body-focused repetitive behavior in which the patient compulsively pulls out their own hair, resulting in noticeable hair loss. It is classified under obsessive-compulsive and related disorders in DSM-5-TR. The scalp is the most common site (75 percent of cases), followed by eyebrows, eyelashes, and pubic hair. The clinical presentation is distinctive: irregular, bizarrely shaped patches of alopecia with hairs of varying lengths (broken and regrowing hairs at different stages), without the scarring, inflammation, or scaling seen in alopecia areata or tinea capitis. Trichoscopy (dermoscopy of the scalp) shows broken hairs at different lengths, V-sign (two hairs broken at the same level from the same follicle), flame hairs (hair residues that resemble a flame shape), coiled hairs, and black dots — but no exclamation point hairs (which are pathognomonic for alopecia areata). The hair-pull test is negative (unlike telogen effluvium). Biopsy shows trichomalacia (distorted, pigment-laden hair shafts in the dermis), the absence of peribulbar inflammation (distinguishing from alopecia areata), and increased catagen and telogen hairs. Treatment includes cognitive-behavioral therapy (habit reversal training — the first-line intervention), SSRIs, clomipramine, and N-acetylcysteine. In children under 5 years, trichotillomania is often a benign, self-limited habit that resolves without intervention.

EVIDENCE: The landmark randomized controlled trial by Grant and colleagues (2009) demonstrated that N-acetylcysteine (NAC), a glutamate-modulating agent, was significantly more effective than placebo for trichotillomania in adults. At 12 weeks, 56 percent of NAC-treated patients were rated as much or very much improved compared to 16 percent with placebo. NAC is well-tolerated, inexpensive, and available over the counter — making it an attractive adjunct to cognitive-behavioral therapy. The proposed mechanism involves normalization of glutamatergic signaling in the corticostriatal circuit, which is implicated in habit-based, compulsive behaviors. Subsequent studies have explored NAC for other body-focused repetitive behaviors (skin picking, nail biting) with promising but less robust evidence.

Clinical Case: Recurrent Pruritic Eruption With Specimen Collection

A 62-year-old retired accountant presents to the dermatology clinic with a 14-month history of intense pruritus and a sensation of crawling insects on his skin. He has seen four dermatologists and two infectious disease specialists, none of whom found evidence of infestation. He brings a plastic bag containing tissue paper with collected skin debris, fibers, and crusts, which he insists are the remains of parasites emerging from his skin. On examination, there are scattered excoriations, erosions, and shallow ulcerations on the forearms, shoulders, upper back, and legs — all consistent with self-inflicted damage from picking. No primary dermatologic lesions (vesicles, papules, wheals, burrows) are present. The areas between the excoriations show normal skin. Microscopic examination of the collected specimens reveals only skin debris, dried blood, and clothing fibers — no organisms.

The clinical reasoning identifies this presentation as delusional infestation: the fixed belief in cutaneous parasitosis despite multiple negative evaluations, the matchbox sign (specimen presentation), self-inflicted excoriations without primary lesions, and the inability of reassurance or negative workup results to alter the belief. However, before diagnosing a primary psychiatric disorder, secondary causes must be excluded. Laboratory evaluation includes complete blood count (to exclude eosinophilia suggesting true parasitosis or lymphoma), comprehensive metabolic panel (hepatic and renal function), thyroid function tests, vitamin B12 level, HIV testing, and RPR. Urine drug screen is performed to exclude stimulant use. All results return within normal limits. The patient is not on any medications known to cause formication. A careful trial of permethrin cream is offered (both to treat the possibility of missed scabies and as a therapeutic gesture of good faith). After the permethrin trial produces no improvement, the diagnosis of primary delusional infestation is confirmed. Treatment with low-dose risperidone is initiated — introduced as medication that helps the skin heal faster and reduces the sensation of crawling, avoiding the word antipsychotic. The patient is also prescribed emollients and a mild topical corticosteroid for the excoriations. Follow-up at 8 weeks shows partial improvement in both the delusion and the self-inflicted skin damage.

Paraneoplastic AN vs. Benign Insulin-Resistant AN: The discriminating features are onset (benign — gradual; paraneoplastic — sudden and rapidly progressive), extent (benign — flexural only; paraneoplastic — flexural plus mucosal and palmar involvement, tripe palms), patient profile (benign — young, obese, insulin-resistant; paraneoplastic — older, non-obese), and associated findings (paraneoplastic — weight loss, sign of Leser-Trelat, GI symptoms). Cognitive trap: dismissing new-onset AN in a non-obese older patient as cosmetic delays malignancy diagnosis.

SJS/TEN vs. Generalized Bullous FDE: The discriminating features are mucosal involvement (SJS/TEN — prominent in greater than 90%; GBFDE — absent or minimal), lesion morphology (SJS/TEN — confluent necrotic sheets; GBFDE — discrete, well-demarcated round plaques), post-inflammatory hyperpigmentation (marked in GBFDE), and timeline (GBFDE — hours on re-exposure; SJS/TEN — 1 to 4 weeks). Cognitive trap: missing early SJS/TEN by calling it a fixed drug eruption delays critical supportive care.

Summary and Key Concepts

Cutaneous signs of endocrine disease provide diagnostic clues to the underlying systemic disorder: necrobiosis lipoidica and diabetic dermopathy signal microvascular disease in diabetes; pretibial myxedema is specific to Graves disease; wide violaceous striae suggest Cushing syndrome; and diffuse hyperpigmentation with palmar crease accentuation suggests Addison disease.

Paraneoplastic dermatoses — including sudden-onset acanthosis nigricans with mucosal involvement, the sign of Leser-Trelat, dermatomyositis (15 to 30 percent malignancy risk in adults — anti-TIF1-gamma antibodies guide screening intensity), and necrolytic migratory erythema (glucagonoma marker) — may precede the diagnosis of internal malignancy and mandate comprehensive cancer workup.

Drug eruptions are classified by morphology and severity: morbilliform eruptions are the most common (7 to 14 day latency), SJS/TEN is the most life-threatening (SCORTEN predicts mortality), DRESS has the longest latency (2 to 8 weeks) and causes organ damage, and AGEP has the shortest latency (1 to 5 days). HLA-B*5801 screening before allopurinol initiation prevents SJS/TEN in high-risk populations.

Hepatic disease produces spider angiomas, palmar erythema, jaundice, and pruritus of cholestasis; renal disease produces uremic pruritus, half-and-half nails, and calciphylaxis; and gastrointestinal disease produces erythema nodosum and pyoderma gangrenosum (IBD), dermatitis herpetiformis (celiac disease), and mucocutaneous lentigines (Peutz-Jeghers syndrome).

Psychodermatology disorders — delusional infestation (matchbox sign, fixed belief, antipsychotics), dermatitis artefacta (geometric self-inflicted lesions, denied by patient), neurotic excoriations (acknowledged compulsive picking, CBT and SSRIs), and trichotillomania (irregular alopecia with broken hairs at different lengths, habit reversal training) — require integrated dermatologic and psychiatric management.

CHAPTER 23: PIGMENTARY DISORDERS AND DISORDERS OF MELANOCYTES

Learning Objectives

1. Explain the pathogenesis of vitiligo as an autoimmune melanocyte destruction process mediated by CD8+ cytotoxic T cells and the IFN-gamma-CXCL10-CXCR3 axis, and apply the Vitiligo Area Scoring Index (VASI) to guide treatment decisions.
2. Classify pigmentary disorders by mechanism — melanocyte destruction (vitiligo, albinism), melanin overproduction (melasma, post-inflammatory hyperpigmentation), and melanocyte proliferation (lentigines, cafe-au-lait macules) — and implement evidence-based management strategies for each.
3. Recognize the clinical and dermoscopic features that distinguish benign pigmentary conditions from melanocytic neoplasms, and apply appropriate diagnostic algorithms including Wood lamp examination, dermoscopy, and biopsy.
4. Address the unique diagnostic challenges of pigmentary disorders in skin of color (Fitzpatrick IV to VI), including the differential diagnosis of dermatosis papulosa nigra, the increased risk of post-inflammatory hyperpigmentation, and the importance of culturally sensitive counseling.

Vitiligo: Pathogenesis, Classification, and Evidence-Based Treatment

Pathogenesis and Immunology

Vitiligo is an acquired, chronic depigmenting disorder resulting from the autoimmune destruction of melanocytes. It affects 0.5 to 2 percent of the global population across all races and skin types, with onset typically before age 30 in more than half of patients. The pathogenesis involves the convergence of genetic susceptibility (multiple susceptibility loci including NLRP1, CTLA-4, HLA-A2, PTPN22 — many shared with other autoimmune diseases), cellular stress in melanocytes (oxidative stress, unfolded protein response, heat shock proteins released as danger signals), and an autoimmune effector response. The IFN-gamma-CXCL10-CXCR3 axis is central: stressed melanocytes release danger signals that activate innate immunity, which produces IFN-gamma, which induces keratinocytes to secrete CXCL10 (a chemokine that recruits CXCR3-expressing CD8+ cytotoxic T cells into the skin). These melanocyte-specific CD8+ T cells are the direct effectors of melanocyte killing. This axis has become the target of new therapies — ruxolitinib, a JAK1/JAK2 inhibitor, interrupts IFN-gamma signaling and is the first FDA-approved topical treatment specifically for vitiligo repigmentation (2022).

Classification and Clinical Features

Vitiligo is classified into two major forms. Non-segmental vitiligo (the most common form, approximately 85 to 90 percent of cases) is a chronic, progressive, autoimmune-mediated process that typically presents as bilateral, symmetric, well-demarcated, chalk-white macules and patches. It favors periorificial areas (perioral, periocular, perianal, genital), extensor surfaces (dorsal hands, elbows, knees), and trauma-prone sites (Koebner phenomenon). Acrofacial vitiligo (face and distal extremities) and vitiligo universalis (greater than 80 percent BSA depigmentation) are subtypes. Non-segmental vitiligo has a strong association with other autoimmune diseases — autoimmune thyroid disease (Hashimoto thyroiditis and Graves disease) is the most common (15 to 25 percent), followed by pernicious anemia, type 1 diabetes, Addison disease, alopecia areata, and rheumatoid arthritis. Segmental vitiligo (approximately 10 to 15 percent of cases) presents as unilateral, dermatomal or quasi-dermatomal depigmented patches that develop rapidly, stabilize within 1 to 2 years, and do not progress to generalized involvement. It has a weaker autoimmune association and a stronger association with ipsilateral leukotrichia (white hair within the lesion — which indicates destruction of the melanocyte reservoir in the hair follicle and carries a poorer repigmentation prognosis). The diagnosis is clinical in most cases; Wood lamp examination enhances the contrast between depigmented and normal skin (vitiligo fluoresces bright white under Wood lamp, which is particularly helpful in fair-skinned patients where lesions may be subtle in ambient light).

Evidence-Based Treatment

The treatment of vitiligo aims to halt disease progression (stabilization) and restore pigmentation (repigmentation). Topical therapies are first-line for limited disease (less than 10 percent BSA): topical corticosteroids (medium to high potency for the body; low potency for the face — 3-month courses with monitoring for atrophy), topical calcineurin inhibitors (tacrolimus 0.1 percent and pimecrolimus — preferred for facial and intertriginous vitiligo to avoid steroid side effects, particularly in children), and topical ruxolitinib 1.5 percent cream (the first FDA-approved topical JAK inhibitor for non-segmental vitiligo in patients aged 12 years and older — applied twice daily, it produces facial repigmentation in approximately 30 percent of patients at 24 weeks, with continued improvement through 52 weeks). Phototherapy is the mainstay for extensive disease (greater than 10 percent BSA): narrowband UVB (NB-UVB, 311 nm) administered 2 to 3 times weekly for at least 6 to 12 months is the gold standard — it stimulates melanocyte migration from the hair follicle reservoir and promotes melanocyte differentiation and melanogenesis. The face and neck repigment most readily; the acral areas (fingers, toes, lips) respond poorly because they lack hair follicles and thus lack the melanocyte stem cell reservoir. Surgical options for stable segmental vitiligo unresponsive to medical therapy include melanocyte-keratinocyte transplant procedures (MKTP — a cell suspension is prepared from a donor site and applied to a dermabraded recipient site) and suction blister grafting. Combination therapy (NB-UVB plus topical calcineurin inhibitors or topical corticosteroids) achieves higher repigmentation rates than either modality alone.

EVIDENCE: The pivotal TRuE-V1 and TRuE-V2 phase 3 randomized controlled trials (2022) demonstrated the efficacy of topical ruxolitinib cream 1.5 percent for vitiligo repigmentation. At 24 weeks, significantly more ruxolitinib-treated patients achieved at least 75 percent improvement in the Facial

Vitiligo Area Scoring Index (F-VASI75) compared to vehicle (approximately 30 percent vs. 8 percent). Continued treatment through 52 weeks showed progressive improvement, with approximately 50 percent of patients achieving F-VASI75. The most common adverse effects were application site acne and pruritus. These trials led to the FDA approval of topical ruxolitinib as the first targeted therapy for vitiligo repigmentation — a milestone that translated the understanding of the IFN-gamma-CXCL10-CXCR3 axis directly into clinical practice.

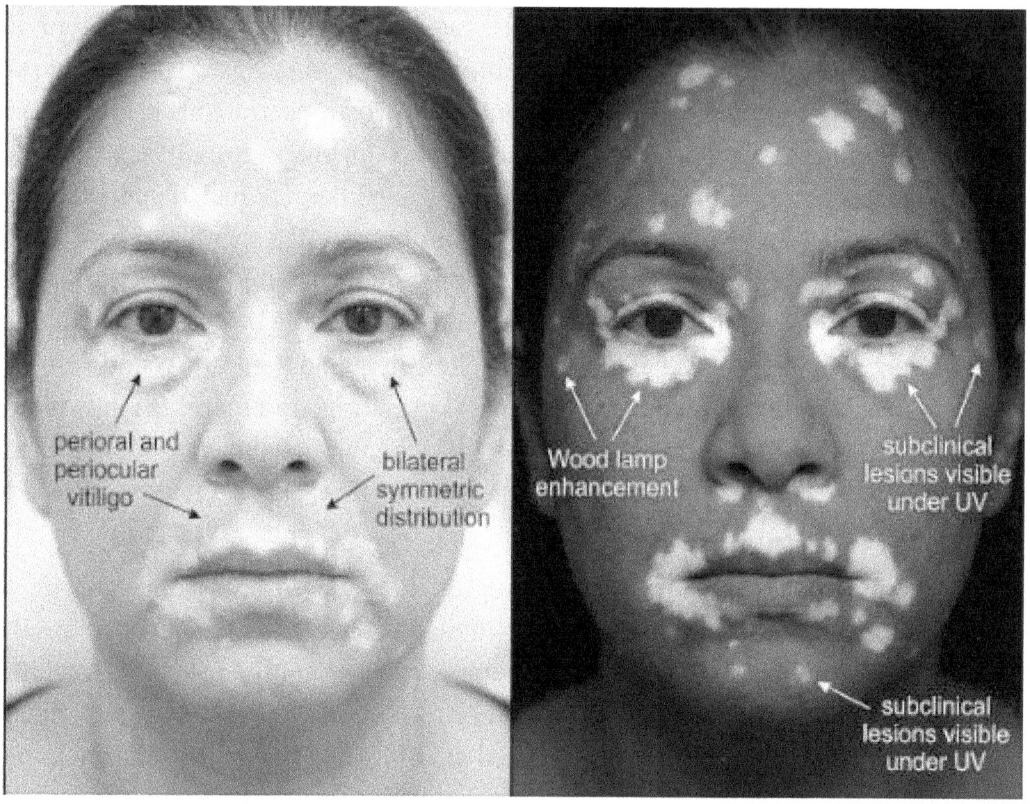

Melasma: Hormonal Influences, Diagnosis, and Multimodal Management

Pathogenesis and Risk Factors

Melasma is an acquired, chronic disorder of hyperpigmentation that disproportionately affects women (90 percent of cases) with Fitzpatrick skin types III to V. It presents as symmetric, irregular, brown to grey-brown macules and patches on the face, with three recognized distribution patterns: centrofacial (the most common — forehead, cheeks, nose, upper lip, chin), malar (cheeks and nose only), and mandibular (jawline). The pathogenesis is multifactorial: ultraviolet radiation is the most important exacerbating factor (UV stimulates melanogenesis through multiple pathways including p53-mediated upregulation of proopiomelanocortin and its cleavage products, including alpha-MSH), and hormonal influences are central — estrogen and progesterone receptors are overexpressed in melasma skin, explaining the strong association with pregnancy (chloasma, the mask of pregnancy), combined oral contraceptive use, and hormone replacement therapy. Recent research has identified that melasma involves not only epidermal hyperpigmentation but also a significant dermal component: increased vascularity, mast cell infiltration, solar elastosis, and basement membrane disruption — which explains why melasma is often treatment-resistant and recurrent. Visible light (400 to 700 nm, particularly blue light from screens and indoor lighting) can trigger and worsen melasma, especially in darker skin types, because visible light activates opsin-3 receptors in melanocytes and stimulates melanogenesis independently of UV exposure.

Diagnosis and Management

The diagnosis of melasma is clinical. Wood lamp examination helps distinguish epidermal melasma (pigment enhanced under Wood lamp — more responsive to topical therapy) from dermal melasma (pigment NOT enhanced — less responsive) and mixed melasma (mixed enhancement). Dermoscopy shows a reticular pattern of brown pigment in epidermal melasma and a blue-grey pattern in dermal melasma. Biopsy is rarely needed but is indicated when the diagnosis is uncertain — histopathology shows increased melanin in the epidermis (epidermal type) or melanophages in the dermis (dermal type), with solar elastosis and increased dermal vascularity. Management follows a multimodal approach: (1) strict photoprotection is the foundation — broad-spectrum sunscreen with SPF 30 or higher, containing iron oxide (which blocks visible light — standard chemical and mineral sunscreens do not adequately block the visible light spectrum), reapplied every 2 hours, combined with wide-brimmed hats and sun avoidance. (2) First-line topical therapy is triple combination cream (hydroquinone 4 percent, tretinoin 0.05 percent, and fluocinolone acetonide 0.01 percent — the modified Kligman formula) — this combination targets melanin synthesis (hydroquinone inhibits tyrosinase), promotes epidermal turnover (tretinoin), and reduces inflammation (corticosteroid). Hydroquinone is used in 3-month cycles to avoid ochronosis (paradoxical blue-grey discoloration from prolonged use). (3) Second-line agents include tranexamic acid (an oral or topical plasminogen inhibitor that reduces melanogenesis by blocking the interaction between keratinocytes and melanocytes), azelaic acid (a tyrosinase inhibitor that also has anti-inflammatory properties), cysteamine, and vitamin C (an antioxidant that inhibits melanin oxidation). (4) Procedures include chemical peels (glycolic acid, salicylic acid — superficial peels only; deep peels risk post-inflammatory hyperpigmentation in darker skin types) and laser therapy (used with extreme caution — the risk of rebound hyperpigmentation and PIH is significant, particularly in darker skin types; low-fluence Q-switched Nd:YAG laser has shown some efficacy but results are inconsistent).

THE CUTANEOUS MIMICKER RECOGNITION ATLAS — Melasma versus Post-Inflammatory Hyperpigmentation

The Clinical Pattern: Melasma presents as symmetric, bilateral, ill-defined brown to grey-brown macules and patches in a characteristic facial distribution — centrofacial (forehead, cheeks, nose, upper lip, chin), malar, or mandibular. The pigmentation is typically uniform within each patch and darkens with sun exposure. The patient is usually a woman of reproductive age with Fitzpatrick III to V skin, and there is often a history of hormonal trigger (pregnancy, OCP use). There is no preceding inflammatory event — the pigmentation appears de novo.

The Mimicker: Post-inflammatory hyperpigmentation (PIH) on the face can closely resemble melasma, particularly when it results from a diffuse inflammatory dermatosis (such as acne, eczema, or contact dermatitis) that affects the same facial regions. PIH, however, is asymmetric or follows the distribution of the preceding inflammatory process (e.g., along the jawline in hormonal acne, on the cheeks where eczema was most active). There is always a history of a preceding inflammatory event — the patient can often describe the rash, acne, or injury that preceded the dark spots.

Trap Logic: Treating facial PIH with the aggressive hydroquinone and retinoid regimens appropriate for melasma without addressing the underlying inflammatory condition may worsen irritation and perpetuate the cycle of inflammation and hyperpigmentation — especially in darker skin types. **Conversely, attributing melasma to a preceding inflammation that did not occur** leads to a search for a non-existent trigger while missing the hormonal and UV-driven pathogenesis. The treatment approach differs: PIH requires treatment of the underlying cause plus anti-pigment therapy; melasma requires long-term photoprotection plus multimodal anti-pigment therapy and hormonal modification if applicable.

The Decision Anchor: The discriminating features are **symmetry (melasma — bilateral and symmetric; PIH — follows the pattern of the preceding inflammation), history (melasma — no preceding inflammatory event; PIH — always preceded by an identifiable rash, acne, or injury), distribution (melasma — centrofacial, malar, or mandibular; PIH — matches the distribution of the prior dermatosis), and response to hormonal changes (melasma worsens with pregnancy and OCPs; PIH does not)**. Both conditions are worsened by UV exposure, but only melasma is worsened by visible light. Wood lamp may help: epidermal PIH enhances under Wood lamp similarly to epidermal melasma, but the asymmetry and history distinguish them clinically.

Condition	Mechanism	Color	Wood Lamp	Distribution	Key Differentiating Feature
Vitiligo	Autoimmune melanocyte destruction	Chalk-white (complete depigmentation)	Bright white fluorescence	Periorificial, acral, symmetric; Koebner phenomenon	Complete depigmentation; may have associated autoimmune diseases
Pityriasis versicolor	Malassezia yeast overgrowth	Hypopigmented (lighter than surrounding, not white)	Pale yellow-green fluorescence	Trunk, shoulders, proximal arms	Fine powdery scale; KOH shows spaghetti and meatballs
Pityriasis alba	Mild eczematous dermatitis	Hypopigmented with fine scale	Slight enhancement	Face (cheeks) in children	Associated with atopy; self-limited; fine scale
Post-inflammatory hypopigmentation	Temporary melanin production inhibition	Lighter than surrounding skin	Variable enhancement	Matches distribution of prior dermatosis	History of preceding inflammatory event;

					repigments spontaneousl y
Idiopathic guttate hypomelanos is	Age-related melanocyte loss	Porcelain-white, 2–5 mm macules	White enhancement	Shins, forearms (sun-exposed)	Multiple discrete small macules; elderly patients
Ash-leaf macule (TSC)	Focal melanocyte dysfunction in hamartoma	White, lance-ovate or polygonal	Bright white (like vitiligo)	Trunk, extremities; present from birth	Associated with tuberous sclerosis complex; polygonal or ash-leaf shape

Post-Inflammatory Hyperpigmentation and Hypopigmentation

Pathogenesis and Clinical Features of PIH

Post-inflammatory hyperpigmentation (PIH) is the most common pigmentary disorder encountered in dermatologic practice, disproportionately affecting individuals with darker skin types (Fitzpatrick III to VI). It results from increased melanin production and transfer to keratinocytes (epidermal PIH — brown color, enhanced under Wood lamp) or from melanin dropped into the dermis following basal layer damage (dermal PIH or pigmentary incontinence — grey-blue color, NOT enhanced under Wood lamp, carried by dermal melanophages). Any cutaneous inflammation can trigger PIH: acne vulgaris (the most common cause), eczema, psoriasis, lichen planus, contact dermatitis, and iatrogenic causes (laser procedures, chemical peels, cryotherapy — particularly in darker skin types). The severity of PIH does not always correlate with the severity of the preceding inflammation — even mild acne can produce pronounced PIH in susceptible individuals. PIH can persist for months to years, particularly the dermal component, which is resistant to topical therapy.

Management of PIH and Post-Inflammatory Hypopigmentation

The cornerstone of PIH management is treatment and prevention of the underlying inflammatory condition — PIH will recur if the inflammatory trigger is not controlled. Strict sun protection is essential, as UV exposure darkens and prolongs PIH. Topical depigmenting agents include hydroquinone (the most effective — 2 to 4 percent, applied to affected areas for 3-month cycles with monitoring for exogenous ochronosis), retinoids (tretinoin, adapalene — promote epidermal turnover and accelerate melanin dispersion), azelaic acid (15 to 20 percent — both anti-pigment and anti-inflammatory, useful when PIH coexists with acne or rosacea), niacinamide (inhibits melanosome transfer from melanocytes to keratinocytes), alpha-hydroxy acids (glycolic acid, lactic acid — exfoliate and promote turnover), and vitamin C (an antioxidant that inhibits tyrosinase). Chemical peels (superficial glycolic or salicylic acid peels) accelerate resolution but must be performed cautiously in darker skin types because the peel itself can cause PIH if too aggressive. Post-inflammatory hypopigmentation (PIHypo) presents as well-demarcated, lighter patches at the sites of prior inflammation — caused by temporary inhibition of melanin production (not melanocyte destruction, distinguishing it from vitiligo). PIHypo is most visible in darker skin types and is commonly seen after eczema, psoriasis, pityriasis alba (a mild eczematous dermatitis in children presenting as hypopigmented patches on the cheeks), and cryotherapy-induced hypopigmentation. PIHypo is usually self-limited and repigments spontaneously over months, though targeted phototherapy (excimer laser 308 nm) can accelerate repigmentation.

CLINICAL PEARL: Pityriasis alba — a common, mild eczematous dermatitis in children — presents as ill-defined, hypopigmented, slightly scaly patches on the cheeks that are most noticeable in darker-skinned children after sun exposure (the surrounding tanned skin accentuates the contrast). It is a frequent source of parental concern and is the most common cause of facial hypopigmentation in the pediatric population. Pityriasis alba is associated with atopic dermatitis and is self-limited — the hypopigmentation results from temporary suppression of melanin transfer (not melanocyte destruction), so full repigmentation occurs over months to years. Treatment is emollient therapy and mild topical corticosteroids or calcineurin inhibitors if eczematous features are present. The key reassurance for parents is that this is NOT vitiligo — the pigment WILL return. Wood lamp helps confirm: pityriasis alba shows mild, off-white enhancement (not the bright, chalk-white fluorescence of vitiligo), and the borders are ill-defined (not sharply demarcated as in vitiligo).

Clinical Case: Progressive Facial Depigmentation in a Young Woman

A 24-year-old woman with Fitzpatrick IV skin presents with a 6-month history of progressively enlarging white patches on her face. She first noticed a small pale area around her right eye, which has gradually expanded to involve the periorbital skin bilaterally, the perioral area, and the dorsal hands. She has no history of preceding rash, injury, or topical product use on the affected areas. Family history is notable for autoimmune thyroid disease in her mother and type 1 diabetes in a sibling. On examination, there are well-demarcated, chalk-white, completely depigmented macules and patches in a bilateral, symmetric, periorificial distribution. Under Wood lamp, the lesions fluoresce bright white and are sharply enhanced. Several additional subclinical depigmented patches are visible on the neck under Wood lamp that were not apparent in ambient light. There is no scaling, no inflammation, and no palpable abnormality. KOH scraping is negative. Hair within the periocular patches remains pigmented (no leukotrichia).

The clinical reasoning begins with the distribution and morphology: bilateral, symmetric, periorificial depigmentation in a young woman with a family history of autoimmune disease is classic for non-segmental vitiligo. The complete depigmentation (chalk-white, not merely lighter), sharp demarcation, Wood lamp enhancement, and absence of scale distinguish it from pityriasis versicolor, pityriasis alba, and post-inflammatory hypopigmentation. The absence of leukotrichia is prognostically favorable — it indicates that the melanocyte reservoir in the hair follicle is preserved, which predicts better repigmentation with treatment. Baseline laboratory evaluation includes thyroid function tests (TSH, free T4, anti-thyroglobulin and anti-TPO antibodies — given the 15 to 25 percent association with autoimmune thyroid disease), CBC (to screen for pernicious anemia), fasting glucose and HbA1c (to screen for type 1 diabetes), and ANA. TSH returns mildly elevated with positive anti-TPO antibodies, consistent with early Hashimoto thyroiditis — she is referred to endocrinology. Treatment is initiated with topical ruxolitinib 1.5 percent cream twice daily to the facial patches (approved for non-segmental vitiligo in patients aged 12 and older) and NB-UVB phototherapy three times weekly for the hands and body. Periocular repigmentation begins perifollicularly at 12 weeks — small islands of pigment appear around each hair follicle and gradually expand and coalesce.

Albinism: Types, Ocular Findings, and Skin Cancer Risk

Classification and Clinical Features

Oculocutaneous albinism (OCA) is a group of autosomal recessive disorders caused by mutations in genes encoding enzymes involved in the melanin biosynthesis pathway, resulting in reduced or absent melanin production in the skin, hair, and eyes. OCA type 1 (OCA1 — mutations in the TYR gene encoding tyrosinase, the rate-limiting enzyme in melanin synthesis) is the most severe form: OCA1A (complete absence of tyrosinase activity) presents with snow-white skin, white hair, and translucent irides at birth, while OCA1B (reduced activity) presents with minimal pigmentation that may increase slightly with age (yellow mutant albinism). OCA type 2 (the most common form worldwide — mutations in the OCA2 gene encoding the P protein, which regulates melanosomal pH and tyrosinase processing) presents with variable pigment reduction — patients typically have light-brown to yellow hair, blue or hazel irides, and reduced but present skin pigmentation that may tan slightly. OCA type 3 (mutations in TYRP1 — tyrosinase-related protein 1) produces a reddish-brown phenotype (rufous albinism), most commonly described in sub-Saharan African populations. OCA type 4 (mutations in SLC45A2) resembles OCA2 clinically and is more common in East Asian populations.

Ocular Findings and Skin Cancer Risk

All forms of OCA produce characteristic ocular abnormalities: reduced visual acuity (from foveal hypoplasia — the fovea fails to develop normally without melanin during embryogenesis), nystagmus (involuntary, rhythmic eye movements — present from infancy), photophobia (from iris transillumination — reduced iris pigment allows light to pass through, causing glare), and misrouting of optic nerve fibers at the chiasm (an excess of contralateral projections, detectable by visual evoked potential testing). Strabismus is common. These ocular findings are present even in milder OCA subtypes and are often the presenting concern. The skin cancer risk in OCA is dramatically elevated: patients with OCA1A (complete absence of melanin) have no photoprotection and develop extensive actinic damage, actinic keratoses, and early-onset non-melanoma skin cancer (squamous cell carcinoma — the most common malignancy in albinism, often aggressive — and basal cell carcinoma) if not rigorously protected from UV radiation. In sub-Saharan Africa, where access to dermatologic care and sunscreen is limited, SCC in patients with albinism is a major cause of morbidity and mortality, with many patients developing advanced, metastatic SCC by their third or fourth decade. Management centers on lifelong strict photoprotection (high-SPF broad-spectrum sunscreen, protective clothing, sun avoidance), regular dermatologic surveillance for actinic damage and skin cancer, and low-vision aids and educational accommodations for visual impairment.

Lentigines, Ephelides, and Cafe-au-Lait Macules

Ephelides and Solar Lentigines

Ephelides (freckles) are small (1 to 3 mm), well-demarcated, uniformly tan to light-brown macules that appear on sun-exposed areas (face, arms, shoulders) in childhood, darken with UV exposure, and fade during winter months. Ephelides reflect increased melanin production by a normal number of melanocytes (stimulated by UV in the setting of MC1R variants — the same gene associated with red hair and fair skin). They are benign and require no treatment. Solar lentigines (liver spots, sun spots, age spots) are larger (3 mm to 2 cm), uniformly brown, well-demarcated macules that develop on chronically sun-exposed skin (dorsal hands, forearms, face, upper chest) in middle-aged and older adults. Unlike ephelides, solar lentigines reflect an increased number of melanocytes (melanocytic hyperplasia) in the epidermis and do NOT fade in winter. Histologically, solar lentigines show elongation of rete ridges with increased melanocyte density at the tips, producing the club-shaped or bulbous rete ridge pattern. Solar lentigines are benign but must be distinguished from lentigo maligna (melanoma in situ on sun-damaged skin) — lentigo maligna presents as an irregularly pigmented, asymmetric macule with color variation (tan, brown, black) and irregular borders on the face of an elderly patient. Dermoscopy helps: solar lentigines show a homogeneous fingerprint pattern, moth-eaten borders, and uniform brown color, while lentigo maligna shows asymmetric pigmented follicular openings (annular-granular pattern), rhomboidal structures, and obliterated follicles.

Cafe-au-Lait Macules and Syndromic Associations

Cafe-au-lait macules (CALMs) are well-demarcated, uniformly light-brown (coffee-with-milk-colored) macules or patches that can occur anywhere on the body. Isolated CALMs are common (10 to 20 percent of the general population has 1 to 2 CALMs), are benign, and have no clinical significance. However, multiple CALMs are a hallmark of neurofibromatosis type 1 (NF1 — 6 or more CALMs greater than 5 mm prepubertal or greater than 15 mm postpubertal is one of the NIH diagnostic criteria), McCune-Albright syndrome (large, unilateral CALMs with jagged, coast of Maine borders, polyostotic fibrous dysplasia, and precocious puberty), and Legius syndrome (a milder NF1-like syndrome caused by SPRED1 mutations — multiple CALMs and axillary freckling without neurofibromas or optic gliomas). The border morphology provides a clinical clue: NF1 CALMs have smooth, regular borders (coast of California), while McCune-Albright CALMs have jagged, irregular borders (coast of Maine). Becker nevus — a large, unilateral, hyperpigmented patch with hypertrichosis on the shoulder or upper trunk of adolescent males — enters the differential of large CALMs but is distinguished by its characteristic location, associated hair growth, and lack of systemic associations. Becker nevus is not a CALM but an androgen-sensitive hamartoma.

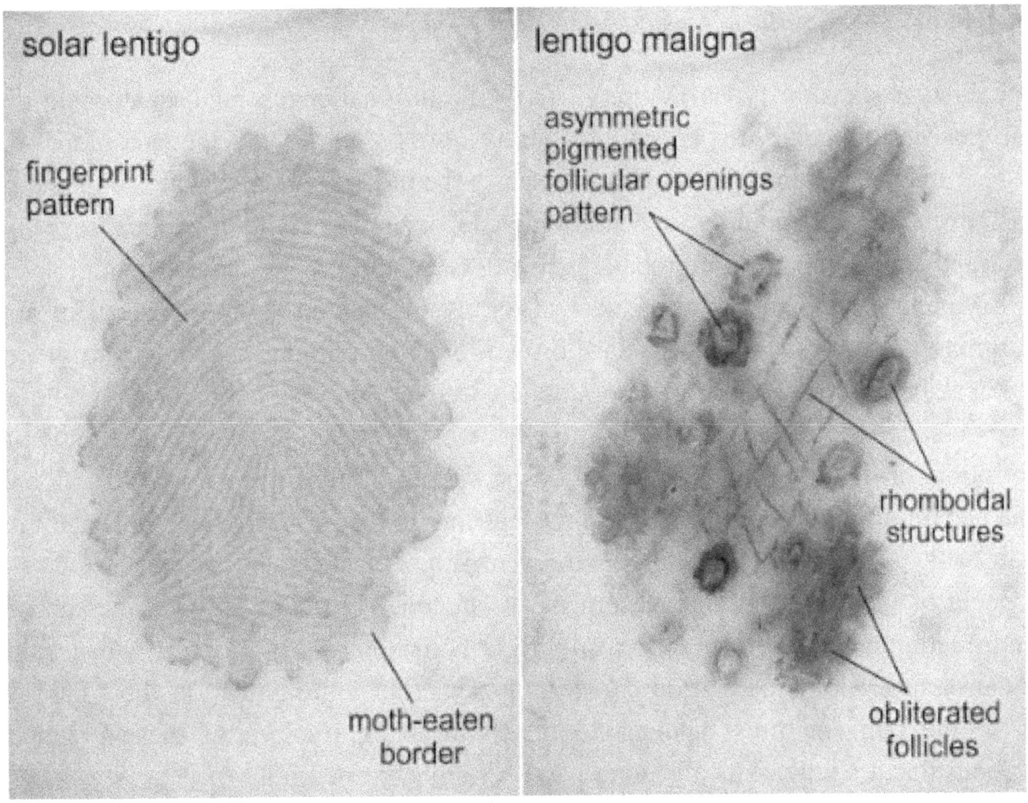

Dermatosis Papulosa Nigra and Pigmentary Conditions in Skin of Color

Dermatosis Papulosa Nigra

Dermatosis papulosa nigra (DPN) is a common, benign condition characterized by multiple small (1 to 5 mm), pedunculated, dark-brown to black papules on the face — particularly the malar cheeks, temples, forehead, and periorbital areas — and neck. It occurs in approximately 35 percent of Black adults and is more common in women and increases in number with age. DPN lesions are histologically identical to seborrheic keratoses (acanthotic, papillomatous epidermis with horn pseudocysts) and are considered a clinical variant of seborrheic keratosis in darker skin types. DPN is entirely benign and requires no treatment, but patients frequently request removal for cosmetic reasons. Treatment options include electrodesiccation (gentle, low-power settings to minimize the risk of post-inflammatory hyperpigmentation and scarring — the most common complication of treatment in darker skin types), curettage, cryotherapy (used very cautiously — cryotherapy carries a high risk of PIH and hypopigmentation in Fitzpatrick IV to VI skin), and laser ablation (CO2 or erbium:YAG — with similar caveats about pigmentary complications). The key principle in treating DPN is that the treatment must not cause a cosmetic outcome worse than the original condition.

Pigmentary Challenges in Skin of Color

Patients with Fitzpatrick skin types IV to VI face unique challenges in dermatologic diagnosis and management. Post-inflammatory hyperpigmentation is more common, more severe, more prolonged, and more distressing in darker skin types — it is frequently the chief complaint that brings the patient to the dermatologist, even when the underlying condition (acne, eczema) is mild by clinical severity scales. The psychological and social impact of pigmentary disorders in skin of color is substantial and must not be minimized. Erythema is difficult to appreciate in darkly pigmented skin — instead of appearing red, inflammation may present as violaceous, dark brown, or hyperpigmented, leading to diagnostic delay. Dermoscopy in skin of color requires attention to the vascular patterns visible through pigmented skin — glomerular vessels, dotted vessels, and linear vessels can be identified but their colors may differ from the classic descriptions in lighter skin. Conditions with particular relevance to skin of color include acne keloidalis nuchae (chronic folliculitis and keloidal scarring on the posterior neck in Black men — related to curved hair follicles and close shaving), central centrifugal cicatricial alopecia (CCCA — progressive scarring alopecia of the vertex in Black women, associated with hair care practices and PADI3 gene variants), and traction alopecia (from chronically tight hairstyles — tight braids, weaves, and ponytails cause follicular damage along the hairline). Culturally sensitive communication about hair care practices is essential — the clinician must understand the cultural significance of these practices and offer recommendations that are both clinically sound and culturally respectful.

KEY POINT: The diagnosis of inflammatory skin conditions in skin of color (Fitzpatrick IV to VI) requires recalibration of the clinical eye: erythema appears violaceous or dark brown rather than red, the clinical severity of inflammation may be underestimated by scales validated predominantly on lighter skin (PASI, EASI), and the chief concern is frequently the post-inflammatory pigmentary change rather than the inflammatory disease itself. Dermoscopy in skin of color is an evolving field — normal dermoscopic patterns (such as the parallel ridge pattern on acral skin, which is a red flag for melanoma in lighter skin) may be a normal finding in darkly pigmented skin, and the clinician must be aware of these differences to avoid both false positives and missed diagnoses.

Laser and Light-Based Treatments for Pigmentary Disorders

Principles of Selective Photothermolysis

Laser and light-based treatments for pigmentary disorders operate on the principle of selective photothermolysis: selecting a wavelength preferentially absorbed by the target chromophore (melanin), delivering the energy in a pulse duration shorter than the thermal relaxation time of the target, and using sufficient fluence to destroy the target while sparing surrounding tissue. Melanin absorbs broadly across the visible and near-infrared spectrum, with peak absorption in the shorter wavelengths (UV and blue-green). The challenge in treating pigmentary disorders — particularly in darker skin types — is that melanin is present in BOTH the lesion and the surrounding normal epidermis, creating a competition for laser energy. This epidermal melanin competition is the reason pigmentary treatments carry a higher risk of adverse effects (blistering, PIH, hypopigmentation) in darker skin types. Longer wavelengths (Nd:YAG 1064 nm) penetrate deeper and are less absorbed by epidermal melanin, making them safer in Fitzpatrick

IV to VI skin, while shorter wavelengths (ruby 694 nm, alexandrite 755 nm) are more strongly absorbed by melanin and are more effective in lighter skin types but carry higher risk in darker skin.

Specific Laser Systems for Pigmented Lesions

Q-switched lasers (ruby 694 nm, alexandrite 755 nm, Nd:YAG 532/1064 nm) deliver extremely short pulse durations (nanoseconds) that produce photomechanical disruption of melanosomes — the melanin-containing organelles are shattered by the rapid thermal expansion, and the debris is cleared by macrophages. Q-switched lasers are the standard of care for benign pigmented lesions (solar lentigines, cafe-au-lait macules, nevus of Ota, nevus of Ito) and for tattoo removal. Picosecond lasers (alexandrite 755 nm, Nd:YAG 532/1064 nm) deliver even shorter pulses (picoseconds), producing more efficient photomechanical fragmentation with less thermal damage — theoretically reducing the risk of PIH and scarring. For melasma, low-fluence Q-switched Nd:YAG (1064 nm) laser toning has been used in some Asian dermatology practices, but results are inconsistent and there is a risk of rebound hyperpigmentation and mottled depigmentation (confetti-like hypopigmentation from melanocyte destruction). Intense pulsed light (IPL) delivers broad-spectrum light (500 to 1200 nm) with cut-off filters and is effective for solar lentigines and diffuse photodamage on Fitzpatrick I to III skin, but is NOT safe in darker skin types (the broad-spectrum energy is absorbed by epidermal melanin, causing burns and PIH). The excimer laser (308 nm) delivers targeted UVB to depigmented patches and is used for vitiligo repigmentation and localized psoriasis — it achieves higher fluences than NB-UVB phototherapy booths, allowing treatment of resistant areas.

CAUTION: Laser and light-based treatments for pigmentary disorders in Fitzpatrick IV to VI skin carry significant risks of post-inflammatory hyperpigmentation, hypopigmentation, and scarring. The mantra is start low, go slow: use lower fluences, longer pulse durations, and longer wavelengths (Nd:YAG 1064 nm preferred over ruby or alexandrite), and always perform a test spot in an inconspicuous area before treating the full lesion. IPL is generally NOT safe for darker skin types due to its broad-spectrum absorption by epidermal melanin. Pre-treatment with hydroquinone or a topical retinoid for 2 to 4 weeks may reduce the risk of PIH. Post-treatment photoprotection is essential. In melasma, laser treatment should be considered a last resort — the risk of rebound hyperpigmentation is substantial, and topical therapy plus strict photoprotection remains first-line.

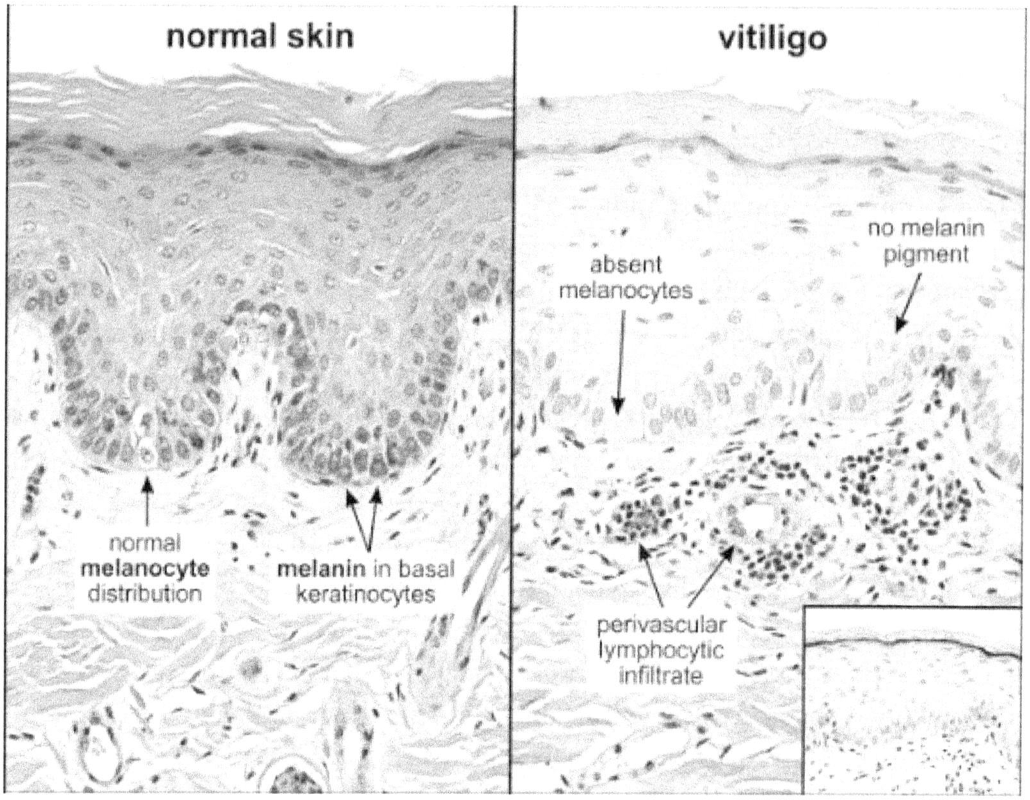

THE CUTANEOUS MIMICKER RECOGNITION ATLAS — Vitiligo versus Pityriasis Versicolor

The Clinical Pattern: Vitiligo presents as well-demarcated, chalk-white (completely depigmented), symmetric macules and patches in periorificial and acral distribution, with positive Wood lamp enhancement (bright white fluorescence). The depigmentation is complete — there is no residual pigment within the lesion. The patient may have a personal or family history of autoimmune disease. The course is chronic and progressive in non-segmental vitiligo.

The Mimicker: Pityriasis versicolor (tinea versicolor — caused by Malassezia yeast) presents as hypopigmented (NOT depigmented — lighter than surrounding skin but not chalk-white), finely scaling macules and patches on the trunk, shoulders, and proximal arms. Under Wood lamp, pityriasis versicolor fluoresces a pale yellow-green (not bright white like vitiligo). The patches have fine, powdery scale that is accentuated by stretching the skin (the stretch sign or Zireli sign). KOH preparation shows the characteristic spaghetti and meatballs pattern (short hyphae and round yeast clusters).

Trap Logic: Treating pityriasis versicolor as vitiligo and initiating immunosuppressive therapy or phototherapy is unnecessary and wasteful — pityriasis versicolor is a superficial yeast infection that responds to topical or oral antifungals. **Conversely, treating vitiligo as a fungal infection with repeated courses of antifungals** delays appropriate immunomodulatory therapy and allows progressive melanocyte destruction. The distinction is particularly confusing when vitiligo involves the trunk (atypical distribution for vitiligo but typical for pityriasis versicolor) or when pityriasis versicolor is extensive.

The Decision Anchor: The discriminating features are **degree of pigment loss (vitiligo — complete depigmentation, chalk-white; pityriasis versicolor — hypopigmentation, lighter than surrounding skin but not white), scale (vitiligo — no scale; pityriasis versicolor — fine powdery scale accentuated by stretching), Wood lamp (vitiligo — bright white fluorescence; pityriasis versicolor — pale yellow-green fluorescence), distribution (vitiligo — periorificial, acral, symmetric; pityriasis versicolor — trunk, shoulders, proximal arms), and KOH (vitiligo — negative; pityriasis versicolor — spaghetti and meatballs)**. A KOH preparation is the simplest definitive test.

THE CUTANEOUS MIMICKER RECOGNITION ATLAS — Pigmentary Disorder Diagnostic Arcs

---

Melasma vs. PIH: The discriminating features are symmetry (melasma — bilateral and symmetric; PIH — follows the pattern of the preceding inflammation), history (melasma — no preceding inflammatory event; PIH — always preceded by an identifiable rash or injury), hormonal association (melasma worsens with pregnancy and OCPs; PIH does not), and visible light sensitivity (melasma worsens with visible light; PIH does not). Cognitive trap: treating facial PIH aggressively with depigmenting agents without controlling the underlying inflammation perpetuates the cycle.

Vitiligo vs. Pityriasis Versicolor: The discriminating features are degree of pigment loss (vitiligo — complete depigmentation; pityriasis versicolor — hypopigmentation), scale (vitiligo — none; pityriasis versicolor — fine powdery scale), Wood lamp (vitiligo — bright white; pityriasis versicolor — yellow-green), and KOH (vitiligo — negative; pityriasis versicolor — spaghetti and meatballs pattern). Cognitive trap: treating vitiligo as a fungal infection with antifungals delays immunomodulatory therapy and allows progressive melanocyte destruction.

Summary and Key Concepts

Vitiligo is an autoimmune melanocyte destruction disorder driven by the IFN-gamma-CXCL10-CXCR3 axis. Topical ruxolitinib 1.5 percent cream (the first FDA-approved targeted therapy) and narrowband UVB phototherapy are the mainstays of treatment. Acral areas respond poorly because they lack the hair follicle melanocyte stem cell reservoir. Segmental vitiligo with leukotrichia has a poor repigmentation prognosis.

Melasma involves both epidermal hyperpigmentation and a dermal component (increased vascularity, solar elastosis, basement membrane disruption). Strict photoprotection with iron oxide-containing sunscreen (to block visible light) is the foundation. Triple combination cream (hydroquinone, tretinoin, fluocinolone) is first-line topical therapy; hydroquinone is cycled to avoid ochronosis.

PIH disproportionately affects darker skin types, can be more distressing than the underlying condition, and requires treatment of the inflammatory trigger as the cornerstone of management. Epidermal PIH (brown, Wood lamp-enhanced) responds better to topical therapy than dermal PIH (grey-blue, not enhanced).

Oculocutaneous albinism produces characteristic ocular findings (reduced visual acuity from foveal hypoplasia, nystagmus, iris transillumination, strabismus) and dramatically elevated skin cancer risk — SCC in patients with albinism in sub-Saharan Africa is a major cause of morbidity and mortality, underscoring the importance of lifelong photoprotection and surveillance.

Laser and light-based treatments for pigmentary disorders carry significant risks in Fitzpatrick IV to VI skin — longer wavelengths (Nd:YAG 1064 nm) are safer than shorter wavelengths; IPL is generally contraindicated; and the mantra is start low, go slow with test spots before full treatment. In melasma, laser therapy is a last resort due to the risk of rebound hyperpigmentation.

CHAPTER 24: DERMATOLOGIC THERAPEUTICS AND PROCEDURES

Learning Objectives

1. Apply the principles of topical therapy — vehicle selection (ointment, cream, lotion, gel, foam, solution), potency classification, and the fingertip unit system — to select the appropriate formulation and strength for the patient's condition, body site, and skin type.
2. Classify topical corticosteroids by the 7-class potency system, implement steroid-sparing strategies for chronic dermatoses, and recognize the adverse effects of inappropriate corticosteroid use including skin atrophy, striae, perioral dermatitis, and hypothalamic-pituitary-adrenal axis suppression.
3. Compare the mechanisms, indications, monitoring requirements, and safety profiles of systemic immunosuppressive agents (methotrexate, cyclosporine, azathioprine, mycophenolate) and biologic therapies (TNF-alpha inhibitors, IL-17 inhibitors, IL-23 inhibitors, IL-4/IL-13 inhibitors, JAK inhibitors) used in dermatology.
4. Describe the principles of selective photothermolysis and apply them to select the appropriate laser or energy-based device for vascular lesions, pigmented lesions, hair removal, and skin resurfacing.

Principles of Topical Therapy: Vehicle Selection, Potency, and Application Techniques

Vehicle Selection and Bioavailability

The vehicle in which a topical medication is delivered determines its bioavailability, patient acceptability, and clinical efficacy. Ointments (greasy bases — petrolatum, mineral oil) provide the highest bioavailability because their occlusive nature enhances hydration of the stratum corneum and drug penetration — they are preferred for dry, lichenified, and hyperkeratotic dermatoses and for application to thick-skinned areas (palms, soles). Creams (oil-in-water emulsions) are cosmetically elegant, well-accepted by patients, and appropriate for most body sites and most acute and subacute dermatoses. Lotions and solutions are thin, easily spread formulations ideal for hairy areas (scalp, chest) where ointments and creams are impractical. Gels (transparent, semisolid) and foams are lightweight, dry quickly, and are preferred for acne therapy and scalp applications. The general principle is that the vehicle should match the condition: wet (acute, oozing) conditions are treated with wet formulations (solutions, compresses) — the drying effect is therapeutic; dry (chronic, lichenified) conditions are treated with occlusive formulations (ointments) — the moisturizing and penetration-enhancing effects are therapeutic.

Application Techniques and the Fingertip Unit

The fingertip unit (FTU) system standardizes the amount of topical medication applied: one FTU is the amount of cream or ointment squeezed from a standard tube onto the volar surface of the distal phalanx of the index finger (from the tip to the distal interphalangeal crease), which covers approximately 2 adult palms of skin surface area (roughly 2 percent BSA). A standardized dosing guide based on FTUs helps ensure adequate (but not excessive) application: face and neck require 2.5 FTU, one arm requires 3 FTU, one leg requires 6 FTU, trunk (front or back) requires 7 FTU. Frequency of application is typically twice daily for most topical corticosteroids and calcineurin inhibitors. The soak-and-seal technique — applying the topical medication immediately after bathing (within 3 minutes) to hydrated skin — enhances penetration and is the standard recommendation for atopic dermatitis management. Occlusion (covering the treated area with plastic wrap or hydrocolloid dressings) dramatically increases drug penetration (up to 10-fold for topical corticosteroids) and is used for recalcitrant, thick plaques, but increases the risk of adverse effects and must be used with caution.

Topical Corticosteroids: Classification, Appropriate Use, and Adverse Effects

The 7-Class Potency System

Topical corticosteroids are classified by potency into 7 classes (Class I — superpotent to Class VII — least potent) based on the vasoconstriction assay. The choice of potency is guided by the condition being treated, the body site, the patient's age, and the chronicity of the dermatosis. Class I (superpotent — clobetasol propionate 0.05 percent, betamethasone dipropionate in optimized vehicle 0.05 percent) is reserved for thick-skinned areas (palms, soles), recalcitrant plaques (psoriasis, lichen simplex chronicus), and short-term use (2 to 4 weeks). Classes II and III (high potency — fluocinonide 0.05 percent, betamethasone dipropionate 0.05 percent cream) are appropriate for moderate-to-severe dermatoses on the trunk and extremities. Classes IV and V (medium potency — triamcinolone acetonide 0.1 percent, fluticasone propionate 0.05 percent) are the workhorse potencies for most inflammatory dermatoses on the trunk and extremities. Classes VI and VII (low potency — desonide 0.05 percent, hydrocortisone 1 to 2.5 percent) are used for the face, eyelids, intertriginous areas, genital skin, and in infants and young children — sites where the thin epidermis increases drug penetration and the risk of atrophy. The same active ingredient in a different vehicle may change its effective potency: betamethasone dipropionate in ointment is more potent than the same concentration in cream.

Adverse Effects and Steroid-Sparing Strategies

Local adverse effects of topical corticosteroids result from the catabolic effects of glucocorticoids on dermal collagen and the epidermis. Skin atrophy (thin, transparent, fragile skin with visible dermal vessels — cigarette paper skin) is the most common local adverse effect and is more likely with higher potency, longer duration, occlusion, and use on thin-skinned areas. Striae (stretch marks) from topical corticosteroid use are irreversible and occur in high-risk areas (axillae, groin, inner thighs). Steroid rosacea (perioral and periocular erythema, papules, and pustules — worsened by steroid withdrawal, creating a dependency cycle), steroid acne (monomorphic papulopustules without comedones), and telangiectasias are additional local effects. Perioral dermatitis — grouped erythematous papulopustules around the mouth, nose, and eyes — is triggered or perpetuated by topical corticosteroid use on the face and treated by corticosteroid withdrawal (which initially worsens the eruption — the rebound flare) followed by topical metronidazole or oral tetracyclines. Systemic absorption and hypothalamic-pituitary-adrenal (HPA) axis suppression can occur with prolonged use of superpotent topical corticosteroids over large body surface areas, particularly under occlusion and in infants (whose higher BSA-to-body-weight ratio increases systemic exposure). Steroid-sparing strategies include proactive maintenance therapy (twice-weekly application to previously affected areas), topical calcineurin inhibitors for sensitive areas, and weekend-only therapy for chronic dermatoses.

Topical Calcineurin Inhibitors, PDE4 Inhibitors, and JAK Inhibitors

Mechanism and Clinical Applications

Topical calcineurin inhibitors (TCIs — tacrolimus 0.03 percent and 0.1 percent ointment, pimecrolimus 1 percent cream) inhibit calcineurin-mediated T-cell activation and cytokine production, reducing cutaneous inflammation without the atrophogenic effects of topical corticosteroids. They are first-line steroid-sparing agents for the face, eyelids, intertriginous areas, and genital skin — sites where chronic topical corticosteroid use causes atrophy, telangiectasias, and perioral dermatitis. TCIs are approved for atopic dermatitis (second-line after topical corticosteroids for moderate-to-severe AD in patients aged 2 years and older for tacrolimus, 3 months and older for pimecrolimus). The most common adverse effect is a transient burning and stinging sensation at the application site during the first few days of use — patients should be counseled that this typically subsides with continued use. The FDA black-box warning (theoretical risk of malignancy based on animal data with systemic calcineurin inhibitors) remains controversial and has not been supported by long-term human safety data — multiple large cohort studies and systematic reviews have found no increased risk of lymphoma or skin cancer with topical calcineurin inhibitor use. Topical PDE4 inhibitors (crisaborole 2 percent ointment) inhibit phosphodiesterase 4, reducing inflammatory cytokine production, and are approved for mild-to-moderate AD in patients aged 3 months and older. Topical JAK inhibitors represent the newest class: ruxolitinib cream 1.5 percent (JAK1/JAK2 inhibitor) is approved for AD (aged 12 and older) and vitiligo (aged 12 and older — the first FDA-approved treatment for vitiligo repigmentation).

Safety Monitoring and Special Populations

Long-term safety data for topical calcineurin inhibitors now span over two decades of post-marketing surveillance. The APPLES study (a 10-year prospective pediatric safety study of pimecrolimus) demonstrated no increased risk of malignancy, and large pharmacovigilance database analyses have consistently confirmed the safety profile. For topical JAK inhibitors, application site area should not exceed 20 percent BSA to minimize systemic absorption — monitoring for hematologic and immunologic effects is not routinely required at approved topical doses but should be considered in patients applying to large body surface areas or under occlusion. Pediatric considerations are particularly relevant: pimecrolimus is approved from 3 months of age and tacrolimus from 2 years, making them essential options for infantile AD involving the face and diaper area where topical corticosteroids carry the greatest atrophy risk. In immunosuppressed patients (organ transplant recipients, HIV-positive individuals), the theoretical malignancy risk requires individualized assessment, though current evidence does not support withholding TCIs based on immune status alone.

Systemic Immunosuppressives: Methotrexate, Azathioprine, Mycophenolate, and Cyclosporine

Methotrexate and Cyclosporine

Methotrexate (MTX) is a folate antagonist that inhibits dihydrofolate reductase and purine synthesis, producing anti-inflammatory and immunosuppressive effects at the low doses used in dermatology (7.5 to 25 mg per week). Indications include moderate-to-severe psoriasis (one of the oldest systemic therapies for psoriasis), psoriatic arthritis, and off-label use in severe atopic dermatitis, bullous pemphigoid, dermatomyositis, sarcoidosis, and morphea. Monitoring requirements include baseline CBC, comprehensive metabolic panel (hepatic and renal function), hepatitis B and C serologies, and chest radiograph. Ongoing monitoring includes CBC and liver function tests every 1 to 3 months. Hepatotoxicity is the most serious chronic adverse effect — the risk of hepatic fibrosis and cirrhosis increases with cumulative dose and concomitant alcohol use. Folic acid supplementation (1 mg daily, held on MTX day) reduces gastrointestinal and hematologic toxicity without compromising efficacy. MTX is absolutely contraindicated in pregnancy (category X — causes neural tube defects and craniofacial anomalies) and must be discontinued at least 3 months before conception in both men and women. Cyclosporine (a calcineurin inhibitor that blocks T-cell activation and IL-2 production) is used for severe, rapidly flaring dermatoses requiring rapid control — including severe atopic dermatitis, severe psoriasis (bridging to biologic therapy), and pyoderma gangrenosum. Nephrotoxicity (dose-dependent decline in GFR) and hypertension are the principal toxicities — serum creatinine and blood pressure must be monitored every 2 weeks initially, then monthly. Duration should be limited to 1 to 2 years due to the risk of cumulative nephrotoxicity.

Azathioprine and Mycophenolate

Azathioprine (a purine synthesis inhibitor that suppresses lymphocyte proliferation) is used as a steroid-sparing agent in autoimmune blistering diseases (pemphigus vulgaris, bullous pemphigoid), dermatomyositis, and severe atopic dermatitis. TPMT (thiopurine methyltransferase) genotyping or phenotyping must be performed before initiation — patients with low or absent TPMT activity are at high risk for severe myelosuppression (potentially fatal pancytopenia) at standard doses. Monitoring includes CBC every 1 to 2 weeks initially, then every 1 to 3 months. Mycophenolate mofetil (an inosine monophosphate dehydrogenase inhibitor that selectively suppresses lymphocyte proliferation) is used for the same indications as azathioprine and has a more favorable side effect profile — gastrointestinal symptoms (nausea, diarrhea) are the most common adverse effects. Both agents are teratogenic (category D) and must be discontinued before conception.

Biologic Therapies: Mechanism, Indications, Monitoring, and Safety

Biologic Classes in Dermatology

Biologic therapies have transformed the management of moderate-to-severe psoriasis, atopic dermatitis, and hidradenitis suppurativa. TNF-alpha inhibitors (adalimumab, infliximab, etanercept, certolizumab) were the first biologic class approved for psoriasis and remain important for psoriatic arthritis and hidradenitis suppurativa. Pre-treatment screening includes tuberculosis testing (TB skin test or interferon-gamma release assay — TNF-alpha inhibitors can reactivate latent TB), hepatitis B serologies, and assessment for heart failure (TNF-alpha inhibitors are contraindicated in NYHA class III-IV heart failure). IL-17 inhibitors (secukinumab, ixekizumab, brodalumab, bimekizumab) target the IL-17 pathway — the central cytokine axis in psoriasis — and achieve PASI 90 or PASI 100 responses in a majority of patients. They carry a small increased risk of mucocutaneous candidiasis (oral thrush, vulvovaginal candidiasis) due to the role of IL-17 in mucosal antifungal immunity. Brodalumab carries a boxed warning for suicidal ideation. IL-23 inhibitors (guselkumab, risankizumab, tildrakizumab) target the p19 subunit of IL-23, achieving durable responses with less frequent dosing — risankizumab is administered every 12 weeks after induction. IL-4/IL-13 inhibitors (dupilumab — anti-IL-4 receptor alpha, blocking both IL-4 and IL-13 signaling) are approved for moderate-to-severe atopic dermatitis (aged 6 months and older), asthma, and chronic rhinosinusitis with nasal polyps. The most common adverse effect is conjunctivitis (in approximately 10 to 25 percent of AD patients). Oral JAK inhibitors (upadacitinib, abrocitinib — JAK1 selective; baricitinib — JAK1/JAK2; deucravacitinib — TYK2) represent the newest class of targeted oral therapies for psoriasis and atopic dermatitis, with rapid onset and oral convenience but a boxed warning for major adverse cardiovascular events, malignancy, thrombosis, and serious infections based on the class-wide ORAL Surveillance trial findings with tofacitinib in rheumatoid arthritis.

KEY POINT: Before initiating any biologic therapy, a standardized pre-treatment screening protocol is mandatory: tuberculosis testing (TST or IGRA — biologic-associated TB reactivation carries high morbidity), hepatitis B serologies (HBsAg, anti-HBs, anti-HBc — risk of reactivation, particularly with TNF-alpha inhibitors), hepatitis C serologies, HIV testing, CBC, comprehensive metabolic panel, and age-appropriate cancer screening. Live vaccines must be administered at least 4 weeks before starting biologic therapy and are contraindicated during treatment. For IL-17 inhibitors, assess for history of inflammatory bowel disease (IL-17 inhibition may exacerbate IBD). For JAK inhibitors, add lipid panel and consider cardiovascular risk assessment.

Comparative Efficacy and Treatment Selection

Treatment selection among biologics is guided by disease severity, comorbidities, patient preference, and comparative efficacy data. In moderate-to-severe psoriasis, network meta-analyses consistently rank IL-17 and IL-23 inhibitors as the most efficacious classes, with risankizumab and bimekizumab achieving the highest PASI 100 (complete clearance) rates. IL-23 inhibitors offer the advantage of infrequent dosing (every 8 to 12 weeks after induction), improving adherence for patients who find frequent injections burdensome. For patients with concomitant psoriatic arthritis, IL-17 inhibitors and TNF-alpha inhibitors have stronger evidence for joint disease than IL-23 inhibitors. In atopic dermatitis, dupilumab remains the first-line biologic with the longest safety record, while tralokinumab (anti-IL-13) provides an alternative for patients who develop dupilumab-associated conjunctivitis. Oral JAK inhibitors (upadacitinib, abrocitinib) achieve faster onset of itch relief than dupilumab but require ongoing cardiovascular and malignancy risk monitoring. Treatment switching — from one biologic class to another when efficacy wanes — is common, and understanding the mechanistic differences between classes is essential for rational sequencing.

EVIDENCE: The ORAL Surveillance trial (a postmarketing safety study comparing tofacitinib with TNF-alpha inhibitors in rheumatoid arthritis patients aged 50 and older with cardiovascular risk factors) demonstrated higher rates of major adverse cardiovascular events and malignancies with tofacitinib, leading to a class-wide boxed warning for all JAK inhibitors. However, the applicability of these findings to younger, healthier dermatology populations remains debated — the trial enrolled an inherently high-risk population (older, with pre-existing cardiovascular risk factors) that does not represent typical psoriasis or AD patients starting JAK inhibitors. Ongoing post-marketing surveillance studies in dermatologic populations are addressing this evidence gap.

Retinoids: Topical and Systemic Applications

Topical and Systemic Retinoids

Retinoids (vitamin A derivatives) modulate keratinocyte proliferation, differentiation, and apoptosis through nuclear retinoid receptors (RAR and RXR). Topical retinoids (tretinoin, adapalene, tazarotene, trifarotene) are first-line therapy for acne vulgaris — they normalize follicular keratinization, prevent microcomedone formation, and have mild anti-inflammatory activity. Tretinoin is also used for photoaging (reducing fine wrinkles, dyspigmentation, and surface roughness over months of use). Topical retinoid-associated irritation (retinoid dermatitis — erythema, peeling, dryness, burning) is the most common reason for non-adherence and can be minimized by starting with a lower concentration, applying every other night initially, and using a moisturizer. Systemic isotretinoin (13-cis-retinoic acid) is the most effective treatment for severe, nodular, and scarring acne — it is the only acne therapy that addresses all four pathogenic factors (sebum production, follicular hyperkeratinization, Cutibacterium acnes proliferation, and inflammation). Isotretinoin is absolutely teratogenic (category X) and is dispensed under the iPLEDGE risk management program: female patients of reproductive potential require two negative pregnancy tests before starting, two forms of contraception, and monthly pregnancy testing throughout treatment. Common adverse effects include mucocutaneous dryness (cheilitis in nearly 100 percent of patients, xerosis, epistaxis, dry eyes), hypertriglyceridemia, elevated liver transaminases, and musculoskeletal symptoms. Acitretin (a systemic retinoid used for psoriasis — particularly pustular and erythrodermic psoriasis) has a prolonged teratogenic window: it must be discontinued at least 3 years before conception in women because acitretin can be converted to etretinate (which has a half-life of 120 days and is stored in adipose tissue) when combined with alcohol.

Monitoring and Adverse Effect Management

Isotretinoin requires a structured monitoring protocol: baseline and monthly fasting lipid panels and liver function tests throughout the treatment course. Hypertriglyceridemia (the most common laboratory abnormality) is managed by dietary modification and, if severe (triglycerides exceeding 500 mg/dL — 5.65 mmol/L), dose reduction or discontinuation to prevent pancreatitis. The association between isotretinoin and depression remains controversial — large population-based studies have not demonstrated a causal relationship, and some data suggest that severe acne itself is a stronger predictor of depression than isotretinoin treatment. Nonetheless, clinicians should screen for mood changes at each visit. The isotretinoin initial flare (temporary worsening of acne during the first 2 to 4 weeks) can be mitigated by starting at a lower dose (0.25 to 0.5 mg/kg/day) and escalating. For acitretin, monitoring includes lipid panels and liver function tests at baseline, 1 month, and every 3 months thereafter, with particular attention to hepatotoxicity in patients with pre-existing liver disease or concomitant alcohol use.

Phototherapy: Narrowband UVB, PUVA, and Targeted Phototherapy

Phototherapy Modalities and Indications

Phototherapy delivers controlled doses of ultraviolet radiation to treat inflammatory and pigmentary skin diseases. Narrowband UVB (NB-UVB, 311 nm) is the most widely used phototherapy modality and is first-line for moderate-to-severe psoriasis, vitiligo, mycosis fungoides (early-stage CTCL), atopic dermatitis, and pruritus of chronic kidney disease. NB-UVB produces immunomodulatory effects (inducing T-cell apoptosis, shifting the cutaneous immune response from Th1/Th17 toward Th2) and stimulates melanocyte proliferation and migration (the basis for its use in vitiligo). Treatment is administered 2 to 3 times weekly, with dosing based on minimal erythema dose (MED) testing or Fitzpatrick skin type. PUVA (psoralen plus UVA) combines oral or topical psoralen (a photosensitizing agent — methoxsalen, 8-MOP) with UVA radiation (320 to 400 nm). Psoralen intercalates into DNA and, upon UVA activation, forms cross-links that inhibit DNA replication and cell proliferation. PUVA is more effective than NB-UVB for thick plaque psoriasis and palmoplantar dermatoses but carries higher risks: phototoxicity, nausea (with oral psoralen), and a long-term dose-dependent risk of squamous cell carcinoma and melanoma — cumulative PUVA sessions must be tracked and limited. The excimer laser (308 nm — targeted UVB) delivers focused high-fluence UVB to localized lesions, sparing uninvolved skin. It is used for localized psoriasis, vitiligo, and alopecia areata.

Safety, Adverse Effects, and Patient Education

Acute adverse effects of phototherapy include erythema (the phototoxic threshold must be carefully titrated — sunburn is the most common reason for treatment interruption), pruritus, and xerosis. Long-term risks include photoaging and cutaneous carcinogenesis — the carcinogenic risk is substantially higher with PUVA than with NB-UVB, and patients receiving PUVA should have a lifetime cumulative dose tracked (exceeding 200 PUVA treatments is associated with a significantly increased squamous cell carcinoma risk). NB-UVB is preferred over PUVA for most indications because of its more favorable long-term safety profile. Patient education is critical for treatment adherence: patients must protect non-target skin and eyes during treatment (UV-blocking goggles are mandatory — PUVA-associated ocular toxicity includes cataracts), apply broad-spectrum sunscreen to non-treated areas, avoid additional UV exposure on treatment days, and understand that clinical response typically requires 20 to 30 sessions. For PUVA patients, psoralen-induced photosensitivity persists for 24 hours after ingestion — patients must wear wrap-around UV-blocking sunglasses and avoid sun exposure for the remainder of the treatment day. Home phototherapy units (NB-UVB) are an increasingly important option for patients who cannot attend in-office sessions 2 to 3 times weekly, with comparable efficacy to in-office treatment when properly supervised.

Procedural Dermatology: Cryotherapy, Electrodesiccation, Curettage, and Chemical Peels

Destructive Techniques

Cryotherapy uses liquid nitrogen (at a temperature of negative 196 degrees Celsius) to freeze and destroy tissue through intracellular ice crystal formation, cell membrane disruption, and vascular stasis. It is used for actinic keratoses (the most common indication), common warts, seborrheic keratoses, and selected superficial skin cancers (superficial BCCs in non-critical sites in patients who are not surgical candidates). The freeze-thaw-freeze (double freeze) cycle produces deeper tissue destruction than a single freeze. Adverse effects include pain, blistering, and post-inflammatory hypopigmentation (particularly in darker skin types — melanocytes are highly sensitive to cold injury). Electrodesiccation and curettage (ED&C) is a combined technique used for superficial and nodular BCCs in non-critical sites (trunk, extremities), actinic keratoses, and benign tumors. The lesion is curetted (scraped with a sharp curette — the softer tumor tissue is distinguishable from the firm surrounding dermis by the gritty feel of the curette reaching the tumor margin), then the base is electrodesiccated to destroy residual tumor cells and achieve hemostasis. The cycle is typically repeated 2 to 3 times. ED&C heals by secondary intention, producing a hypopigmented, atrophic scar. Chemical peels (glycolic acid, salicylic acid, trichloroacetic acid — TCA) cause controlled chemical destruction of the epidermis and superficial dermis. Superficial peels (glycolic 20 to 50 percent, salicylic 20 to 30 percent) treat acne, melasma, and photoaging by promoting epidermal turnover. Medium-depth peels (TCA 35 percent, or Jessner solution plus TCA 35 percent) treat moderate photoaging and actinic keratoses. Deep peels (phenol-based) produce dramatic rejuvenation but carry risks of cardiac arrhythmia from phenol absorption and permanent depigmentation.

Patient Selection and Complications

Patient selection for destructive procedures requires assessment of skin type, wound healing capacity, and cosmetic expectations. Cryotherapy is relatively contraindicated in patients with Fitzpatrick skin types IV through VI for cosmetically sensitive areas because melanocyte cold sensitivity produces conspicuous and potentially permanent hypopigmentation. For dark-skinned patients requiring treatment of actinic keratoses, topical field therapy (5-fluorouracil, imiquimod, ingenol mebutate) may be preferred over cryotherapy to avoid dyspigmentation. ED&C is not appropriate for morpheaform or infiltrative BCC subtypes (the lack of a defined tumor margin means the curette cannot distinguish tumor from stroma), recurrent tumors, or tumors in high-risk anatomic locations where tissue conservation and margin assessment are critical. Chemical peel depth must be calibrated to the patient's skin type — deeper peels carry a higher risk of post-inflammatory hyperpigmentation in darker skin and a risk of permanent hypopigmentation in any skin type. Wound care counseling (petrolatum ointment application, avoidance of crusting, strict photoprotection during re-epithelialization) is essential for optimal healing outcomes after all destructive procedures.

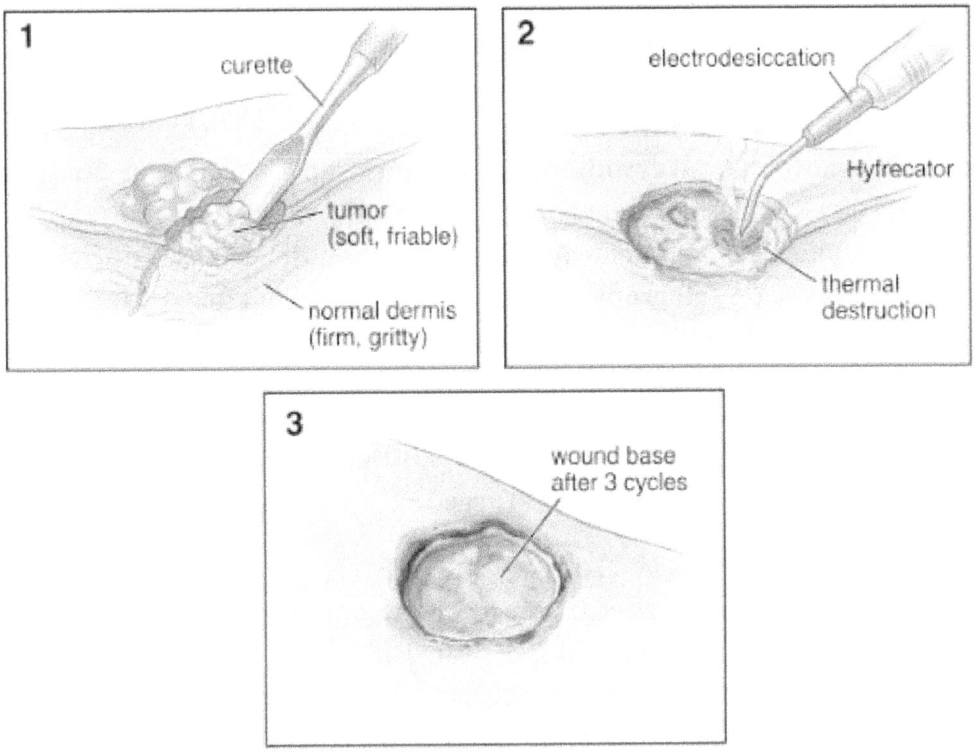

THE CUTANEOUS MIMICKER RECOGNITION ATLAS — Cryotherapy-Induced Hypopigmentation versus Vitiligo

The Clinical Pattern: Vitiligo presents as well-demarcated, depigmented (not hypopigmented) macules and patches with a chalky-white color that is accentuated under Wood lamp examination (bright blue-white fluorescence). The lesions are typically bilateral and symmetric, favor the periorificial areas (around eyes, mouth, nostrils), acral sites (fingertips, dorsal hands), and areas of trauma or friction (Koebner phenomenon). The depigmentation is complete — melanocytes are absent from the lesional epidermis — and the surface texture is normal (no scale, no atrophy).

The Mimicker: Cryotherapy-induced hypopigmentation (or depigmentation) occurs at sites of prior liquid nitrogen treatment, producing well-circumscribed, pale to white macules that mimic vitiligo. Melanocytes are among the most cold-sensitive cells in the skin, and even a single freeze-thaw cycle can permanently destroy melanocytes in the treated area, producing depigmentation that may persist indefinitely. In patients with Fitzpatrick skin types IV through VI, the contrast between the depigmented treatment site and the surrounding normally pigmented skin is particularly conspicuous and cosmetically distressing.

Trap Logic: Initiating vitiligo therapy (topical calcineurin inhibitors, phototherapy) for post-cryotherapy depigmentation is futile — the depigmentation is iatrogenic, not autoimmune, and the melanocyte reservoir may be permanently depleted at that site. **Conversely, dismissing new depigmented patches as cryotherapy scars in a patient with a history of cryotherapy** may delay the diagnosis of early vitiligo — particularly if the depigmentation extends beyond the boundaries of previously treated sites or appears in anatomically typical vitiligo distributions.

The Decision Anchor: The discriminating features are **history and location (cryotherapy depigmentation is confined to the exact footprint of a previously treated lesion with a clear temporal relationship to the procedure; vitiligo extends beyond treatment sites and favors characteristic distributions), lesion morphology (cryotherapy sites may show concurrent atrophic scarring or textural change; vitiligo skin has normal texture), Wood lamp pattern (cryotherapy sites may show incomplete depigmentation — hypopigmentation rather than the complete, bright fluorescence of vitiligo), and clinical course (cryotherapy depigmentation is stable after the initial post-procedural period; vitiligo is progressive and may demonstrate the Koebner phenomenon at new sites of trauma)**.

Laser and Energy-Based Devices: Principles, Indications, and Safety

Selective Photothermolysis and Chromophore Targeting

Selective photothermolysis (Anderson and Parrish, 1983) is the foundational principle of laser dermatology: a specific wavelength is selected to match the absorption spectrum of the target chromophore (melanin, oxyhemoglobin, water, or tattoo ink), delivered in a pulse duration shorter than the thermal relaxation time of the target, at sufficient fluence to achieve the desired effect while minimizing collateral thermal damage. For vascular lesions (port-wine stains, hemangiomas, telangiectasias, rosacea), pulsed dye laser (PDL, 585 to 595 nm) is the gold standard — it targets oxyhemoglobin, producing selective photothermolysis of blood vessels. For pigmented lesions, Q-switched and picosecond lasers (ruby 694 nm, alexandrite 755 nm, Nd:YAG 1064 nm) target melanin, producing photomechanical disruption of melanosomes. For hair removal, alexandrite (755 nm) and diode (810 nm) lasers target melanin in the hair follicle matrix — multiple sessions are required because only hairs in the anagen (growth) phase are susceptible; hair removal is most effective for dark hair on light skin and is less effective or ineffective for blonde, grey, and white hair (insufficient melanin). For skin resurfacing (wrinkles, scars, photoaging), ablative lasers (CO_2 10,600 nm, erbium:YAG 2940 nm) target water in the epidermis and dermis, vaporizing tissue layer by layer — fractional ablative lasers (which deliver energy in a pixelated microcolumn pattern, leaving untreated bridges of skin between the columns) have largely replaced fully ablative treatment because they achieve significant resurfacing with faster healing and fewer complications.

Complications and Post-Procedural Care

Laser complications are classified as immediate (pain, edema, erythema, purpura — expected and self-limited), early (blistering, crusting, infection — typically within 1 to 2 weeks), and delayed (dyspigmentation, scarring — weeks to months). Post-inflammatory hyperpigmentation (PIH) is the most common delayed complication and is more frequent in patients with darker skin types (Fitzpatrick IV through VI) — it is managed with strict photoprotection, topical hydroquinone, and time (most cases resolve within 3 to 6 months). Post-inflammatory hypopigmentation may also occur and is typically transient but can be permanent after aggressive ablative treatments. Scarring (hypertrophic or atrophic) is rare with appropriate settings but can result from excessive fluence, improper pulse duration, or treatment of actively infected skin. Herpes simplex virus reactivation is a recognized risk after perioral or full-face laser treatment — prophylactic antiviral therapy (valacyclovir) is standard practice for patients with a history of herpes labialis. Post-procedural wound care for ablative procedures includes petrolatum application, gentle cleansing, strict avoidance of sun exposure, and delayed introduction of topical retinoids and active ingredients until re-epithelialization is complete.

THE CUTANEOUS MIMICKER RECOGNITION ATLAS — Topical Steroid Withdrawal versus Rosacea Flare

---

The Clinical Pattern: Rosacea (papulopustular subtype) presents as central facial erythema with inflammatory papules and pustules on the cheeks, nose, chin, and forehead. The erythema is persistent (not transient flushing) and the papulopustules lack comedones (distinguishing rosacea from acne vulgaris). Triggers include UV exposure, hot beverages, alcohol, spicy foods, and temperature extremes. The background erythema and telangiectasias are chronic and progressive.

The Mimicker: Topical steroid withdrawal (TSW, also called red skin syndrome or steroid addiction) occurs after prolonged use of topical corticosteroids on the face, producing a rebound eruption of intense erythema, burning, papulopustules, and edema that mimics a severe rosacea flare. The patient reports that the condition initially improved with the topical steroid but worsened each time the steroid was stopped, requiring higher potency or more frequent application — the dependency cycle. The eruption extends beyond the typical rosacea distribution and involves the periocular skin, forehead, and neck.

Trap Logic: Prescribing more topical corticosteroids for what appears to be a rosacea flare perpetuates the TSW cycle — the temporary improvement is followed by a worse rebound, escalating potency requirements, and progressive skin damage. **Conversely, abruptly stopping topical corticosteroids in a patient with genuine steroid-dependent rosacea** produces a severe rebound flare that the patient cannot tolerate, leading them to restart the steroid on their own and deepening the dependency.

The Decision Anchor: The discriminating features are **medication history (TSW requires a history of prolonged or inappropriate topical corticosteroid use on the face; primary rosacea does not), distribution (TSW extends beyond the central face to involve the periocular area, forehead, and neck; rosacea is centrofacial), burning quality (TSW produces intense burning and heat**

intolerance; rosacea papulopustules are less symptomatic), and response to steroid cessation (TSW — initial severe worsening followed by gradual improvement over weeks to months; rosacea — stable worsening without the rebound pattern). Management of TSW is gradual corticosteroid taper (not abrupt cessation), transition to non-steroidal anti-inflammatory agents (tacrolimus, ivermectin), and supportive care with bland emollients and cooling techniques.

Surgical Dermatology: Excision, Flaps, Grafts, and Mohs Micrographic Surgery

Excisional Surgery and Margin Assessment

Standard excision with predefined clinical margins is the workhorse of surgical dermatology. The recommended clinical margins depend on the diagnosis and tumor characteristics: for basal cell carcinoma (nodular type, less than 2 cm), 4 mm clinical margins achieve histologic clearance in approximately 95 percent of cases; for squamous cell carcinoma (well-differentiated, less than 2 cm), 4 to 6 mm margins are recommended; for melanoma, excision margins are determined by Breslow thickness (melanoma in situ — 5 mm; Breslow 1.0 mm or less — 1 cm; Breslow 1.01 to 2.0 mm — 1 to 2 cm; Breslow greater than 2.0 mm — 2 cm). Excision specimens are processed with standard bread-loaf sectioning (vertical cross-sections at 2 to 3 mm intervals) — this method examines less than 1 percent of the actual margin, which is why clinical margins must be generous to compensate for the sampling limitation.

Mohs Micrographic Surgery

Mohs micrographic surgery (MMS) achieves the highest cure rate for skin cancer (approximately 99 percent for primary BCC, 97 percent for primary SCC) because it examines 100 percent of the surgical margin — in contrast to the less than 1 percent examined by standard bread-loaf processing. In Mohs surgery, thin layers of tissue are excised, mapped, and processed with horizontal frozen sections that allow complete peripheral and deep margin evaluation. If tumor is identified at any margin, another layer is taken only in the direction of the positive margin, and the process is repeated until all margins are clear. This complete margin control allows the surgeon to remove the entire tumor with maximum tissue conservation — sparing the maximum amount of normal tissue, which is critical in cosmetically and functionally sensitive areas. Indications for Mohs surgery include skin cancers in high-risk anatomic locations (face — nose, eyelids, lips, ears, periorbital area; genitalia; hands; feet), recurrent tumors, tumors with aggressive histologic subtypes (morpheaform/infiltrative BCC, poorly differentiated SCC), tumors with perineural invasion, and tumors in immunosuppressed patients.

Flaps, Grafts, and Wound Reconstruction

After tumor excision or Mohs surgery, the resulting defect requires repair. The reconstructive ladder progresses from simplest to most complex: secondary intention healing (allowing the wound to granulate and epithelize — appropriate for concave surfaces such as the medial canthus, temple, and conchal bowl where secondary intention produces excellent cosmetic results), primary linear closure (direct side-to-side closure — preferred when adequate tissue laxity permits tension-free approximation along relaxed skin tension lines), local flaps (advancement, rotation, and transposition flaps that recruit adjacent tissue to fill the defect while preserving blood supply and matching skin color, texture, and thickness), and skin grafts (full-thickness grafts — FTSG — from the preauricular, postauricular, supraclavicular, or inguinal donor sites for facial defects; split-thickness grafts — STSG — for larger defects where cosmesis is less critical). The bilobed flap is the workhorse transposition flap for nasal tip and alar defects. The melolabial (nasolabial) interpolation flap provides excellent tissue match for alar and lateral nasal defects, performed as a two-stage procedure with pedicle division at 3 weeks. Graft survival requires a well-vascularized recipient bed — grafts will not take on exposed cartilage, bone, or tendon without periosteum or perichondrium.

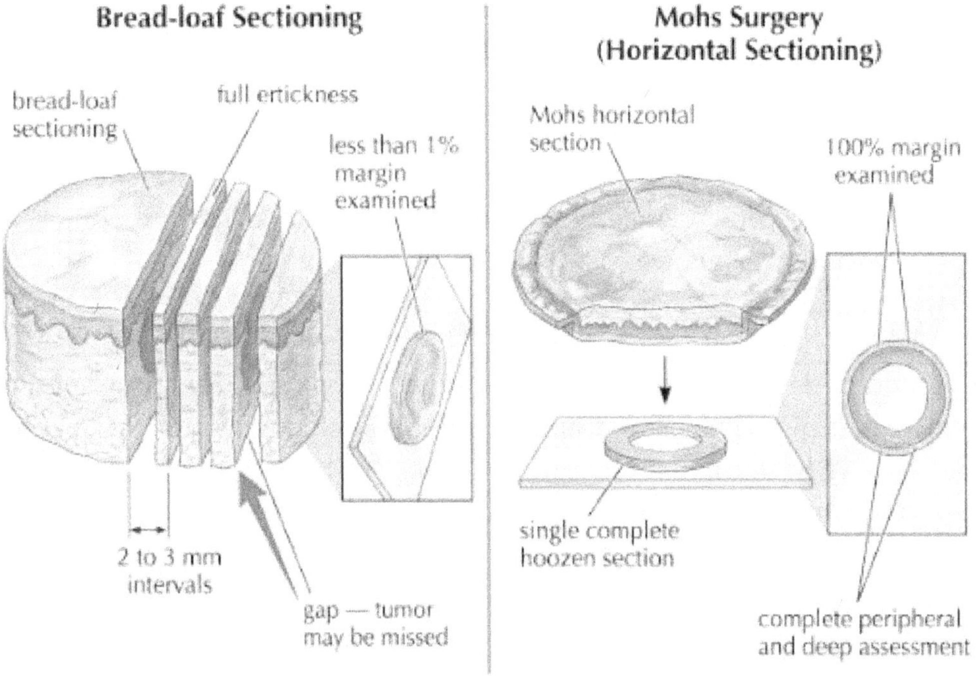

A 19-year-old male presents to the dermatology clinic with severe nodulocystic acne of the face, chest, and back that has been present for 3 years and has failed multiple courses of oral antibiotics (doxycycline, minocycline), topical retinoids, and benzoyl peroxide. Examination reveals numerous inflammatory papules, pustules, deep tender nodules, and draining sinus tracts on the bilateral cheeks and jawline, with extensive atrophic and hypertrophic scarring. The chest and upper back show confluent inflammatory papules, nodules, and post-inflammatory hyperpigmentation. The patient reports significant psychosocial distress, including avoidance of social situations and declining academic performance.

The clinical presentation — severe nodulocystic acne with scarring, sinus tracts, and failure of conventional therapies — meets the criteria for systemic isotretinoin. Pre-treatment evaluation includes a comprehensive metabolic panel, fasting lipid panel, and CBC. Given the patient is male, iPLEDGE registration is required but the pregnancy prevention requirements do not apply. Isotretinoin is initiated at 0.5 mg/kg/day for the first month (to minimize the initial flare that can worsen severe nodular disease) and titrated upward to 1 mg/kg/day. At the 1-month follow-up, the patient reports expected mucocutaneous dryness (cheilitis managed with petroleum-based lip balm, xerosis managed with bland emollients) and mild epistaxis. Triglycerides are mildly elevated but below the threshold for intervention. By month 3, inflammatory lesions have decreased by approximately 70 percent and no new nodules have formed. The treatment course continues for a total of 6 months, targeting a cumulative dose of 150 mg/kg. At completion, the patient has achieved near-complete clearance with no active inflammatory lesions and is counseled on long-term maintenance with topical retinoids and benzoyl peroxide.

CAUTION: Topical corticosteroids are the most prescribed medications in dermatology — and the most commonly misused. The two most dangerous patterns of misuse are: (1) inappropriate potency on sensitive sites (superpotent corticosteroids on the face, eyelids, or intertriginous areas — producing irreversible striae, atrophy, telangiectasias, glaucoma, and cataracts), and (2) prolonged unsupervised use without a defined endpoint (producing steroid dependency, rebound flares on cessation, and cumulative skin damage). Every prescription for a topical corticosteroid should specify: the correct potency for the body site, the duration of the treatment course, and a clear plan for tapering or transitioning to a steroid-sparing agent. Class I (superpotent) corticosteroids should NEVER be used on the face, eyelids, axillae, or groin except for very brief, closely monitored courses in exceptional circumstances.

THE CUTANEOUS MIMICKER RECOGNITION ATLAS — Therapeutic Decision Arcs

Cryotherapy-Induced Hypopigmentation vs. Vitiligo: The discriminating features are history and location (cryotherapy depigmentation is confined to the exact footprint of a previously treated lesion; vitiligo extends beyond treatment sites and favors characteristic periorificial and acral distributions), lesion morphology (cryotherapy sites may show concurrent atrophic scarring; vitiligo skin has normal texture), Wood lamp pattern (cryotherapy sites may show incomplete depigmentation; vitiligo shows bright, complete fluorescence), and clinical course (cryotherapy depigmentation is stable; vitiligo is progressive with Koebner phenomenon). Cognitive trap: initiating vitiligo therapy for post-cryotherapy depigmentation is futile because the mechanism is iatrogenic melanocyte destruction, not autoimmune.

Topical Steroid Withdrawal vs. Rosacea Flare: The discriminating features are medication history (TSW requires prolonged facial corticosteroid use; primary rosacea does not), distribution (TSW extends beyond the central face; rosacea is centrofacial), symptom quality (TSW — intense burning and heat intolerance; rosacea — less symptomatic papulopustules), and the dependency cycle (TSW worsens with each steroid cessation; rosacea does not follow a rebound-escalation pattern). Cognitive trap: treating the TSW rebound with more corticosteroid perpetuates the cycle.

Mohs Surgery vs. Standard Excision — Decision Framework: Mohs micrographic surgery is indicated when margin control must be complete and tissue conservation is critical: high-risk anatomic locations (face, particularly nose, eyelids, ears, lips), recurrent tumors, aggressive histologic subtypes (morpheaform BCC, poorly differentiated SCC), perineural invasion, and immunosuppressed patients. Standard excision with predefined clinical margins is appropriate for low-risk tumors on the trunk and extremities where tissue conservation is less critical. Cognitive trap: applying standard excision to a morpheaform BCC on the nasal ala risks incomplete removal because bread-loaf sectioning examines less than 1 percent of the margin.

Summary and Key Concepts

Topical therapy effectiveness depends on vehicle selection (ointments for highest bioavailability, creams for cosmetic elegance, solutions for hairy areas) and the fingertip unit system for standardized application. The soak-and-seal technique and occlusion enhance drug penetration.

Topical corticosteroids are classified into 7 potency classes. Site-appropriate potency selection prevents adverse effects: low potency for the face, eyelids, and intertriginous areas; superpotent agents reserved for thick skin and recalcitrant plaques with defined treatment courses. Steroid-sparing strategies (calcineurin inhibitors, PDE4 inhibitors, proactive maintenance) prevent chronic toxicity.

Systemic immunosuppressives (methotrexate, cyclosporine, azathioprine, mycophenolate) require pre-treatment screening, ongoing laboratory monitoring, and awareness of organ-specific toxicities. All are teratogenic. TPMT testing is mandatory before azathioprine initiation.

Biologic therapies have transformed psoriasis and atopic dermatitis management: IL-17 and IL-23 inhibitors achieve PASI 90 to 100 in psoriasis; dupilumab is approved for AD from age 6 months; JAK inhibitors offer oral convenience but carry class-wide boxed warnings. Pre-treatment TB and hepatitis screening is mandatory for all biologics.

Mohs micrographic surgery examines 100 percent of the surgical margin (vs. less than 1 percent with bread-loaf sectioning), achieving the highest cure rates for skin cancer with maximum tissue conservation — indicated for high-risk locations, recurrent tumors, aggressive subtypes, and immunosuppressed patients.

THE CUTANEOUS MIMICKER MASTER ATLAS

The Cutaneous Mimicker Master Atlas consolidates every mimicker pair introduced across the twenty-four chapters of this textbook into a structured, indexed reference designed for rapid clinical decision-making. Each mimicker pair names two conditions that can be confused at the bedside, and the atlas supplies the discriminating features — the clinical, dermoscopic, histopathologic, or laboratory findings that separate one from the other. The atlas is organized in four complementary ways: by morphologic category (Section I), by body site (Section II), by skin-tone considerations for Fitzpatrick IV through VI (Section III), and by master alphabetical index cross-referenced to chapter location (Section IV). Use any entry point that matches how you are encountering the diagnostic question — by what the lesion looks like, where it is, or whose skin you are examining.

Section I: Mimicker Pairs Indexed by Morphologic Category

Papulosquamous and Scaly Dermatoses

- **Pityriasis Rosea vs. Secondary Syphilis (Chapter 4)** Serologic testing (RPR/VDRL with confirmatory FTA-ABS) is mandatory in every sexually active patient with a papulosquamous eruption resembling pityriasis rosea. The herald patch does not reliably exclude syphilis, and the condylomata lata of secondary syphilis mimic the collarette scale of pityriasis rosea. Syphilis serologies, not clinical morphology, are the decision anchor.
- **Plaque Psoriasis vs. Nummular Dermatitis (Chapter 4)** Distribution (extensor, symmetric for psoriasis vs. scattered, non-symmetric for nummular), scale character (thick silvery micaceous for psoriasis vs. thin crusted for nummular), and Auspitz sign (pinpoint bleeding after scale removal — specific to psoriasis) are the discriminating features.
- **Nummular Dermatitis vs. Tinea Corporis (Chapter 3)** KOH preparation showing branching, septate hyphae is the definitive discriminator. Central clearing occurs in both conditions. KOH must be performed before prescribing topical corticosteroids — treating tinea with corticosteroids produces tinea incognito, masking the infection and delaying diagnosis.
- **Tinea Corporis vs. Nummular Eczema (Chapter 11)** The active border is the clinical clue (tinea has a raised, scaly, advancing border; nummular eczema is uniformly inflamed). KOH from the active border confirms dermatophyte infection. Bilateral symmetric distribution favors nummular eczema.
- **Lichen Planus vs. Lichenoid Drug Eruption (Chapter 6)** A thorough medication history with attention to drugs started within the preceding 12 months is the discriminating approach. The 5 Ps (pruritic, planar, polygonal, purple papules) overlap between the two conditions, and photodistribution favors drug-induced lichenoid eruption.
- **Discoid Lupus vs. Tinea Faciei (Chapter 19)** Follicular plugging and the carpet-tack sign (keratotic spicules on the undersurface of a removed scale) are present in DLE and absent in tinea. DLE produces

atrophic scarring and permanent pigmentary change; tinea resolves without scarring. KOH and DIF separate the two.

- **Patch-Stage Mycosis Fungoides vs. Chronic Eczema (Chapter 16)** Sun-protected bathing trunk distribution favors MF; flexural and atopic distribution favors eczema. Clinically, fixed patches (stable location over months), poikiloderma (atrophy, telangiectasia, dyspigmentation), and failure to respond to topical corticosteroids mandate biopsy for MF.
- **Mycosis Fungoides Plaque vs. Psoriasis Plaque (Chapter 16)** Distribution (sun-protected, flexural for MF; extensor for psoriasis), scale quality (fine, thin in MF; thick, silvery in psoriasis), and pruritus pattern (persistent, refractory pruritus disproportionate to clinical findings in MF) are the discriminating features. Skin biopsy with immunophenotyping is definitive.

Vesiculobullous and Erosive Dermatoses

- **Pemphigus Vulgaris vs. Bullous Pemphigoid (Chapter 7)** Blister tension (flaccid in PV, tense in BP), Nikolsky sign (positive in PV, negative in BP), mucosal involvement (early and prominent in PV, uncommon in BP), and DIF pattern (intercellular fishnet IgG in PV, linear BMZ IgG and C3 in BP) are the discriminating features.
- **Dermatitis Herpetiformis vs. Linear IgA Bullous Dermatosis (Chapter 7)** DIF is definitive: granular IgA at dermal papillae (DH) versus linear IgA at the BMZ (LAD). DH requires lifelong GFD and celiac disease screening; LAD requires evaluation for drug-induced etiology (vancomycin is the most common trigger).
- **Herpes Zoster vs. Zosteriform Herpes Simplex (Chapter 1)** Recurrence in the same dermatomal distribution is the discriminating feature. Zoster virtually never recurs in the same dermatome in immunocompetent patients; recurrent vesicles in the same dermatome are zosteriform HSV until proven otherwise.
- **Herpes Zoster vs. Contact Dermatitis (Chapter 10)** Symptom quality (pain and prodrome in zoster vs. pruritus without prodrome in contact dermatitis) and distribution quality (strictly dermatomal in zoster vs. geometric or linear in contact dermatitis reflecting external exposure) are the discriminating features. Viral PCR or DFA confirms.
- **Erythema Multiforme vs. Stevens-Johnson Syndrome (Chapter 5)** Lesion morphology (raised three-zone targets in EM vs. flat two-zone atypical targets in SJS), distribution (acral vs. central), and mucosal involvement severity separate the two. EM is typically HSV-associated; SJS is drug-associated.
- **SJS/TEN vs. Generalized Bullous Fixed Drug Eruption (Chapter 22)** Mucosal involvement (prominent in SJS/TEN, absent or minimal in GBFDE), lesion morphology (widespread atypical targets in SJS/TEN vs. round, well-demarcated plaques with central bullae in GBFDE), and recurrence at identical sites upon re-exposure (pathognomonic for FDE) are the discriminating features.
- **SSSS vs. Toxic Epidermal Necrolysis (Chapter 9)** Level of epidermal cleavage is definitive: SSSS cleaves within the granular layer (superficial, subcorneal); TEN cleaves at the dermoepidermal junction (full-thickness). Age (SSSS in neonates and young children; TEN in adults) and mucosal

involvement (absent in SSSS; prominent in TEN) further separate them. Frozen section biopsy provides rapid diagnosis.

- **Erosive Oral Lichen Planus vs. Oral Squamous Cell Carcinoma (Chapter 6)** Induration, verrucous change, fixation, failure to respond to previously effective topical therapy, and a change in pain character mandate biopsy. OLP itself carries a small malignant transformation risk, and SCC arising within OLP is indistinguishable clinically without tissue sampling.

Pigmented Lesions and Melanocytic Mimickers

- **Melanoma vs. Seborrheic Keratosis (Chapter 2)** The ugly duckling sign combined with dermoscopic absence of seborrheic keratosis structures (comedo-like openings, milia-like cysts, brain-like fissures) is the discriminating finding. Any pigmented lesion lacking typical seborrheic keratosis dermoscopic features must be biopsied.
- **Seborrheic Keratosis vs. Melanoma (Chapter 13)** Dermoscopic confirmation of milia-like cysts, comedo-like openings, and the cerebriform pattern is diagnostic of seborrheic keratosis. Irritated or inflamed seborrheic keratoses lose their characteristic features — biopsy is indicated when dermoscopic reassurance is incomplete.
- **Nodular Melanoma vs. Seborrheic Keratosis (Chapter 15)** Blue-white veil, polymorphous vascular pattern, and asymmetric pigment distribution on dermoscopy distinguish nodular melanoma. The stuck-on appearance clinically attributed to seborrheic keratosis is unreliable for nodular melanoma — dermoscopy or biopsy is mandatory for any rapidly growing pigmented nodule.
- **Acral Melanoma vs. Acral Nevus (Chapter 15)** The parallel ridge pattern on dermoscopy is pathognomonic for acral melanoma; the parallel furrow pattern indicates a benign acral nevus. Any pigmented lesion on the palms, soles, or nail bed with a parallel ridge pattern or irregular pigmentation requires biopsy.
- **Subungual Melanoma vs. Subungual Hemorrhage (Chapter 18)** Migration with nail growth separates the two: hemorrhage migrates distally and grows out; melanonychia remains fixed with new pigment continuously deposited at the proximal nail fold. The Hutchinson sign (periungual pigment extension) is specific to subungual melanoma.
- **Actinic Keratosis vs. Bowen Disease (Chapter 14)** Border quality (AKs are poorly demarcated; Bowen disease is sharply demarcated), texture (AKs are rough and gritty; Bowen disease is flat and erythematous with a stuck-on scale), and histologic extent (AK is partial-thickness atypia; Bowen disease is full-thickness SCC in situ) are the discriminating features.
- **Basal Cell Carcinoma vs. Intradermal Nevus (Chapter 14)** Dermoscopic vascular pattern is discriminating: arborizing tree-like vessels are pathognomonic for BCC; comma-shaped vessels and cobblestone pattern characterize intradermal nevi. Pearly translucence with surface telangiectasias favors BCC over nevus.
- **Pyogenic Granuloma vs. Amelanotic Melanoma (Chapter 13)** Dermoscopic vascular pattern separates the two: homogeneous red with white collarette favors pyogenic granuloma; polymorphous vessels with structureless areas suggest amelanotic melanoma. Any rapidly growing vascular nodule in an adult must be biopsied to exclude amelanotic melanoma.

Erythematous and Inflammatory Dermatoses

- **Atopic Dermatitis vs. Cutaneous T-Cell Lymphoma (Chapter 3)** Persistent fixed patches in non-flexural distribution with poikiloderma, epidermotropism of atypical lymphocytes on biopsy, and failure to respond to standard AD therapy discriminate MF from refractory AD. Fixed non-migrating patches in bathing trunk distribution mandate skin biopsy.
- **Allergic Contact Dermatitis vs. Irritant Contact Dermatitis (Chapter 2)** Patch testing is the definitive discriminator. No clinical feature reliably separates the two in every case. Chronic, recurrent, or refractory hand dermatitis in particular requires patch testing before attributing the dermatitis to irritant exposure.
- **Cellulitis vs. Stasis Dermatitis (Chapter 9)** Laterality (cellulitis is unilateral; bilateral erythema is almost always stasis dermatitis), chronicity (acute progression vs. chronic stable or fluctuating course), and hemosiderin staining (brown discoloration from prior venous hypertension, specific to stasis) are the discriminating features.
- **Chronic Spontaneous Urticaria vs. Urticarial Bullous Pemphigoid (Chapter 5)** Lesion persistence beyond 24 hours at the same site, peripheral eosinophilia, and DIF showing linear BMZ IgG and C3 deposition discriminate urticarial BP from CSU. Urticarial BP is often misdiagnosed as refractory urticaria for months before the correct diagnosis is made.
- **Scabies vs. Eczema (Chapter 12)** Interdigital web space, wrist, genital, and periumbilical involvement strongly favors scabies — sites rarely involved in eczema. Household contacts with pruritus and the presence of linear burrows are diagnostic clues. Skin scraping with mineral oil preparation confirms the diagnosis.
- **Infantile AD vs. Seborrheic Dermatitis (Chapter 21)** Pruritus (AD — intense itch; seborrheic — non-pruritic), distribution (AD — cheeks with nose sparing, extensors; seborrheic — scalp cradle cap, nasolabial folds, diaper area), and scale quality (AD — dry, rough, xerotic; seborrheic — greasy, yellowish, adherent) are the discriminating features.
- **Paraneoplastic Acanthosis Nigricans vs. Benign Acanthosis Nigricans (Chapter 22)** Onset (benign — gradual; paraneoplastic — sudden and rapidly progressive), extent (benign — flexural only; paraneoplastic — extensive, involving mucosal surfaces and atypical sites), and associated findings (florid cutaneous papillomatosis, tripe palms, sign of Leser-Trelat) discriminate the two. Sudden-onset AN mandates malignancy screening.
- **Topical Steroid Withdrawal vs. Rosacea Flare (Chapter 24)** Medication history (TSW requires prolonged facial corticosteroid use; rosacea does not), distribution (TSW extends beyond the central face to periocular area and neck; rosacea is centrofacial), and the dependency cycle pattern (TSW worsens with each steroid cessation; rosacea does not follow a rebound-escalation pattern) are the discriminating features.
- **Hidradenitis Suppurativa vs. Recurrent Furunculosis (Chapter 1)** Recurrence in apocrine-gland-bearing skin with architectural change (double-ended comedones, sinus tracts, bridging scarring) discriminates HS from furunculosis. Furunculosis produces discrete, non-connected abscesses; HS produces interconnected tunnels visible on ultrasound.

Granulomatous and Papulonodular Lesions

- **Granuloma Annulare vs. Tinea Corporis (Chapter 8)** Surface scale is the key: tinea has a scaly advancing border (KOH-positive) while GA is smooth and non-scaly (KOH-negative). KOH must be performed before attributing an annular plaque to granuloma annulare.
- **Necrobiosis Lipoidica vs. Granuloma Annulare (Chapter 8)** The quality of the plaque center discriminates: NL has an atrophic, transparent center with visible telangiectasias and ulceration risk; GA has a normal or slightly depressed center without atrophy or telangiectasias. Pretibial location strongly favors NL. Diabetes association is present in both but stronger for NL.
- **Molluscum Contagiosum vs. Disseminated Cryptococcosis (Chapter 10)** In immunocompromised patients (particularly advanced HIV), dome-shaped, umbilicated papules may represent disseminated cryptococcosis rather than molluscum. Skin biopsy showing Henderson-Patterson bodies confirms molluscum; encapsulated yeast with a clear halo on mucicarmine stain confirms cryptococcosis.
- **Cutaneous Leishmaniasis vs. Squamous Cell Carcinoma (Chapter 12)** Travel or endemic area exposure history is essential for CL. Age and chronic actinic damage profile (SCC favors elderly, sun-damaged skin), tempo (CL develops over weeks to months after exposure; SCC develops insidiously), and tissue sampling (touch preparation showing amastigotes for CL; histology showing keratinocyte atypia for SCC) are discriminating.

Purpuric and Vascular Lesions

- **Palpable Purpura (LCV) vs. Thrombocytopenic Purpura (Chapter 20)** Palpability (LCV is raised; thrombocytopenic purpura is flat), distribution (LCV is gravity-dependent on the legs; thrombocytopenic is diffuse including mucosal), and platelet count (normal in LCV; reduced in thrombocytopenic) are the discriminating features. Palpable purpura always warrants skin biopsy.
- **Venous Ulcer vs. Pyoderma Gangrenosum (Chapter 20)** Border morphology (PG is undermined and violaceous; venous is flat and irregular), surrounding skin (venous shows hemosiderin staining and lipodermatosclerosis; PG has a violaceous, boggy border), and pathergy (PG worsens with debridement; venous ulcers improve with compression) are the discriminating features. Debridement of suspected PG is contraindicated.
- **Mongolian Spots vs. Non-Accidental Bruising (Chapter 21)** Color evolution (bruises change color over days — red to purple to yellow-green; Mongolian spots are stable blue-grey), tenderness (bruises may be tender; spots are non-tender), location (Mongolian spots favor the lumbosacral area and buttocks; non-accidental bruises favor unusual sites — ears, neck, torso), and photographic documentation from birth or early infancy are discriminating.

Depigmented and Hypopigmented Lesions

- **Vitiligo vs. Pityriasis Versicolor (Chapter 23)** Degree of pigment loss (vitiligo — complete depigmentation; pityriasis versicolor — hypopigmentation), scale (vitiligo — no scale; PV — fine powdery scale on scraping), Wood lamp pattern (vitiligo — bright blue-white fluorescence; PV — yellow-green fluorescence), and KOH (PV — spaghetti and meatballs; vitiligo — negative) are the discriminating features.
- **Pityriasis Versicolor vs. Vitiligo (Chapter 11)** Fine powdery scale on scraping, yellow-green Wood lamp fluorescence, and KOH showing short hyphae and clusters of round spores (spaghetti-and-meatballs pattern) confirm pityriasis versicolor. The hypopigmentation of PV is incomplete (hypopigmented, not depigmented) and repigments with treatment.
- **Melasma vs. Post-Inflammatory Hyperpigmentation (Chapter 23)** Symmetry (melasma — bilateral and symmetric in centrofacial, malar, or mandibular patterns; PIH — follows the distribution of the preceding inflammation), history (melasma — hormonal triggers, sun exposure; PIH — preceding dermatitis, acne, or trauma), and chronicity (melasma is chronic and recurrent; PIH improves with time if the inciting cause resolves) are the discriminating features.
- **Cryotherapy-Induced Hypopigmentation vs. Vitiligo (Chapter 24)** History and location (cryotherapy depigmentation is confined to the exact footprint of a previously treated lesion; vitiligo extends beyond treatment sites), lesion morphology (cryotherapy sites may show concurrent atrophic scarring; vitiligo skin has normal texture), and clinical course (cryotherapy depigmentation is stable after the procedure; vitiligo is progressive with Koebner phenomenon) are the discriminating features.

Sclerosing Dermatoses, Hair, and Nail Disorders

- **Morphea vs. Lichen Sclerosus (Chapter 19)** Depth of involvement (morphea is deep, firm, and bound-down; LS is superficial and thin), the lilac ring (active morphea border), and genital involvement (LS strongly favors anogenital skin; morphea does not) are the discriminating features. Biopsy location and depth are critical: a superficial shave biopsy may miss the deep dermal sclerosis of morphea.
- **Alopecia Areata vs. Tinea Capitis (Chapter 17)** Scalp surface (smooth and scale-free in AA; scaling in tinea), hair shaft appearance (exclamation point hairs in AA; comma hairs and corkscrew hairs in tinea), and KOH/fungal culture (negative in AA; positive in tinea) are the discriminating features. Tinea must be excluded before diagnosing AA in children.
- **Frontal Fibrosing Alopecia vs. Traction Alopecia (Chapter 17)** Trichoscopy at the hairline margin discriminates: perifollicular scaling and erythema with loss of follicular ostia in FFA (scarring); preserved ostia with short broken hairs in traction alopecia (early non-scarring). Eyebrow loss strongly favors FFA. Continued traction causes eventual scarring, but the fringe sign (retained vellus hairs at the original hairline) is specific to FFA.
- **Nail Psoriasis vs. Onychomycosis (Chapter 18)** Pitting (regular pitting is specific to psoriasis), oil drop sign (specific to psoriasis), concurrent skin psoriasis on other body sites, and KOH/fungal culture (positive in onychomycosis, negative in psoriasis) are the discriminating features. The two conditions

coexist frequently — fungal culture must be performed even in known psoriasis patients before starting systemic antifungals.

Section II: Mimicker Pairs Indexed by Body Site

Face and Perioral Region

- **Central face** Topical Steroid Withdrawal vs. Rosacea Flare (Ch. 24); Discoid Lupus vs. Tinea Faciei (Ch. 19); Infantile AD vs. Seborrheic Dermatitis (Ch. 21, cheeks); Melasma vs. PIH (Ch. 23, malar and centrofacial).
- **Perioral and periocular** Topical Steroid Withdrawal — extends to periocular and perioral (Ch. 24); Erosive Oral Lichen Planus vs. Oral SCC (Ch. 6, perioral and intraoral).

Scalp

- **Alopecic patches** Alopecia Areata vs. Tinea Capitis (Ch. 17); Frontal Fibrosing Alopecia vs. Traction Alopecia (Ch. 17, frontotemporal hairline).
- **Scaly scalp** Psoriasis Plaque vs. MF Plaque (Ch. 16); Infantile Seborrheic Dermatitis — cradle cap (Ch. 21).

Trunk

- **Diffuse trunk eruption** Pityriasis Rosea vs. Secondary Syphilis (Ch. 4); Patch-Stage MF vs. Chronic Eczema (Ch. 16, bathing trunk); Scabies vs. Eczema (Ch. 12); SJS/TEN vs. Generalized Bullous FDE (Ch. 22).
- **Annular trunk lesions** Granuloma Annulare vs. Tinea Corporis (Ch. 8); Tinea Corporis vs. Nummular Eczema (Ch. 11); Nummular Dermatitis vs. Tinea Corporis (Ch. 3).
- **Pigmented trunk lesions** Melanoma vs. Seborrheic Keratosis (Ch. 2); Seborrheic Keratosis vs. Melanoma (Ch. 13); Nodular Melanoma vs. Seborrheic Keratosis (Ch. 15).

Extremities

- **Lower extremities** Cellulitis vs. Stasis Dermatitis (Ch. 9); Palpable Purpura (LCV) vs. Thrombocytopenic Purpura (Ch. 20, gravity-dependent); Venous Ulcer vs. Pyoderma Gangrenosum (Ch. 20, medial malleolus and pretibial); Necrobiosis Lipoidica vs. Granuloma Annulare (Ch. 8, pretibial); Plaque Psoriasis vs. Nummular Dermatitis (Ch. 4, extensors).
- **Upper extremities** Lichen Planus vs. Lichenoid Drug Eruption (Ch. 6, flexural wrists); Allergic Contact Dermatitis vs. Irritant Contact Dermatitis (Ch. 2, hands).

Hands, Feet, and Acral Sites

- **Palms and soles** Acral Melanoma vs. Acral Nevus (Ch. 15); Erythema Multiforme — acral target lesions (Ch. 5); Secondary Syphilis — condylomata lata on palms and soles (Ch. 4).
- **Nails** Subungual Melanoma vs. Subungual Hemorrhage (Ch. 18); Nail Psoriasis vs. Onychomycosis (Ch. 18).

Intertriginous and Genital Regions

- **Axillae and groin** Hidradenitis Suppurativa vs. Recurrent Furunculosis (Ch. 1); Paraneoplastic AN vs. Benign AN (Ch. 22, flexural); Morphea vs. Lichen Sclerosus (Ch. 19, anogenital for LS).
- **Diaper area** Infantile AD vs. Seborrheic Dermatitis (Ch. 21, diaper area involvement favors seborrheic); Scabies — nodular scabies on genitalia (Ch. 12).

Dermatomal and Linear Distribution

- **Dermatomal** Herpes Zoster vs. Zosteriform Herpes Simplex (Ch. 1); Herpes Zoster vs. Contact Dermatitis (Ch. 10).

Lumbosacral and Buttocks

- **Blue-grey patches** Mongolian Spots vs. Non-Accidental Bruising (Ch. 21). Mongolian spots favor the lumbosacral area and buttocks; bruises in this distribution in infants require clinical context and documentation.

Section III: Mimicker Pairs With Skin-Tone Considerations (Fitzpatrick IV–VI Diagnostic Modifiers)

Clinical diagnosis in patients with Fitzpatrick skin types IV through VI requires awareness that erythema appears violaceous or hyperpigmented rather than red, that depigmented and hypopigmented lesions are more conspicuous, and that several dermatoses present with morphologic variants not emphasized in standard references. The following mimicker pairs carry specific diagnostic modifiers for darker skin.

- **Vitiligo vs. Pityriasis Versicolor (Ch. 23)** Both conditions produce high-contrast lesions in dark skin. Wood lamp is essential — vitiligo produces bright blue-white fluorescence (complete depigmentation); pityriasis versicolor produces yellow-green (hypopigmentation with retained melanocytes). KOH is confirmatory. Post-treatment repigmentation of PV may be slow, mimicking treatment failure.
- **Melasma vs. PIH (Ch. 23)** Both are disproportionately prevalent in Fitzpatrick IV through VI. Wood lamp helps determine depth: epidermal hyperpigmentation is accentuated; dermal hyperpigmentation is not. Treatment of PIH requires treatment of the underlying cause (e.g., acne) to prevent recurrence, while melasma requires indefinite photoprotection.
- **Cryotherapy-Induced Hypopigmentation vs. Vitiligo (Ch. 24)** Melanocytes in darker skin types are more sensitive to cryotherapy-induced destruction, and the resulting depigmentation is more

conspicuous and potentially permanent. In Fitzpatrick IV through VI patients, topical field therapy may be preferred over cryotherapy for actinic keratoses to avoid iatrogenic depigmentation.

- **Acral Melanoma vs. Acral Nevus (Ch. 15)** Acral melanoma constitutes a disproportionately high percentage of melanomas in patients of African and Asian descent (60 to 70 percent of melanomas, compared with less than 5 percent in White patients). The parallel ridge pattern on dermoscopy is pathognomonic regardless of skin type. Any new or changing pigmented lesion on the palm, sole, or nail bed in a patient of color warrants urgent evaluation.
- **Subungual Melanoma vs. Subungual Hemorrhage (Ch. 18)** Melanonychia striata is common and benign in Fitzpatrick V and VI — present in up to 77 percent of Black patients over age 20. The challenge is identifying the rare subungual melanoma among benign melanonychia. Width greater than 3 mm, Hutchinson sign, rapid change, and single-digit involvement warrant biopsy.
- **Patch-Stage MF vs. Chronic Eczema (Ch. 16)** Hypopigmented MF is a distinct variant that disproportionately affects children and young adults of African and Asian descent. Hypopigmented patches in a bathing trunk distribution that fail to respond to emollients and topical corticosteroids should be biopsied — hypopigmented MF is often misdiagnosed as pityriasis alba or vitiligo for years.
- **Cellulitis vs. Stasis Dermatitis (Ch. 9)** Erythema is difficult to detect in dark skin — it appears as hyperpigmentation, violaceous discoloration, or increased warmth without visible color change. Palpation for warmth and tenderness, rather than visual assessment of redness alone, is critical for diagnosing cellulitis in Fitzpatrick V and VI.
- **Mongolian Spots vs. Non-Accidental Bruising (Ch. 21)** Mongolian spots are present in more than 80 percent of Asian, African, and Native American neonates and can be extensive. Photographic documentation at birth is essential. Clinicians unfamiliar with Mongolian spots in diverse populations may misidentify them as bruises, potentially triggering inappropriate child abuse investigations.
- **Palpable Purpura (LCV) vs. Thrombocytopenic Purpura (Ch. 20)** Purpura is more difficult to visualize in darker skin — use diascopy (pressing a glass slide against the skin; purpura does not blanch) and palpation (LCV is raised; thrombocytopenic purpura is flat) to confirm. In dark skin, purpura may appear dark brown or black rather than the classic violaceous color.
- **Lichen Planus vs. Lichenoid Drug Eruption (Ch. 6)** LP is more common and often more severe in patients of African descent. Post-inflammatory hyperpigmentation from LP is more pronounced and long-lasting in darker skin types. Oral LP can present with distinctive reticulate hyperpigmentation on the buccal mucosa in dark-skinned patients.
- **Scabies vs. Eczema (Ch. 12)** Nodular scabies (persistent, pruritic, red-brown nodules on the genitalia, axillae, and buttocks) is more common in patients of color and can persist for months after successful scabicidal treatment. These nodules are a hypersensitivity reaction to mite antigens, not active infestation.
- **Infantile AD vs. Seborrheic Dermatitis (Ch. 21)** In infants with darker skin, the erythema of AD may be subtle — the predominant finding may be follicular accentuation (perifollicular papules) and lichenification rather than the classic red, oozing plaques seen in lighter-skinned infants. Seborrheic dermatitis in dark-skinned infants may present with hypopigmented patches rather than the classic erythematous, greasy scale.

Section IV: Master Alphabetical Index — Every Mimicker Pair Cross-Referenced to Chapter Location

Herpes Zoster vs. Contact Dermatitis	Vesiculobullous	10
Herpes Zoster vs. Zosteriform Herpes Simplex	Vesiculobullous	1
Hidradenitis Suppurativa vs. Recurrent Furunculosis	Inflammatory	1
Infantile AD vs. Seborrheic Dermatitis	Inflammatory	21
Lichen Planus vs. Lichenoid Drug Eruption	Papulosquamous	6
Melasma vs. Post-Inflammatory Hyperpigmentation	Depigmented	23
Molluscum Contagiosum vs. Disseminated Cryptococcosis	Papulonodular	10
Mongolian Spots vs. Non-Accidental Bruising	Purpuric	21
Morphea vs. Lichen Sclerosus	Sclerosing	19
Mycosis Fungoides Plaque vs. Psoriasis Plaque	Papulosquamous	16
Nail Psoriasis vs. Onychomycosis	Nail	18
Necrobiosis Lipoidica vs. Granuloma Annulare	Papulonodular	8
Nodular Melanoma vs. Seborrheic Keratosis	Pigmented	15
Nummular Dermatitis vs. Tinea Corporis	Papulosquamous	3
Palpable Purpura (LCV) vs. Thrombocytopenic Purpura	Purpuric	20
Paraneoplastic AN vs. Benign Insulin-Resistant AN	Inflammatory	22
Patch-Stage MF vs. Chronic Eczema	Papulosquamous	16
Pemphigus Vulgaris vs. Bullous Pemphigoid	Vesiculobullous	7
Pityriasis Rosea vs. Secondary Syphilis	Papulosquamous	4

Pityriasis Versicolor vs. Vitiligo	Depigmented	11
Plaque Psoriasis vs. Nummular Dermatitis	Papulosquamous	4
Pyogenic Granuloma vs. Amelanotic Melanoma	Pigmented	13
Scabies vs. Eczema	Inflammatory	12
Seborrheic Keratosis vs. Melanoma	Pigmented	13
SJS/TEN vs. Generalized Bullous FDE	Vesiculobullous	22
SSSS vs. Toxic Epidermal Necrolysis	Vesiculobullous	9
Subungual Melanoma vs. Subungual Hemorrhage	Pigmented	18
Tinea Corporis vs. Nummular Eczema	Papulosquamous	11
Topical Steroid Withdrawal vs. Rosacea Flare	Inflammatory	24
Venous Ulcer vs. Pyoderma Gangrenosum	Purpuric	20
Vitiligo vs. Pityriasis Versicolor	Depigmented	23
Melanoma vs. Seborrheic Keratosis	Pigmented	2

CONCLUSION: THE INTEGRATIVE DERMATOLOGIST

The twenty-four chapters and the Cutaneous Mimicker Master Atlas that precede this conclusion represent a single argument: that clinical dermatology is, at its core, a discipline of pattern recognition disciplined by mechanism. The skin is the only organ system that presents its pathology to the unaided eye — and that visibility is both its gift and its trap. What the eye sees is morphology; what the clinician must understand is the pathophysiologic process that produced it. This textbook has been built around the conviction that the distance between seeing and understanding is where diagnostic errors live, and that closing that distance requires not just factual knowledge but a structured approach to the mimicker pairs that populate every dermatologic differential.

From Pattern to Mechanism to Decision

Every chapter in this textbook has followed a consistent architecture: foundational science (the molecular, cellular, and immunologic mechanisms that drive disease), clinical presentation (the morphologic patterns those mechanisms produce on the skin surface), diagnostic reasoning (the systematic approach to distinguishing one pattern from its mimickers), and management (the therapeutic interventions that target the underlying mechanism, not merely the visible eruption). This architecture reflects the way clinical dermatology is actually practiced — the clinician who understands why a plaque of psoriasis is silvery and micaceous (because the accelerated epidermal turnover produces parakeratotic scale that reflects light) is the clinician who will not confuse it with the thin, crusted scale of nummular eczema, and who will select a therapy that targets the IL-23/IL-17 axis rather than merely suppressing the surface inflammation.

The Cutaneous Mimicker Recognition Atlas — integrated into every chapter as a Rhythm Layer and consolidated in the Master Atlas — embodies this principle. Each of the forty-eight mimicker pairs names a specific diagnostic trap: two conditions that look alike at the bedside but diverge at the level of mechanism, and therefore diverge at the level of treatment. The four-part structure of each mimicker entry — the Clinical Pattern, the Mimicker, the Trap Logic, and the Decision Anchor — is designed to train the eye and the mind simultaneously. The Clinical Pattern teaches what to see. The Mimicker teaches what else could produce the same appearance. The Trap Logic names the cognitive error that leads to the wrong diagnosis. And the Decision Anchor supplies the discriminating feature — the one finding, test, or clinical detail that separates the two conditions and commits the clinician to a management pathway. This is not a memorization exercise; it is a framework for clinical reasoning that becomes more powerful with each patient encounter.

The Evolving Landscape of Dermatology

The therapeutic transformation that has reshaped dermatology over the past two decades — from broad immunosuppression to targeted cytokine blockade, from empiric topical therapy to mechanism-driven biologic selection — shows no sign of slowing. IL-23 inhibitors achieve complete psoriasis clearance in a majority of patients. Dupilumab and JAK inhibitors have redefined the management of moderate-to-severe atopic dermatitis. Ruxolitinib cream has become the first FDA-approved treatment for vitiligo repigmentation. Each of these advances was made possible by a deeper understanding of cutaneous immunology — the same mechanistic knowledge that this textbook foregrounds in every chapter. The clinician who understands the IL-4/IL-13 axis understands not only why dupilumab works in atopic dermatitis but also why it causes conjunctivitis, why it does not work in psoriasis, and why tralokinumab (which blocks IL-13 alone) may be preferred in specific clinical scenarios. Mechanism is not background knowledge; it is the operating system of modern therapeutic decision-making.

Emerging frontiers — artificial intelligence in dermoscopy and histopathology, teledermatology as a triage and access tool, pharmacogenomic-guided drug selection, and the expanding role of the skin microbiome in inflammatory disease — will continue to reshape how dermatology is practiced. But no technology replaces the clinician's ability to integrate what is seen on the skin with what is known about the patient, the mechanism, and the mimicker. The structured clinical reasoning that this textbook teaches — see the pattern, name the mimicker, identify the trap, anchor the decision — is as relevant in the era of AI-assisted diagnosis as it was in the era of the hand lens.

A Note to the Reader

Medicine is practiced one patient at a time, and every patient's skin tells a story that no textbook can fully anticipate. The knowledge in these pages is a foundation, not a ceiling. Use it to build clinical confidence, to sharpen diagnostic reasoning, and to approach each new eruption with the disciplined curiosity that is the mark of an excellent dermatologist. When in doubt, return to the mechanism — it will not mislead you. And when the clinical pattern and the mimicker look identical at the bedside, trust the Decision Anchor: the one finding that separates the two is almost always available if you know to look for it.

www.ingramcontent.com/pod-product-compliance
Lightning Source LLC
LaVergne TN
LVHW060439061126
851857LV00016B/1670
* 9 7 8 1 1 0 5 0 3 4 7 7 0 *